ESSENTIALS OF
VETERINARY PRACTICE

ESSENTIALS OF VETERINARY PRACTICE

Dr. Debasis Jana
Dr. Nilotpal Ghosh

2026

Daya Publishing House®

A Division of

Astral International Pvt. Ltd.

New Delhi – 110 002

First Published, 2011

Reprinted, 2026

ISBN: 978-81-7035-744-5 (HB)

Published by : **Daya Publishing House®**
A Division of
Astral International Pvt. Ltd.
– ISO 9001:2015 Certified Company –
4736/23, Ansari Road, Darya Ganj
New Delhi-110 002
Ph. 011-43549197, 8130496929
E-mail: info@astralint.com
Website: www.astralint.com

Printed at : Replika Press Pvt. Ltd.

— Dedicated to —

All those veterinarians who love their profession and are proud of being a veterinarian with a pledge to serve the farmers

Acknowledgement

It is our immense pleasure that this book ultimately came to light. The information received from various sources is gratefully acknowledged. The relevant reference books are cited at the end of this book to give due credits to the authors and/or publishers. In this occasion, we extend our thanks to our teachers, relatives, friends and colleagues for their inspiration and motivation to complete this work. Our sincere thanks are also due to Mr Anil Mittal, Daya Publishing House, New Delhi for accepting the manuscript and quick publishing this book. We shall be grateful for any suggestion and constructive criticism from readers regarding the text and presentation of the book so that the 2nd edition may be more informative and useful for the veterinary professionals. Observations may please be sent to the author's e-mail address: drdebasisjana@rediffmail.com or gnilotpal@yahoo.com.

Dr. Debasis Jana

Dr. Nilotpal Ghosh

Bidhan Chandra Krishi Viswavidyalaya
P.O. Krishi Viswavidyalaya, Mohanpur -741252
District - Nadia, West Bengal
Website: www.bckv.edu.in
Office: 033-25879772
03473-222666
Fax: 03473-222275
E-mail: bckvvc@gmail.com
sarojsanyal@yahoo.co.in

Prof. Saroj Kumar Sanyal
M. Sc. (IARI), Ph.D. (Cambridge)
FISSS, FNAAS
Vice-Chancellor

No. VC/BCKV/33/231
Date: January 3, 2011

Foreword

Veterinary is primarily concerned with health care of animals, and a veterinarian is a physician of animals and a practitioner of veterinary medicine. The job of a veterinary practitioner is very daunting, keeping in view the wide range of animals, which are unable to express their suffering. Besides treating various ailments of animals, a veterinarian is the person who is entitled to ensure production of safe and hygienic animal food products including milk, meat and egg for human consumption. Another important activity of veterinary professionals is to prevent zoonotic diseases that are transmitted from animals to human beings like Bird flu, Swine flu, Rabies, Anthrax, Mad Cow Disease *etc*. These make the veterinary science a vast and interesting subject. The demand of veterinary professionals is on the rise mainly in view of huge livestock population vis-à-vis demand of quality animal food products.

Keeping these in view, the present book entitled *'Essentials of Veterinary Practice'* is written by Dr. Debasis Jana and Dr. Nilotpal Ghosh, which deals with diagnosis as well as treatment of a large number of livestock diseases. All the essential subject matters are systematically presented in six sections, *viz.*, Diagnostic section, Medicine section, Gynaecology and Obstetrics section, Surgery section, Veterinary pharmaceuticals and Miscellaneous information pertaining to veterinary practice. The veterinary drug index chapter is unique and requires a special mention. The photographs of various diseases are important assets of this book. The proforma of various certificates and list of instruments/equipment used in veterinary practice are nicely compiled. The language is very simple and lucid. This book is a good reference material as it covers a wide spectrum of topics of veterinary practice. Efforts have been made to facilitate easy reading and help students as well as neo-vets gather important information of veterinary science in a single volume.

I am hopeful that this book will be of great use to the students as well as practitioners of veterinary medicine.

I extend my best wishes to the authors for the work they undertook to the cause of their profession.

S.K. Sanyal

Preface

- The book *'Essentials of Veterinary Practice'* is actually composed of six parts, *viz.*, (1) Diagnostic section, (2) Medicine section, (3) Gynaecology and Obstetrics section, (4) Surgery section, (5) Veterinary pharmaceuticals, and (6) Miscellaneous information pertaining to veterinary practice. The total text is divided into 22 chapters.
- This book has been compiled in the simplest and most lucid form giving emphasis to modern technologies of animal health management and veterinary therapeutics with complete information on animal diseases of varied etiology.
- Most characteristic features of this book are description of clinical as well as laboratory diagnosis of animal diseases, large number of common systemic as well as infectious and/or contagious diseases and incorporation of commonly used surgical procedures in curing various diseases. Every disease has been presented in the most precise and systematic manner aiming to serve the need of animal health practitioners. The veterinary drug index chapter indicating medicines and vaccines available in the market is unique, which is presented in a very systematic manner to link up with the modern art of treatment to be utilized under Indian farms and veterinary fields.
- Vast field experiences of the authors on livestock production management and treatment as a clinician as well as an academician, have been utilized to bring out this publication. Large numbers of photographs of various diseases and disease conditions for recognition of important diseases have been incorporated in this book which would be of immense help to the neo-vets and obviously to the budding veterinarians.

- ☆ One thing should be kept in mind that the use of trade names in this book is solely for the purpose of providing specific information. It is not a guarantee or warranty of the products named, and does not signify that they are approved to the exclusion of others of similar/suitable composition.

WHO WILL BE BENEFITED?

- ☆ This book is primarily meant for the *veterinary students* in India who are undergoing Internship training at the end of the 5-year integrated course (B.V. Sc. & A.H.).
- ☆ It will also help the concerned *teachers/demonstrators* for offering this course to the veterinary students.
- ☆ The book shall also be useful for the neo-vets and budding veterinarians, practicing veterinary clinicians, livestock development officers, animal health workers, *Pranibandhu* and progressive animal farmers in India and other tropical countries.

Dr. Debasis Jana

Dr. Nilotpal Ghosh

Contents

Acknowledgement vii

Foreword ix

Preface xi

PART – I DIAGNOSTIC SECTION

1. **Clinical Diagnosis of Diseases** 3

1.1 Introduction 1.2 History taking 1.3 Signs and symptoms of ill health 1.4 Clinical examination of patients 1.4.1 What to do before examining a patient? 1.4.2 Inspection of different body parts 1.4.3 Various methods of clinical examination 1.4.3.1 Recording of rectal temperature 1.4.3.2 Recording of pulse rate 1.4.3.3 Recording of respiration rate 1.4.3.4 Examination of visible mucous membrane 1.4.3.5 Examination of eyes 1.4.3.6 Palpation 1.4.3.7 Percussion 1.4.3.8 Auscultation.

2. **Laboratory Diagnosis of Diseases** 11

2.1 Laboratory tests 2.1.1 Examination of blood 2.1.1.1 Routine haematological examination of a blood sample 2.1.1.2 Blood smear examination 2.1.2 Faecal examination 2.1.3 Urine analysis 2.1.4 Examination of cerebrospinal fluid (CSF) 2.1.5 Examination of rumen fluid 2.1.6 Examination of skin scrapings 2.1.7 Other diagnostic aids 2.2 Post mortem examination 2.3 Collection, preservation and transportation of samples for laboratory diagnosis 2.3.1 Histopathology 2.3.2 Haematology 2.3.3 Serology 2.3.4 Microbiology 2.3.5 Parasitology 2.4 Important bacterial and viral diseases of livestock and poultry and clinical samples/specimens for laboratory diagnosis 2.5 Transport media for bacteriological specimen 2.6 Transport media for virological specimen 2.7 Tips for diagnosing foreign body in reticulum 2.8 Fine needle aspiration cytology 2.9 Biological tests for metabolic disorders

PART – II MEDICINE SECTION

3. Classification of Animal Diseases **51**

3.1 Health and Disease 3.2 Classification of diseases

4. Systemic Diseases and their Treatment **55**

4.1 Diseases of alimentary system 4.1.1 Stomatitis 4.1.2 Pharyngitis 4.1.3 Parotitis 4.1.4 Choke 4.1.5 Colic 4.1.6 Rumen dysfunction 4.1.7 Ruminal acidosis/Lact acidosis/Grain poisoning 4.1.8 Simple indigestion 4.1.9 Bloat 4.1.10 Vagus indigestion 4.1.11 Ruminal fermentative disorders in ruminants 4.1.12 Diseases of liver 4.1.13 Jaundice or Icterus 4.1.14 Hepatitis 4.2 Diseases of respiratory system 4.2.1 Rhinitis 4.2.2 Laryngitis, Tracheitis and Bronchitis 4.2.3 Pulmonary emphysema 4.2.4 Pulmonary oedema 4.2.5 Pneumonia 4.2.6 Epistaxis 4.2.7 Snoring disease 4.3 Diseases of reproductive system 4.3.1 True venereal diseases (transmitting through sexual contact) 4.3.2 Specific infections of reproductive system 4.3.3 Inflammation of specific organs caused by various agents 4.3.4 Trichomoniasis 4.3.5 Foetal maceration 4.4.1 Anuria 4.4.2 Oliguria 4.4.3 Polyuria 4.4.4 Haemoglobinuria 4.4.5 Haematuria (Red urine) 4.4.6 Nephritis 4.4.7 Pyelonephritis 4.4.8 Cystitis 4.4.9 Urinary incontinence 4.4.10 Urethral rupture (Urolithiasis) 4.4.11 Balanoposthitis 4.5 Diseases of cardiovascular system 4.5.1 Pericarditis 4.5.2 Foreign body syndromes 4.5.3 Cardiac arrest 4.5.4 Congestive cardiac failure 4.5.5 Peripheral circulatory failture (PCF) 4.5.6 Diseases of blood and blood forming organs 4.5.7 Haemorrhage 4.5.8 Oedema 4.6 Diseases of nervous system 4.6.1 Incordination of gait 4.6.2 Polyneuritis 4.6.3 Motor disturbances 4.6.4 Epilepsy/Epileptic seizure 4.6.5 Brain trauma 4.7 Diseases of locomotor system and muscles 4.7.1 Sprains 4.7.2 Myositis 4.7.3 Myopathy 4.7.4 Arthritis 4.7.5 Radial nerve paralysis 4.7.6 Rickets (Infantile tetany) 4.7.7 Osteomalacia/Adult rickets 4.7.8 Osteoporosis 4.8 Diseases of the eye 4.8.1 Examination of the eye 4.8.2 Conjunctivitis 4.8.3 Keratitis and Kerato conjunctivitis 4.8.4 Corneal opacity 4.8.5 Otitis 4.9 Diseases of skin 4.9.1 Urticaria 4.9.2 Eczematous dermatoses 4.9.3 Pyderma 4.9.4 Photosensitization 4.9.5 Ring worm 4.9.6 Para keratosis 4.9.7 Hypodermatosis 4.9.8 Mange.

5. Metabolic Diseases: Their Treatment and Control **126**

5.1 Introduction 5.2 Impact of metabolic disorders and nutritional disharmony in animal production 5.3 How do the metabolic diseases precipitate? 5.4 Important metabolic diseases of livestock 5.4.1 Parturient paresis (Milk Fever) 5.4.2 Bovine Ketosis 5.4.3 Downers Syndrome 5.4.4 Hypomagnesaemia 5.4.5 Post-parturient Haemoglobinuria 5.4.6 Fatty cow syndrome in cow–Lipid mobilization syndrome

6. Common Poisonings and their Management **139**

6.1 Introduction 6.2 Common symptoms of poisoning 6.3 General principles of treatment of poisoning 6.4 Common poisonings and their management 6.4.1 Chlorinated hydrocarbon poisoning 6.4.2 Organophosphorus compound poisoning 6.4.3 Lead poisoning 6.4.4 Nitrates and nitrites poisoning 6.4.5 Mercury poisoning 6.4.6 Arsenic poisoning 6.4.7 Urea poisoning 6.4.8 Cyanide poisoning 6.4.9 Lantana camera poisoning 6.4.10 Plant toxicity 6.5 Materials to be sent for chemical analysis in poisoning cases

7. Bacterial Diseases: Their Treatment and Control **147**

7.1 Introduction 7.2 Anthrax 7.3 Black Quarter 7.4 Haemorrhagic Septicaemia 7.5 Brucellosis 7.6 Tuberculosis (TB) 7.7 Tetanus 7.8 Actinobacillosis 7.9 Actinomycosis (Lumpy Jaw) 7.10 Botulism 7.11 Colibacillosis 7.12 Contagious Bovine Pleuro Pneumonia (CBPP) 7.13 Contagious Caprine Pleuro Pneumonia (CCPP) 7.14 Enterotoxaemia 7.15 Listeriosis 7.16 Leptospirosis 7.17 Paratuberculosis

8. Viral Diseases: Their Treatment and Control **158**

8.1 Introduction 8.2 Foot and Mouth Disease 8.3 Rinderpest (RP) 8.4 Bovine Ephemeral Fever 8.5 Blue Tongue 8.6 Pox 8.7 Peste Des Petits Ruminants (PPR) 8.8 Contagious Ecthyma 8.9 Cutaneous Papillomatosis 8.10 Hydrophobia (Rabies) 8.11 Hog Cholera (Classical Swine Fever)

9. Protozoan Diseases: Their Treatment and Control **173**

9.1 Introduction 9.2 Anaplasmosis 9.3 Babesiosis (Piroplasmosis) 9.4 Trypanosomiasis (Surra) 9.5 Coccidiosis 9.6 Drugs acting against haemoprotozoan parasites 9.6.1 Diminazine diaceturate 9.6.2 Quinapyramine sulphate/chloride

10. Parasitic Diseases: Their Treatment and Control **179**

10.1 Introduction 10.2 Internal parasites: the worms 10.2.1 Nematodes (round worms) – Ascarids, Gastro-intestinal worms, Lung worm, Nodular worm, Heart worm, Hook worm, 10.2.2 Trematodes (Flukes) – Fascioliasis and Distomiasis, Paramphistomiasis, Amphistomes, Nasal schistosomiasis 10.2.3 Cestodes (Tapeworms) 10.3 Deworming schedule of animals 10.3.1 Deworming schedule for cattle and buffalo 10.3.2 Deworming schedule for sheep and goat 10.3.3 Deworming schedule for pig 10.3.4 Deworming schedule for dog 10.4 Ecto parasitism (diseases caused by ectoparasites) 10.4.1 Types of ectoparasites of veterinary importance 10.3.2 Medicines used for ectoparasitic control

11. Nutritional Diseases: Their Treatment and Control **193**

11.1 Vitamins deficiency diseases 11.1.1 Hypovitaminosis A (Vitamin A deficiency disease) 11.1.2 Polyneuritis 11.1.3 Polyencephalomalacia 11.2 Mineral deficiency diseases 11.2.1 Macromineral deficiency 11.2.1.1 Deficiency of calcium and phosphorus 11.2.2 Micro/trace mineral deficiency 11.2.2.1 Zinc deficiency 11.2.2.2 Copper deficiency 11.2.2.3 Iron deficiency 11.2.2.4 Iodine deficiency 11.2.2.5 Selenium deficiency 11.2.2.6 Manganese deficiency 11.2.2.7 Cobalt deficiency

12. Common Ailments and their First Aid Treatment **203**

12.1 Pneumonia 12.2 Fever 12.3 Diarrhoea 12.4 Constipation 12.5 Anaemia 12.6 Thelitis 12.7 Anorexia 12.8 Pica 12.9 Simple indigestion 12.10 Enteritis in Sheep and Goat 12.11 Neonatal Calf Diarrhoea 12.12 Neonatal Calf Pneumonia 12.13 Salmonellosis in Calves 12.14 Mycoplasma in Calves 12.15 Agalactia 12.16 Blood in Milk 12.17 Udder Oedema 12.18 Parturient Paresis 12.19 Acute Pulmonary Emphysema 12.20 Retention of Urine 12.21 Torticolis 12.22 Parotitis 12.23 First Aid in Bleeding 12.24 Cuts and Wounds 12.25 Horn Injuries 12.26 Burns and Scalds 12.27 Tail Gangrene 12.28 Fracture 12.29 Yokegall 12.30 Abscess 12.31 Broken Horn (Horn Fracture) 12.32 Avulsion of Horn 12.33 Snake Bite

13. Common Control Measures Against Infectious Diseases **232**

13.1 Tips for controlling infectious diseases of animals 13.2 Prophylactic vaccination schedule for various species of animals

PART – III GYNAECOLOGY AND OBSTETRICS SECTION

14. Reproductive Characteristics of Animals **245**

14.1 Reproductive system of animals 14.1.1 Male reproductive system 14.1.2 Female reproductive system 14.2 Reproductive characteristics of livestock 14.3 Forecasting of date of parturition

15. Breeding Policy, Andrological Examination of Bull and Artificial Insemination **249**

15.1 Breeding policies for cattle and buffalo in India 15.2 Andrological examination of bull 15.3 Collection, processing, cryopreservation and evaluation of semen 15.4 Reproductive biotechniques for improving fertility of dairy cattle and buffaloes 15.5 Requirements for field insemination units 15.6 Records to be maintained at the artificial insemination (AI) unit

16. Reproductive Disorders and Post Parturient Diseases: Their Treatment and Control **264**

16.1 Reproductive disorders 16.1.1 Anoestrus 16.2 Post parturient diseases 16.2.1 Retention of placenta 16.2.2 Metritis-Pyometra 16.2.3 Prolapse of genetalia 16.2.4 Mastitis 16.2.5 Agalactia and Hypogalactia

PART - IV SURGERY SECTION

17. Elementary Veterinary Surgery 277

17.1 Surgical pack for various operations 17.1.1 Common surgical pack for large animal 17.1.2 Surgical pack for small animal 17.2 Suture materials 17.3 Suture technique 17.4 Suture size 17.5 Sterilization 17.6 Preparation of site for operation 17.7 Anaesthesia 17.7.1 Local anaesthetic drugs 17.7.1.1 Lignocaine HCl 17.7.1.2 Procaine HCl 17.7.1.3 Hexacycloine (Cyclaine) 17.7.1.4 Butacaine (Butyne) 17.7.2 General anaesthetic drugs 17.7.2.1 Anaesthetic gases 17.7.2.2 Anaesthetic agents 17.7.2.3 Inhalation anaesthetics 17.7.2.4 Xylazine hydrochloride 17.7.3 Tranquilizer 17.7.3.1 Chlorpromazine 17.7.3.2 Triflupromazine 17.7.3.3 Thiopentone sodium 17.7.3.4 Pentothal sodium injection 17.7.3.5 Ketamine HCl Injection/Ketamil Injection (Helpro Health) 17.7.4 Medicines for sedation, analgesia and restraining animals 17.7.5 Epidural anaesthesia 17.8 Restraint of animals for surgical procedures 17.9 Common surgical cases 17.9.1 Castration (Vasectomy) 17.9.2 Atresia ani 17.9.3 String halt (Medial pattelar dysmotomy) 17.9.4 Amputation of tail 17.9.5 Surgical management of Ranula 17.9.6 Caesarean operation 17.9.7 Hernia 17.9.8 Surgical management of Urolithiasis/Urinary calculi 17.9.9 Penile retraction (Paraphimosis) 17.9.10 Common surgical conditions of horns 17.9.11 Euthanasia

PART - V VETERINARY PHARMACEUTICALS

18. Veterinary Pharmacy 299

18.1 Common terminologies 18.2 Pharmacological preparation 18.3 How drug acts? 18.4 General idea about prescription 18.5 Latin phrases and abbreviations used in prescription writing 18.6 Weights and measures in prescription 18.7 Commonly used drugs(chemicals/pure herbal products) in veterinary first aid 18.8 Common topical preparations 18.8.1 Ointment 18.8.2 Paste 18.8.3 Lotion 18.8.4 Solution for topical use 18.8.5 Antiseptic 18.8.6 Liniment 18.8.7 Dressing oil 18.8.8 Carron oil 18.8.9 Astringent powder 18.9 Drug delivery systems/ methods of administration of medicines 18.9.1 Common routes of drug administration 18.9.2 Various enteral dose forms 18.9.3 Oral route of drug administration 18.9.4 Other routes of drug administration

19. Veterinary Drug Index 319

19.1 Therapeutic/Pharmacological list of drugs/medicines used in veterinary practice 19.2 Antibiotics 19.2.1 Ampicillin 19.2.2 Amoxycillin 19.2.3 Oxytetracycline 19.2.4 Ampicillin + Cloxacillin combipack 19.2.5 Enrofloxacin 19.2.6 Ciprofloxacin 19.2.7 Cephalexin 19.2.8 Pefloxacin 19.2.9 Ceftriaxone 19.2.10 Ceftiofur 19.2.11 Penicillin 19.2.12 Streptopenicillin 19.2.13 Cefotaxime sodium 19.2.14 Chloramphenicol 19.2.15 Neomycin 19.2.16 Amoxycillin + Cloxacillin 19.2.17 Gentamicin 19.2.18 Amikacin 19.2.19 Lincomycin 19.3 Sulphonamides 19.3.1 Sulphadimidin 19.3.2 Gut acting Sulphonamides 19.3.3

Oral Sulphonamide bolus 19.3.4 Sulphonamide combination (Co-Trimoxazole) 19.3.5 Oral Broad Spectrum Antidiarrhoeals for Calf, Sheep and Goat 19.3.6 Herbal Antidiarrhoeals 19.4 Electrolytes/Oral Rehydration Solution (ORS) 19.5 Anthelmintics (Dewormers) 19.5.1 Albendazole 19.5.2 Fenbendazole 19.5.3 Mebendazole 19.5.4 Oxfendazole 19.5.5 Levamisole 19.5.6 Closantel (Ectendoparasiticidal) 19.5.7 Ivermectin oral 19.5.8 Parenteral Ivermectin (A friendly dewormer of animals) – Ivermectin Injection (1 per cent w/v) 19.5.9 Triclabendazole (Flukicide) 19.5.10 Oxyclozanide (Flukicide) 19.5.11 Dichlorophen 19.5.12 Piperazine Hexahydrate solution 19.5.13 Levamisole (Parenteral preparation as Immunomodulator and broad spectrum worm eradicator) 19.5.14 Combined Broad Spectrum Dewormer for the treatment of mixed worm infestation/Dual Power Anthelmintic 19.5.15 Ayurvedic Anthelmintic 19.6 Non Steroidal Anti-inflammatory and Analgesic Drugs (NSAID) 19.6.1 Paracetamol 9.6.2 Meloxicam 19.6.3 Meloxicam with Paracetamol Combination (Injectable Preparations) 19.6.4 Ketoprofen (Safe and Effective NSAID) 19.6.5 Nimesulide Injection 19.6.6 Analgin 19.5.7 Meloxicam Group (with or without Paracetamol) 19.6.8 Nimesulide + Paracetamol Combination (NSAID) 19.6.9 Phenyl Butazone and Analgin Combination 19.7 Antispasmodic Drug (for Colic) 19.7.1 Dicyclomine HCl 19.7.2 Valthamate Bromide 19.8 Corticosteroids 19.8.1 Prednisolone 19.8.2 Dexamethasone 19.8.3 Triamcenolone 19.9 Parenteral Antihistaminic 19.10 Haemostat 19.10.1 Ethamsylate/Adenochrome Monosemicarbazone 19.11 Parenteral Vitamins and Minerals 19.11.1 Vitamin-A 19.11.2 Vitamin-AD$_3$ Injection 19.11.3 Injectable Vitamin B-Complex 19.11.4 Neurotropic B-Vitamins (B$_1$, B$_6$, B$_{12}$) 19.11.5 Vitamin-E Injectable Preparation 19.11.6 Liver Extract with Vitamin B-Complex Injection 19.11.7 Power Packed Injection of Calcium, Vitamin D$_3$ and B$_{12}$ (Injectable Calcium for IM use) 19.11.7.1 Preparations containing Calcium Levulinate 19.11.7.2 Preparations containing Calcium Gluconolactobionate with Vitamin D$_3$ E B$_{12}$ 19.11.7.3 Parenteral Calcium (IV and SC use) 19.11.8 Phosphorous 19.12 Hormones for Fertility Management 19.12.1 Diethyl Stilbosterol 19.12.2 Hydroxy Progesterone 19.12.3 LH Preparation 19.12.4 Chorionic Gonadotrophin 19.12.5 Synthetic Analogue to GnRH 19.12.6 Pregnant Mare Serum Gonadotrophin (PMSG) 19.12.7 Cloprostenol (Synthetic PG F$_2\alpha$) as Fertility Solution 19.12.8 Dinoprost Trimethiamine 19.13 Non-Steroidal (Non Hormonal) Synthetic Chemical for Subfertility/Infertility Management 19.13.1 Clomifene Citrate 19.13.2 Valethamate Bromide 19.14 Uterine Tonic and Ecbolic 19.15 Mastitis Care : Intra Mammary Infusion Tubes 19.16 Herbal Veterinary Medicine 19.16.1 Herbal Digestive and Stomachic 19.16.2 Antiflatulents (Antizymotics) 19.16.2.1 Anti Bloat Suspension (Oral Liquid) Medicines 19.16.2.2 Herbal-Anti Bloat/Anti Tympany Preparation (for prompt relief of Tympany or Bloat) 19.16.3 Herbal Liver Tonic 19.16.4 Herbal Cough Mixture (Expectorant) 19.16.5 Galactogogue – for better milk production 19.16.6 Herbal Antistress Medicine 19.16.7 Antiseptic Herbal Dressing Oil 19.16.8 Herbal Ointments 19.16.9 Non Herbal and Herbal Aerosol Spray for Topical Wound Cure 19.16.10 Non Hormonal Herbal Heat Inducer 19. 16.11 Herbal Immunomodulator 19.17 Mineral Mixtures 9.17.1 Common Mineral

Mixtures 19.17.2 Mineral Mixtures with Vitamins 19.17.3 Vitamin-Mineral Mixtures for better milk production 19.17.4 Oral Calcium Syrup (Tonic)/ Supplement 19.17.4.1 Herbal Preparation 19.17.4.2 Non-Herbal Calcium Oral Tonic 19.18 Reproduction Formula 9.18.1 Non Hormonal Preparation 19.18.2 Vaginal Pessuries (for uterine treatment) 19.18.3 Intra Uterine Medicines – for effective uterine wash Atibiotics/Antibacterials/Antiseptics 19.19 Ectoparasiticides 19.20 Vaccines and Vaccination

PART – VI MISCELLANEOUS INFORMATION PERTAINING TO VETERINARY PRACTICE

20. Common Instruments/Equipment Used in Veterinary Practice 441

21. Proforma of Various Certificates 461

21.1 Certificate of soundness of animal 21.2 Consent form for surgery 21.3 Consent form for euthanasia 21.4 Proforma for post mortem report 21.5 Proforma for sending samples to laboratory 21.6 Proforma of fit certificate for slaughter 21.7 Proforma of certificate for transport of dog 21.8 Record card for vaccination 21.9 Recording of a case history

22. Miscellaneous Information 470

22.1 Important physiological norms and longevity of various animals 22.2 Important physiological data of common laboratory animals 22.3 Normal haematology of animals 22.4 Normal serum biochemistry of animals 22.5 Physiological norms of some zoo animals in captivity 22.6 List of teratogenic drugs 22.7 List of drugs contra-indicated in lactation 22.8 List of drugs safe in lactation 22.9 List of potentially hazardous drugs in pregnancy 22.10 List of potentially hazardous drugs in neonates 22.11 List of drugs not recommended in particular species of animals 22.12 Relative production efficiencies and economy of different meat producing animals 22.13 Contents of a veterinary emergency kit

References **477**

Index of Animal Diseases **479**

Index of Generic and Trade Names of Medicines/Drugs Used in Veterinary Practice **485**

Part – I
Diagnostic Section

Chapter 1
Clinical Diagnosis of Diseases

1.1 INTRODUCTION

Diagnosis of the disease in animals which cannot express complaints is a very difficult task. Recognition and determination of the nature of disease is vital, for adopting proper line of treatment. History taking is the key for an accurate diagnosis in veterinary practice, based on asking suitable questions to the animal owner. After that signs and symptoms of ill health of animals are to be noted, which may be followed by clinical and laboratory examinations for proper diagnosis of animal diseases.

1.2 HISTORY TAKING

History pertaining to *present illness*

(*a*) Onset of the disease and its duration (acute or chronic nature of the disease).

(*b*) Normal behaviour and expression of animal – any change or abnormality noted – like change of voice, continuous bellowing *etc.*

(*c*) Symptoms noticed by the farmers.

(*d*) Appetite and water intake (thirst), any change in diet, feed intake.

(*e*) History of calving, milk production, grazing history, feed history, access to pasture sprayed with insecticide.

(*f*) History of any forced feeding, drenching (possibility of drenching pneumonia).

(*g*) Any other animal in the herd or flock affected (possibility of common cause of infections or contagious disease).

(*h*) History of any prophylactic vaccination, routine deworming and medication.

(*i*) Information about past illness (previous illness) if any and its relation with the present ailment.

(*j*) Any outbreak of any disease in the locality.

(*k*) Whether any treatment given earlier or initiated.

For making a diagnosis of disease general inspection of the animal is the 2nd most important task. General inspection includes general appearance, condition, posture, gait, conformation, surface and body coat.

Condition of the Patient

Physical examination of the animal whether healthy, weak, debilitated, emaciated, physiological status of the animal *viz.* rumination, lactation, respiration urination, defecation *etc.* behaviour of the animal, position of standing, posture and gait, evidence of any localized lesions *viz.* injuries, fractures, abscess, tumors, should be inspected or properly known. There are some specific conditions in specific diseases like septicaemia along with crepitating of muscle, as the indication of Black Quarter, arched back condition in traumatic pericarditis, tucked up abdomen in bloat or in tympanitis, taking unusual feed in pica, hide bound cachectic condition in T.B., sweet smell in Ketosis, circling in goat (Gid).

Posture and Behaviour of Animals

Normal posture of the animal may be changed in some disease or disease conditions like walking in circle (in Gid, Surra), abduction of elbows in chest pain, arched back condition in traumatic pericarditis, keeping the head on flank region in milk fever.

Abnormal postures in animals are observed in paralysis, dislocation of hip, fracture, neuritis, pain, sprain, injury, oedema, trauma and inflammation. Animal with tucked up abdomen may stand with an extended head and stretched out feet, stiff gait and lock jaw (trismus) in tetanus. Change in behaviour of animal may be indicative of some diseases like excitement in cystitis, nephritis, difficulty in defecation indicative of constipation, impaction, colitis *etc.*

Behavioural Anomalies of Animals

Abnormal behaviour of an animal is considered to be an imbalance between animal and its environment.

Cattle

Hair licking, drinking of urine, milk sucking, sucking own milk (vices of animal).

Buffalo

Thudding, Head rotation.

Goat

Licking, self-milk sucking, viciousness in bucks, throwing feed out of manger, masturbation and homosexual behaviour in bucks, holding up of milk in does, inter sucking in kids (kids suck various body parts especially navel sheath and ears of other kids during sucking period). Behaviour of an animal during lameness and injury can vary from normal actions and can be used for diagnosis. Corrective management and handling can be planned once the abnormal behaviour is observed in time.

Pig

Chewing or licking objects or performing empty chewing.

Dog

Chewing objects, attacking without provocation, urinating indoors, howling.

Skin Condition

Skin abnormalities as a whole with or without lesions including changes in hair or wool *etc.* are the indication of either skin diseases or some systemic diseases like cow pox, sheep pox, goat pox and buffalo pox *etc.* There may be scales, crusts, fissures, papules, macules, vesicles, nodules and diffuse lesions – indicative of skin disease and dermatitis.

Scales – Excess keratinous debris heaped up on the skin.

Crusts – Dried exudates containing serum, blood, pus, scales.

Fissure – Deep linear cleavage on the skin.

Lichenification – Thickening and hardening of skin.

Leukoderma – Lack of pigmentation.

Hair loss or falling called alopecia may be the indication of parasitic infestations, mineral deficiency and some other skin diseases. Look for general lusture, pliability of skin, oedema, dehydration and loss of pigmentation (rough harsh body coat) in deficiency diseases.

1.3 SIGNS AND SYMPTOMS OF ILL HEALTH

1. Off fed, hypophagia, loss of appetite, anorexia *etc.*
2. Fever, pyrexia, hypothermia (subnormal temperature) *etc.*
3. Suspended rumination, ceased rumination (no rumination).
4. Reduced or absence of ruminal motility, atony of rumen.
5. Abnormalities in respiration – frequency and breathing pattern (deep, shallow), respiratory distress, dyspnoea, gasping.
6. Altered normal physiological parameters like – temperature, pulse and respiration.
7. Depression, drowsiness, dullness, unthriftiness, torticollis, anxious expression, excitation, hyperaesthetia.
8. Abnormalities in behaviour, appearance and expression.
   (*a*) Walking in circle, showing abnormal gait and posture, incoordination, trembling, ataxia, convulsion, seizure, fit, muscular weakness and tremor, sway back, arched back, and torticolis.

(*b*) Pushing head against wall, head pressing.

(*c*) Charging at various objects and acting aggressively.

9. An abnormal gait associated with pain in the legs, chest or abdomen or is an indication of nervous diffuse.
10. Abnormal posture – standing with an extended head and stretched out feet (in tucked up abdomen/abdominal distension) lying with head turned along its side, unable to rise (Downers syndrome, hypocalcaemia/milk fever).
11. Abnormal secretions and excretions (discharges or protrusions from the body).

    (*a*) Discharge from nose – rhinitis, serous discharge, catarrhal, mucoid, mucopurulent, blood stained discharge, fresh blood (epistaxis).

    (*b*) Excessive saliva from mouth (hypersalivation).

    (*c*) Discharges from eye – lacrimation, excessive tear, sticky mucous, pusy secretion.

    (*d*) Protruding from the vulva – (prolapse, tumour).

    (*e*) Abnormal discharges from genitalia (pus, blood, foul smelling discharges) – pyometra, metritis.

    (*f*) Abnormal urine – scanty urination, anuria, urinary incontinence, blood in urine, haemoglobinurea, haematuria, red urine.
12. Abnormality in visible mucosae : pale mucous membrane (anaemia), blood shot, rose red appearance, congested mucous membrane, yellowish discoloration of mucosae (ecterus/jaundice), bluish discoloration of mucosae (Cyanosis).
13. Abnormalities in structures:

    (*a*) Swellings (neoplasms, cysts, haematoma, abscesses).

    (*b*) Enlarged joints, joint pains, swelling (arthritis, synovitis).

    (*c*) Abdominal distension (bloated abdomen).

    (*d*) Growth on eye.
14. Defecation – Constipation, loose motion/diarrhoea, blood in faeces (malena), bloody diarrhoea, hard stool (fecocolith) *etc.*
15. Abnormal colour: Black areas on horse and swine, red areas on light coloured skin, dark blue areas on the skin or udder (Gangrene).
16. Odour – Foul smelling rotten odour (FMD), a medicinal odour/odour of poison (accidental ingestion of chemicals or poison), stink weed or an acetone odour (ketosis).
17. Milk secretion: Reduction in milk yield, watery milk, blood in milk, milk leakage, curds and flakes in milk, hot painful udder, swollen teats and udder with changes in colour, physical and physiological abnormalities of milk, consistency of milk *etc.* are indication of mastitis.

1.4 CLINICAL EXAMINATION OF PATIENTS

1.4.1 What to Do Before Examining a Patient?

The following points are to be considered before going to examine a patient for diagnosis and treatment.

(*a*) Species

(*b*) Breed

(*c*) Age

(*d*) Sex

(*e*) Colour

(*f*) Management practices like stall fed or grazing *etc.*

(*g*) Prevalence of certain disease according to geographical location by parasitic disease, vector borne disease, endemic nature of disease.

(*h*) Soil micronutrient status to rule out deficiency disease, plant poisoning and toxicity *etc.*

1.4.2 Inspection of Different Body Parts

It is most relevant for diagnosing a disease and to pinpoint the location of illness.

Head

Softening and thinning of skull (cranial bones locally) with circling symptom indicative of gid (sturdy) in goats. Abnormal facial expression indicates the sign of various diseases like poisoning, rabies *etc.* Enlargement of mandible or maxilla (jaw bones) is seen in actinomycosis (Lumpy jaw). Submandibular oedema or swelling below the jaw is indicative of hypoproteinemia, fluke infestation, haemonchosis in goats, actinobacillosis in cattle. Nasal and oral froth or discharge with ocular lacrimation, dry muzzle are the indications of some diseases of animals. Examination of neck and thorax is important in disease diagnosis, *viz.* enlargement of throat, swelling at the ventral part of neck, swelling of lymph nodes (in Haemorrhagic Septicaemia), thyroid enlargement (in Goitre) *etc.*

The rate, rhythm, depth and types of respiration should be noted. Throat swelling, with soaring sound and dyspnoea with nasal, oral and ocular sensation is clear indication of Haemorrhagic Septicaemia or acute laryngitis. The respiration is painful, quick and shallow in pneumonia. Cough may be observed in bronchitis and pneumonia, collapsed and consolidation of one lung may lead to deficient or abnormal movement of chest. Chest movement is decreased bilaterally in bronchitis and in pneumothorax. Chest movement is decreased in the affected side. Brisket oedema invariably seen in cattle and buffaloes suffering from traumatic pericarditis, Haemorrhagic Septicaemia, endoparasitic infestation, hepatic insufficiency, asepsis during parenteral drug administration and protein loosing nephropathy.

Abdomen

Variation in abdominal size or volume is appreciated at general inspection of the animal. Distension of abdomen or its increase in size could be due to excess food, fluid, fat, or for the presence of foetus. Differentiation is possible with close examination. Distension of abdomen may occur in tympany, impaction, ascites, internal obstruction, choke *etc*.

Decrease in abdominal size may be due to starvation, diarrhoea and even in rabies. Umbilical hernia, navel ill, omphalitis, omphalocele *etc* are observed on close inspection.

External Genitalia

Vulval myiasis, maggot wound, orchitis are noticed from a distance. Discharges of pus or blood from urinary passage indicate the infection of urinary tract.

Udder

Abnormality of udder and teats or mammary glands characterized by disproportionate size of quarter and swelling, udder abscess or hypertrophy can be seen from out side and by palpation.

1.4.3 Various Methods of Clinical Examination

1.4.3.1 Recording of Rectal Temperature

Recording of body temperature of animal is most important in clinical diagnosis. Temperature should be recorded while the animal is at rest. Generally rectal temperature is recorded in animals by inserting the bulb of a clinical thermometer in the rectum, placed in contact of the rectal mucosae and keeping it for one to two minutes. The temperature is to be recorded twice in a day in ailed animal to know the type of fever (biphasic, continuous, intermittent, recurrent fever *etc.*). High fever is a first sign in most of the diseases.

1.4.3.2 Recording of Pulse Rate

Usually the pulse rate is equal to the rhythmic contraction and expansion of heart. Increased pulse rate is common and occurs in most cases of septicaemia, toxaemia, circulatory failure, excitement and in pain striken condition. Marked slowing of heart beat (bradycardia) is common in traumatic reticulo peritonitis in cattle.

Site for Recording Pulse

Cattle: Middle coccygeal artery, ventral coccygeal artery under the tail, facial artery, maxillary and median artery; femoral arteries (in case of calf).

Dog: Femoral artery on the inner side of thigh.

1.4.3.3 Recording of Respiration Rate

In cattle average respiration rate per minute is 12-16. Variation occurs due to high ambient temperature, after exercise and it is normal. Respiratory rate is accelerated during fever and respiratory distress due to disease. Respiration rate should be noted when the animal is at rest. The type of respiration like costal, intercostal, abdominal, jerkey *etc.* are also to be noted. There is a ratio of 1 : 3 between respiration rate and pulse rate in healthy animals. Examination of respiration rate of animals is indicated for primary respiratory disease as well as secondary respiratory disease due to cardiac involvement, allergy and anaphylaxis.

1.4.3.4 Examination of Visible Mucous Membrane

This includes the examination of conjunctiva, buccal, nasal, vulval, vaginal and rectal mucosae. In normal and healthy condition of animals, the mucous membrane is moist and rosy in colouration. The following changes of mucous membrane are seen in unusual conditions of animals.

- *Congestion:* Signs of fever and inflammation, systemic diseases and allergic sensitization.
- *Paleness:* Revealing anaemia, internal haemorrhage, hypoproteinaemia, excessive blood loss and shock.
- *Yellow discolouration:* Signs of ecterus and hepatic disorder, jaundice.
- *Pin point/Petecheal haemorrhages:* Indicates septicaemia, surra, phosphorus and arsenic poisoning.
- *Cyanotic changes:* Bluish discolouration owing to dyspnoea, hypoxia, venous stasis, congestive cardiac failure, pleurisy, HCN and nitrate poisoning.
- *Ulcerations:* Typical ulcers on oral mucous membrane seen in FMD, PPR and RP.
- *Pinkish:* Equine infectious anaemia.

1.4.3.5 Examination of Eyes

Ophthalmic examination gives some clues in diagnosing some diseases.

- *Sunken appearance:* Indicates chronic wasting disease and dehydration.
- *Pupillary reflex:* Loss of pupillary reflex and pupillary response to light are seen in toxaemia and shock, poisoning and CNS disease.
- *Dilatation of pupil:* Seen in poisoning and shock.
- *Corneal opacity, ulcers:* Commonly occurs in mechanical injury or trauma. In canine it could also be due to canine distemper.

Normal Colour of Conjunctiva of Various Animals

- *Cattle and Buffalo* – Pale pink
- *Horse* – Pale roseate
- *Sheep and Goat* – Pale pink
- *Pig* – Reddish tinged
- *Dog* – Roseate
- *Cat* – Pale.

1.4.3.6 Palpation

Consistency of an organ or tissues or a part of the body can be felt by lying hand with gentle pressure. Tips of fingers and flat of the hand are mostly used for handling the tissues or organs.

When tissue appears firm, hard, solid like muscle, that could be a neoplasm (tumour).

When structure appears bone like consistency – it could be the exostosis or ossification of cartilage. Hot and painful swelling, hard or soft could be the abscess (hard in initial stage, soft in maturity/ripened abscess).

Doughy – Where soft tissues retain finger points, or causes pits on pressure – oedema and impaction of rumen.

Cold and painless (fluctuating) – could be the cyst distended with gas (bloat), distended with food (impaction), distended with fluid (ascites), crepitating sound (Black Quarter or Subcutaneous emphysema).

Abnormalities of abdominal and urogenital organs can be felt by rectal palpation.

1.4.3.7 Percussion

Striking of any part of the body with a short, sharp blow that enables underlying organs to vibrate and generate an audible sound is called percussion. Drum like sound audible from rumen indicates tympanitis, dull resonance in impaction. Hyper resonant sound is observed while the lungs are filled with excessive air. Increased amount of gases will emit tympanic sound in abdomen.

This method is useful in small animals than the large animals.

1.4.3.8 Auscultation

It means listening of various functional sounds produced by some thoracic and abdominal organs by use of stethoscope for ascertaining the pathological condition of lungs, pleura, heart and certain parts of alimentary tract.

It is useful for hearing peristaltic sounds during ruminal and intestinal contractions, listening sounds produced in course of normal functioning of trachea and lungs (dry rales in congestion and moist rales in exudation), cardiac sounds like cardiac murmurs in valvular disease, splashing sounds in pericarditis and hydro pericardium *etc.*

Chapter 2
Laboratory Diagnosis of Diseases

2.1 LABORATORY TESTS

Laboratory tests and interpretation of results help in confirmatory diagnosis of animal diseases. Various laboratory tests which can be done for this purpose are haematological examination, blood smear test for haemoprotozoan infestation or other bacteria, faecal examination for worm infestation, urine analysis, examination of rumen fluid, examination of skin scrapings for fungal infestation *etc.*

2.1.1 Examination of Blood

2.1.1.1 Routine Haematological Examination of a Blood Sample

Site of Blood Collection

For routine haematological exanimation, generally venous blood is collected. The site of collection of blood in different species of animal may vary, as depicted below.

Species of Animal	*Site of Blood Collection*
Cattle, Buffalo, Sheep, Goat, Horse	Jugular vein
Pig	Anterior vena cava
Dog	Cephalic vein (Fore limb) and recurrent tarsal vein (Hind limb)
Cat	Ear vein
Rabbit	Ear vein and heart
Rat and Mouse	Heart or by sniping of a piece of tail
Fowl	Wing vein

Anticoagulants for Blood Sample

Different types of anticoagulants are used for different types of estimation related to blood. The following is the list of common anticoagulants used in veterinary laboratory.

Anticoagulants	*Quantity Required for 10 ml Blood Sample*
EDTA – 1 per cent solution	1 ml
Double oxalate mixture – 10 per cent solution (1.2 g Ammonium oxalate + 0.8 g Potassium oxalate in 100 ml distilled water)	0.3 ml
Sodium citrate – 4 per cent solution	1 ml
Sodium fluoride – 1 per cent solution	1 ml
Heparin – 1 per cent solution	0.1 ml (the vial or syringe is to be rined with it)

(i) Determination of Haemoglobin (Hb)

(*a*) Acid Haematin method.

(*b*) Cyanmethaemoglobin method

(*c*) Spectrophotometric method.

Significance: Decrease in Hb concentration in blood below normal values indicates anaemia of animal.

(ii) Determination of Haematocit

Methods: (1) Wintrobe Method; (2) Capillary Method.

Significance: It is a reasonable index of R.B.C. (Red cell) population. The value of haematocrit is used along with Hb concentration and R.B.C. count for the calculation of the MCH, MCV and MCHC, the three important red blood cell indices used in diagnosing anaemia.

(iii) Total Erythrocytic Count (TEC)

Method: Haemocytometric method by using Neubauer chamber.

(iv) Total Leucocytic Count (TLC)

Method: Haemocytometric method by using Neubauer chamber.

(v) Differential Leucocytic Count (DLC)

Method: Examination of stained blood smear.

Interpretation of Hematological Findings

Decrease in haemoglobin percentage indicates anaemia. Causes could be the haemorrhage, excessive blood loss, blood sucking parasitic load, haemolysis due to toxins, haemoprotozoan infection like Babesiosis. *Increase in its beyond normal range* indicates haemoconcentration occurring in dehydration.

Alteration in Leukocyte Picture

(*i*) *Leukopenia* mainly characterized by reduction in total leukocyte count (TLC), which indicates possible viral diseases CD, ICH, RP, Bovine malignant catarrh,, terminal stages of fatal bacterial infection and possible drug interaction like sulpha drugs, analgesics and steroids.

(ii) *Leukocytosis* – Characterized by increase in TLC giving possibility of bacterial infections, traumatic reticulitis, pericarditis, peritonitis, metritis *etc*.

(iii) *Eosinophilia* is observed in parasitic infestations, allergic conditions *etc*.

2.1.1.2 Blood Smear Examination

In cattle and buffaloes the ear vein is the convenient site for taking blood for preparation of blood smear. Blood smear in animals can also be prepared from blood taken from 'jugular vein'. At least two good films/smears are to be prepared for laboratory diagnosis. The blood film is to be air dried and fixed with 95 per cent alcohol or methylated spirit for one minute. After proper drying, the slide is to be wrapped in clean paper after proper marking and to be sent the same to the laboratory for diagnosis.

Examination for Haemoprotozoan Infestation and Other Bacteria

Case history and clinical symptoms are helpful in making a tentative diagnosis of protozoal diseases like Babesiosis, Trypanosomiasis, Anaplasmiosis *etc*. Confirmation can be made by microscopic examination.

In pyrexial phase when trypanosomes are present in large numbers in the peripheral blood, both the wet film and stained preparations may reveal trypanosomes but detection of light or chronic infection is almost impossible with a microscope.

Thick blood film examination may give better diagnosis. Blood film with simple water *i.e.*, wet film and stained after dehaemoglobinising by 1-2 per cent formalin may show trypanosomes more definitely. Trypanosomes can be concentrated by centrifuging the suspected blood and examining the supernatant fluids.

Peripheral blood (from ear tips), lymph node aspirate and or aqueous fluid smears and smears prepared from the EDTA blood using centrifuge techniques can be stained with Giemsa and should be examined for the presence of extra cellular flagellate.

(a) For Detection of Blood Protozoa

The simplest procedure is blood smear examination by Leishman's stain under microscope.

Procedure of Leishman's Stain

1. Make blood smear (collecting blood from ailed animals at its febrile stage from the eartips) and dry in air.
2. Pour undiluted Leishman's stain over the smear and allow the stain to act for 1 minute.
3. Add double volume of distilled water on the slide with a pipette and mix with the stain. Allow it for 10 minutes.
4. Wash in distilled water for 30 seconds.

(b) For Detection of Blood Protozoa (Mainly Intracellular Haemoparasites)

Giemsa's stain is used to detect the intracellular haemoparasites.

Procedure of Giemsa's Stain

1. Make a thin smear, dry in air and fix in methyl alcohol for 3 minutes.
2. Dip the slide in a jar (1 : 10 stain) and keep it for 20 minutes.
3. Wash in water, blot, dry in air and observe under miscroscope (In case of 1 : 20 dilution, stain for 45 minutes).

Ear tip blood smears stained with Giemsa if found positive for intracellular piroplasms that suggests Babesiosis.

(c) Detection of Acid Fast Bacteia

It is done by Ziehl-Neelsen's method. Certain bacteria *e.g.* Mycobacterium tuberculosis and Leprosi bacilli are resistant to staining, but when they are stained by strong stains like carbol fuchsin they resist decolorisation by acid. Ziel-Neelsen procedure is the reliable staining method of such acid alcohol fast bacteria.

Procedure of Ziehl-Neelsen Staining

1. Make a smear, dry in air and fix it by flaming, and for histopathological staining – (*i*) Deparaffinize tissue sections with xylene; (*ii*) Take section to water.
2. Flood the smear/slide with carbol fuchsin, heat to steaming and leave for 10 minutes and for tissue sections stain in carbol fuchsin at 37°C for 1 hour or at 56°C (Wax oven – for histopathological sections) for 30 minutes.
3. Rinse well in tap water.
4. Decolourize with 3 per cent HCl in 70 per cent alcohol (or 1 per cent aqueous sulphuric acid) until the smear/sections are pale pink for 1 to 5 minutes. Decolourization should not be attempted in one step, intermittent washings in water and reapplication of acid alcohol mixture is good for this purpose.
5. Wash in water and counter stain in 1 per cent Methylene blue for 10-30 seconds or in light green for 1 minute.
6. Rinse in water.
7. Dehydrate in two changes each of 95 per cent and absolute alcohol. See under oil immersion focus.
8. Clear in xylene (2 changes for tissues).
9. Mount in balsam or permount (for histopathological sections).

Result: Acid fast bacilli – bright red, tissue – blue, caseous material – pale grayish blue.

Erythrocytes (RBC) – slight reddish tint.

(d) Detection of Gram Positive and Gram Negative Organisms

Procedure

1. Make the microscopic slide grease free.
2. Make a smear with discrete bacterial colony, dry in air and fix by flaming.

3. Cover the slide with 1 per cent aqueous crystal violet for 3 minutes.
4. Tip off the stain and treat with Gram's iodide solution (GIS) for one minute.
5. Counter stain with diluted (1 : 10) carbol fuchsin for 30 seconds to one minute.
6. Wash under slow running tap water and make it air dry and focus under oil immersion lens.
7. Observe (Gram Positive – Violet colour and Gram negative – Pink colour).

Note: Gram's iodine serves the mordant function and alcohol as decolourizer.

(e) Detection of Haemoprotozoan Infection by Knott Method

Procedure of Knott Method

Stained blood smear is helpful for detection of haemoprotozoan infection after staining by Geimsa stain.

The blood smear is to be fixed in methanol for 3-5 minutes. After fixation undiluted Geimsa stain is to be poured on it and kept for 5 minutes.

Add double the volume of phosphate buffer saline (pH 7.2) (NaCl 8 g, KH_2PO_4 0.2 g, KCl 0.2 g and Na_2HPO_4 1.15 g in 1000 ml of distilled water) and keep it for 20 minutes.

Pour off the stain, wash under thin stream of running water and observe under high power magnification.

(f) Special Stains for Capsulated Organisms (Bacteria)

Presence or absence of capsule with bacteria leads to designate the organism as pathogenic or non-pathogenic. This is well applicable for the capsulated bacteria and the lucid example is *Bacillus anthracis*.

The staining can be accomplished by

(*a*) Polychrome Methylene blue (Mac Fadyan Reaction) Method.

(*b*) Giemsa stain method.

(i) Mac Fadyan Reaction (Polychrome Methylene Blue) Method

1. Make the slide grease free.
2. Prepare the smear ready with heat fixation.
3. Flood the smear with 1 per cent Polychrome methylene blue (matured, filtered) and allow to stand for 3 to 5 minutes.
4. Wash with distilled water until all the coloured artifacts are removed.
5. Air dry and focus with oil immersion facility.

Observation: The capsulated virulent organism will give the light pink to red blue surrounding their body wall whereas their body mats will take the blue colour.

(ii) Giemsa Stain Method

1. Make a film on a grease free slide and make it air dried. Fix the smear with methanol by immersing the air dried film for 3 minutes in absolute methanol.

2. Flood the film with Giemsa stain and allow to hold for 3-4 minutes.
3. Add 0.01 M-phosphate buffer (pH 7) to the stain and stand for 30 seconds and repeat the wash subsequently.
4. Examine under oil immersion lens.

Observation: Bacterial cells appear as blue purple rods surrounded by pink to red hue (if capsule is present).

(iii) Staining of Spore

Method-I

1. Stain with Ziehl – Neelsen's carbol fuchsin for 3 to 5 minutes, heating the preparation until steam rise.
2. Wash with water.
3. Treat with 0.25 or 0.5 per cent sulphuric acid for one to several minutes, the period being determined by trial for each culture. Alternatively luminous result can be obtained by decolourizing in a 2 per cent solution of Nitric acid in ethanol. The slide should be dipped once rapidly in the solution and immediately washed in water.
4. Wash under slow flow of tap water.
5. Counter stain with 1 per cent aqueous methylene blue for 3 minute.
6. Wash in water, blot and dry.

Observation: The spores are stained bright red and the protoplasm of the bacilli blue.

Method-II

1. Flood the smear with 5 per cent aqueous malachite green and steam for 1 minute.
2. Wash under running water and counter stain with 0.5 per cent aqueous Safranin for 15-30 seconds.
3. Wash in water, air dry or blot and examine under oil immersion lens.

Observation: Bacterial bodies stain red and spores green.

Method-III

1. Flood the film with strong carbol fuchsin and allow to steaming for 3 to 5 minutes.
2. Wash well in water. Decolourize with absolute alcohol (ethanol) until all tracts of red have been removed.
3. Wash thoroughly in water.
4. Counter stain with Loeffler's Methylene blue for 1 to 2 minutes.
5. Wash and drain, air dry or blot and examine under oil immersion lens.

Observation: Bacterial bodies stain blue and spores red.

(*N.B:* This method is very similar to Ziehl Neelsen's method. Instead of acid alcohol mixture, here absolute alcohol alone is used as decolourizer).

2.1.2 Faecal Examination

It is indicated for endoparasitic infestation mainly for worm infestation and coccidiosis in animals.

For dispatch of faecal sample to a distant laboratory about 5 g of stool may be collected directly from the rectum and it should be mixed with formal saline (10 per cent formalin) for preservation.

Procedure

1. *Direct Method:* Take a very little quantity of feaces and make a uniform suspension with little water. Take a drop of that homogenized suspension on the glass slide and put a cover slip on it to see under low power followed by high power microscope.
2. *Concentration method:* These are (a) Floatation method and (b) Sedimentation method.

(a) Floatation Method

Make the faecal suspension in sugar solution or sodium nitrate solution of greater density so that the parasitic ova of lower density may float on the surface.

General Methodology

To make a uniform suspension of test sample (faecal sample 2-3 g) 20 ml of either sugar solution or sodium nitrate solution to be added on the faecal material. Remove the fibrous content of the sample using a filter. Then pour the suspension in the centrifuge tube at 600-1000 rpm for 3-5 minutes and in absence of centrifuge machine, keep the tube in the tube rack for resting proper sedimentation for 20 minutes. Collect the surface layer using the headed glass road and transfer a drop on the slide. Put a cover slip and see under microscope. Light eggs and coccidian oocysts are easily detected by floatation method.

For this purpose different floatation fluids are in vogue which is dependent on species of parasite expected to be present.

(i) Saturated Salt Solution

Sodium chloride (NaCl) – 400 g

Water–1000 ml.

(Specific gravity: 1.18-1.20; this solution may distort eggs).

(ii) Salt and Sugar Solution

Sodium chloride – 400 g

Sugar – 500 g

Water – 1000 ml

(Dissolve the salt in water to make a saturated solution. Add the sugar to the saturated salt solution. Stir until the sugar is dissolved).

(iii) For Stronglyes

Sodium Nitrate solution

Sodium Nitrate – 400 g

Water–1000 ml.

This solution is used for Stronglyes eggs but may form crystals and distort eggs if left for longer than 20 minutes.

(iv) Magnesium Sulphate Solution

Magnesium sulphate – 370 g

Water – 1000 ml

This is used for the recovery of Fasciola eggs.

Direct Floatation of Nematode Eggs, Coccidian Oocysts and Moniezia Eggs

1. Take small amount of fresh faeces (2 g).
2. Add 10 ml of floatation solution.
3. Prepare suspension and pour in a test tube.
4. Add more solution to fill the tube to the top.
5. Place a coverslip on the top of the liquid.
6. Remove the cover slip and place it on a glass slide and examine under microscope.
7. Use centrifuge to accelerate the flotation of eggs.

(b) Sedimentation Method

It is very much useful for heavier parasitic ova like nematode ova and other operculated ova. Prepare a faecal suspension in water (2 g faeces in 20 ml water), filter it and centrifuge at 1000 rpm for 2-3 minutes. Discard the supernatant and examine the thick sediment.

Interpretation of Faecal Examination

Qualitative Assay

No. of Ova per Low Power Field	*Indication*
1 to 2 ova	Mild/light infestation (+), which may not manifest clinically.
3 to 4 ova	Moderate infestation (++)
More than 5 ova	Heavy infestation (++++)

NB: For quantitative assay *i.e.*, for more accurate judgment, McMaster technique may be followed.

Quantitative Estimation of Worm Infestation

Direct floatation method does not give idea about parasite load. Quantitative estimation is the best guide for deworming treatment. The egg per gram of faeces is indicative for anthelmentic treatment. The faecal samples are to be examined every 4-8 weeks to monitor the worm load in animals.

(a) Modified McMaster Method

Take 1 gram of faecal sample and triturate it in 14ml of distilled water. Then strain it. Insert 0.3ml of saturated sucrose solution in Mc Master slide. Mix 0.3ml of homogeneous faecal suspension with saturated sucrose solution. Keep it for few minutes to float the eggs or oocysts. Examine under low power of microscope nearly at plane of air bubble. Conversion: Egg per gram/Oocyst per gram

or EPG/OPG = Y X 50 where Y = No. of eggs/Oocysts per slide.

(b) Modified Wisconsin Sugar Floatation Method

This method is the most accurate as in this floatation method little debris interferes with the count.

Method: Fill a 15 ml test tube with 10 ml of Sheathers' solution.

Take 3 g of faeces in a cup. Pour sheathers solution from the test tube into the cup and mix well. Place a funnel into the test tube, place a strainer into the funnel and pour the faecal sugar solution mixture through the strainer into the test tube. Using a tongue depressor, squeeze the liquid out of the faeces that is left in the strainer. Centrifuge the tube for 2-4 minutes.

Fill the tube to its top and place a coverslip onto a meniscus. Remove the coverslip after 15 minutes and place it on a slide. Examine the entire coverslip and count the number of eggs that you find.

The number of eggs counted is the number per three grams of faeces, so divide by 3 to find the EPG.

(c) Quantitative Examination for Trematode Egg

Faeces to be mixed with 0.4 (N) NaOH (1.6 g NaOH) in 100ml distilled water. (For sheep and goat take 10 g faeces and for cattle and buffalo take 30 g of faeces). This suspension should be kept overnight (10 hours) at room temperature.

Next day morning add 200ml of 0.4 (N) NaOH solution and shake it vigorously.

Take out 7.5 ml and 5ml mixtures (sheep and goat and cattle and buffalo respectively) and subsequently spin it at 2000-2500 rpm for 10 minutes.

Discard supernatant and add saturated NaCl and centrifuge it.

Wash thrice with the same solution and finally strain the sediment and watch for the presence of trematode eggs (*e.g.* Fasciola).

Conversion Factor

For sheep and goat one egg = 4 eggs per g of faeces and for cattle one egg = 2 eggs per gram of faeces.

Zinc sulphate ($ZnSO_4$) solution can also be used in this technique and that would be helpful for enumeration of Fasciola eggs.

(d) Ethyl Acetate Sedimentation Technique

Pass a piece of faeces (5 x 5 mm approx) through a sieve into about 9ml of water, then pour solution into a 15ml centrifuge tube.

Add 3 ml of ethyl acetate and plug the tube with a rubber stopper. Shake the tube vigorously and centrifuge it.

Using a stick 'ring' the plug of fat at the water ethyl acetate interface (where the plug adheres to the side of the tube and that must be detached before the liquid contents of the tube can be poured off).

Pour off the supernatant, taking due care to leave the pellet at the bottom of the tube intact.

Use two sticks to remove some of the pellet and smear it on a slide. This technique is preferred for formalin fixed samples.

2.1.3 Urine Analysis

Routine examination of urine sometimes becomes essential for diagnosing some of the diseases of animals. Urinalysis can yield much valuable informations with regard to functions of urinary system as well as other organs or system. For the purpose of chemical analysis of urine, cellular castes, calculi *etc.* urine needs to be collected in clean containers. For cultural examination urine should be collected aseptically and kept in sterilized container.

A complete urinalysis is indicated for the following conditions.

1. Kidney (Renal) diseases – Proteinuria, casts, leucocytes and erythrocytes.
2. Bladder infections and neoplastic diseases – Proteinuria, leucocytes, bacteria, blood and exfoliated neoplastic cells.
3. Liver diseases – Billirubin crystals and bilirubinuria.
4. Diabetes – Ketonuria, glycosuria.
5. Acidosis – Low pH.
6. Alkalosis – Increased pH.

Collection and Preservation of Urine

Urine must be collected in aseptic manner as well as in clean condition. Early morning sample is preferred for the presence of constituents of diagnostic value. First part of the urine should be discarded as it may contain cellular debris and some undesirable constituents flushed from the urethra, prepuce and genitalia. Catheterization and cystocentesis are followed for urine collection for bacteriological investigation. Fresh urine sample is preferred to avoid possible contamination with urea splitting bacteria from urethra which may result in alkalising the urine and dissolving casts and cells.

Urine sample can also be preserved by refrigeration and can be analysed within 2 to 3 hours. The following preservatives can be used for the preservation of urine sample :

1. Small crystal of Thymol
2. One drop of formalin in 30ml of urine (but it may interfere with glucose reaction).
3. Few drops of Chloroform.

4. Boric acid approx. 1 gram in 24 hours urine sample (collected) can be used for hormone analysis as and when required.

Physical Examination of Urine

Volume: Urine volume is inversely related to the specific gravity of urine. Urine volume is increased in Polyuria and urine volume decreases in Oliguria (*e.g.* shock, dehydration, acute renal disease). High volume with low sp. gravity. Low volume with high sp. gravity.

Transparency: Change in transparency of urine may occur in some disease conditions. It may be thick and cloudy in Nephritis.

Smell: Normal smell of urine is uraemic. In abnormal conditions the sample may give a smell of ammonia, fetid or acetone (in Ketosis).

Colour: The colour of urine varies from almost colourless to amber colour. In diseased condition urine may be red (red urine in Babesiosis and Hematuria, deep yellow in Icterus or Jaundice).

Colour of urine may be changed according to parts of urinary system affection.

Sl.No.	*Abnormal Colour*	*Indication/Conditions*
1.	Thick grayish colour	Pus in urine
2.	Dark yellow, brown or greenish yellow	Bile pigment present in urine (Jaundice/Liver dysfunction)
3.	Red colour	Haematuria (intact erythrocytes in urine)
4.	Reddish brown	Haemoglobinuria and Myoglobinuria (Presence of free haemoglobine in urine)
5.	Dark red	Beat/turnip feeding
6.	Pale urine	Pyometra, diabetes
7.	Greenish colour	Methylene blue therapy

Haemoglobin produces a clear brown red colour in urine. Haemorrhage into the urinary tract and extra urinary haemolysis cause the presence of haemoglobin in urine. Myoglobin is an abnormal brown urinary pigment derived from severely damaged muscles. It is encountered in urine, in case of equine azoturia and crushing injuries. However, normal horse urine is cloudy and thick due to presence of mucus and crystals.

Chemical Examination of Urine

(1) Hydrogen Ion Concentration (pH) or Reaction of Urine

pH of urine varies in different species and it depends on the diet and metabolism. Range of pH of urine is given in Table 1.

(2) Determination of Protein (Albumin)

Urinalysis in healthy animals revealed absence of protein in urine. Protein may be present in urine of diseased animals (in urinary system affections) and that can be estimated by acid precipitation test by following method.

Roberts reagent concentrated nitric acid (HNO_3) 1 part and saturated magnesium sulphate 5 parts *i.e.* 770 g/litre of distilled water.

Methodology: Take 2ml of Robert's reagent in a test tube and layer 2ml of clean urine on the reagent gently inclining the tube. A (+)ve test is indicated by the formation of white ring at the zone of contact. Negative test – No ring in the contact.

Example: Proteinuria is common in Enzootic bovine haematuria.

Table 1: Nature/Reaction of Urine with pH of Livestock Species

Species	*Nature*	*pH*
Bovine	Alkaline	7.4-8.2
Bubaline	Alkaline	7-8.4
Horse	Alkaline	8
Sheep	Alkaline	8.07
Goat	Alkaline	
Pig	Acidic or alkaline	
Dog	Acidic	6-7
Cat	Acidic	6-7

(3) Determination of Glucose

Normal urine is devoid of glucose and its significance is of great value in cats and dogs than that of ruminant livestock. Glucose can be estimated by Benedict's test.

Benedicts' Reagent:

- ☆ Copper sulphate – 17.30 g
- ☆ Sodium citrate – 17.3 g
- ☆ Anhydrous sodium carbonate – 100 g
- ☆ Distilled water -1 litre

Test

Take 5 ml of Benedict's reagent into a test tube and add 8 drops of urine in it. Boil the mixture for 2 minutes and allow cooling slowly.

A (+) ve test is shown by the presence of greenish yellow to orange red precipitate.

Reducing sugars present in urine react with copper sulphate to reduce cupric ions to cuprous oxide, giving a colour change depending upon the amount of sugars present in urine.

A slight green colour, a small bluish precipitate or faint turbidity may be caused owing to the presence of urates and other non-sugar reducing materials.

Urine is found positive for sugar in diabetes, enzootic bovine haematuria.

(4) Determination of Bilirubin (Bile Pigment)

Presence of bilirubin in urine is confirmatory to liver dysfunction and jaundice. It may be detected by Foam test and Hay's test.

- ☆ *Foam test:* Take few ml of urine in a test tube and shake it vigorously for few minutes. Bile pigment present in urine would produce a brown or yellowish green colour that would be imparted to the foam.

☆ *Hay's Test:* Take few ml of urine in a test tube and sprinkle small amount of sulphur granules on top surface of urine sample. If sulphur sinks down in the bottom, it indicates the presence of bile salts.

(5) Determination of Ketone Bodies

The specific test for acetone or Ketone bodies, Rothera's test to be carried out with the following procedure. In a test tube take 3 ml of urine sample and Rothera's reagent amounting to 1 ml to be added gently into the urine sample. Then with a dropper add 1 ml of liquor Amn. fortis over the solution for the development of a strong permanganate colour at the zone of contact that develops within a minute indicating positive (+ve) reaction.

(6) Determination of Blood/Blood Pigment

The test needs Benzidine solution as reagent. Take 2 ml of saturated solution of benzidine in glacial acetic acid in a test tube. To this add 2 ml of urine and mix it properly. Appearance of blue colour indicates the presence of blood or blood pigment (Haemoglobin).

Interpretation of Urine An alysis

Observation/Result	*Interpretation*
Increased specific gravity	Specific gravity of urine is increased in fever, nephritis, cystitis, dehydration and diabetis mellitus *etc.*
Decreased specific gravity	Seen in chronic nephritis, excessive water intake *etc.*
Albuminuria/proteinuria	Seen in cystitis, nephritis, toxic nephrosis, drugs and chemical toxicosis.
Haematuria	Renal congestion, acute nephritis, pyelonephritis, Bracken Fern poisoning, cystitis, urethritis, urolithiasis, crystaluria due to sulpha drugs and some other nephro toxic chemicals, trauma *etc.*
Haemoglobinuria	Piroplasmosis (Red urine), Leptospirosis, Anaplasmosis (occasionally), post parturient haemoglobimuria, poisoning and toxicity.

Microscopic Examination of Urine

Fresh samples of urine to be used for microscopic examination. In urinary system affection microscopic structures like casts, erythrocytes, leucocytes, bacteria, crystals *etc.* may be seen with microscopic examination of urine.

Method

Agitate the whole urine sample and fill the centrifuge tube for low speed. Centrifugation at 2000-3000 rpm for 3-5 minutes. Collect the sediment and mix the sediment with little volume of urine. Put a drop on a glass slide and covering with cover slip and examine under microscope both with low power objective and high power objectives to identify smaller objects. If necessary stain urine smear with methylene blue or Giemsa stain.

- *Epithelial cells:* Round to oval or spindle shaped, transitional cells.
- *Erythrocytes:* Yellow to orange or may be colourless if haemoglobin is dissolved out, smaller than leucocytes or pus cells with no internal structure.
- *Leucocytes/Pus cells*: Smaller than epithelial cells, appear as granular amoeboid cells.
- *Crystals:* Presence of crystals in urine is of great importance in urolithiasis and metabolic disorders. Amorphous phosphates, calcium oxalate and triple phosphate crystals may be present in urine sediment.

2.1.4 Examination of Cerebrospinal Fluid (CSF)

Examination of C.S.F. is of immense diagnostic value in brain and C.N.S. diseases, cerebral syndrome, cerebellar syndrome, spinal syndrome including bacterial meningitis, metastatic carcinoma, purulent or suppurative meningitis, canine distemper (CD) and other viral disease affecting brain.

Collection of Samples

Lumber puncture in between 3rd and 4th lumber vertebrae is the usual site for CSF sample collection in case of dog. Besides lumber puncture, approach through cistern magna can be tried.

Examination of Samples

Smear examination: For bacteria and Trypanosomiasis.

(a) Physical Examination

Colour

Normal CSF is transparent and colourless and any deviation indicates cerebral pathology. It becomes turbid where there is excessive presence of cells in CSF.

Coagulation

As a rule CSF does not coagulate but it coagulates in some inflammatory conditions *e.g.* purulent or acute supportive meningitis.

- *Specific gravity:* 1.003-1.008.
- *Reaction:* Alkaline.

(b) Chemical Examination

Protein

CSF is examined for protein contents (Pandy's test).

(1) Foam Test

In normal case C.S.F. is clear, colourless and does not produce foam if it is agitated. If slight foam is produced at all it disappears after few minutes automatically. But the foam will be more when protein content is more in CSF in diseased condition.

(2) Sulphosalicyclic Acid

Take 0.1 ml of CSF in a test tube. Add 3 ml of 3 per cent sulphosalicyclic acid. Mix it properly and keep it for 5 minutes. Turbidity is read visually.

Enzymes

Lactate dehydrogenase (LDH), creatine phosphokinase, and transminases are increased in inflammatory conditions of CNS.

Cytology

(1) Total Cell Count

1. Fill the leucocyte counting pipette to mark by diluting fluid and then with CSF to mark eleven (11).
2. Mix it properly and discard 1st 2-3 drops.
3. Fill the haemocytometer chamber on one of both the sites as for blood count and left for 2 minutes till cells settle down.
4. The cells are counted in all the ruled areas on both the sites of the counting chamber and multiply it by 0.6 to obtain the no. of cells/Cu mm.

(2) Differential Cell Count

Centrifuge the spinal fluid for 5 minutes and discard the supernatant. Then a smear to be made out of the sediment, air dried and stained with Wright's or Giemsa stain. Count 100 cells.

Principles of Treatment of CNS Syndrome

1. Specific treatment in specific diseases (*e.g.* Trypanosomiasis, Listeriosis, Ketosis *etc.*).
2. Antibiotics for control of infections.
3. Intracranial pressure of fluid can be relieved by IV injection of hypertonic solutions.
4. CNS depression.
5. CNS stimulants.

2.1.5 Examination of Rumen Fluid

Analysis and examination of rumen fluid is very much important for rational treatment of ruminants. Change in colour, smell, viscosity, pH, floatation, sedimentation gives important clues for diagnosing ruminal disorder.

Technique of Collection

Paracentesis ruminis – Trocarisation is done at the middle of the left paralumber fossa with long sterilized needle and aspiration of ruminal fluid is made with glass syringe.

Intubation of stomach tube: The animal has to be restrained properly and then by pulling out the tongue to one side the mouth has to be opened widely. The head of the animal is then held high to facilitate stomach tube with suction strainer. As it reaches the cardia, some resistance will be felt and again it has to be passed further until a firm resistance is felt denoting its entry into the ventral sac of the rumen.

Important Points for Consideration

1. Rumen fluid is to be collected up to 500ml for conducting various tests.

2. Rumen fluid can be kept at room temperature for 9 hours and in refrigerator for 24 hours.
3. Rumen fluid container should be closed air tight soon after collection.
4. To avoid error in pH, first 200 ml of rumen fluid should be discarded and after that rumen liquor is to be collected about ½ litre.

Preservation of Rumen Liquor

Saturated solution of $HgCl_2$ (@ 1 drop/5 ml of rumen fluid) is used as preservative. The fluid should be kept in a test tube with a layer of liquid paraffin to preserve the anaerobic environment and to be stored in refrigerator for 3-4 hours.

Common Field Test for Diagnosis

1) Colour

Normal colour of rumen fluid depends upon the diet.

Grass fed: grey to olive green.

Straw fed: Grey brown or yellowish brown.

Abnormal Colours	*Indications*
Blackish green	Rumen putrefaction
Dark brown	Simple inactivity of flora and fauna
Dark brown/green	Rumen alkalosis (slightly ammoniacal smell)
Slightly milky or brown	Chronic latent rumen acidosis.
Milky green	Acute rumen acidosis/Lactacidosis.
Grayish green	Bloat
Olive to brownish green	T.R.P.
Dark olive	Latent hydrochloric acidosis.
Relatively dark	a) Posterior stenosis
	b) Functional or anatomical gastric stenosis
	c) Left side abomasal displacement.

2) Smell/Odour

Rumen fluid is normally aromatic in nature.

Abnormal Colours	*Indications*
Acid or sour	Acute Rumen acidosis, Lactacidosis.
Faecal odour	Rumen putrefaction protein decomposition.
Slightly ammonical	Urea poisoning, Rumen alkalosis.
Musty/sour	HCl acidosis
Putrid	Protein over feeding
Fairly abnormal	TRP
Smell of abomasal contents	Gastric stenosis, pyloric obstruction.
Stale/musty odour	Inactive rumen juice

3) Viscosity/Consistency

Abnormal Viscosity/Consistency	*Indication*
Extremely viscous	Saliva mixed
Foaming	Frothy bloat
Mixture of water foam	Rumen putrefaction (*E. coli, Proteus* species)
Watery	Inactive rumen fluid (Bloat, lactacidosis)
Shining pulp	Over feeding
Variable	Rumen alkalosis

4) Sedimentation Activity Times (SAT)

Freshly collected rumen liquor about 100ml to be passed through a sterilized gauge for primary filtration and observed as it settles in a glass cylinder.

Normal Stratification	*Indication*
Fine food particles and infusoria	Settle at once/starts settling immediately.
Larger and more fibrous particles	Form a broad upper layer as they are carried upward.
Complete sedimentation and floatation	Takes 4-8 minutes.

Abnormal S.A.T. (stratification)	*Indication*
Slow floatation and rapid sedimentation	Reflux of abomasal fluid into the forestomach
Rapid sedimentation and retarded floatation or absence of floatation	In appearance, Hypophagia, Acidosis
Rapid floatation with abundant foam	Rumen decomposition (Decomposed ruminal contents), solid particles remain in suspension for a long time
Variable activity	Rumen alkalosis
Scanty SAT or absence of stratification (SAT)	Functional atony or Ruminal stasis
Pulpy to firm above and fluid below/ arranged in horizontal layer	TRP (Traumatic reticulo pericarditis)

5) pH (Hydrogen Ion Concentration)

Avoid unnecessary delay in examination of pH. pH should be measured soon after rumen fluid collection. It can be measured by using indication paper (pH paper), Grip pH meter (in field condition) and digital pH meter in laboratory condition.

Normal pH of Rumen liquor is 5.5 (Range 5.5-7.0).

Hydrogen Ion Concentration/pH

Condition	pH shifts/pH Change
Ration rich in crude protein (CP) and or crude fibre (C.F.)	Higher range 6.5-7.0.
Ratio rich in sugar or starch	Lower range – 5.5-6.0
After withdrawal of food for 24 hour or more inactivated fore stomach	Up to 8.5
Urea poisoning	8 – 9.5
Rumen decomposition	7.5-8.5
HCl acidosis (Hydrochloric acidosis)	4.3-7.0
Lactacidosis (Rumen acidosis)	May reach less than 4
Reflux of abomasal juice	Pyloric stenosis, Abomasitis, Abomasal ulceration

6) Laboratory Tests

(A) Cellulose Digestion Test

Cellulose digestion within 48-50 hours indicates disturbances. Glass bead will fall to the bottom of the tube within 48-54 hours in normal cases (indicative of active rumen liquor).

Test: 10 ml of rumen fluid is taken in which 0.3 ml of 16 per cent glucose solution is to be added in a test tube. Then suspend a cellulose thread or a pure cotton thread in rumen fluid and at the lower end of which a glass bead is tied and incubate at 39°C or keep it adjacent to a light bulb for 24 hours. See the fall of glass bead to the bottom (48-54 hrs. is indicative of normal condition).

(B) Glucose Fermentation Test

The test is carried out in a fermentation Saccharometer. Take 10 ml of strained rumen fluid to which add 0.5ml of 16 per cent glucose solution in fermentation Saccharometer and incubate at 39°C for 30-60 minutes. Read the result after incubation.

Importance

Normal rumen liquor with active flora	Glucose is fermented resulting in gas formation
Rumen liquor containing inactive microflora	No gas is formed
Foamy bloat	More gas is formed with pronounced foaming
Rumen decomposition	Increased gas formation
Latent rumen acidosis	Normal-increased gas formation
Rumen alkalosis, clinical rumen acidosis, Reflux of abdomasal fluid into fore stomach	Reduced gas formation

(C) Methylene Blue Reduction Test (MBRT)/Methylene Blue Reduction Time (Redox potential test)

Take 20 ml of freshly collected rumen fluid. To this add 1 ml of 0.03 per cent Redox dye solution (Methylene blue solution) and mix. Measure the time required for decolouration of the test sample, using a plain rumen fluid as a basis for comparison.

Importance

Microbial Status

	Time for reduction
a) Highly active microflora	
i) Animals maintained on hay and concentrate	3 minutes
ii) Only concentrate ration	1 minute
iii) Only hay ration	3-6 minutes
b) Inactive flora due to	
i) Ration poor in structure	3 minutes
ii) Inappetance	More than 15 minutes
Rumen acidosis (pH less than 5.0)	Considerable delay Less than 5 minutes up to pH 5.2, more than 5 minutes for below pH 5.2.
Hydrochloric acidosis	More than 5 minutes

(D) Nitrite Reduction Test

Take three test tubes and in each tube pour 10 ml of strained rumen fluid. Add 0.2 ml and 0.7 ml of 0.025 per cent potassium nitrite solution in Tube-2 and Tube-3 respectively and keep in water bath at 39°C. At every 5 minute 1 drop from each tube is placed in the small wells of a ceramic plate and to each well 2 drops of test reagent (*i.e.* 2 ml of sulphanilic acid, 140 ml distilled water). Samples that still contain Nitrite are coloured.

Significance

(*a*) Animals on mixed ration – 5-10 min – Tube – 1
20 min – Tube- 2
30 min – Tube-3

(*b*) Green fodder, rumen alkalosis – Rapid reduction, ruminal decomposition, bloat.

(*c*) Deficient ration, lack of appetite, clinical lactacidosis – slow reduction.

(E) Chloride Test

To 0.1 ml of the chloride standard solution, add deionized water 1ml and pour 0.2 ml of indicator. Then titrate the standard with mercuric nitrate solution. The end point is obtained when permanent violet colour appears. This is the standard. Repeat the same with rumen liquor sample.

Calculation: Test reading/Standard reading x 100 = in microgram (μgm).

This is useful in distinguishing hydrochloride acidosis from lactic acidosis.

Normal – 15-25 m Val/litre.

Abnormal – Lactacidosis – Less than 40 m Val/litre

Hydrochloric acidosis – More than 25-30 m Val/litre; may increase 30-100 m Val/litre in supplementation of ration with sodium chloride., abomasitis, abomasal ulcer, sand in stomach or intestine, abomasal displacement, paralytic ileus and reflux of abomasal contents.

(F) Protozoal Count

Protozoa, both ciliates and flagellates are present in rumen of which ciliate have physiological importance by virtue of their mass and number. Greater the protozoal density more active is the rumen fluid.

Place a drop of rumen fluid on a slide and cover it with a cover glass and examine under low power (80 or 100 magnification).

Study the Following Characters

1. Density : Vigorous + + + +

   Abundant + + + (more than 30 protozoa/LPF)

   Moderate + + (10-30 protozoa LPF)

   Few + (1-10 protozoa/LPF)

   Greater the protozoal density more active is the rumen fluid. Simple inactivity of microflora and fauna → -/+

   Rumen decomposition → -/+

   Latent lactacidosis → + + +

   Clinical lactacidosis → -
2. Proportion of dead to live protozoa

   Rumen acidosis → dead microfauna

   HCl acidosis → death is still earlier

   Moderate digestive disorders – Proportion of dead to live protozoa increases.
3. Iodophilic activity

   Add a drop of Lugol's iodine to 2-3 drops of rumen fluid on a glass slide and cover it with a cover slip and examine under the microscope.

   Iodophilic activity is recognized by black colouration of starch contents of protozoa.

   It is graded as :

   (0), (+), (+ +), (+ + +), depending on the starch quantity contained.

Total Protozoal Count

Take 5 ml of strained rumen liquor and dilute into 20 ml with 10 per cent formal saline. From this 10 ml of mixed rumen liquor is taken and 10 drops of 2 per cent. Eosin is added to stain the protozoa. The diluted rumen liquor is charged in a Neubaure's slide with Neutoaeu rulling 8 sq. mm and the results is expressed as total counts per ml (X x 10^5).

Normal Protozoan Count–1.66 × 10^5 to 2.56 × 10^5/ml.

Normal Counts

Mixed ratio diet → 10^{5}/ml

Concentrate diet → 10^{6}/ml

In diseased condition → Decreased or nil

Bloat → Decreased total protozoal count.

Disappearance of Holotrichs.

Acidosis → Nil; if present only a few entodinomorphs.

Bacteria

An air dried rumen fluid smear is stained by Gram's staining technique and observed as 10x and 45 x under the microscope.

Gram (+ ve) organism → Violet colour appearance.

Gram (- ve) organism → Red or pink colour.

Composition of smear from sick animal with that from healthy one, both maintained on same ration.

2.1.6 Examination of Skin Scrapings

Skin scraping is to be mixed with 10 per cent KOH and heat until keratinized tissues dissolve; then

- ✰ Centrifuge it at 1500 rpm for 10 minutes.
- ✰ Examine the sediment under 10x and high power magnification.

Diagnosis of Fungal/Mycotic Infection on Skin

Collection of Material

Before collection of skin scrapings the affected parts of animal body are cleaned with 70 per cent alcohol to avoid contamination. Deep skin scrapings, invaded hairs are to be collected from the border of the lesions with the help of sterilized blunt scalpel blades. The samples are to be kept in sterilized cotton plugged small glass tubes.

a) Direct Examination of Fungal Bodies

One drop of 10 per cent KOH and a pinch of specimen is to be taken on a clean glass slide. Put a cover slip on it and examine the digested material under 100x/400x magnification.

b) By wood's Lamps

Positive samples show green fluorescence.

c) Isolation of Fungi

(*i*) *Primary isolation*: Sabouraud's Dextrose Agar (SDA) medium fortified with cyclohexamide and chloramphenicol is used. The sample is inoculated in the medium under aseptic conditions and is incubated aerobically at 27°C and 37°C for a period of one month.

(*ii*) *Subculture and maintenance of fungal isolates*: Positive isolates are picked up after primary isolation, subcultured and maintained in SDA medium for further characterization.

(*iii*) Use selective medium for characterization of fungal isolates.

(*a*) Boiled rice medium (BRM) – It is used for isolation of *Microspora* sp. and *Trichophyton* sp.

BRM: Unfortified rice – 8 g

Tap water – 25 ml.

(*b*) Corn Meal Agar (CMA) – It is used for isolation of *T. rubrum* and *T. terrestre.*

Composition : (CMA) : brewer powder – 65 g, corn meal agar, Dextrose – 200 mg Tween – 80-10 ml, Distilled water – 1000 ml.

(*c*) Trichophyton agar: It is used for isolation and characterization of Trichophyton species. There are 7 types of trichophyton agar.

1. *Trichophyton Agar No. 1 (TA-1)*

Casamirno acid – 2.5 g

Dextrose – 40 per cent

Monopotassium phosphate – 1.8 g

Agar – 15 g

Distilled water – 100 ml.

2. *Trichophyton Agar No. 2*

TA No. 1 + 50 mg inositol and 200 mg thiamine.

3. *Trichophyton Agar No. 3*

TA No. 1 with 50 mg inositol and 200 mg thiamine.

4. *Trichophyton Agar No. 4*

TA No. 1 with 200 mg thiamine.

5. *Trichophyton Agar No. 5*

TA No. 1 with 2 mg nicotinic acid.

6) *Trichophyton Agar No. 6*

Amonium nitrate – 1.5 g

Magnessium sulphate – 0.1 g

Monopotassium phosphate – 1.8 g.

Agar – 1.5 g, Distilled water – 100 ml.

7. *Trichophyton Agar No. 7*

TA No. 6 with 30 mg

Histidine HCl.

Study of Micromorphology of Fungal Bodies

The fungal bodies are stained by Lactophenol cotton blue to record structures of fungal bodies. One drop of Lactophenol cotton blue is mixed with one loopful of isolated organism on a glass slide. The stained material is observed under microscope after putting one cover slip under low and high power microscope.

Composition

Lactophenol cotton blue.

- ☆ Phenol crystal – 20 g
- ☆ Lactic acid – 20 ml
- ☆ Glycerine – 40 ml
- ☆ Cotton blue – 0.05 mg
- ☆ Distilled water – 20 ml

2.1.7 Other Diagnostic Aids

In addition to above parameters, sometimes other specialized methods or tests are required for diagnosing the diseases of animals.

For confirmation of some of the tentative diagnosis – X-ray examination, radiographic imaging, rectal examination, exploratory puncture (to differentiate hygroma, haemotoma, abscess, cyst), examination of faeces, urine, milk, blood, bacteriological examination, serological tests (laboratory tests), allergic test, tissue biopsy, biochemical tests and other diagnostic tests including E.C.G., endoscopy, laparoscopic examination *etc.* are done.

Cultural examination and antibiotic sensitivity test have become valuale diagnostic aids in successful therapeutic management of mastitis, metritis and urinary tract infection.

2.2 POST MORTEM EXAMINATION

Detail post mortem examination (PM) of animals can give the proper avenue to investigate the actual cause of death. PM examination or autopsy should be carried out in bright day light, and not in artificial light or at night.

The P.M. examination needs to be carried out for the following findings to correlate it with the manifested signs or symptoms as revealed by the animal in the course of its sufferings or ailments. The specific findings in this regard are the condition of carcass, condition of visible mucosae, secretion or excretion from mouth, nostrils and other natural orifices if any, any wound on the body surface, nature of injury or type of wound, bullet holes, trauma, bruishes, abrasions, laceration, fractures, burns and scalds, alopecia, cyanosis, haemorrhage, congestion of organs, colour and smell of stomach contents, oedema, post mortem staining, colour of blood and subcutaneous tissue, ejection of blood, condition of organs *etc.*

Requirements for Necropsy

1. Measuring Tape.
2. Small animal P.M. Set/Large animal P.M. Set.
3. Empty vials/bottles for collecting viscera (if poisoning is suspected)

4. Glass slides and clean papers for wrapping. Prepare heart blood smears and impression smears from liver, lungs, and spleen *etc.* for laboratory examination.
5. A small note book and a pencil to note down every points and detail findings on the spot.

How to Write Post Mortem Report

1. A correct and complete description of the animal is to be given (*e.g.* bloated, emaciated, hide bound, cachectia, injuries, wounds, fractures, burns *etc.*)

   Condition of the skin coat

   Secretions and excretions from the natural orifices

   Condition of various regions like head, neck, chest *etc.*

   Condition of the external genitalia

   Condition of visible mucous membrane

   Condition of perineal region.

   If there is an injury – that should be noted down in detail with the following.

   Nature of injury, type of wounds or fracture, size, length, depth, direction, situation *etc.* Arrow shot wound, gun shot/bullet holes and marks of burning at entry and exit of bullets should be noted.
2. For autopsy – cut the carcass to open it and to see the lesions if any (find out the pathognomonic lesions – suspected for infectious diseases). This is also known as necropsy.
3. The following changes are usually noticed after death – which should be borne in mind for giving diagnosis out of autopsy. *e.g.* Rigor mortis, PM Staining, PM Softening (after death the tissues are softened by the action of autolytic enzymes and proteolytic ferments of the infecting bacteria), PM Clotting of blood (PM clot is soft and elastic, does not attach to the endothelium, but ante mortem clot is friable and non-elastic), P.M. bloat, hypostatic congestion, P.M. imbition of bile around gallbladder *etc.* In Anthrax no clot forms because the bacteria liquefy the fibrin. In sweet clover poisoning clotting does not occur since prothrombin activity is inhibited.
4. Open the carcass starting from the ventral abdomen along the course of linea alba and extend cranio dorsally till to the buccal cavity and caudally till to the perineum (anus). Examine the carcass – as per body cavity *e.g.* abdominal cavity, pelvic cavity, thoracic cavity, buccal cavity, cranial cavity and note down the abnormalities or changes organ wise and structure wise.
5. Examine the organs properly for detectable abnormalities, cyanosis, congestion, haemorrhage of organs, colour and smell of stomach content, oedema. Post mortem staining, colour of blood and subcutaneous tissue, ejection of blood, condition of organs *etc.*

6. For suspected case of poisoning – collect secretions and excretions if available – *e.g.* saliva, stool, urine, vomit, remnants of feed and fodder, ingesta, stomach content; collect different organs *e.g.* intestine, liver, lung, kidney, stomach with its contents *etc.*
7. Preservation of materials – the collected materials should be preserved either in rectified spirit and or in saturated salt solution (45 g NaCl in 100 ml water). For forensic laboratory examination formalin should never be used. Samples after proper labelling *e.g.* the information *viz.* species, sex, age, weight, PM No, PM date, contents of the jar *e.g.* liver, lungs, spleen, kidney *etc.* preservatives used and signature with date, needs to be sent to the forensic laboratory after packing in a container with proper sealing. No necropsy is complete without histopathological examination of tissues.
8. For histopathological examination and diagnosis – the organ specimen with active lesion alongwith some healthy portion needs to be collected and preserved in 10 per cent formalin solution. The visceral organs are liver, kidney, lung, spleen, lymph node, intestine *etc.* The tissues fixed in 10 per cent formal saline may be replaced by the 5 per cent strength of the same after a week.
9. Collection of specimen for laboratory diagnosis. Collection of specimens for specific diseases should be done most aseptically. Suitable materials should be collected and after proper fixation and preservation needs to be submitted for laboratory diagnosis.
10. Blood smears should be prepared from the carcass under necropsy studies for the demonstration of blood protozoa and microfilarae. The search of microfilarae should be conducted by direct examination of whole blood or of centrifuged blood samples in which haemolysis has been produced by addition of acetic acid.
11. On routine necropsy examination the most commonly sought worms are those located in the gastro intestinal tract and since the gastro intestinal tract contains most of the internal parasites, it is preferable to examine the contents of each portion separately.
12. Examine all the organs thoroughly for appreciable changes, for the presence of lesions like nodules, tumors, cysts, ulcers, necrosis, hemorrhage *etc.*

Post Mortem report format is given in Chapter 21 (Part-VI) of this book.

2.3 COLLECTION, PRESERVATION AND TRANSPORTATION OF SAMPLES FOR LABORATORY DIAGNOSIS

There are various diagnostic activities which includes histopathology, haematology, serology, microbiology (virus, bacteria, fungi, rickettsia *etc.*), parasitology and toxicology *etc.* For various diagnostic activities various specimen are collected and they are sent to the laboratory with different preventives or directly with cold chain maintenance. A general guideline is being given in this regard for the transportation of samples for diagnostic purpose.

2.3.1 Histopathology

Sample: Tissue from the lesions needs to be collected. Preservative to be used – 10 per cent buffered formalin.

Type of container: Leak proof glass or plastic jar.

Comments: Tissue less than 1 cm thick.

Ratio of formalin to tissue is 1 : 10.

2.3.2 Haematology

Sample: Whole blood.

Preservative: In anticoagulant under refrigeration.

Container: Glass or plastic vial.

Comments: Gently rotate vial to mix anticoagulant.

Don't keep for a long time.

Transport with ice packing.

2.3.3 Serology

Sample: Serum.

Preservative: Refrigeration or freezing with Marthiolate (1 : 10,000 dilution) or 5 per cent phenol.

Container: Glass or plastic vial.

Comments: Blood to be handled gently, so that while separating the serum it is not haemolysed and transport with ice packing.

2.3.4 Microbiology

Samples: Organs, tissue, swabs, exudates, intestinal loops, body fluids, urine, milk.

Preservative: Usually refrigeration or freezing and for virological investigation, 50 per cent phosphate buffer glycerine can be used as preservative.

Comments: Avoid contamination, collect and dispatch appropriate samples and sample varies in different diseases. Transport with ice packing.

2.3.5 Parasitology

For the detection of parasitic infestation the following samples are generally collected.

1. Faecal samples
2. Blood
3. Skin scrapings
4. Collection of parasites.

Faecal Samples

Faecal sample should be collected from rectum and if it is to be collected from ground it should be from the top of the freshly passed out faeces.

At least 5 g of faeces is to be collected and kept in air tight and water tight container and to be labelled properly. Sample should be examined within 12 hours after collection. If more than 2-3 days elapsed between collection and examination, equal part of 5 per cent formalin is to be added. (In case of suspected Eimeriasis or Cryptosporidiosis – faecal sample is to be preserved in 2.5 per cent potassium dichromate solution).

Blood Samples

(*a*) *For microfilaria*: For its detection by Knott method atleast 1 ml venous blood is to be collected in anticoagulant (Heparin/EDTA) and to be stored in room temperature before sending it to the laboratory for examination.

(*b*) *For haemoprotozoa*: For its detection blood smear is to be prepared from fresh blood. Fresh blood is to be smeared and air dried on a slide and then despatched. Blood smear should not be made from blood collected in anticoagulant.

Collection of Skin Scrapings

(*a*) For skin lesions with minimal epidermal hyperplasia and lesions caused by deeply burrowing mites (*e.g.* Sarcoptes) or in hair follicles (*e.g.* Demodex mange): Scalpel blade is to be dipped in glycerine/mineral oil. Periphery of the lesions at right angles to the skin is to be scrapped until and unless pinpoint haemorrhages occur. The sample should be pink in colour.

(*b*) For lesions with marked epidermal hyperplasia and exfoliation (*e.g.* lice and Chorioptes mites): Dried exudates and debris are scrapped and kept in a small container. Vaccum cleaner fitted with an in line filter may be used to collect epidermal dermis and various ectoparasites (fleas, lice, Demodex, Psoroptes, Sarcoptes *etc.*)

(c) For ear mites: Cotton swab is to be used.

Collection of Parasites

(*i*) Ectoparasites

Lice, ticks, fleas, kids *etc.* can be collected with forcep or fingers. Ticks with their intact mouth part should be collected carefully for proper species identification.

Lice and fleas may also be collected from recently dead or morbid animals by placing the animal in a closed plastic bag.

Large ectoparasites is to be preserved in 70 per cent alcohol and for long time storage 70 per cent ethanol or 5 per cent glycerol is recommended. Mites can be preserved in 70 per cent isopropyl alcohol.

(*ii*) Endoparasites

Preservation is recommended in 70 per cent ethanol or 5 per cent glycerol. If live worms are collected they should be relaxed in tap water or saline prior to killing in hot water (65°C) or formalin.

Lung worm detection in lung tissue: The material is to be submitted immediately to the referred laboratory for detection of Dictyocolus larvae by Bearmann technique.

For Nematodes, fresh gut scrapings/portion of gut (intestines) is to be submitted after fixing in 10 per cent formalin or in 70 per cent alcohol. Each section of the intestines or gut scrapings should be submitted in individual containers to prevent mixing and confusion.

2.4 IMPORTANT BACTERIAL AND VIRAL DISEASES OF LIVESTOCK AND POULTRY AND CLINICAL SAMPLES/ SPECIMENS FOR LABORATORY DIAGNOSIS

Bacterial Diseases

Name of the Disease	*Etiology*	*Host/Species Primarily Affected*	*Clinical Specimen of Samples of Choice for Lab. Diagnosis*
Anthrax	*Bacillus anthracis*	Cattle, Buffaloes, pigs	Peripheral blood smear, smears from heart blood and spleen, smears from the swollen lymph node (in case of swine).
Brucellosis	*Brucella abortus, B. melitensis, B. suis*	Cattle, Sheep, Goat, Pig	Placenta, aborted foetus, vaginal swab, milk, semen samples, swabs from the male reproductive organs.
Campylobacter infection	*Campylobacter foetus*	Cattle	Cervical mucous, Prepucial wash
Clostridial infection	*Clostridium chauvoei*	Cattle	Smear from the local tissue, (affected muscle smear), Muscle pieces
	C. novi	Sheep	Liver
	C. perfringens	Sheep, Goats and Cattle	Swabs from the exudates and pieces of small intestines
Pasteurellosis	*Pasteurella multocida*	Cattle and Buffalo	Smears from peripheral blood
	Pasteurella haemolytica	Bison, Cattle and Sheep and Goat	Swabs from exudates, heart blood and pieces of liver, spleen and kidney
	Pasteurella anatipestifer	Ducklings	Do
Leptospirosis	*Leptospira icterohaemorrhagica*	Cattle	Whole blood
	L. pomona	Dogs	Urine, Pieces of kidney and liver
	L. canicola	Pigs	
	Leptospira monocytogenes	Cattle, Pig	

Contd...

Contd...

Name of the Disease	*Etiology*	*Host/Species Primarily Affected*	*Clinical Specimen of Samples of Choice for Lab. Diagnosis*
Listeriosis	*Listeria monocytogenes*	Cattle, pigs	Medulla and portion of spinal cord, uterine discharges, foetal membrane and abnormal content of aborted foetus
Tuberculosis	*Mycobacterium tuberculosis var. bovis, M. tuberculosis var. avium*	Cattle Poultry	Nasal swabs, bronchial lymph nodes biopsy, pieces of lung and bone marrow (poultry)
Paratuberculosis	*Mycobacterium paratuberculosis*	Cattle and buffaloes	Faecal sample, intestinal biopsy, terminal part of ileum and mesenteric lymph node.
Glanders	*Pseudomonas mallei*	Equine	Swabs from nose, cutaneous nodules, smears from the nasal septum and lung pieces.
Erisipeiothrix	*Erysipelothrix rhusiopathiae*	Pig, sheep and cattle	Whole blood, synovial fluid and heart blood
Salmonella infections			
(a) Fowl typhoid	*Salmonella gallinarum*	Poultry	Heart blood, liver, spleen, serum
(b) Pullorum disease	*S. pullorum*	Poultry	Heart blood, pieces of liver, spleen and serum
(c) Paratyphoid	*Salmonella* species	Different species of animal and birds	Pieces of liver, gall bladder, intestines
Collibacillosis	*Escherichia coli*	Young animals and birds	Pieces of intestine and heart and blood.
Mastitis	Different species of bacteria	Cattle, sheep, goats and pigs	Milk samples from the affected quarters
Staphylococcal infection	*Staphylococcus aureus*	Different species of animals and birds	Swabs from the localized lesions.
Streptococcal infection	*Stphylococcus* species	Animals and birds	Heart blood and pieces of lungs.
Strangles	*Staphylococcus equi*	Equine	Swabs from the localized suppurative lesions
Contagious bovine Pleuropneumonia (CBPP)	*Mycoplasma mycoides*	Cattle	Pieces of lungs, pleural fluid and serum
Contagious caprine pleuropneumonia (CCPP)	*Mycoplasma capri*	Sheep, Goat	Pieces of lungs, pleural fluid and serum

VIRAL DISEASES

Name of the Disease	*Etiology*	*Host/Species Primarily Affected*	*Clinical Specimen of Samples of Choice for Lab. Diagnosis*
FMD	*Apthovirus* (Picorna)	All cloven hoofed animals	Epithelia covering the vesicles, vesicular fluid and serum
Blue tongue	*Orbi virus*	Sheep, goats and cattle	Whole blood and serum
Infectious Bovine Rhinotracheitis (IBR)	*Herpes virus*	Cattle	Swabs from nasal passage, vulval mucosa, conjunctiva, pieces of liver, spleen and lymph nodes
Neonatal Diarrhoea	Rota virus	Calves and piglets	Rectal swabs and faeces
ORF/Contagious Ecthyma	Parapox virus	Sheep and goat	Scab material
Sheep pox	Sheep pox virus	Sheep	Scab material
Bovine viral Diarrhoea (BVD)	Pestivirus	Cattle	Whole blood, pieces of liver, spleen and lymph nodes
Rabies	Lyssa virus (Rhabdo virus)	All warm blooded animals	Brain (Hipocampus)
Rinder Pest	Morbilli virus	Cattle, buffalo, Pig and other animals	Whole blood, pieces of spleen, mesenteric lymph node and serum
Ephemeral fever	Rhabdo virus	Cattle	Whole blood
Adeno virus infection	Adeno virus	Cattle	Rectal swabs, Nasal and eye swabs, pieces of lungs, mesentric lymph nodes
Peste des petits ruminants (PPR)	*Morbilli virus*	Sheep and goat	Mesenteric lymph nodes, spleen and serum
Malignant catarrhal fever	*Herpes virus*	Cattle	Whole blood and lymph nodes
Visna-Maedi	*Lenti virus*	Sheep and goat	Brain tissue, pieces of lungs, Bronchial and mediastinal lymph node
Swine vesicular disease	*Entero virus*	Pigs (Swine)	Vesicular fluid and vesicular epithelium
Swine fever (Hog cholera)	*Toga virus* (*Pantropic RNA virus*)	Pigs	Whole blood, pieces of spleen, mesenteric lymph node, pancreas and spleen
Parvo virus infection	*Parvo virus*	Pigs	Pieces of liver, spleen, and kidney, vaginal mucous and serum
Swine pox	*Swine pox virus*	Pigs	Scab material
Pseudo Rabies	*Herpes virus*	Pigs	Pieces of brain and spinal cord, serum
Canine distemper	*Morbilli virus*	Dogs	Whole blood, conjunctival swab, pieces of lungs, stomach and bladder

Contd...

Contd...

Name of the Disease	*Etiology*	*Host/Species Primarily Affected*	*Clinical Specimen of Samples of Choice for Lab. Diagnosis*
Infectious canine Hepatitis	*Adeno virus*	Dogs	Pieces of liver and kidney
Parvo *virus* disease	*Parvo virus*	Dogs	Rectal swab, faecal sample, pieces of heart muscle, and mesenteric lymph node.
Infectious laryngo tracheitis (ILT)	*Herpes virus*	Poultry	Larynx and Trachea
Infectious Bronchitis (IB)	*Corona virus*	Poultry	Trachea, bronchi, lung, air sacs and kidney
Fowl pox	*Avipox virus*	Poultry	Scab material, larynx and trachea.
Inclusion body Hepatitis	*Adeno virus*	Poultry	Liver, cloacal swabs, lungs and trachea
Egg drop syndrome (EDS)	EDS virus	Poultry	Cloacal swab, reproductive organs
African Horse sickness	Orbi *virus*	Horses	Liver of aborted foetus and neural tissue
Equine infectious anaemia	Lenti *virus*	Horses	Whole blood and spleen

2.5 TRANSPORT MEDIA FOR BACTERIOLOGICAL SPECIMEN

1. Nutrient Broth

Peptone – 10 g

Beef extract – 10 g

Sodium chloride – 5 g

Distilled water -1000 ml.

2. Dextrose Broth

1 per cent Sodium dextrose or Glucose in nutrient broth.

3. Peptone water

Peptone – 10 g

Sodium chloride – 5 g

Distilled water – 1000 ml

The mixture is sterilized by autoclaving, distributed in small volume in sterilized test tubes or vials and stored in a refrigerator for future use.

2.6 TRANSPORT MEDIA FOR VIROLOGICAL SPECIMEN

Hank's balanced salt solution	8.6 ml
Bovine serum albumin solution	10.0 ml
Sodium bicarbonate 5 per cent solution (pH 5.6)	1.5 ml
Penicillin 10,000 IU/ml	1 ml
Streptomycin 10 mg/ml	1ml
Nystatin 2,500 mg/ml	1ml
Phosphate buffer solution	1 ml
Phenol red solution (0.4 per cent)	0.5 ml

All the ingredients should be mixed and distributed in sterilized screw cap vials and stored in a refrigerator for use whenever required.

Phosphate Buffer Glycerine (50 per cent)

Phosphate buffer solution.

Solution (A) Disodium hydrogen phosphate – 7.13 g

Distilled water – 500 ml

Solution (B) Sodium bihydrogen phosphate -2.27 g

Distilled water – 500 ml.

Solution-A and Solution-B – mixed and the pH is adjusted at 7.4 to 7.6. Equal quantities of a neutral glycerine buffer solution and the phosphate buffer solution are added together, sterilized by autoclaving, distributed in sterilized screw cap vials and stored in refrigerator for use whenever necessary.

2.7 TIPS FOR DIAGNOSING FOREIGN BODY IN RETICULUM

Diagnosis for foreign body in reticulum is based on history, clinical finding, physical examination, clinical pathology, laboratory findings and post mortem examination.

History

1. Recent parturition.
2. An abrupt and drastic fall in milk yield (40-50 per cent).
3. Reduced appetite.
4. Reluctance to walk or get up or lie down or doing so with caution.
5. Standing for longer periods.
6. Gradual development of oedematous swelling in neck, fall or brisket.

These could give the suspicion in occurrence of traumatic pericarditis and or traumatic peritonitis.

Clinical Findings

1. Animals would be dull and depressed.
2. Complete anorexia at terminal stage.
3. Reluctance to move and does slowly.
4. Kyphosis (arching of back with head kept down).
5. Animal would appear gaunt or tucked up and with abducted elbows and trembling of triceps muscles.
6. Moderate temperature reaction (103-104°F).
7. Respiration-shallow or jerky.
8. Prominent jugular pulse.
9. Muffled heart sound.
10. Mild tympany.
11. Brisket oedema with the release of clear fluid without flakes on aspiration.
12. Constipation or scant faeces.
13. In defecation and urination there could be pain. There may be granting during defecation or urination.
14. Walking particularly downhill may accompany grunting.

Physical Examination

External palpation being not possible for its intra thoracic position and tension of the abdominal wall around the xiphoid cartilage, acoustic percussion can be made which would reveal extensively damp sound at the level of 6th to 8th ribs.

Auscultation

William's auscultation or William's reticular grunt test can be made at 6th or 7th ribs where reticular movements are audible and that would reveal rumbling gurgle, accompanied or followed by a liquid pouring sound. Cattle with traumatic injury to the reticulum may emit a grunt or tinkling sound when reticulum contracts.

Test for Foreign Bodies

Pole test and wither pinch test are sufficient to confirm foreign body syndrome. The basis of these tests is that indirect pressure exerted over the site of the reticulum may cause the animal to grunt if pain persists in reticulum.

Pole Test

It is done taking a-pole (preferably bamboo) 1-1.5 meters long placing under the animals body and being held at each end by two persons where the pole is pulled upwards slowly and allowed to fall suddenly, starting at the xiphoid region and proceeding backwards at intervals of a hand breadth without injuring penis in case of male and gravid uterus in case of pregnant cows. The animal would hold its back and belly arched while test is done and such posture can be corrected by carrying out a back grip. Pain percussion can be carried out with a fist and hammer, having a rubber head applied with short strokes starting with light blows and progressing to heavier blows.

Wither Pinch Test

It is also known as back grip test where a fold of skin over the withers is pulled up so that animals back is suddenly pressed down. This helps in displacing organs in the region of the xiphoid cartilage. If the animal is very big and strong, it may be necessary to use a padded pole instead of a hand grip. Failure to ventriflex the spine may be an indication of pain in upper thoracic area or in the anterior abdomen.

Laboratory Examination

Blood should be collected in a sterilized test tube for hemogram which would reveal leukocytosis, neutrophilia and monocytosis. In acute diffuse peritonitis there may be degenerative left shift, leucopenia and lymphopenia.

Generally animals in most of the cases do not respond to treatment and collapse within a week or so.

Other Valuable Diagnostic Methods

1. Abdominocentasis
2. Right flank laparoscopy (using flexible fiberoptic laparoscope).
3. Radiological examination of reticulum with animal in dorsal
4. Ferroscopy
5. Ultrasonography.

Abdominocentesis

Abdominocentesis and peritoneal fluid analysis can be valuable diagnostic aid. The site for abdominocentesis is 10-12 cm caudal to xiphisternum and 10-15cm lateral to midline. A blunt end teat canula or 16 gauge long hypodermic needle may be used to derive peritoneal fluid. The changes as observed could be of diagnostic value. Macrophages may predominate in chronic peritonitis. Physical appearance of peritoneal fluid may be amber to pink and turbid.

Ferroscopy

It involves the use of a metal detector (or a Ferroscope), applied at the ventral and ventrolateral parts of chest and abdomen to detect the foreign body (*viz.* iron, steel or nickel).

Radiography

Radiography of the reticulum can provide information on the shape and size of an opaque foreign body and may show if it is penetrating the wall of the reticulum and in case there is traumatic pericarditis (TRP). It is best suited for visualization of radio dense foreign bodies.

Conventional radiography of the reticulum is conducted with the animal in standing position. The horizontal beam is centered on the reticulo-diaphragmatic caudal pericardial region and includes the area confined ventrally by the sternum and dorsally by the caudal venacava.

The purpose of this examination is to determine whether there are radio-dense (metallic) or radio-lucent (non-metallic) foreign bodies.

Lateral view with the animal in lateral recumbent position or dorsal recumbent position with the fore limbs stretched forward. Will show in normal radiograph, the part of sternum; cardiac outline, reticulum and a portion of lung more clearly.

Ultrasonography

The reticulum can be visualized by using a 3.5 MHZ linear transducer applied to the ventral midline of the thorax over the 6th and 7th intercostals spaces. The contour of reticulum, reticular contractions can be imaged. In cows with disturbed reticular motility, the number of biphasic contractions is reduced and indistinct. Foreign bodies cannot be visualized ultrasonographically.

Post Mortem Examination

In dead animals post mortem examination can be performed to determine the cause and the extent of the damage caused by the foreign body. In most of the cases the foreign body is found perforating the cranioventral aspect of the reticulum or a perforating fibrinous tract is evident. There may be extensive fibrinous adhesions between the cranioventral aspects of reticulum, ventral abdominal wall and diaphragm.

Animals with oedematous swelling on opening of that carcass may reveal accumulation of huge amount serosanguineous fluid beneath the skin in the neck and the thoracic region. On gross examination the heart may be enlarged. Foul smelling grayish fluid may be accumulated in the pericardial sac. Heart may reveal a typical shaggy appearance. A piece of wire, sewing needle or even nails is usually found lying in the reticulum which is the main culprit in animals causing death of affected animal (owing to foreign body in reticulum and its penetration).

2.8 FINE NEEDLE ASPIRATION CYTOLOGY

Cytologic or histologic evaluation can be done by needle aspiration or surgical biopsy. Fine needle aspiration cytology has become an important diagnostic aid in diagnosis of tumour or neoplasms, hyperplasia, haematoma, cysts, abscess *etc*. The techniques of aspiration consisted of inserting a fine needle into target organ and aspirating cells with syringe. The material in the needle is expressed on glass slide and smears are prepared. Wet fixation in 95 per cent alcohol and staining with haematoxylin eosin. Cytological diagnosis by this technique can be obtained rapidly.

Fine Needle Aspiration Cytology of Prostrate in Canines

The digital rectal palpation is an essential examination in the diagnosis of prostatic diseases. But it is not sufficiently accurate in tumour diagnosis. For this purpose transrectal aspiration biopsy cytology of prostrate can be done.

Aspiration of prostrate can be done using locally available different instruments *e.g.* long needle for lumber puncture (22 No.) a piece of plastic tube (approx 3 inch length). This plastic tube can be an intravenous catheter or a scalp vein cannula. Disposable plastic aspiration syringe (5/10 ml), syringe gun (Cameco) *etc.* are required The apparatus should be routinely sterilized.

Technique of Trans-rectal Aspiration of the Prostrate

Before performing the respiration biopsy, rectum and bladder needs to be completely evacuated. The dog should be placed in standing position and careful digital examination of the prostrate can be done to assess the size of prostrate and consistency of lesion. The glove in the left hand is replaced and instrument is arranged on the gloved left index finger. The piece of plastic tube to be used as a needle guide is fixed to the gloved left index finger by means of adhesive tape. The syringe, fine lumbar puncture needle attached is taken in the right hand and needle is passed through the proximal end of the plastic needle guide till the needle point reaching the distal end of the guide with gloved right hand, a finger is put over the left index. This fixes the guide more firmly on the palpating finger and minimizes contamination when the finger is introduced into the rectum.

The index finger of the left hand with this arrangement is then well lubricated with jelly and is slowly inserted into the rectum. The tumour suspect area is again palpated with the left index finger and good contact with the biopsy target is established. The needle should pass through the finger coat and via the rectal mucosa into the lesion. The plunger of the syringe is then retracted with the help of syringe gun (Cameco syringe gun) to create a negative pressure in the barrel of the syringe. The needle is then moved back and forth in the biopsy target three or four times by quick movements. Throughout this procedure, a negative pressure must be maintained by keeping the plunger retracted.

When the aspiration is completed, the pressure in the syringe is to be equalized by allowing the plunger slowly to return to its normal position. The needle is then pulled back into the plastic tube which is used as a needle guide. Then the index finger is withdrawn from the rectum.

After withdrawing the index finger, syringe is disconnected, filled with air and connected to the needle. The material in the needle is expressed on the clean glass slide as a single drop and the smear is prepared as like as blood smear. As soon as the smears are made, these are fixed in 95 per cent alcohol for minimum of 30 minutes. The smears are stained with haematoxylin and Eosin and Papanicaau.

This technique is safe and convenient. Trans-rectal aspiration cytology of prostrate gives rapid cytological diagnosis.

2.9 BIOLOGICAL TESTS FOR METABOLIC DISORDERS

Biological tests are useful in supporting problems found in nutritional management, ration formulation and disease incidence on herd basis.

Ruminal pH Testing

It is the definitive test for ruminant acidosis. However, ruminal pH may vary from day to day and time to time within herd. Hence, single sampling of a group of cow is vulnerable error. pH paper is not accurate enough for the said purpose because it is influenced by the green colour of ruminal fluid.

For field use Cardy Twin pH meter – (Spectrum Technologies 23839W) is ideal. It requires only a small volume of ruminal fluid. It has automatic calibration routine and compensates for the temperature of the sample.

The cut point of ruminal pH is 5.5. If it is 3 to 5 animals are tested for a group of 15 animals having a ruminal pH of 5.5, the group is considered to be at high risk for subacute ruminal acidosis.

Serum-β-Hydroxy Butyric Acid (BHBA)

The 'gold standard' test for subclinical ketosis is serum BHBA.

This ketone body is more stable in blood than acetone or acetoacetate. Canadian research has defined a cut point of 1400 mmol/l (14.4 mg/dl) BHBA for subclinical ketosis. At above this value, cattle are at increased risk for displaced abomasitis, clinical ketosis and decreased milk production. This test can be performed on serum samples. Serum BHBA concentration typically increases after feeding. Extremely high BHBA concentration above 30 mg/dl is meant for clinical ketosis.

Urinary pH Testing for Dosing Anions (for milk fever prevention)

Dietary cation-anion difference (DCAD) and milk fever prevention are optimal at urinary pH values of about 6.0 to 6.5. The mean urinary pH value below about 6.0 is uncommon and indicates over acidification diet. High chloride content in one of the forages can contribute to the low urinary pH.

Urea Nitrogen Testing (UNT)/(Blood urea nitrogen and milk urea nitrogen testing)

Blood UN (BUN) and milk UN (MUN) are indirect measures of protein and energy nutrition in lactating cows. High urea nitrogen is a risk factor for infertility and body condition score loss due to the energy cost of detoxifying excessive ruminal ammonia into urea by the liver.

Bulk tank milk urea nitrogen (MUN) is attractive because it provides a mean value for a large group of lactating cows with a single test without concerns of getting and adequate sample size. Bulk tank MUN testing is inexpensive and accurate and because UN is evaluated on a basis of the group mean, bulk tank MUN screening is a reasonable procedure to conduct on a routine basis.

Part – II
Medicine Section

Chapter 3
Classification of Animal Diseases

3.1 HEALTH AND DISEASE

Normal physiological, anatomical and mental conditions of animal body are called health. Any deviation from normal physical, mental or physiological conditions will be considered as disease.

3.2 CLASSIFICATION OF DISEASES

Animal diseases can be classified on the basis of the following criteria.

(*a*) According to mode of origin or genesis of disease
(*b*) According to the involvement of system
(*c*) According to changes in the organ
(*d*) According to causes or etiology
(*e*) According to mode of infection
(*f*) According to clinical manifestation and course of the disease
(*g*) According to the intensity and spread of the disease
(*h*) According to place of origin
(*i*) According to source of infection

(a) According to Mode of Origin or Genesis of Disease

(*i*) *Hereditary disease*: Diseases which are transmitted to the offsprings through sire or dam

e.g.. Haemophilia, Epilepsy *etc.*

(*ii*) *Congenital disease*: Development defects or anomaly either structural, functional or both, acquired during intra uterine life and appreciable at birth.

e.g. Atresia ani, Atresia vulvi, Congenital hydrocephalus. Schistosomus reflexus, Crooked calf disease *etc.*

(*iii*) *Acquired disease*: Diseases that are contracted during the entire life span of an animal.

e.g. Senile cataract.

(*b*) According to the Involvement of System

(*i*) *Localised disease*: Disease or lesions confined to a particular spot or organ.

(*ii*) *Generalised disease*: Disease involving most of the systems or body parts.

e.g. Septicaemia, Toxemia *etc.*

(*c*) According to Changes in the Organ

(*i*) *Structural disease:* Disease which affects the structure of an organ and brings about pathological changes.

e.g. Rickets, Orchitis, Nephritis, Osteomalacia, *etc.*

(*ii*) *Functional disease:* Disease affecting functional efficiency of an organ. *e.g.* Cardial arrhythmia, Vulvular inefficiency *etc.*

(*d*) According to Causes or Etiology

(*i*) *Bacterial disease, caused by Bacteria*

e.g. Anthrax, Haemorrhagic Septicaemia, Black Quarter, Brucellosis *etc.*

(*ii*) *Viral disease, caused by Virus*

e.g. Rinderpest (RP), Foot and Mouth Disease (FMD), *Peste des petits ruminants* (PPR), Blue tongue *etc.*

(*iii*) *Ricketsial disease, caused by Ricketsia*

(*iv*) *Chlamydial disease, caused by Chlamydia*

(*v*) *Fungal/Mycotic disease, caused by Fungus*

e.g. Aspergillosis, Fusariotoxicosis, Candidiasis *etc.*

(*vi*) *Parasitic disease or Worm infestation, caused by parasites*

e.g. Fasciolisis, Amphistomiasias, Schistosomiasis *etc.*

(*vii*) *Protozoan disease, caused by Protozoa*

e.g. Babesiosis, Theileriosis, Trypanosomiasis *etc.*

(*viii*) *Microfilarial disease, caused by Microfilaria*

e.g. Filariasis, Hump Sore *etc.*

Besides this classification, according to etiology disease can be divided into (*a*) Contagious disease and (*b*) Infectious disease.

(*a*) *Contagious disease:* Disease spreads by intimate contact.

e.g. FMD, PPR *etc.*

(*b*) *Infectious disease:* Disease caused by microbes or infecting organisms. *e.g.* Viral disease, Protozoan disease, Mycotic disease *etc.*

(*c*) *Non-specific disease:* Diseases which are caused by multiple etiologies or multiple factors.

e.g. Diarrhoea, Dysentery, Pneumonia, Bronchitis, Colic *etc.*

(*e*) According to Mode of Infection

(*i*) *Primary disease:* Disease that occurs independently and not influenced by another disease. *e.g.* FMD, Canine Distemper, Rabies *etc.*

(*ii*) *Secondary disease:* Super imposed disease that supervene out of already prevailing primary disease. *e.g.* Secondary Pneumonia due to secondary bacterial invasion after a viral disease.

(*iii*) *Intercurrent disease:* Disease occurs as a sequence to primary disease. *e.g.* disturbed thermoregulation as a sequele of FMD, chorea as a sequele to Canine Distemper.

(*f*) According to Clinical Manifestation and Course of the Disease

(*i*) *Acute Disease:* Such disease is characterized by a sudden on set and a short course with severe manifestation. *e.g.* FMD, PPR, HS, BQ.

(*ii*) *Per acute disease:* Sudden onset with a very severe course with a very short spans than acute disease. *e.g.* Per acute anthrax, Per acute HS, Per acute septic mastitis.

(*iii*) *Sub acute disease:* Disease whose onset and severity is lesser than acute is called sub acute disease. Usually the disease runs a course of 2 to 4 weeks *e.g.* Sub acute mastitis.

(*iv*) *Chronic disease:* Disease runs a protracted course with less severity but may terminate fatally. *e.g.* Brucellosis, Paratuberculosis, Tuberculosis *etc.*

(*v*) *Carrier:* It is an interrelationship between the microorganism and the animal body without obvious clinical manifestation of the disease. *e.g* Surra in cattle, highly pathogenic Avian influenza in duck.

(*g*) According to the Intensity and Spread of the Disease

(*i*) *Sporadic disease:* Disease which affects a single animal but not spreads to others in the same flock or hard. *e.g.* Polyencephalomalacia, Sporadic bovine encephalomyelitis *etc.*

(*ii*) *Enzootic disease:* It is a kind of outbreak of disease affecting animals in a definite area or district. *e.g.* Enzootic haematuria in cattle (hill region), Anthrax *etc.*

(*iii*) *Epizootic disease:* Diseases which affects a large population of animals in a wide spread manner (covering in large area). *e.g.* RP, PPR and FMD.

(*iv*) *Endemic disease:* Diseases which is retained for a long time in some areas or locality years together affecting a large number of animals under same species. *e.g.* Anthrax, HS, BQ *etc.*

(*v*) *Panzootic disease:* When an epidemic spreads over many countries or even continents is called a Panzootic disease; *e.g.* Bird flu (Avian Influenza).

(*h*) According to Place of Origin

(*i*) *Indigenous disease:* Disease prevalent as native one. *e.g.* Malaria, Filaria, TB, Leprosy, Degnala.

(*ii*) *Exotic disease:* Disease that has been acquired from foreign countries. *e.g.* Japanese encephalitis, South African Horse Sickness.

(*iii*) *Emerging disease:* Disease which are not in existence but may be introduced at any time. *e.g.* Louping ill in sheep.

(*i*) According to Source of Infection

(*a*) *Endogenous disease:* It is otherwise known as auto infection where disease originates as a result of activation of the residential organisms in the host's system owing to lowered resistance and stresses. *e.g.* Shipping fever, Pharyngitis, Laryngitis.

(*b*) *Exogenous disease:* Disease which animals get infected from other animals, feed stuffs, water, air, soil, secretions and excretions *etc.*

Chapter 4
Systemic Diseases and their Treatment

4.1 DISEASES OF ALIMENTARY SYSTEM

4.1.1 Stomatitis

It may be defined as the inflammation of buccal (oral) mucosa associated with glossitis (inflammation of tongue), gingivitis (inflammation of the gum) and inflammation of palate (palatitis). The lesions may spread to teeth (odontitis) or lips (chelitis).

Etiology

- ☆ The causes of this disease are many. It may be due to physical agents *e.g.* traumatic injuries of oral mucosae, trauma during mastication of roughages like hay, fodder, spine of plants, thorns *etc.*, laceration or injury by sharp foreign objects.
- ☆ Chemical agents like – acid, alkali, corrosive chemicals, irritant drugs *etc.*
- ☆ Infective agents – causing bacterial stomatitis due to Actino bacillus lignieresi, Streptococus, Staphylococci *etc.*
- ☆ Viral etiology – *e.g.* RP, FMD, Mucosal disease, Vesicular stomatitis, Vesicular exanthema, Blue tongue, PPR in small ruminants *etc.*
- ☆ Mycotic etiology – *e.g. Monizia* species, *Candida* species *etc.*

Symptoms

Stomatitis is manifested by painful mastication, partial or complete loss of appetite, profuse salivation accompanied with smacking sound of lips. Swelling of face, bad breath, foul smell from mouth, and oral lesions may be seen (*e.g.* vesicular lesions, ulcerative or necrotic lesions). These may be white velvety deposits on tongue (*e.g.* in PPR).

Stomatitis is of different types as per lesions. These are catarrhal stomatitis, papular stomatitis, vesicular stomatitis, ulcerative stomatitis, necrotic stomatitis *etc.*

Treatment

1. Boro glycerine (1-2 per cent)

   Boro glycerine may be applied over the lesions.
2. Mouth washing using 1 : 10,000 Potassium permanganate solution, 2 per cent Copper sulphate solution, 5 per cent Sodium bicarbonate solution, 2 per cent Alum solution.

   Gentian violet 1 per cent solution can also be painted over lesions.
3. Supportive treatment
   - (*a*) Vitamin B-Complex, *e.g.* Inj. Hivit, Inj. Conciplex, Inj. X-L-plex, Inj. Pinkojet, Inj. Tribivet @ 5-10 ml by IM route on alternate day for 3 occasions.
   - (*b*) Liver extract with B-Complex, *e.g.* Inj. Belamyl, Inj. Livron, Inj. Livobex, Inj Pepcid, Inj. Stronic @ 5-10 ml by IM route on alternate day for 3 occasions.
   - (*c*) Vitamin-A injection, *e.g.* Inj. Veta-A, Inj. Intavita, Inj. Vitacept, Inj. Vet ADE @ 5-10 ml by IM route at 3 days interval can be advocated.
4. If necessary, parenteral antibiotic (broad spectrum) *e.g.* Inj. Oxytetracycline, Inj. Enrofloxacin can be given by IM route for 3 days.

4.1.2 Pharyngitis

It denotes the inflammation of the pharyngeal mucosa and submucosa which may extend to soft palate and tonsil. It is characterized by coughing, salivation and painful swallowing of feed.

Etiology

Injury from thorns, foreign bodies, faulty instrumentation in oral cavity, irritation by smokes, gas, fumes, irritant drugs and ingestion of too hot or too cold feed. Besides these, infective causes (*e.g.* virus and bacteria) like *Actinobacillus lignieresi* in cattle may be responsible for this disease.

Symptoms

Dull and depression, off fed, stretching of neck and head, inspiratory dyspnsea, painful cough, regurgitation of food and water through nostrils, mucopurulent nasal discharge, oedema and congestion of soft palate *etc.* The animal may suffer from respiratory distress with high rise of temperature, rapid heart rate.

Treatment

1. Withheld all the feed until the animal is relieved.
2. Keep the animal in well ventilated, clean warm premises.

3. Parenteral fluid therapy in case of off fed conditions *e.g.* IV DNS, 5 per cent Dextrose, Rintose, Intalyte *etc.*
4. Correction of primary causes with proper measures, Broad spectrum Antibiotics or sulphur drugs can be judiciously used.
5. NSAID *e.g.* Inj. Meloxicam, Inj. Zobid-M, Inj. Neoprofen, Inj. Oxalgin NP can be used by IM route.
6. Local paint with Mandel's solution. Composition of this solution is Iodine 600 mg, Potassium iodide 1 g, Pepermint oil 250 mg and Glycerine 30 ml.
7. Carminative and antispasmodic mixture. Purgatives for cattle can be used *e.g.* Papazyme syrup, Carmizen symp (Nugen) P-Zyme vet (Oxford) @ 50-100 ml BID can be drenched.
8. Supportive treatment
   (*a*) Rumenotoric bolus, *e.g.* Rumentus, Ecotus, Provisac, Floraboost, AD_3, Floratone, Gofeed, Feed on bolus, Pachoplus @ 2 boli BID.
   (*b*) For impaction of rumen, Gastina liquid, Blotocil, Tymplex, Tyral 50-100 ml BID can be drenched.
   (*c*) Liver extract with B-complex injection by IM route can be administered *e.g.* Inj. Belamyl, Inj. Livobex, Inj. Livron, Inj. Stronic @ 5-10 ml by IM route on alternate day.
9. A course of antihistaminic preparation to be given to reduce pharyngeal oedema *e.g.* Inj. Chloril, Inj. Zeet, Inj. Anistamin, Inj. Chlorazin @ 5-10 ml by IM route daily for 3 days.
10. Inhalation of Tr. Benzoin to soften the viscid/mucoid exudates.

4.1.3 Parotitis

Inflammation of the parotid gland is known as parotitis. It may be acute or chronic in nature, characterized by glandular abscess, painful swallowing and salivation. The condition is fairly common in cattle owing to some infectious diseases like Tuberculosis, Actinobacillosis *etc.*

Etiology

External tramma, extension of infection from pharyax, salivary calculi, inflammation of glandular tissues, inflammation of submaxillary and sublingual salivary glands, lymph node abscess, irritation from grass or awn on the glandular duct.

Symptoms

Intense painful swelling of the glands and adjoining areas, pyrexia, oedemotous swelling may extend over the base of the ear, swelling may be hot and painful. Dysphasia, salivation, painful mastication and disinclination to open mouth out of pain.

Treatment

1. Magsulph hot formentation or Boric acid hot compress can be given on the swollen area.

2. Surgical drainage with proper care should be made for abscession.
3. Tr. Iodine paint on the swelling can be done.
4. A course of antibiotic can be given. *e.g.* Procaine Penicillin 20-40 lakhs (Inj. F.P.P. 20, 40 lakhs for large animal, 4-10 lakhs for small animals), Streptopenicillin 2.5 g (Inj. Bistrepen, Inj. Biostrep, Inj. Munomycin Fort) through IM route daily for 5-7 days.. Or Broad spectrum antibiotic *e.g.* Oxytetracycline (Inj. Intamycin, Inj. Loxy, Inj. Terramycin), Inj. Ampicillin, Inj. Ampicillin-Cloxacillin (Inj. Acvet, Inj. Inclox, Inj. Cilclox), Inj. Enrofloxacin (Inj. Enrocin, Inj. Floxidin, Inj. Enrored, Inj. Enrovet) through IM route daily for 5-7 days.
5. The wounds should be dressed with local antibiotic or antiseptic solution or multipurpose herbal ointments (Topicure, Sorine, Himax *etc.*).
6. In chronic cases, Lugol's iodine 2-5 ml may be injected directly to the gland to make it atrophied.

4.1.4 Choke

It is the sudden closure or obstruction of oesophagus by foreign body or food mass characterized by hypersalivation, inability of deglutination and regurgitation. In ruminants bloat is the pathognomonic manifestation of choke.

Etiology

Cattle and buffalo due to their greedy nature of feed intake suffer from choke with the solid objects like potatoes, apple, guava, mango seed, beet, turnip, cabbage, watermelon *etc.* which stuck up in the oesophagas while swallowing.

Space occupying lesions on the oesophageal wall *e.g.* papilloma, neoplasm, any granutomatous lesion may cause obstruction of the oesophageal passage. Chronic obstruction may result from stenosis after oesophagitis, external pressure by tubercular and neoplastic lymph nodes at the base of the lungs.

Symptoms

Choke may be partial or incomplete and full or complete.

In partial choke, bloat is not well marked, gas and liquid may pass but there is regurgitation of the solid food.

In acute choke, there is complete closure of oesophagus. Salivation, restlessness, distress, grunting, bloat, coughing, protrusion of tongue, regurgitation, fatal tympany and respiratory distress are common. Colic like symptoms, cough, regurgitation of food and saliva are seen in early stage but if the condition persists for long time death occurs due to inhalation pneumonia.

Diagnosis

- ☆ Palpation of cervical oesophagus for foreign bodies.
- ☆ Use of mouth gag to examine pharyngeal obstruction.
- ☆ Clinical signs.

☆ The obstruction may be located by passing probang or stomach tube.

☆ Surgical exploration for prompt diagnosis and repair may also be made.

Treatment

1. Attempt may be made to push the obstruction onward with great care with the help of lubricated stomach tube or probing.
2. In small animals remove the foreign body through mouth with long handled forceps.
3. In acute cases with much discomfort or distress sedate the animal by tranquilizers *e.g.* Siquil (Triflupromezine), Largactil (Chlorpromazine); Doses for large animal is 0.5 to 2.2 mg/kg and for small animal 0.5 to 1.5 mg/kg body weight of 2.5 per cent solution by IM route.
4. To relax oesophageal spasm Inj. Atroprine sulphate 16-32 mg for large animals (like cattle, buffalo and horse) by SC route can be administered.
5. Solid obstruction at the pharyngeal region can be removed by opening the mouth by gag and through digital manipulation or with the help of a wire loop to pull the object entangled in it.
6. Palpable food *e.g.* watermelon, potato *etc.* may be crushed by physical means from outside.
7. If all measures fail, obligatory surgical intervention should be carried out to save the life by removing the hurdle by oesophagotomy.

4.1.5 Colic

Colic may be defined as severe pain in stomach and intestine. It is one of the most important complications in equine species. It also occurs in all other species of animals. Precisely colic indicates pain in the colon and in broader connotation it is the painful condition of any abdominal organs. Colic is of different types:

1. True colic – pain originating from gastrointestinal tract.
2. False colic – Pain originating from other than G.I. tract. *e.g.* Renal colic, uterine colic.
3. Physical colic – Owing to obstruction of G.I. tract or any physical agents causing distension of stomach *e.g.* Enterolith.
4. Spasmodic colic – Owing to spasmodic contraction of the intestine, *e.g.* Drinking of cold water after rigorous work, heavy parasitic infestation like Strongylosis.
5. Tympanic colic – Owing to over production and accumulation of gases in GI tract. *e.g.* Flatulent colic.
6. Obstructive colic – It is otherwise known as impactive colic. *e.g.* Impaction of caecum, colon *etc.*
7. Extraluminal colic – *e.g.* Volvulus, torsion, hernia *etc.*

Etiology

Intestinal parasites, intestinal twist (volvulus, strangulation), poisoning, drinking of too cold water, sudden excitement. Intaking irritants drugs and chemicals, intake of mouldy feed (Fusariotoxicosis), damaged feeds and hay, heavy viral and bacterial infections in the gut *etc.*

Symptoms

Severe intense abdominal pain, rolling on the ground, kicking at the abdomen, restless condition looking at the flank region or towards the site of pain involvement, stamp and kick on the ground, lie down and get up, increased thirst, anorexia, perspiration, anorexia and angry look.

Treatment

1. For spasmodic colic, use spasmolytic drugs, *e.g.* Pethidine HCl @ 1 mg/Ib body weight, Inj. Atropine sulphate – 15-30 mg by SC or IM depending on the body weight, Inj. Valethamate bromide (*e.g.* Valginate, Epidosin) 20-30 ml by IM route can be given.
2. Use analgesic injection and or antispasmodics, *e.g.* Inj. Epidosin (TTK) 1 per cent Valethamate bromide @ 8 to 10 ml for cattle and horse, 2 to 5 ml for sheep and goat, and 1 to 2 ml for dog by IM route. (It is most effective in intestinal sparms, renal colic, uterine colic *etc.*). Inj. Meloxicam (*e.g.* Inj. Melonex, Inj. Meloxi, Inj. MPS, Inj. Melobest (TTK), Inj. A_3 vet, Inj. Zobid-20 *etc.*) @ 10-15 ml depending on the body weight, Inj. Ketoprofen (*e.g.* Inj. Ketop, Inj. Neoprofen), Inj. Analgin, Inj. Oxalgin, Inj. Vetalgin @ 8-10 ml/100 kg body weight by IM route.
3. Oral bolus *e.g.* Spasmonim (Excell) 2 boli BID along with rumenotoric *e.g.* Pachoplus, Provisace, Yeasacc, Rumentus @ 2 boli BID can be tried.
4. Oral drench *e.g.* Chloral hydrus – 25 ml

   Oil Turpentine – 30 ml

   Oil Linseed – 450 ml

   Mft. Haust

   Sig. Administer by stomach tube.
5. For Bloat and tympanic reason, drench Gastina, Tymplex, Debloat, Blotocil, Bloatcon, Tympex liquid or Herbal antibloat Timpol powder, Gasnil *etc.*

4.1.6 Rumen Dysfunction

Ruminal dysfunction results in the production of common diseases of rumen, like simple indigestion, bloat (tympany), lactacidosis, ruminal stasis and ruminal parakeratosis *etc.* Besides a good numbers of nutritional, environmental infections and metabolic diseases, some other conditions like ammonia toxicity, para amphistomiasis, traumatic reticulo-peritonitis, vagus indigestion *etc.* may lend to the development of rumen and reticulum dysfunctions.

Symptoms

Anorexia, abdominal distension, diarrhoea, constipation and abdominal pain.

Diagnosis

Ruminal dysfunction can be examined and evaluated by palpation, percussion, auscultation or ballotment. Besides physical examination by Rumenotomy, diagnostic imaging, metal detector will be of immense value in diagnosis.

Treatment

The principles of treatment of rumen dysfunction are:

1. Correction of ruminal pH.
2. Release of excess gas (by using trocar and canula).
3. Restoration of fluid and electrolytes imbalance (isotonic fluid, sodium carbonate 0.8 per cent, DNS).
4. Replacement of microorganisms (fresh rumen liquid or transplant).
5. Supply of co-factors like phosphorus, calcium, magnesium, cobalt, copper, manganese, zinc, iron to keep rumen environment in healthy state.

The commercial preparations used for treating rumen dysfunction are:

- ☆ Stomachic powder (herbal preparations like H.B. strong, Catone, Natural Batisa, Himalayan Batisa).
- ☆ Rumenotorics like Floratone, Rumentas, Floraboost, Yeasace, Bovirum bolus, Rumen bolus, Provisac bolus *etc.*
- ☆ For tympany (bloat) antibloat preparations, *e.g.* Gasnil liquid (Vet Med) 50 ml BID for large animal and 25 ml BID for small animal), Tympex, Tymplex, Bloatocil, Bloatcon *etc.* or herbal antibloat pulv preparations like Timpol, Gastina *etc.*
- ☆ Antihistaminic injection like Avil, Chloril, Zeet, Chlorazin, Antilar *etc.*
- ☆ As a metabolic booster and rejuvenator the neurotropic B-vitamins (parenteral preparations) like Inj. Tribivet (Intas), Inj. Polyvet (Excell) *etc.* or oral preparations stimulating ruminal function and digestion like Papazyme, Carmigen, Digecon, P-Zymevet (Oxford Gem) can be recommended.
- ☆ Systemic liver extract injection with vitamin B-complex like Inj. Belamyl, Inj. Levadex, Inj. Livron, Inj. Stronic, Inj. Pepcid, Inj. Livobex (TTK) @ 5-10 ml IM on alternate day for 3-5 occasions can be administered.
- ☆ For restoring fluid and electrolyte balance DNS (5 per cent Dextrose normal saline) should be administered if there is dehydration with electrolyte imbalance.
- ☆ For impaction, vegetable oil (½-1 litre) can also be drenched.
- ☆ Fresh rumen liquor transplantation can be started in severe rumen dysfunction due to lactacidisis. For alkalosis Liq. Vinegar @ 2 ml/kg body weight mixed in 2 to 5 litres of water can be placed intraruminally gives better result.
- ☆ Purgative like Magnesium sulphate @ 250-500 ml/day for two days for impaction.

- ☆ Parenteral administration of calcium boroglucanate (IV and SC) can be recommended because hypocalcaemia reduces the ruminal motility leading to ruminal stasis or slagish rumination and ruminal impaction. Parenteral calcium like Inj. Calborol, Inj. Calgonate (Indian Immunologicals), Inj. Calmax (Vetnex) 150-200 ml through IV or SC route give excellent result.
- ☆ Supplementation of mineral mixtures like Agrimin (Glaxo Smithkline), Ranmix (Vetnex), Floraboost AD_3 powder (Excell), Minirex-L powder (Excell) @ 30 g/day also can reduce ruminal dysfunction and associated problems in cattle.

4.1.7 Ruminal Acidosis/Lact Acidosis/Grain Poisoning

Ruminal acidosis which constitutes 18 per cent of indigestion cases in India is a major managemental disease of ruminants. Greedy nature of animals especially goats and cow, mostly suffer from the disease owing to excessive consumption of readily fermentable carbohydrate rich diet. This becomes very fatal and thus causes significant economic loss if proper diagnosis and treatment is not done in time.

Etiology

Ingestion of large quantities of highly fermentable carbohydrate rich feeds.

Symptoms

Moderate acidosis: Inappetance, complete absence of rumination, distended rumen, watery rumen consistency, atony of rumen, abdominal pain, grinding of teeth, reduced rectal temperature, congested visible mucous membranes and moderate constipation.

Severe acidosis: Anorexia, absence of rumination, distended rumen, watery rumen consistency, absence of ruminal motility, abdominal pain, lateral recumbency, anuria, reduced rectal temperature and diarrheoa. Continuous gurgling sound on auscultation of rumen, dyspnoea but accelerated respiration and increased pulse rate.

Mild acidosis: Inappetance, partially suspended rumination, decreased rumen motility, moderate constipation thick, firm and doughy condition of rumen and dull sound on percussion.

Treatment

For Mild Acidosis

- ☆ Sodium bicarbonate OD for 2-3 days in fresh water (sheep and goat @ 3-5 g in 50 ml of fresh water).
- ☆ Stomachic bolus like Rumbion (Indian Herbs), Pachoplus (Dabur Ayurvet), Provisacc bolus (Vetnex), Yeasacc (Vetnex) cattle 2 boli BID, sheep and goat 1 bolus BID for 3 days.
- ☆ Anigest powder (Sarabhai), Digestovet, Herbogastrin (Vetmed) 25 g BID for large animal and 5-10 g BID for small animal orally for 3 days.
- ☆ Vitamin syrup *e.g.*, Ambiplex (Brihans), Lysovit (Oxford), Livolysin syrup (Pharmacon) @ 5 ml BID for small animal and @ 10-15 ml for calf, colt and others orally for 8 days.

For Moderate Acidosis

- ☆ Antihistaminic injection like Inj. Avil, Inj. Chloril, Inj. Zeet, Inj. Chlorazine @ 5-10 ml for large animal and @ 1-2 ml for small animal IM daily for 3 days.
- ☆ Dexamethasone sodium veterinary preparation, Inj. Dexona (Sarabhai Zydus), Inj. Brisone (Brihans), Inj. Enidex (Excell) 1st day 1-1.5ml, 2nd day 0.75-1 ml and 3rd day 0.5 ml for small animal; for large animal first day 2-3 ml, 2nd day 1-2 ml and 3rd day 1 ml by IM route
- ☆ Combination mixture of Sodibicarb and Pachoplus (Dabur), Rumbion bolus (Indian Herbs), Rumentus (Intas) Provisacc bolus (Vetcare), Yeasac bolus (Vetnex) @ 2 boli BID (for large animal) and 1 bolus BID for small animal for 3 days
- ☆ Besides, oral vitamins like Ambiplex, Vimeral, Lysovit, Livolys *etc.* may be given.
- ☆ Sodibicarb (7.5 per cent) 25 ml by IV route for small animal, single dose can be given and for large animal 100-150 ml by IV.
- ☆ Liver extract with B-complex injection like Inj. Livobex (TTK), Inj. Belamyl (Sarabhai Zydus), Inj. Stronic (Vetnex) @ 5-10 ml on alternate day for large animal and @ 2 ml IM for small animal by 3 injections on alternate day should be given.

For Severe Acidosis

- ☆ Antihistaminic injection.
- ☆ Dexamethasone sodium injection.
- ☆ Inj. Sodibicarb 7.5 per cent (Bengal Chemicals) @ 50 ml IV OD for 2 days followed by 5 g sodibicarb orally in 50 ml of fresh water BID for next 2 days for small animal. Combination of stomachic bolus like Provisacc, Rumentus, Rumbion, Floratone *etc.* with Digestovet, Herbogastrin, Himalayan Batisa along with Neodox bolus, Steclin or Cycline (Excell) @ 1 bolus BID for 3 days for small animal and for large animal 2 boli BID and 25-30 g powder for large animal.
- ☆ Normal saline solution by IV route @ 100 ml daily for 3 days for small animal, @ 100 ml-1.5 litres for 3 days for large animal.
- ☆ Liver extract with vitamin B-complex injection, like that of moderate acidosis and from 3rd day onwards oral liver tonic or vitamin syrup can be fed orally for a week. When rumen pH would be improved, then fresh rumen cud transplantation from healthy goats @ 150-200 ml/day for small animal and 500 ml-1 litre on large animal orally on 3-4 days.

4.1.8 Simple Indigestion

Rumen indigestion could be either alkaline indigestion, acid indigestion or indigestion without change in normal pH. Seasonal variations play role in the occurrence of particular type of indigestion depending on the availability of fodders and grasses in the areas in different seasons. Feeding exclusively dry fodders like rice straw, wheat straw *etc.* When greens are not available usually leads to alkaline indigestion (with rumen pH above 7.5); and overfeeding of greens, silages, grain engorgement might lead to acid indigestion (with rumen pH below 6.0). Putrefaction of protein rich diets in the rumen releases toxic amides and amines causing ruminal atony. Simple indigestion is common in stall fed dairy cattle especially when fed with concentrate rich diet. In field conditions, indigestion also occurs when animal gains accidendental access to large quantities of grain or when they are fed a little more concentrate than they can digest adequately.

Symptoms

Reduction in the appetite is the first clinical sign. The rumen of the affected animals may be firm and doughy without obvious distension, and ruminal movement may be depressed. Heart rate, body temperature and respiration rate may remain within the normal range.

Treatment

1. A wide variety of oral preparations containing rumenotorics can be used. Preparations containing Nux vomica, ginger, tarmeric *etc.* can also be used.
2. Stomachic powder like Herbogastin, Catone, Digestovet, Himalayan Batisa, @ 25 g twice daily for 3-5 days for large animal.
3. Rumenotoric bolus *e.g.* Bovirum bolus, Rumentus, Rumen bolus, Provisacc, Yeasacc bolus @ 2-4 boli/day for 3 days for large animal, and 1-2 boli/day for small animal for 2-3 dys.
4. Administration of antihistaminic drugs *e.g.* Inj. Anistamin, Antilar, Allervil, Avil, Chlorazin @ 5 to 10 ml for large animal, 1-2 ml for small animal may reverse the atony in rumen.
5. Good quality B-complex vitamin *e.g.* Inj. Tribivet, Inj. Polyvet, Inj. Neuroxin-12, Inj. Neurovet @ 5-10 ml IM daily for 3-5 days can be used. During indigestion there is inactivity of ruminal microflora and there is shortage of vitamin that affect cellular metabolism. Hence administration of B vitamin plays beneficial effect in curing indigestion in animals.
6. Liver extract with vitamin B-complex *e.g.* Inj. Belamyl, Inj. Livron, Inj. Livobex, Inj. Stronic *etc.* @ 5-10 ml IM on alternate day can be administered.
7. Rumen buffering agents can be supplemented to enrich microbial status in acidotic rumen *e.g.* sodium bicarbonate alone or sodium bicarbonate with yeast and minerals (*e.g.* Bufzone) @ 100 ml as a drench. The dose of Bufzone (Intas) is in case of large animal 200 g daily for 3-4 days, and in case of small animal 50 g daily for 3-4 days.

4.1.9 Bloat

Accumulation of gas in the rumen is called bloat, which is otherwise known as ruminal tympany. Bloat may be acute or chronic. Normally animal passes away the gases produced in the rumen by eructation or ructus that will occur in every 40-50 seconds. Bloat occurs either due to too rapid formation of gas than the normal or due to eructation failure. Acidity of the rumen will lead to gas formation and finally tympany. Ruminal impaction leading to atony and constipation can also be attributed to indigestible coarse feed, lack of drinking water, hot environment, may result into rumino reticular paralytic effect and tympany.

Acute Bloat

Acute bloats maximally occur as man made reasons either due to faulty feeding or due to excess feeding of highly fermentable legumes. Acute bloat is of two types:

1. Dry bloat
2. Frothy bloat.

Dry bloat is less harmful than frothy bloat and most of the frothy bloats end in death.

Etiology

Some green plants contain saponin which leads to frothy bloat. Some green fodders contain HCN, like Sorghum, tapioca leafs which are toxic and paralyse the ruminal muscles and eructation failure results in acute bloat.

Natural saliva is very good antifoaming agent because it contains mucin that prevents froth formation. If froth formation is in quick rate, that will end in acute frothy bloat. In frothy bloat, the froth may obstruct the Cardia and there are no chances of ructus or eructation.

Treatment

1. In more severe and acute cases, to relieve pressure on thoracic cavity, gases in rumen may be relieved by using Trocar and Cannula but is aware of the risk of negative pressure (try to release the gas very slowly).
2. If the bloat is due to alkalinity – ammonium odour will present in rumen gas. In that case Kitchen Vinegar (weak acetic acid) at the dose rate of 2 ml/kg body weight mixed in 2 to 5 litres of water can be drenched.
3. If the bloat is due to acidity alkalinizing agent like sodium bicarbonate @ 1 g/kg body wt. mixed in 2-5 litres of water should be drenched.
4. Antihistaminic injection like Inj. Anistamin, Inj. Antilar, Inj. Allergo, Inj. Allervil, Inj. Chloril *etc.* @ 5-10 ml by I/M route and in severe bloat when the animal is in lateral recumbancy steroid injection *e.g.* Inj. Dexamethasone, Inj. Dexona, Inj. Enidex 2-5ml I/V should be administered.
5. If the bloat is froathy in nature any antifoaming preparation (as per index) *e.g.* Gastina 200 ml, Tyrel 120 ml, Bloatocil 100 ml may be used orally or any vegetable oils @ 300-500 ml orally to increase the surface tension and to reduce the froth formation should be used. Besides this herbal antibloat preparation Gasnil liquid (Vetmed) @ 50 ml BID for large animal, 25 ml BID for small animal can be done.
6. Follow up and supportive treatment should be the restoration of normal digestion. Orally rumentorics, stomachics and good vitamin B-complex preparations should be given parentally. Helping rumen to restore normal

digestion by providing essential minerals with yeast *e.g.* bolus Minotas (Intas) 1-2 boli daily for 5 days. And rumenotorics and microflora rejuvenator *e.g.* bolus Provisacc (Vetcare), Floraboost bolus (Excell), Floratone (Concept,) Rumentous (Intas) 2 boli twice daily for 3 days can be used, good B-complex like Inj. Polyvet (Excell) Inj. Neurovet (Alved) Inj. Tribivet (Intas) @ 5-10 ml IM for 3-5 days.

7. If necessary, broad spectrum, oral antibiotics like Steclin 500 mg, Neocyclin 500 mg, Cyclin 500 mg boli or oral Amoxycillin (Amoxinum) may be given to destroy unfavourable gas producing rumen microbes.

Chronic Bloat

Chronic bloat in ruminants especially in bovines is very common. It is not fatal to animal life but harmful to animal owners as it adversely affects the production performance (milk yield).

Faulty diet or unbalance diet usually lead to chronic bloat. Diet containing more protein and less sugar, too wet feeding of concentrates and greens and less or without dry fodder like hay or straw usually lead to chronic bloat owing to less salivary stimulation and less buffering action. This may result in chronic mild acidosis which in turn lead to chronic and recurrent bloat. Chronic and recurrent bloat may occur in subclinical hypophosphatemia, subclinical hypocalcemia, ruminitis, reticulitis and abomasitis. Besides thesem vegus nerve dysfunction, tumour around cardia, abscess around cardia, diaphramatic hernia may cause chronic or recurrent tympany.

Treatment

The principles of treatment for chronic bloat are:

1. Remove the primary cause (provide well balanced feed). Avoid sudden changes of diet. Stop the unbalanced faulty diet.
2. Restore normal digestion by treatment.
3. Supportive treatment.

Commercial preparations for treating chronic bloat are:

1. Use rumenotorics and microflora rejuvenator *e.g.* Rumentas (Intas), Yeas acc (Vetnex), Feed on bolus, Gofeed bolus (legend), Floraboost bolus (Vets Farma) @ 1-2 boli BID for 3-5 days.
2. Use herbal stomachic powder like Catone (CRIL), Herbogastrin (Vetmed), HB Strong powder (Indian Herbs), Himalayan Batisa *etc.* @ 20-25 g orally BID with warm water.
3. Provide essential minerals with yeast *e.g.* Minotas (Intas) @ 1-2 boli orally daily for 5 days for helping the rumen to restore normal digestion.
4. Broad spectrum oral antibiotic like Tetracycline bolus (*e.g.* Steclin, Neocyclin, Cyclin 500 mg), Amoxycillin bolus (like Amoxicillin, Glaxo) can be fed orally to destroy unfavourable gas producing microbes.

5. Inj. Liver extract with B-complex like Inj. Belamyl, Inj. Feroliv, Inj. Stronic, Inj. Livobex @ 5-10 ml on alternate day.
6. Good vitamin-B complex mainly neurotropic B vitamins *e.g.* Inj. Tribivet, Inj. Neuroxin-12 vet, Inj. Polyvet (Excell) @ 10 ml daily for 3-5 days by IM route is beneficial to restore normal digestion and rumen function.

4.1.10 Vagus Indigestion

It is a disease condition affecting the digestive system of ruminants characterized by chronic indigestion, tympany and apple shaped abdomen and is also known as Hoflund's syndrome. It is a functional disorder which may be either reticulo-omasal transfer failure (cranial functional disorder) or pyloric outflow failure (caudal functional disorder). Simply it means paralysis or relaxation of these sphincters.

Etiology

Injury to vagus nerve, traumatic reticulitis, reticuler abscess, adhesion be tween rumen and abomasums liver abscess, actinobacillosis of the rumen, fibropapilloma of the cardia, diaphragmatic hernia, enlargement of lymphnodes in tuberculosis and lymphomatosis or it may be due to secondary toxaemia and septicemia.

Symptoms

Anorexia, chronic indigestion, dehydration, abdominal distension, scanty and pastey faeces, agalactia, weakness and recurrent tympany.

Treatment

Prognosis of this condition is poor in most of the cases.

1. Intravenous infusion of Hypertonic saline to provide chloride in greater amount (Hypertonic saline solution consisting of 2.7 per cent NaCl and total 8.0gram potassium chloride (in 5 liters of solution) to be administered I/V for crossbred and pure bred exotic large animals). This treatment is given to correct the rumen hypokalemic and hypochloremic alkalosis.
2. Antibiotics to be administered to take care of possible infection if any in the body *viz.* Amoxicillin and Cloxacillin combination or Enrofloxacin by IM route.
3. NSAID like Ketoprofen *e.g.*, Inj. Neoprofen (Vetnex), Ketop (Alembic), Analgin injection or Meloxicam *e.g.*, Inj. Melonex (Intas), Inj. MP3 (Vetnex).
4. Vitamin B complex *e.g.*, Inj. Tribivet (Intas) or Neurotropic B vitamins *e.g.*, Inj. Neuroxin 12, Inj. Neurovet (Alved) @ 10 ml IM for large animal and 2-3 ml for small animal by IM route.
5. Parenteral Calcium Magnesium borogluconate with dextrose *e.g.*, Inj. Mifex (Novartis), Inj. Calmex M (Vetnex), Inj. Miphocal (Indian Immunologicals) @ 150-200 ml IV and SC route on alternate day for 2-3 occassions.
6. Antiflatulent/anti bloat preparations like Tymplex, Gastina, Gasnil liquid, Bloatocil, D-bloat @ 50 ml orally BID for large animal and @ 20-25 ml BID for small animal can be recommended.

7. Stomachic and yeast bolus like Rumentus (Intas), Ecotus (Intas), Provisacc (Vetcare), Yeasacc (Vetnex), Floraboost (Excell) 2 boli BID for large animal and 1 bolus BID for small animal can be recommended.

4.1.11 Ruminal Fermentative Disorders in Ruminants

This complication as a whole occurs mainly due to dietetic errors characterized by general metabolic disturbances, diarrhea, tympany, depressed appetite, hypophagia, paresis, staggering gait, colic signs, watery diarrhoea, acidosis alkalosis, ruminal atony, intoxication followed by acetonuria *etc.*

The important dietetic errors which cause reticulo-rumen fermentative disorders in animals are as follows:

1. Sudden change of feeds and fodder (ration)
2. Too much of fine feed
3. Too much feeding of leguminous fodder
4. Diet with lack of protein and sugar at the same time
5. Diet with too much of proteins combined with lack of sugar
6. Diet with too much of easily digested carbohydrates
7. Deficient fiber content in the fodder
8. Contaminated feeds and water
9. Starvation
10. Too much of fat.

(a) Sudden Change of Ration (Feeds and Fodder)

Digestion of ruminant animals entirely depends upon the resident microflora in the rumen. The rumen microorganisms also require small quantities of carbohydrate and protein to promote the digestion in the rumen. Sudden change in feed may produce serious digestive disturbances as the rumen microorganisms cannot adopt themselves. Hence gradual transition is to be made from one type of diet to another.

Symptoms

Digestive disorders, indigestion and diarrhoea.

Treatment

1. Stomachic powders like Catone (CRIL), H.B. strong (IH), Herbogastrin (Vetmed).
2. Rumenotoric bolus *viz.* Floraboost (Vets Farma), Floratone (Concept), Rumentus (Intas), Provisacc (Vetmed).
3. Microflora rejuvenator *e.g.* Rumicare (Intervet) for large animal 125 g BID and for small animal 30 g once daily as drench.
4. Fresh rumen cud transplantation.
5. Oral supplementation of acid sodium phosphate with B-complex.

6. Injection Polyvet (Intas), Inj. Neurovet (Alved), Inj. Hivit (Vetnex), Inj. Conciplex (Concept) for large animal @ 10-15 ml IM for 3-5 days and for small animal 3-5 ml daily by IM route.

(*b*) Sugar and Protein Deficient Diets

Late harvested hay, damaged hay and hay from phosphate deficient land are deficient in protein and sugar alongwith 'P' (Phosphorus) and when such feeds are offered to animals for a long time that results in impaired cellulose digestion and adversely affects the synthesis of amino acids and vitamins.

Symptoms

Wasting of body condition, loss of body weight and reduction in milk yield and other symptoms of wasting disease types.

Treatment

1. Fresh rumen cud transplantation.
2. Oral supplement of acid sodium phosphate with B-complex and molasses.
3. Inj. Uremin (Glaxo), Inj. Alphos-40 (Alved), Inj. Tonophosphan (Intervet) @ 10 ml to large animal, and for small ruminant @ 2-5 ml IM thrice in a week by IM or SC route.
4. Injection ND Plex Fort (Nandini), Inj. XL Plex (Alved), Inj. Pepcid (Concept) @ 10 ml IM on alternate day to large animal and 3-5 ml for small animal by IM route can be administered.
5. Microfloral rejuvenator *e.g.* Rumicare (Intervet) @ 125 g (1 sachet) for adult cattle once in 12 hours as drench in 1 litre water. Young animal – ½ sachet (60-65 g) twice daily in ½ to 1 litre water. Sheep and goat – 31-32 g (1/4th sachet) in ½ to 1 litre water.

(*c*) Rumen Alkalosis

Diet with too much of protein combined with lack of sugar may develop rumen alkalosis.

Symptoms

Tympany, depressed appetite, suspended rumination or depressed rumination, recurrent tympany, diarrhoea, paresis, staggering gait and recumbancy *etc.*

Rumen fluid pH is 7 to 8.5 and ammonic smell.

Treatment (for large animals)

1. 2.5 per cent Kitchen Vinegar – 1 to 2 litres mixed in water or Lactic acid 50 to 70 ml in 8-10 litres of water by stomach tube to neutralize rumen alkalinity or sodium proprionate @ 50 g BID orally.
2. Parenteral Calcium-Magnesium preparation *viz.* Inj. Calvib (Glaxo SmithKline) or Inj. Calbim (Glaxo), Inj. Lactovet (Intas), Inj. Calmax-M (Vetnex) @ 300-450 ml IV or SC.

(*d*) Rumen Acidosis

1. Acute rumen acidosis
2. Sub acute rumen acidosis
3. Chronic latent rumen acidosis

Diet with too much of easily digested carbohydrates causing rapid formation of lactic acid and dropping of the rumen pH and results in development of rumen acidosis.

(*i*) Acute Rumen Acidosis

It develops due to consumption of large quantity of easily digested Carbohydrates either accidentally causing acute grain engorgement or feeding out of ignorance.

Symptoms

Sudden off fed, sudden drop in milk yield, colic signs, watery diarrhoea, tympany, recumbancy leading to coma and death. Rumen pH goes below 5 and rumen liquour turning milky gray discoloration. Mostly the affected animals die unless they are attended in time.

Treatment

1. IV infusion of DNS and 2-5 per cent solution of sodium bicarbonate.
2. Oral administration of Magnesium carbonate 200-400 g in water for large ruminants and for small ruminants 50-100 g in water to be done or drenched for neutralizing rumen acidity.
3. Antihistaminic preparation such as Inj. Antilar, Anistamin, Chloril, Zeet 5-10 ml by IM route can be administered because histamine level is invariably increased in rumen.
4. Stomachic bolus like Rumen bolus (Alembic), Rumentus (Intas) Provisacc (Vetcare) 2 boli BID for large animal and 1 bolus BID for small animal.
5. Stomachic powder like Catone Powder (Cattle Remedies), Rumicare (Intervet) 125 g BID with water, Harbogastrin (Vetmed) @ 25-50 g orally BID can be fed. Oral administration of Gasnil liquid (Vetmed) 50 ml for cattle and buffalo BID is beneficial.
6. As supportive treatment, liver extract with B complex like Inj. Livobex (TTK), Inj. Bivital forte (Alembic), Inj. Stronic (Vetnex), or Phosphorus Inj. *viz.* Inj. Alphosh 40 (Alved), Inj. Tonophosphan (Intervet) @ 15-20 ml IM for large animal and 3-5 ml for small animal by IM route can be administered.
7. Injectable Metaclopromide monohydrate like Inj. Reglan @ 60-80 mg (6- 8 ml) IM followed by oral dosing of Reglan 5-10 tablets BID for 2 days can be tried in case of acidosis alongwith impaction, which increases tone and contractions of stomach and helps in relieving ruminal stasis.

(*ii*) Chronic Latent Rumen Acidosis

When milched animals are fed with grains for better milk production, the lactic acid produced in the rumen may not be upto the level of producing acute acidosis but this may affect other organs adversely causing:

1. Sub clinical ketosis.
2. Fat cow syndrome
3. Parakeratosis of rumen
4. Low milk fat syndrome.
5. Chronic laminitis
6. Cerebrocortical necrosis *etc.*

The rumen pH may range from 5 to 5.5.

Prevention and Control

To prevent chronic latent acidosis and its associated adverse effects and or complications buffers like sodium bicarbonate and magnesium oxide or commercially available buffer *viz.* Buffer (Excell) or Bufzone (Intas) may be fed alongwith concentrates.

Treatment

Oral feeding of buffer is recommended.

1. Feeding of magnesium oxide and sodi bicarb.
2. Rumennotonics.
3. Supportive therapy Inj. Pepsid, Belamyl, Polyvet, Tribivet @ 5-10 ml daily of 3-5 days.

(*iii*) Sub Acute Rumen Acidosis

It is a most harmful nutritional disease of dairy cattle and is shortly known as SARA or sleeper disease owing to excessive accumulation of VFA (Volatile fatty acids) especially lactic acid due to excess production. Low fiber feed, wet feeding, inability to remove VFA especially lactic acid via absorption leads to development of Sub acute rumen acidosis (SARA).

Symptoms

Loss of appetite, poor rumen motility, intermittent-mild diarrheoa, deterioration of health, simple respiratory infections etc. Rumen pH may be 5-5.5. Laminints may develop when the animal is kept much time on concentrate feeding.

Prevention and Treatment

1. Feed greens and fodders prior to concentrate feeding.
2. Buffers *viz.* Sodium bicarbonate, Magnesium oxide along with concentrates to be fed.
3. Avoid wet ration, for natural buffering by saliva.
4. Administer liver extract with B-complex *e.g.* Inj. Belamyl, Inj. Feroliv (Excell), Inj. Livron (Vets Farma), Inj. Levobex (TTK), Inj. Levadex (GSK), Inj. Stronic (Vetnex) @ 5-10 ml daily for 5-6 occasions by IM route.
5. Administer neurotropic B-vitamins *e.g.* Inj. Polyvet (Excell), Inj. Neurovet (Alved), Inj. Neuroxin-12 (Sarabhai Zydus), Inj. Tribivet (Intas) @ 5-10 ml IM on alternate day for 3-5 occasions.

6. Rumenotonics bolus like Rumentas (Intas), Ecotas bolus (Intas), Floraboost (Vets Farma), Feed on bolus (Glaxo), Yeasacc bolus (Vetnex) @ 2-4 boli BID for 3-5 days. If possible rumen cud transplantation should be done.
7. Oral vitamins and mineral miztures *e.g.*, Vitaprotein DS (Pharmacon), Ranmix Total (Vetnex), Minfa (Intervet) @ 25-30 g once daily for 10-15 days.

(*e*) Ruminal Indigestion Due to Moulds and Toxins

Normally paddy straws and wheat straws are stacked in open area and are exposed to various seasonal changes. High humidity, winter rains *etc.* enhance the development of moulds on straw. Feeding of such mould infested straw releasing mycotoxins causes mycotoxicosis. Feeding of contaminated paddy straw causes putrefaction of rumen contents and causes disturbances of ruminal digestion due to moulds and their toxins.

Treatment

Mostly symptomatic, transfaunation by rumen cud transplantation and supplementation of vitamin B-complex are suggested.

Inj. Hivit (Vetnex), Inj. Conciplex (Concept), Inj. Pinkojet (Brihans), Inj. Stronic (Vetnex), Inj. Livobex (TTK) @ 5-10 ml IM on alternate day is recommended. Parenteral antibiotics *e.g.* Inj. Enrocin, Inj. Meriquin, Inj. Enrovet, Inj. Floxidin @ 10-15 ml IM daily for 5 days.

Intravenous calcium, magnesium solution *e.g.* Inj. Calmax M (Vetnex), Inj. Lactomag (Intas) may be given.

Oral administration of Herbogastrin liquid and Gasnil liquid @ 50 ml BID for large animal and @ 25 ml BID for small animal can be done.

(*f*) Rumen Putrefaction

Feeding of contaminated feeds, perished feed, dirty feeds, contaminated and foul drinking water causes decomposition of rumen content and emits foul smellings. The pH value may rise up to 7.5 to 8.8 or even higher. Hence synthesis of Vitamin B and K is also suppressed.

Symptoms

Depressed appetite, decreased rumen activity, recurrent tympany, intermittent diarrheoa, paresis and spasticity. Rumen fluid turned black green in colour and foul smelling.

Treatment

Oral antibiotics like Amoxirum bolus, Neodox bolus, 3-Care bolus, Cyclin DT at 12 hours interval for 2-3 days.

Cephalexin (Ledxin, Lixen, Lexin) @ 10-30 mg/kg body weight twice daily. Lavaging of rumen should be done. Rumen cud transplantation 2-3 litres can be done. Mineral mixture and vitamin B-complex Injection *e.g.* Hivit, Conciplex, Pinkojet, XL Plex @ 10 ml daily for 3-5 days should be given. In critical case rumenotomy is suggested.

4.1.12 Diseases of Liver

Liver carries out or performs a wide range of metabolic, secretory and excretory functions. The metabolic functions include carbohydrate, protein and fat metabolism, bile salt secretion, detoxification and excretion. Liver is the biological hub of lipid metabolism and is responsible for lipid homeostasis. It plays a central part in nitrogen metabolism too. Since liver occupies a central position in the metabolism of the cow any hepatic, structural as well as functional disturbance alongwith ruminal dysfunction may result in serious cansequences. Immediately after parturition, the work load of the liver is very much increased for the detoxification of the toxic produces from the uterus. This may lead to liver insufficiency.

Primary diseases of liver in ruminants occur due to Fascioliasis and poisoning and toxicants (in most of the cases). In other animals *viz.*, in dogs it is seen in canine hepatitis (ICH virus), Leptospirosis, secondary bacterial infections and poisoning. Since liver has got tremendous functional reserves, signs of liver disorder or liver diseases are not clinically manifested with mild affections.

Symptoms

1. Anorexia and indigestion (chronic in nature).
2. Constipation followed by loose stool.
3. Dullness, depression and clay coloured fecaces.
4. Weight loss, signs of jaundice, abdominal pain.
5. Anaemia, poor hair coat and rough body coat.
6. Lethergic, emaciation, loss of appetite.
7. Enlargement in size of the liver with or without pain.

Treatment

1. Identification of cause and specific therapy. For Fascioliasis (liver fluke disease) give specific flukicide. In case of poisoning give specific treatment.
2. Give rest and provide easily digestible carbohydrates and protein of higher biological value and fat free diets.
3. IV infusion of Dextrose depending on the species and body weight.
4. Liver tonics herbal preparations (see Livertonics) and Liver extract with B-complex by parenteral route should be done.
5. If liver disorders occur due to bacterial eatiology and if it is associated with fever for preventing secondary bacterial invasion antibiotics should be administered.
6. Vitamin-A injection or supportive therapy can be done.

4.1.13 Jaundice or Icterus

Jaundice is the clinical manifestation of animals when the visible mucous membrane turned into yellowish discolouration (or pigmentation) alongwith yellowish secretions and excretions owing to haemobilirubin or cholebilirubin or both.

The chief forms of jaundice are –

1. Obstructive (post hepatic) jaundice,
2. Haematogenous or haemolyic (prehepatic) jaundice, and
3. Toxic (intra hepatic) jaundice.

Etiology

Causes of jaundice are many. Toxic chemicals and drugs, viral and bacterial infections, obstruction of the bile duct by endoparasites *e.g.* liver flukes pressure upon the duct by tumors, nodules in liver, cirrohosis of liver, invasion of erythrocytes by protozoa (haemoprotozoan parasitic infection) *etc.*

Symptoms

Yellowish discolouration of mucous membrane, intense yellow colour or dark colour urine, anaemia, rise of temperature (in haemolytic and toxic jaundice), nervous signs *e.g.* muscle tremor and weakness may be observed.

Treatment

1. Rest and feeding of good quality and easily digestible carbohydrates.
2. Feeding of fat free diet.
3. Identification of causes and application of specific therapy. In Haemolytic jaundice specific measures to be taken to prevent haemolysis. If due to haemoprotozoa antihaemoprotozoal drug *e.g.* Inj. Berenil/Protonil @ 0.8-1.6 g/100 kg body weight or Inj. Nilbery, Inj. Prozomin liquid @ 1 ml/20 kg body weight by IM route.

In obstructive jaundice – if it is due to migrating larvae of endoparasites-ascaris, liver flukes, fasciola specific dewormers and flukicides *e.g.* Fluzic (Triclabendazole), Oxylozanide (Nilzan, Distodin), Hexanide *etc.* should be fed.

In toxic jaundice IV Dextrose 5 per cent, 10 per cent, 500-1000 ml by slow IV, vitamin B-complex preparation *e.g.* Inj. Tribivet, Inj. Ferolive, Inj. Hivit *etc.* @ 10 ml by IM route can be given. Calcium therapy in toxicities with slow IV infusion of Calgonate, Calmex, Mifocal, Mifex @ 100-300 ml can be done. Administration of any one of the following liver extracts *e.g.* Inj. Belamyl, Inj. Livobex (ITK) Inj. Livron (Vets Farma), Inj. Stronic (Vetnex) *etc* @ 5-10 ml IM on every alternate day should be done.

Oral liver tonics *e.g.* Livol, Vetliv powder or Lifer, Livsee, Liv-52 syrup can be fed orally BID.

4.1.14 Hepatitis

Inflammation of the hepatic cells is known as hepatitis. It is most commonly seen in dogs. It may also occur in other animals too.

Etiology

Toxic causes: Toxic chemicals or drugs, poisonous plants, cresols from coal tar, CTC, Hexachlorethene *etc.*

Bacterial toxins: Salmonellosis, Leptospirosis *etc.*

Virus: Infectious Canine Hepatitis (ICH), Infectious Equine Anaemia.

Parasites: Infestation of liver flukes, ascaris, *Toxocara* species (dog) *etc.*

Inorganic poisons: Arsenic, phosphorus, selenium.

Nutritional causes: Deficiency of cystine, vitamin E, methionine and choline deficient diet in dog.

Symptoms

Anorexia, dullness, depression, enlargement of liver, indigestion, pain in liver, convulsion, jaundice, steatorrhoca, constipation followed by diarrhoea *etc.*

Diagnosis

From clinical symptoms, laboratory examination of blood and urine.

Treatment

1. Identification of specific cause and adoption of specific therapy.
2. Administration of Injectable Liver extract and B-complex vitamins *e.g.* Inj. Livadex, Inj. Pepsid, Inj. Tribivet, Inj. Livron, Inj. Stronic *etc.* @ 5-10 ml on alternate day.
3. Dextrose 25 per cent solution 500-1000 ml for large animal and 50-100 ml for small animal.
4. Calcium therapy in toxicities – *e.g.* Inj. Calborol, Inj. Calgonate, Inj. Mifex, Inj. Intacal *etc.* @ 100-300 ml for large animal.
5. Oral liver tonic powder *e.g.* Livol, Vet liv, or liquid liver tonic *e.g.* Lifer, Livsee, Livonine, Liv fit, Liv 52 as supportive therapy.
6. Antibiotics with corticosteroids in diffuse liver disease to control secondary bacterial infections.
7. Administer Inj. Berenil, Nilbery, Prozomin @ 1 ml/20 kg body weight for haemoprotozoan infection.
8. Apply specific dewormer: flukicides for flukes, *e.g.* Triclabendazole, Oxyclozanide, Hexanide *etc.*

4.2 DISEASES OF RESPIRATORY SYSTEM

Disorders of the respiratory system are one of the prime causes of morbidity and mortality in domestic animals and a major source of economic loss of the farmers.

4.2.1 Rhinitis

Inflammation of the mucous membrane of the nose is called rhinitis. It is characterized by sneezing, running nose with a profuse nasal discharge and dyspnoea. It may be acute or chronic, characterized by sneezing, hyperemia, inflammation and profuse mucoid nasal discharge and mucopurulent nasal discharge in chronic rhinitis. Nature of discharge varies according to the severity and duration of inflammation.

Etiology

Dust, foreign bodies, pollens, irritant chemicals and smokes, bacteria (*e.g. Spherophones, Bordetella, Pseudomonas, Streptococci* and *Staphylococci*), virus (*e.g.* Influenza virus, FMD virus), Fungus (*e.g.* Aspergillus species, Rhinosporidiosis), and parasitic causes *e.g.* Larvae of *Oestrus ovis* in sheep, *Schistosoma nasalis* in cattle *etc.*

Treatment

1. Inhallation with Tr. Benzoin, Oil turpentine or Oil eucalyptus (@ 10-15 ml/ litre of boiling water) as mucolytic agent.
2. Antihistaminic injection *e.g.* Inj. Avil, Inj. Antilar, Inj. Allergon, Inj. Chloril, Inj. Zeet @ 5-10 ml for large animal and 1-2 ml for small animal by IM route 2-3 days.
3. Antibiotics *e.g.* Inj. Oxytetracycline, Inj. Ampicillin, Inj. Ampicillin-Cloxacillin, Inj. Enrofloxacin or Sulfonamides *e.g.* Inj. Bacterisol, Inj. Duaprim, Inj. Oprim can be administered for 3-5 days.
4. For parasitic etiology like in Nasal Granuloma, Anthiomaline or Lithiomony injection and Oxyclozanide bolus should be administered.

4.2.2 Laryngitis, Tracheitis and Bronchitis

Inflammation of larynx, trachea and bronchus are called laryngitis, tracheitis and bronchitis respectively and are characterized by coughing, noisy respiration, dyspnoea or respiratory distress with the extension of infection from the nasal cavity or pharynx to trachea, larynx or bronchus. Nasal discharge may or may not be present depending upon the amount of exudates present in the bronchioles. Moist cough or dry cough may be there owing to irritation of air ways because of the inflammation.

Etiology

Irritant vapours, chemical irritants, infection of upper respiratory tract *e.g.* Calf diphtheria, *Bordetella bronchoseptica, Cryptococus, Streptococcus* and *Staphylococus*, viral disease – Influenza virus, *etc.*

Symptoms

Coughing, respiratory distress, mild to moderate temperature Mucoporulent disease, painful dyspnoea, noisy respiration. Some degree of inspiratory embarrassment.

Diagnosis

Signs and symptoms, examination of nasal swabs for pathogenic organisms.

Treatment

Treatment should be given as per etiology.

1. Antiseptic inhalation with 10-15 ml of Tr. Benzoin, Eucalyptus or Turpentine oil in one litre of boiling water.

2. Antihistaminic preparation *e.g.* Inj. Avil, Chloril, Chlorazin, Anistamin, Antilar, Zeet *etc.* @ 5-10 ml by IM route to Large animal and 1-2 ml by IM route to small animal to be given.
3. Antibiotic and Sulphonamide drugs (vide antibiotic and sulpha drugs) should be administered.
4. Cough expectorant like Coldex Vet (Oxford), Respigen (Nugen) 20-30 ml BID can be drenched or herbal preparations *e.g.* Biocof, Bronchopyrin, Catcough, Cofgon *etc.* (as per index) can be fed as electuary (25-50 g BID).
5. For the treatment of pyrexin, bronchial congestion, pyrexia, bronchitis and cough – Bronchopyrin liquid (Vetmed) can be tried.

4.2.3 Pulmonary Emphysema

It can be defined as abnormal distension of lungs by air due to rupture of alveolar walls or without escape of air into the interstial tissue caused by reduction in air space. It is characterized by the distension of alveoli with rupture of alveolar walls where movement of chest wall is decreased bilaterally. Percussion sound increases and there is short, weak, hollow cough and dysponoea. Percussion sound may be dull and respiratory sound will be decreased.

Pulmonary emphysema may be of two types:

1. Acute alveolar emphysema (common in horse)
2. Acute intensified emphysema (common in cattle and sheep)

Etiology

Perforation of lungs by foreign body, trauma/infighting trauma on lungs, pulmonary strongylosis as sequel of pneumonia, loud bellowing.

Treatment

Treatment should be initiated with antibiotic or sulpha drugs. For relieving pulmonary distress and emphysema antihistaminic injections (Avil, Antilar, Chlorazin, Zeet *etc.*) @ 5-10 ml IM; cough electuary *e.g.* Pot Iodide – 4 g, Codeinephos – 1g, Pot bromide – 3 g, Pulv glycerrhiza – 30 g and Treacle – as per need. Mft. Electuary BID.

Inj. Atropine sulphate 0.25 mg/kg b.wt. by S/C Inj. Melonex, Inj. Meloxicam *etc.* @ 10-15 ml IM for 2-5 days can be given. Besides treatment, care and nursing is essential, give complete rest to the animal and keep the animal in well ventilated shed and airy and hygienic room. Bronchopyrin liquid (Vetmed) @ 20 ml BID for large animal and @ 10 ml BID for small animal can be carefully drenched.

4.2.4 Pulmonary Oedema

It is characterized by accumulation of oedematous fluid in the lungs characterized by moist rales with severe dyspnoea.

Etiology

Passive venous congestion, bacterial toxins, irritant fumes, anaemia and hypoproteinemia.

Symptoms

Dyspnoea, respiratory distress, open mouth breathing, coughing and nasal discharge with increased respiration.

Treatment

1. Administer antibiotics or sulpha drugs (vide antibiotics and sulpha drugs).
2. Inj. Atropine sulphate – 0.25 mg/kg body weight SC. The average dose for large animals is about 75 to 100 mg. Rest and proper ventilation are needed.
3. Bronchopyrin (Vetmed), Resprigen (Nugen), Coldex (Oxford Gem) expectorant syrup @ 20 ml BID for large animal and 10 ml BID for small animal can be given.

4.2.5 Pneumonia

Inflammation of the lung parenchyma is known as Pneumonia. Inflammation may involve bronchial parenchyma leading to a condition known as Broncho-Pneumonia. Broncho-pneumonia is usually accompanied by a moist painful cough, interstitial pneumona by frequent; dry and hacking cough.

Types of Pneumona

1. Croupous pneumonia (Lobur Pneumonia).
2. Lobular Pneumona (Catarrhal/Broncho Pneumonia)

Etiology

1. Exposure to cold, inclement weather, damp and unhygienic shed, sudden exposure to chilled weather.
2. Bacteria *e.g. E. coli, B. bronchoseptica, Klebsiella,* Streptococci, Staphylococci, Corynaebacterium, *B. bronchoseptica,* Klebsiella.
3. Occasionally viral pneumonia.
4. Parasites – Lungs worm (Verminous Pneumonia).
5. Specific diseases *e.g.* CCPP, CBPP, RP, HS.
6. Aspiration: accidental aspiration of liquid, medicines during oral feeding/ drenching – may produce aspiration pneumonia.
7. Fungus – *e.g. Aspergillus* (causing Mycotic Pneumonia/sudden rise of temperature.

Symptoms

Nasal discharge, dyspnoea, sudden rise of temperature, cough. Fever depends on extent of involvement. Adventitious sound on auscultation, moist rales in Bronchopneumonia, cough and decreased respiratory sound, loud bronchial sound because of collapse or filling with inflammatory fluids. Rapid and shallow respiration is the cardinal sign of early pneumonia. Respiratory embarrassment may be attributed to reduced function of lungs tissue in inflammation.

Treatment

1. Medicated inhalation to relieve the expiratory distress. *e.g.*, Creolin, Tr. Benzoin compound, T-oil and oil Eucalyptus in hot water.
2. Massage with Ammonia liniment or camphor.
3. Cantheridine massage to relieve congestion.
4. Expectorants:
   (*a*) Painful cough with tenacious exudates
   Potassium and Ammonium salts and sedative expectorants
   (*b*) Chronic bronchial irritation with soft cough
   Stimulant expectorant *e.g.* Turpentine, Creosote, Eucalyptus
   (*c*) Spasmodic, exhausting and dry cough
   Anodyne expectorant *e.g.* Codeine phosphate, Morphine and Belladona.
5. Antihistaminic – as bronchodilators, in dyspnoea due to spasm of bronchi, in condition of allergic origin.
   e.g. Inj. Avil, Inj. Chloril, Inj. Anistamin, Inj. Antilar, Inj. Zeet, Inj. Chlorazin @ 5-10 ml IM for large animal and 1-2 ml for small animal.
6. Sulpha drugs *e.g.* Inj. Sulphamezathene 33 1/3 per cent @ 1 g/75 kg. Inj. Brimdin, Inj. Biotrim, Inj. Duaprim (see Sulphonanodes in Veterinary Drug Index) or oral bolus *e.g.* Robatran (TTK), Duaprim (Brihans), Sulcoprim (Concept), Genprim (Legend) 1 – 2 boli BID can be tried.
7. Antibiotic *e.g.* Inj. Streptopenicillin (Inj. Bistrepen, Inj. Mucomycin Fort, Inj. Biostrep *etc*); Broad spectrum antibiotic *viz.* Inj. Oxytetracycline (*e.g.* Inj. Intamycin, Inj. Terramycin, Inj. Oxy-LA, Inj. Terramycin LA, Inj. Intamycin LA, Inj. Loxy) ; Inj. Ampicillin-Cloxacillin (*e.g.* Inj. Acvet, Inj. Inclox, Inj. Vetclox, Inj. Cilclox; Inj. Amoxycillin-Cloxacillin (*e.g.* Inj. Lemox, Inj. Intamox, Inj. Inimox, Inj. Mastox, Inj. Moxcell, Inj. Emoxcell); Inj. Enrofloxacin (*e.g.* Inj. Enrocin, Inj. Quinintas, Inj. Floxidin, Inj. Enrored); Inj. Chloramphenicol (*e.g.* Inj. Phenivet, Inj. Enteromycetin, Inj. Neochlor), Inj. Ciprofloxacin (*e.g* Inj. Cflox, Inj. Cflox power), Cephalosporins *e.g* Inj. Intacef, Inj. Britax, Inj. Wocef, Inj. Cefavet, Inj. Cefstan *etc.* for 3-5 days.

Herbal products as cough electuary – *e.g* Bronchopyrin, Coflon, Cat cough, Biocuf *etc.* 30-40 g orally BID can be tried. In case of persistent spasms, Inj. Prednisolone, Inj. Dexamethosone for 3-5 days can be advocated.

Besides cough mixture, cough expectorant *e.g* Bronchopyrin liquid (Vetmed) @ 20 ml BID for 5 days for large animal. Codex syrup (Oxfer and Gem) and Respigen (Nugen) can be used.

4.2.6 Epistaxis

It can be defined as the bleeding from nose or flow of blood from one or both nostrils in drop or profusely as blood stream.

It is fairly common in all animals and sometimes become a very severe problem, particularly in large animals. It is common in hot summer but may occur in any season. Capillaries of the nasal mucosa get burst and bleed profusely. Bleeding may also occur in trypanosomiasis, due to nasal polyp, nasal granuloma, in poisoning, snake bite *etc*.

Etiology

External injuries, trauma, ulcers, granulomatous lesions, nasal catarrah, pressure of jugular vein, blood sucking by leech, inhalation of irritant vapours, polyps and tumours.

Diagnosis

Examine the nostrils and the nasal cavity. See whether unilateral or bilateral. Examine for N.G. Polyps, tumours, presence of leech, injury *etc*. Blood smear examination can be done if it is suspected for Surra (Tryps).

Treatment

1. Cold water irrigation and cold packs (ice packs) application on head.
2. Local application of Adrenaline 1 : 1000 solution by using swab.
3. Local application of astringent preparation *e.g* Tr. Benzoin. Tr. Feriperchlor, Tr. Iodine.
4. Administration of Hemostatics – *e.g* Inj. Chromostat, Inj. Cadichrome, Inj. Styptobion, Inj. Bleed check (Bee Tee Pharma) @ 10 ml for adult large ruminant and 2-4 ml for small ruminant and other small animal by IM. Inj. Botropase with Vitamin K can also be administered.
5. If bleeding due to N.G., in that case Inj. Antheomaline or Lithiomony @ 10-15 ml IM at 2-3 days interval should be given.

   If bleeding due to lung worm and pulmonary strongylosis, in that case Inj. Levamisol HCl (Lemasol 75, Kalmisol, Inj. Helmonil *etc.*) can be tried.

   If due to Surra/Trypanosomiosis), Inj. Nilbery, Inj. Berenil, Inj. Prozomin *etc* (any one) by deep IM route should be advocated.
6. Herbal products *e.g.* Styplon (Himalayan) 10-15 tabs TID for cattle, 5 tabs TID for sheep and goat or Ayapon tabs (Alarsin) 5-15 tabs BID orally until bleeding is controlled can be tried.

4.2.7 Snoring Disease

It is otherwise known as *nasal schistosomosis* caused by *Schistosoma nasale* or *Nasal granuloma* of cattle. It is one of the most important parasitic diseases of bovine. The infection mostly occurs in bovine of three years old and above, more during winter, of course sporadic cases are met with throughout the year. Water lodges, ponds and lakes provide favourable environment for the multiplication of nails that act as intermediate host for *Schistosoma nasale* (the causative parasite of N.G. or snoring disease).

Symptoms

Snoring, semisolid nasal discharges, pin head size (nasal granuloma) with miliary, or pin head size granular lesions, and cauliflower like unilateral or bilateral growth, and respiratory disorders.

Diagnosis

Examination of nasal scrapings reveals eggs of *S. nasale.* The prevalence of the disease is higher in cattle than buffalo.

Treatment

1. Inj. Anthiomaline or Lithium Antimony Thiomalate (*e.g.* Lithiomony) @ 15-20 ml by deep IM injection on 3-5 occasions as an interval of 3-5 days (on alternate side) is effective treatment.
2. Oral anthelmintic *e.g.* Oxyclozanide preparation (*e.g.* Tolzan-F, Nilzan, Zanil, Neozide) give synergestic action.
3. Copper sulphate solution 2 per cent, Tr. Beazoin, Tr. Iodine, Povidone iodine can be applied topically on the nasal lesions.

4.3 DISEASES OF REPRODUCTIVE SYSTEM

Reproductive diseases are the major causes of infertility in animals. For better understanding they have been discussed under 4 subheadings:

1. True veneral disease transmitted by coitus
2. Specific infection of reproductive system.
3. Inflammation of specific reproductive organ by pathogens
4. Debilitating diseases.

4.3.1 True Venereal Diseases (Transmitting through sexual contact)

It is transmitted during mating/breeding, *viz.* Vibriosis, Trichomoniasis – that causes infertility due to abortion and inflammation of reproductive tract.

Vibriosis is defined as early embryonic mortality, repeat breeding causing vaginitis, metritis etc.

Trichomoniasis caused by Trichomonus foetus, responsible for abortion and infertility and cause inflammation and uterine discharge for long period.

Treatment

Antimicrobials are to be used for treatment of reproductive tract infection (vide Table 4.1).

4.3.2 Specific Infections of Reproductive System

The infectious diseases like Brucellosis, Leptoopinsis, IBR and BVD (Bovine viral diarrhoea) can affect reproductive capabilities of cattle. *Brucella abortus* is the largest cause of infectious abortion and infertility in cattle and buffaloes. *B. melitensis* affect goat posing serious zoonotic threat to human beings. Pathogens *e.g.* microbial organisms and the virus has got specific affinity towards uterus causing late abortion, retained placenta and infertility. *Leptospira pomona* (a spirochete) cause abortion, icterus haemoglobinuria is one of the reason for infertility. IBR virus causing vulvovaginitis, abortion and BVD virus causing abortion, weak calves at birth with brain damage are important specific cause of reproductive system infection and affection.

Treatment

Antimicrobials are to be used for treatment of reproductive tract infection (vide Table 4.1).

Table 4.1: Antimicrobial Agents for Treatment of Reproductive Tract Infection

Group	*Name*	*Dosage, Route and Frequency*	*Antimicrobial Spectrum*
Penicillin	Sodium Penicillin-G	10,000-20,000 IU/kg IM, TID	Gram (+ ve)
	Procaine Penicillin-G	10,000-20,000 IU/kg IM BID	Gram (– ve)
	Benzathine Penicillin-G	10,000-40,000 IU/kg IM 48-72 hrs.	Aerobic and
	Ampicillin	5-10 mg/kg b. wt. IM, IV BID	anaerobic
	Amoxicillin	4-7 mg/kg IM, IV BID or TID	organisms
	Sodium Carbencillin	10-20 mg/kg IM, IV TID or TID	
Aminoglyco-	Gentamycin	3-6 mg/kg IM, IV SID to BID	Gram (– ve)
sides	Kananycin	12-15 mg/kg IM BID	aerobic
	Streptomycin	7-12 mg/kg IM BID	
	Amikacin	5-7 mg/kg IM BID	
Quinolones	Enrofloxacin	2.5-5 mg/kg IM BID	Gram (+ ve), Gram (– ve) aerobes, Brucella, Mycoplasma Chlamydia
Sulphona-mides	Sulphathiazole	60-70 mg/kg PO TID	Gram (+ ve), Gram (– ve) both and some protozoan infections
	Sulphamethazine	220 mg/kg PO or IV	
	Sulphadiazine	50 mg/kg PO BID	
	Sulphadiamethoxime	50-60 mg/kg PO BID	
	Sulphaethoxy pyridazine	55 mg/kg PO BID	
	Potentiated Sulonamide (Trimethoprim and sulphadiazine)	15-60 mg/kg PO IV or IM BID	Gram (+ ve) Gram (– ve) aerobes, anaerobes and Mycoplasma
Tetracyclines	Oxytetracycline	5-10 mg/kg IM, IV BID	Gram (+ ve) Gram (– ve) aerobes, anaerobes and Mycoplasma

Contd...

Table 4.1–Contd...

Group	*Name*	*Dosage, Route and Frequency*	*Antimicrobial Spectrum*
Chloram-phenicol	Chloramphenicol	10-20 mg/kg IM or IV BID	Gram (+ ve) Gram (- ve) some anaerobes
Macrolides	Erythromycin	8-15 mg/kg IM, SID to BID	Mainly Gram (+ ve)
	Tylosin	10-20 mg/kg IM SID to BID	Gram (+ ve), Mycoplasma
Lincosamide	Lincomycin	10 mg/kg IM BID	Mainly anaerobic infection
Miscellaneous antimicrobials	Metronidazole	10-20 mg/kg IV or I/U	Mixed infection – Mycoplasma, anaerobic organisms

4.3.3 Inflammation of Specific Organs Caused by Various Agents

Maladies like vaginitis, metritis caused by various opportunistic agents characterized by mild to severe inflammatory changes of vagina, cervix or uterus/ uterine myometrium may cause infertility amd may even cause death in case of septic metritis. Metritis may reduce fertility by preventing normal estrus. Undesirable uterine condition can prevent normal conception. Chronic endometritis needs special attention because of absence of overt clinical signs. It disturbs cyclicity. Retained placenta, unsanitary assistance during calving, abortion and contaminated quarters are the predisposing factors for uterine pathology.

The signs of metritis vary but there is usually a pus flaked vaginal discharge, straining and in general the animal appears ill. Metritis lowers conception rates and creates long calving intervals. (For treatment, see antimicrobial therapy for treatment of reproduction tract infection given in Table 4.1).

Debilitating disease that lowers efficiency of all the body systems.

Chronic wasting disease and nutritional deficiency disease may also reduce the fertility. Antibiotic therapy is an important viable alternative to reduce the infectious clinical problem which requires judicious selection (see the Table 4.1).

Treatment of Reproductive Tract Infection

1. Use of disinfectant douches like Lugol's iodine, chlorhexidine, iodophors for certain infections are beneficial but there are indication that irritating substances may disturb the local immune defense mechanism.
2. Antiseptic solution can be filled in uterus and then to be siphoned off to clean uterus before administration of antibiotic. This may also cause ascending infection to fallopian tube. So precautions must be taken.
3. Two main routes of administration of antimicrobial agents can be followed for treating genital tract infections. These are (1) Intrauterine (Local) and (2) Systemic (IM or IV).

Intrauterine Administration

Judicious selection of appropriate microbial agent and course of treatment to be decided properly to destroy the specific pathogens. Sulphonamide, Tetracycline, Gentamycin, Ampicillin, Enrofloxacin and Chloramphenicol can be used. Enrocin I/U (Vetnex) 5 per cent solution @ 2.5-5 mg/kg body weight I/U is effective against most of the I/U pathogens. Gentamycin in twice a day schedule is very good against uterine pathogen. Sulfonamide and trimethoprim is well distributed in uterine cavity can provide effective antimicrobial coverage with sensitive flora.

Systemic Administration

Aminoglycosides can be a voided in an aerobic infection in uterus. In presence of blood, pus and tissue debris, sulfonamide and amino glycosides do not work properly. Fluroquinolones are extremely useful in uterine infection because of unique mechanism. Systemic administration of Penicillin sodium @ 22,000-45,000 IU per kg is sufficient to combat pathogen sensitive to penicillin. Oxytetracyclines parenterally can also provide adequate. Systemic administration of antimicrobial agents gives a better distribution in the tabular genital tract and the ovaries.

Supportive therapy including NSAID (anti-inflammatory analgesics) antihistaminic (Pheniramine maleate), rehydration therapy and immune modulator drugs (like Levamisol HCl) should also be advocated.

Non antibiotic therapy can also be advocated in case of bacterial resistance to antibiotics and tissue residues in uterus.

(*a*) To increase contractile effect of uterus that would cause evacuation of tubular genital tract.

(*b*) Use of agents which has got (+ ve) effect of Cellular (CMI) and Humoral local defense.

Hormonal agents like Oxytocin, Estrogen, PGF_2 alpha *etc*. can be used. Inj. Oxytocin (10-20 IU IM) 3 to 4 times day can be administered for evacuation of exudates from uterus.

Inj. Estrogen (Estradiol valerate 3-10 mg) IM repeated once or at 3 days interval with or without antibiotic exert uterotonic effect and can enhance local defense mechanism, Inj. Prostaglandin (Lutalase, 12.5-25 mg IM, Cloprosteriol 0.5 mg, Luprostiol 15 mg/IM) can also be used in case of endometritis. Pessaries can also be used in case of retained placenta after manual removal (see the list of pessaries like Uren vet, Uterine bolus *etc*. in the Drug Index of this book).

4.3.4 Trichomoniasis

Trichomoniasis is a major cause of reproductive failure in cattle. It is a veneral disease caused by *Trichomonas foetus* which is again a parasite of G.I. and reproductive tract. It is a pear shaped organism with a single nucleus having a dark coloured costa and three flagella and is visible under low power microscope.

Pathology and clinical symptoms

T. foetus is confined to the reproductive tract of bulls and cows, although may remain in blood circulation. In bulls the parasites care mostly confined to prepuce.

It may produce inflammatory and painful Balanitis with frequent micturation. Mucopurulent discharge may be present with small reddish papule on the prepucial membrane (sheeth) and glans penis. The affected bulls refuse to mount the cow. The bulls may recover spontaneously and serve as the source of infection to female cows. In cows it produces mild vaginitis, mucopurulent discharge. The symptoms remain for 4-18 days and there after disappears.

The infections in cows have varying sequlae.

1. Organism may cause placentitis, detachment of placenta, death of foetus and abortion in between 8-16 weeks after AI which often goes unnoticed.
2. Irregular uterine discharge and heat appears after abortions.
3. Incomplete elimination of foetus and membranes leads to maturation, which may lead to catarrhal or purulent endometritis. This is another cause of permanent sterility in cow.
4. Sometimes cervix becomes closed and may lead to closed and may lead to closed pyometra.

Diagnosis

History of abortion, identification of organism from prepucial samples. Serological tests *e.g.* Indirect haemagglutination and cervical mucous agglutination test.

Treatment

1. Topical treatment of trichomonads infected bulls to be done with Acriflavin (1 per cent) solution.
2. Diminazine Aceturate (Berenil-1 per cent).
3. Bovoflavin, Chlorhexidine and Metronidazole can also be used.
4. Systemic treatment of bulls with imidazoles derivaties is also beneficial.

Control

Breeding rest, Restriction of natural service and to go for artificial insemination (to stop veneral/sexual transmission). Elimination of infection using chemotherapy.

4.3.5 Foetal Maceration

Foetal maceration denotes putrefaction of soft foetal tissue consequent to incomplete abortion and incomplete cervical dilation. Efforts often fail to further dilate the cervix that had undergone the secondary changes. Structureless nature of macerated foetus limits the use of uterotonic drugs.

Treatment

1. Injection oestradiol.
2. Inj. Prostaglandin F_2 alpha *e.g.* Inj. Vetmet, Inj. Clostenol, Inj. Cyclix @ 2 ml IM.
3. Systemic antibiotic coverage *e.g.* Inj. Gentamycin, Inj. Streptopenicillin, Inj. Enrofloxacin, Inj. Ciprofloxacin *etc.* by IM route can be administered.

Surgical Management

If medicinal treatment fails surgical intervention can be made. The animal can be sedated with chlorpromazine by IM route. Analgesia of the incision site can be induced by local infiltration of 2 per cent lignocaine HCl. A 7-10 cm long incision can be made through skin, muscles, sacrosciatic ligament, thick fat and peritoneum. The uterus is then needs to be exteriorized through the incision. Then a required length incision should be given on the body of the uterus and macerated foetal mass should be removed carefully. The uterus is then needs to be flushed with 1 per cent Povidone iodine solution, sutured in cushing pattern with chromic catgut. Then peritoneum and ligaments should be sutured by simple continuous fashion. Muscles can be sutured by lock stitch pattern and the skin should be closed using horizontal matters sutures. IV infusion of DNS, NS or Ringers lactate should be made along with broad spectrum antibiotic *e.g.* Inj. Oxytetracycline, Inj. Enrofloxacin *etc.* should be administered, Enrocin I/V should be administered by I/V route to prevent uterine infection.

4.4 DISEASES OF URINARY SYSTEM

Both large and small animals including pets are most frequently affected with the disease of urinary systems involving kidneys, urethra or urinary bladder.

Micturation process differs to a wide range amongst different species of animals. Frequency of urination may vary due to factors like intake of food and drinks (water), loss of body fluid through defacation, vomition, perspiration *etc.* According to urinary output the condition may be classified as anuria, oliguria and polyuria.

4.4.1 Anuria

Complete stoppage or absence of urination (retention of urine) is called anuria.

Causes: Renal calculi, urinary obstruction, hypovoluaemia, acute fever, poisoning, growth or calculi in urethra.

4.4.2 Oliguria

It's a condition defined to be less urinary output and less flow of urine. This may be due to less blood flow, hypovoluaemia, haemorrhage, burns, oedema, diarrhoea, vomition, fever and poisoning *etc.*

4.4.3 Polyuria

Increased flow and significant increase in urinary output is known as polyuria. It could be due to maximum water intake, hyperaemia of kidney, chronic nephritis, chronic renal failure, chronic interstitial nephritis, diabetes, hypokalaemia *etc.*

Diagnosis

From clinical signs.

Treatment (Conditions for decreased flow of urine)

1. Give adlibitum fresh water to the animal.
2. Surgical intervention is indicated for urethral calculi.

3. Use of diuretics for cattle and buffaloes : *e.g.* Potassium acetate – 15 g

   Disitalis – 15 ml

   Spirit Nitrosiether – 30 ml

   Aqua – QS

   Mft. Mist prepare 4 such doses

   Adv. to give BID
4. Use catheter to release urine (passage of urine)
5. To check dehydration 5 per cent Dextrose through IV route may be given.
6. Massage of urethra, allow bath and swimming in water pool is advised to stimulate urination.
7. Herbal preparations – *e.g.* Cystone (Himalaya) 5-10 tabs BID; stonil powder @ 40-50 g BID with treacle can be advocated. It is a mixture of herbal drugs acts as a good diuretic and helps in dissolving calculi.
8. Injectable diuretics *e.g.* Frusemide *viz.* Inj. Ridema @ 5-10 ml IM or IV, Tab Lasix 0.5-1 mg/kg body weight or Inj. Lasix @ 5-10 ml by IM or IV can be administered. Never use diuretics for complete urethral obstruction in calculi. Surgical remedy is the only treatment.

4.4.4 Haemoglobinuria

It may be defined as the presence of met-haemoglobin in urine. Haemoglobinuria and myoglobinuria have extra renal causes. Haemoglobinuria is usually followed by haemoglobinaemia.

Etiology

1. Haemoprotozoan parasites – *e.g.* Babesiosis in cattle.
2. Streptococcal septicaemia
3. Certain chemicals *e.g.* Potassium chlorate
4. Phenothiazine derivatives.

Symptoms

The colour of the urine may become brown to red or coffee coloured. Temperature may rise, eyes become shrunken, conjunctiva haemmorhagic. There may be haemolysis in haemoprotozoan parasitic infection.

Treatment

1. As per specific cause.
2. Inj. Berenil, Inj. Nilbery for Babesiosis.
3. Parenteral antibiotics owing to bacterial infection (See antibiotics – *e.g.* Gentamycin, Enrofloxacin).
4. IV infusion of fluids – Rintose, Intalyte *etc.* or Inj. Glucose 25 per cent or Dextrose – 25 per cent IV.

4.4.5 Haematuria (Red Urine)

Escape of R.B.C. through urine is called haematuria. Blood may appear in urine owing to haemorrhages from some parts of the urinary apparatus.

Etiology

Causes of haematuria are many.

1. Pre Renal cause: Severe toxaemia or septicaemia.
2. Renal cause : acute nephritis, trauma, renal infarction.
3. Diseases of urinary organs, cystitis, urethritis, nephritis.
4. Hemoprotozoan parasite – *e.g.* Babesiosis.
5. Poisons
6. Broken Fern poisoning
7. Fungus – *e.g.* Enzootic bovine haematuria.
8. Acute septicaemic condition – *e.g.* H.S., Anthrax.
9. Post renal casues *e.g.* Calculi of urinary bladder, tumor, cystitis, urethral calculi, injury to urethra.
10. Chemical irritants – *e.g.* Carbolic acid, turpentine *etc.*

Treatment

1. Systemic alkaliser *e.g.*, Alkasol syrup (Stadmed) @ 10-15 ml BID can be fed orally. For dog 1-2 tsf BID orally is helpful.

2. Urinary sedative

   For dog –

   Pot. Chlor – 2 g

   Sodi bi carb – 2 g

   Tr. Hyociamus – 2 ml

   Syrup – 30 ml

   Aqua – 200 ml

   Mft., Mist. 1 dose TID orally.

   For large animals (cattle and buffalo) –

   Tr. Hyociamus – 30 ml

   Sodium bicarbonate – 30 g

   Aqua – 125 ml

   Mft. Mist BID for 5 days orally.

3. Haemostatics or styptics to be applied to check capillary bleeding *e.g.* Inj. Bleed check (BeeTee Pharma) 2 ml amp @ 10 ml IM for cattle and buffaloes and @ 2 ml IM for small animals.

   Inj. Chromostat–@ 10ml for cattle and buffalo (IM)

   @ 2 ml for small animals (IM)

4. Administer antibiotics – *e.g.* Ampicillin, Gentamycin *etc.*
5. Sulpha drugs – Injectable preparations containing Trimithoprim and Sulpha combination *e.g.* Biotrim, Oriprim, IM are quite effective in urinary tract infection.
6. For trauma and painful condition NSAIDS *e.g.* Inj. Melonex, Inj. Meloxi, Inj. MP3, Inj. Zobid-M or Inj. Analgin, Oxalgin or Inj. Ketop, Inj. Neoprofen (Ketoprofen) can be used.

4.4.6 Nephritis

Inflammation of renal cells (kidney) is termed as nephritis. It may be suppurative and non-suppurative type. Suppurative nephritis is of two types *viz.*, pyemic nephritis and Pyelonephritis.

In terstitial nephritis both acute and chronic are common in dogs.

Etiology

Bacteria and bacterial toxins may cause this disease.

In dogs: Leptospira and *E. coli.*

Virus: ICH virus in canine.

Parasite: Kidney worm (*Dictophyme renali*)

Chemical poisons: *e.g.* turpentine, carbolic acid.

Toxins: Nephrotoxic agents *viz.* lead, arsenic, DDT, mercury.

Symptoms

Anorexia, depression, arched back, painful micturation, stiffness and pain of joint, staggering gait, frequent urination (polyuria). Proteinuria may be a feature of nephritis.

Diagnosis

Clinical findings, presence of urinary sediments *e.g.* cast, high specific gravity, high protein in urine (Albumin).

Treatment

1. Give specific treatment for specific causes.
2. To check dehydration IV infusion of fluids *e.g.* 5 per cent Dextrose, DNS *etc.* can be used.
3. Use specific antibiotics – *e.g.* Ampicillin, Gentamycin, Enrofloxacin.
4. Use sulpha-trimethoprim combination *e.g.* Biotrim, Oriprim *etc.*
5. Use urinary antiseptic.

   The following misture may be used as urinary antiseptic.

   Hexamine powder – 4 g

   Sod. Acid Phos – 30 g

   Treacle – Q.S.

   Mft. Haust. Sig. Stat.

6. Herbal products like Tab. Bangshil (Alarsin) @ 10 tabs TID for large animal for 10-15 days; and 2 tabs TID for dog for 10-18 days.
7. Parenteral B-complex – Inj. Hivit, Inj. Pinkojet, Inj. Conciplex can be tried.
8. Adjustment of pH of urine should be made using appropriate urinary acidifier or alkalizer.

4.4.7 Pyelonephritis

It is common in farm animals characterized by chronic purulent inflammation of the pelvis of kidneys. In dairy cattle the condition is associated with retention of foetal membrane. In case of female history of recent parturition, with retained placenta, dystocia and uterine infections can easily lead to urinary tract infection and nephritis. Usual cause of this condition is *Corynebacterium renalis*.

Symptoms

Pain and dysuria, frequent attempts of micturation, chronic vaginitis, metritis, cystitis, restlessness, arched back. Presence of abnormal constituents in urine particularly albumin, casts, blood, pus cells, crystals, bacteria, oedema and uraemia in terminal stages.

Diagnosis

1. Examination of urine that reveals pus, blood casts.
2. Examination of kidneys that enlarged, felt per rectal palpation.

Treatment

1. Use urinary antiseptics.
2. Use antibiotics – *e.g.* Gentamycin, Ampicillin, Ampicillin Cloxacillin, Enrofloxacin (see the Drug Index).
3. Use NSAID *e.g.* Inj. Melonex, Meloxicam, Inj. Neoprofen *etc.* Besides NSAID Inj. Epidosin (TTK) can also be tried.
4. Use systemic alkalisers *e.g.* Alkasol syrup.

4.4.8 Cystitis

Inflammation of the urinary bladder is known as cystitis. It is characterized by painful urination, urinary incontinence, haematuria and intermittent temperature. It may be acute or chronic type.

Etiology

1. Ascending infections from urethra
2. Descending infection from kidneys, ureters in nephritis, pyelonephritis.
3. Bacteria *e.g. E. coli, Streptococcus, Staphylococcus, Pseudomonas* spp.
4. Urinary calculi (e) Infection from organism present in blood stream and urine.
5. Irritant chemicals – *e.g.* Turpentine, Cantherides *etc.* sometimes infection may spread from infected genitalia.

Symptoms

Painful micturation, incontinence of urine, cattle may show abdominal pain. Palpation of bladder is painful. Urine may look cloudy or dark in colour with offensive smells.

Diagnosis

Urine analysis and isolation of organisms.

Treatment

1. Remove primary cause.
2. Adjust the pH of the urine using systemic alkaliser *e.g.* Alkasol or acidifier (*e.g.* Sod. Acid phosphate @ 40 mg/kg body weight).
3. Carefully use sterile catheter for the passage of urine.
4. Urinary sedative can be used

   Sodium bicarbonate – 10 g

   Pot. Acetas – 10 g

   Tr. Hyocyamus – 15 ml

   Buchusome – 20 ml

   Mft. Mist. Prepare such doses.

   Adv. to give BID.
5. Administer suitable antibiotics (vide list of antibiotics in the Drug Index).
6. Urinary antiseptics –

   Hexamine – 4 g

   Sod. Acid phos – 30 g

   Treacle – Q.S.

   Mft. Haust. Sig. Stat.
7. Cystone power (Himalayan Drugs) @ 40-50 g or Cystone Tabs @ 5-10 tabs TDS or Stonil Powder (Indian Herbs) and 40-80 g for cattle can be given for 10-18 days.
8. A course of neurotropic B-vitamins (vitamin B_1, B_6 and B_{12}) injection can also be given by IM route for 3-5 days (*e.g.* Inj. Tribivet, Inj. Polyvet, Inj. Neurovet).

4.4.9 Urinary Incontinence

This is a common condition seen in dogs. This could be due to incomplete closure of the sphincter of urinary bladder, due to severe infection, trauma, calculi (stone) and growth. Severe urinary infection, irritation and spinal injury causing weakness of sphincter and loss of neuro muscular control are responsible for urinary incontinence or uncontrolled urination.

Treatment

1. Give proper antibiotic (see antibiotics)

2. Give urinary antiseptic and sedatives.
3. A course of neurotropic B-vitamins *e.g.* Neurobian, Tribivet by IM route.

4.4.10 Urethral Rupture (Urolithiasis)

It is a common surgical condition encountered in male bovines. If proper treatment is not advocated in time, this condition may lead to rupture of urinary bladder or urethra.

Symptoms

Retention of urine, urinary incontinence, edematous swelling anterior to the scrotum, off fed, swelling of ventral abdomen, pitting on pressure.

Surgical Treatment

1. Sedation of animal with Siquil injection (Triflupromazine HCl) @ 0.2 mg/kg body weight.
2. Epidural anaesthesis with 2 per cent Lignocaine HCl @ 10-15 ml.
3. Surgical procedure: Area behind the scrotum is to be made ready for operation and under local infiltration anesthesia an incision of about 8-10 cm long can be made ready in the mid line 2-3 inches posterior to the base of the scrotum. The SC tissue needs to be separated by blunt dissection. Then the penis is o be grasped and exteriorized from the incision. Then palpate the urethra to ascerntain the location of calculus. Then incise the urethra at the site of lodgment and remove the calculi. Then close the urethral incision with 1-0 chromic catgut and to maintain the patency of urethra introducing a polythene catheter. Accumulated SC urine should be drained by incising the skin on either side of the penis.

Post Operative Treatment

1. Intravenous infusion of DNS (1-2 litres) for 2-3 days.
2. Systemic antibiotic therapy (by Inj. Intamox, Inj. Moxell, Inj. Emoxell, Inj. Lemox or Inj. Inclox @ 2 g by IM route or Inj. Gentax, Inj. Gentamycin or Inj. Enrocin, Inj. Floxidin, Inj. quinintas *etc.*) daily for 5-7 days.
3. NSAIDS – like Inj. Melonex, Inj. Zobid-M, Inj. Meloxy, Inj. Ketop, Inj. Neoprofen @ 10-15 ml IM for 3-5 days should be administered.

4.4.11 Balanoposthitis

It is the inflammatory condition of both prepuce and glans penis. Both are involved in inflammatory reactions because of their close apposition. It is a common discase of uncastrated animals (bulls) due to trauma and infection. Balamoposthitis may also occur due to urinary obstruction. Balonoposthitis is not only a problem of breeding bulls but also a problem of calves and castrated animals owing to urinary obstruction and prepucial swelling. Trauma, abrasions, lacerations of prepuce and glans penis may result in introduction of organisms and cause balanoposthitis.

Symptoms

Anorexia, fever, phimosis, subcutaneous swelling on ventral abdomen, prepucial swelling, inflammation of prepuce and penis.

The dusts during summer contaminating the abrasions and wounds of prepuce and glans penis may also cause balanoposthitis. This may also lead to adhesions, phimosis and urinary obstruction.

Treatment

Medical management with a broad spectrum antibiotic (*e.g.* Inj. Oxytetracycline, Inj. Streptopenicillin, Inj. Enrofloxacin or Amoxycillin and Cloxacillin combination @ 10 mg/kg body weight IM for 5-7 days. Irrigation of prepucial cavity with antiseptic, application of acetic acid, chalk paste on the swelling to facilitate reduction and to improve free flow of urine. Give sexual rest till complete recovery. Antihistaminic injection *e.g.* Antilar, Avil, Chloril @ 100 mg (total dose) IM OD for 3-5 days. Lesix injection (Frusemide) @ 2 mg/kg body weight IM OD for 3 days can be given.

Surgical Treatment

Where Balanoposthitis and urinary obstruction syndrome occurs and does not respond to medicinal treatment, surgical treatment should be done through prepuciectomy as circumcision opening to allow free flow of urine.

4.5 DISEASES OF CARDIOVASCULAR SYSTEM

4.5.1 Pericarditis

It is defined as the inflammation of the pericardium and depending on the nature of inflammation it may be fibrinous, adhesive and effusive type. Traumatic pericarditis is widely prevalent in grazing cattle.

Etiology

Bacteria *e.g. Streptococcus* sp., *Pasteurella* sp. and virus *e.g.* Canine distemper virus may affect pericardium; trauma and surgical injury may lead to pericarditis. Extension of focus of infection from pulmonary tuberculosis, pleurisy, endocarditis *etc.* may set up pericarditis. Foreign body penetration through reticulum, peritoneum and diaphragm and reaching the heart usually lead to traumatic reticulo pericarditis (TRP).

Symptoms

Pain over the pericardium, Arching back due to pain sensation, brisket oedema, abducted elbow, prominent jugular vein, chronic indigestion and recurrent tympany (in TRP); restricted movement and disinclination to lie down are usual signs. Auscultation reveal feeble and or muffled heart sound. Area of cardiac dullness is increased.

Treatment

1. Give rest and avoid exercise.
2. For infective pericarditis antibiotic therapy should be given (see antibiotics in the Drug Index).

3. Salt restriction should be made.
4. In case of TRP, surgical removal of foreign body through rumenotomy operation is adviced.

4.5.2 Foreign Body Syndromes

Greedy and voracious nature of eating and grazing of cattle and buffalo make the species most vulnerable to ingestion of foreign bodies and development of the disease as

1. Traumatic reticulitis.
2. Traumatic pericarditis
3. Traumatic reticulo Percarditis (TRP)

Sequele

- ☆ Acute local peritonitis
- ☆ Acute Pericarditis
- ☆ Vagus indigestion
- ☆ Diaphragmatic hernia
- ☆ Congestive heart failure
- ☆ Chronic pericarditis

Symptoms

Persistent pyrexia, rapid pulse and respiration. Anorexia, brisket oedema, reluctance to movement, arched back, extended neck, recurrent attacks of tympanitis, embarrassment of heart function etc. The animal gradually looses condition and may suddenly die.

Diagnosis

1. History
2. Clinical findings
3. Metal detector study.

Treatment

1. Restriction of movements.
2. Immobilization of foreign body by magnet administration.
3. Administration of high doses of broad spectrum antibiotics (see antibiotics)
4. Removal of foreign body by rumenotomy.
5. Fluid therapy as per need.

4.5.3 Cardiac Arrest

It is also known as acute heart failure. In this condition there is sudden loss of consciousness, falling with or without convulsion. There will be severe pallor of mucosae followed by either recovery or death of the animal.

Etiology

Rapid introduction of hypertonic solution by IV route *e.g.* Inj. Mifex, Inj. Mifocal, Inj. Calmax-M *etc.* Rapid and excessive administration of anaesthetic. Myocardial infarction, Massive pulmonary embolism, heat stroke, lightening stroke, shock, toxaemia *etc.*

Symptoms

Severe respiratory distress, dyspnoea, increased rate and shallow respiration, irregular pulse, staggering and falling, convulsions, dilation of pupil and coldness of skin, cyanotic changes.

Treatment

1. Intracardiac administration of Adrenaline or Epinephrine 1 : 1000 ml solution, 2 ml.
2. Oxygen therapy (Pulmonary ventilation)
3. Cardiac massage
4. In case of small animals raise hind quarters and lower the head.

4.5.4 Congestive Cardiac Failure

It is defined to be as chronic heart failure characterized by the failure of the heart to pump blood effectively.

Etiology

Any disorders of pericardium, myocardium and endocardium, myocardial infarction, mitral incompetence, acute drug toxicity, aortic incompetence *etc.*

Treatment

1. Rest and salt free diet indicated.
2. Venesection–@ 2-4 ml blood/kg body weight to be withdrawn in emergency.
3. Diuretics (Inj. Ridema/Lasix *etc.*) can be given IM daily or orally (*e.g.* Lasix tab).
4. Inj. Prednisolone may be administered or orally Prednisolone tablet to the small animals.
5. Slow IV infusion of Manitol 200-300 CC can be carried out.
6. Digitalization is necessary. Inj. Digoxin by IV route is beneficial for ruminants. Inj. Digitalin @ 15-60 mg SC or IM to cattle and horse. Digitalis tincture can be fed to dog, horse and pig orally.
7. Sedative or Tranquiliser can be administered for intense pain management *e.g.* Inj. Anicam (Intas), Inj. Sequil *etc.*

4.5.5 Peripheral Circulatory Failure (PCF)

Failure of venous return to heart is called P.C.F. and it occurs due to reduced cardiac output, less calcium level in blood (hypocalcaemia), excessive haemorrhage and dehydration *etc.*

Symptoms

Depression, subnormal temperature, feeble heart rate, skin are cold to touch, pale mucosae, feeble pulse (imperceptible), respiration increased but shallow, coma and clonic convulsion.

Treatment

1. In case of haemorrhage and dehydration restore circulatary blood volume by warm dextrose solution (vide fluid therapy in the Drug Index) or by blood transfusion.
2. If it is due to vasodilatation, vaso constricting drug *e.g.* Inj. Adrenaline (1 : 1000 solution) 2-4 ml IV to be administered. Adrenaline should never be used if there is reduced circulatory blood volume (CBV).
3. To increase CBV, plasma expanders *e.g.* Dextran, Dextraven *etc.* can also be used.

4.5.6 Diseases of Blood and Blood Forming Organs

Normal functions of blood can be hindered or affected greatly owing to (*a*) decrease in circulating blood volume (hypovolumia) (*b*) abnormalities in blood constituents (*c*) abnormalities in circulation.

It may be defined as a disturbance of body fluids in which more fluid is lost from the body that may coincide with the changes in electrolytes and acid base balance of the body (See the table 4.2 for Types of dehydration).

Table 4.2: Type of Dehydration (per cent) and Clinical Findings

Type of Dehydration	*Percent Dehydration*	*Physical Examination Findings*
Mild Dehydration	5-7 per cent	Fluid loss, dryness of mouth and no skin turgor
Moderate Dehydration	8-10 per cent	Moderately decreased skin turgor, dry oral mucous membranes, depression of eyes and cooling of extremities.
Severe dehydration	10-15 per cent	Marked loss of skin turgor, sunken eye balls, involuntary muscle twitening increased capillary refill time and shock.

Etiology

Inadequate fluid intake, excessive loss of fluids and electrolyses from the body (*e.g.* vomiting, polyurea, diarrhoea, persistent fever, excessive salivation). Acute carbohydrate engorgements, ruminal stasis, extensive burn wounds, acute intestinal and gastric obstruction *etc.*

Symptoms

Dryness, wrinkling of the skin, shrunken appearance of body, face, eyes *etc.* Muscular weakness, decreased skin elasticity, lack of appetite, increased thirst, decrease in urine excretion, dryness of the mouth and throat due to less salivary secretion, anhydremia, oligemia, haemoconcentration, shock, coma and finally death.

Diagnosis

History, symptoms, urine analysis revealing high specific gravity and increased plasma NPN.

Treatment

Judicious and timely restoration of fluid therapy for correcting the abnormalities in water, electrolytes and acid base balance. IV injection of Isotonic solution (*e.g.* Dextran, Inj. Sodium lactate, Ringers lactate *etc.*) Ringer's injection 250-300 ml IV or SC for large animals (See table 4.3 for fluid therapy).

Table 4.3: Suggested IV Fluid Therapy for Different Diseases in Veterinary Practice

Name of the Disease	*Suggested IV Fluid*
Calf scour (Neonatal calf Diarrhoea)	Equal mixture of 0.9 per cent normal saline 1.3 per cent sodium bicarbonate and 5 per cent Dextrose (100 ml/kg)
Grain poisoning/carbohydrate engorgement Rumen impaction	Initially 5 per cent Sodium bicarbonate (5 litres/450 kg) followed by balanced electrolyte solution
Acute diarrhoea in horse	5 per cent sodium bicarbonate (3-5 litres/500 kg) followed by high sodium, high potassium alkalinizing solution for correction of hypokalemia following bicarbonate therapy.
Abnormal torsion in cattle and Abnormal impaction	Balanced electrolyse solution or high potassium and chloride acidifying solution for correction of alkalosis.
Heat stroke	0.9 per cent normal saline
Peracute Mastitis	Balanced electrolyte solution in large quantities for hydration and maintenance (100-150 ml kg/24 hours)
Acute Diffuse Peritonitis	Balanced electrolyte solution in large quantities for hydration and maintenance
Shock	Balanced electrolyte solution with sodium bicarbonate to correct acidosis (about 2 litres/cow)
Acute Intestinal Obstruction	Initially 1.3 per cent sodium bicarbonate (3-5 litres/500 kg) followed by balanced electrolyte solution. Potassium chloride if Hypokalemia develops following bicarbonate therapy in horses.

Source: Sheela (2007).

4.5.7 Haemorrhage

Haemorrhage may be defined as the escape of blood from vascular system *e.g.* artery, vein, blood capillaries etc. to the outside of the body (called external haemmrohage) or into the body cavity (called internal haemorrhage). Minute, pinpoint haemorrhage is called petechiae, if still bigger called ecchymoses. Localized extravasion of blood is called haematoma.

Petechial haemorrhages are seen in diseases like Babesiosis, or Piroplasmosis, Trypanosomiasis, H.S., Glanders, phosphorus and arsenic poisoning and any septicaemic condition.

Depending on the discharges of blood from various parts or sites of the body various terms are used *e.g.*

✰ Haematuria	Blood in urine
✰ Haemoptysis	Blood in sputrum
✰ Haematemesis	Blood in vomitus
✰ Haemothorax	Blood in thorax
✰ Haemosalpinx	Bleeding in oviducts
✰ Haematocele	Bleeding into tunica vaginalis
✰ Haemo pericardium	Blood in Pericardium
✰ Epistaxis	Bleeding from nose
✰ Haematoma	Extravasion of blood locally in a tissue
✰ Extra vacation	Extensive haemorrhages in the tissue
✰ Apoplexy	Bleeding into brain
✰ Enterorrhagia	Bleeding from intestine
✰ Metrorrhagia	Bleeding from uterus

Etiology

Accidental trauma, aneurysm, parasitic and bacterial infection, bacterial toxins, plant toxins. Braken fern, snake envenomation, increased blood pressure, deficiency in vitamin K, C *etc.*, surgical procedures, haemoprotozoan diseases.

Treatment

1. Blood transfusion – Fresh or stored whole blood.
2. Packed red cells and fresh frozen plasma as blood components can be transfused.
3. In bovines – for fresh blood transfusion, blood is to be collected from the jugular vein of a healthy animal. Rate of transfusion 10 ml/kg body weight (Average 2 litres in cattle). Regarding blood transfusion, Donor – Recipient blood matching is must. Cross matching and biological screening tests can be done for the said purpose.

   Canine Blood Types: Dogs have at least 13 blood group types known as dog erythrocyte antigens. Canine RBC are either (+ ve) or (- ve) of a blood type.

   Feline Blood Types: Only recognized blood group is Feline AB blood group and contains 3 alleles : type –A, type-B and rare type AB- Type is dominant over type B.

   Blood Transfusion: Blood transfusion is the transfer of homologous blood from one donor (individual) to another (recipient) of the same species. The blood should be infused slowly 80-100 drops per minute by IV route with a sterile, hypodermic needle in dogs. Infusion can also be carried out through intraperitoneal route, of course absorption is slower.

   In dogs blood to be infused to the jugular vein or cephalic vein by IV catheter.

   Dose: The dose is calculated on the basis of per cent hemoglobin present to which it is increased (at least 75 per cent of the normal level).

4. Isotonic solution should also be infused by slow IV infusion (*e.g.* Dextran-70, Dextrose 5 per cent, 10 per cent, Rintose, Intalyte *etc*).
5. Chromostat injection, Inj. Bleed check (Bee Tee Pharma) @ 10 ml for cattle and 2-4 ml for small animal by IM or IV.

4.5.8 Oedema

Oedema denotes abnormal accumulation of fluid in the tissue space and body cavities owing to endocrine, circulatory and hepatic changes.

Oedema could be either inflammatory or non inflammatory origin. In non-inflammatory oedema transudate (a serous fluid) is accumulated in the tissue space.

According to affection of organ the oedema may be hepatic oedema, cardiac oedema, pulmonary oedema, renal oedema, mammary oedema *etc*. Other types are nutritional oedema, allergic oedema and mechanical oedema.

Etiology

Increase in hydrostatic pressure and fall in plasma colloid osmotic pressure (PCOP), local inflammation like boils, cellulitis, trauma, infection, chemical irritants, blockage of lymphatics and capillaries, heart failure, hepatitis, renal disease, vitamin-A deficiency, infectious diseases *etc*.

Some important terminologies or disease conditions owing to the development of oedema according to organs involved.

Hydrothorax – Oedema (accumulation of water in thorax/thorasic cavity).

Hydrosalpinx – Oedema of oviduct/accumulation of fluid in oviduct.

Hydrocephalus – Accumulation of fluid in pericardium.

Ascitis – Accumulation of fluid in peritoneal cavity.

Symptoms

Painless swelling that pits on pressure is oedema, in hydropericardium and hydrothorax there are restrictions in cardiac movements.

Treatment

1. Correction of primary causes.
2. For cardiac oedema, hydrothorax and hydropericardicum – Rest, adequate protein diet, salt free diet, diuretics and digitalization needs to be made.

   Mixture for digitalization

   Tr. Nux Vom – 10 ml

   Tr Digitalis – 8 ml

   Tr. Zingiberis – 25 ml

   Aqua – 65 ml

   Mft. Mist Adv. OD for 8-10 days.

Perenteral administration of diuretics.

e.g. Inj. Ridema 5-10 ml IM or IV for large animals.

Inj. Lasix (2 ml amp) 5-10 ml IM or IV for large animal and 2 ml for small animal.

Oral frusemide – *e.g.* Lasix tab 0.5-1 mg/kg body weight.

Herbal preparations *e.g.* Stonil, Cystone powder/tabs can be used.

For Renal oedema – Salt free diet, amino acids, corticosteroid to be administered.

Hepatitic oedema – Rest, deworming with anthelmentics, antibiotics, liver extract with B-complex and oral liver tonics.

Allergic oedema – Inj. Avil/Chloril/Zeet, and Corticosteroids *e.g.* Inj. Prednisolone, Inj. Dexamethasone.

Table 4.4: Fluid Replacement Therapy in Veterinary Practice

Fluids	*Uses*
0.9 per cent Normal saline (Isotonic solution)	To restore circulating blood volume
7 per cent Normal saline (Hypertonic solution)	To increase intravascular volume (shock)
5 per cent Dextrose (Isotonic solution)	Extracellular fluid diluent (ECF)
1.3 per cent sodium bi-carbonate (Isotonic)	Acidosis
1.3 per cent sodium bi-carbonate in 5 per cent dextrose	Acidosis
5 per cent sodium bi-carbonate	Severe acidosis
Equal mixture of 0.9 per cent normal saline and 1.3 per cent sodium bi-carbonate	Acidosis and dehydration
Lactated ringers solution	Acidosis
Balanced electrolyte solution	Acidosis, alkalosis, electrolyte losses and dehydration
High sodium alkanizing solution (*i.e.* Lactated Ringers solution + sodium bicarbonate 5 g/litre)	Acidosis and hyponatremia
High sodium, high potassium alkanizing solution (Lactated Ringers solution + 1 g/litre potassium chloride solution + 5 g/litre sodium bicarbonate)	Acidosis, hyponatremia and hypokalemia
High Potassium acidifying solution (0.9 per cent normal saline with 2.5 g potassium chloride/litre)	Alkalosis, hypochloremia and hypokalemia.

4.6 DISEASES OF NERVOUS SYSTEM

Before going to deal with nervous disorders or diseases of nervous system functional neuroanatomy and neuro physiology to be known. The different components of the nervous system includes (*i*) Cerebrum (*ii*) Cerebellum (*iii*) Spinal cord (*iv*) Autonomic nervous system (*v*) Peripheral nervous system.

Functions of various components of nervous system in animal body.

Sl.No.	Components	Functions
1.	Cerebrum	Consciousness, sensory motor activities
2.	Brain stem	Motor activity, regulation of vital body functions
3.	Cerebellum	Musculo skeletal co-ordination
4.	Spinal cord	Motor functions of limbs and spinal reflex
5.	Autonomic nervous system	Co-ordination of internal body functions
6.	Peripheral nervous system (*e.g.* cranial and spinal nervous system)	Motor function and reflex to external stimuli or environment.

General Manifestations of Nervous Disorder

1. Incardination (abnormal gait and posture)
2. Excitement (hyperaesthesia), irritability or depression.
3. Functional disturbances affecting entire body when CNS is affected.
4. Loss of consciousness, nervous depression, increased nervous irritability and involuntary contractions.
5. Paralysis and other disturbances of function, stupor *etc.*
6. Muscular tremor, ataxia, convulsions, dullness, mania, paresis and paralysis.
7. Complete loss of consciousness or a state of coma.
8. A bilateral paralysis of the posterior part of the body and hind limbs resulting from injury to the cord-paraplegia.
9. Paralysis arising in the brain cortex and in the peripheral nerves called hemiplegia with unilateral affection.
10. Loss of control on sphinctors of anus, bladder, fecocolith (stony bowels due to vegal injury).

4.6.1 Incordination of Gait

Abnormalities in gait, ataxia and or incordinated gait may occur due to primary disease of the nervous system. Pain in joint, muscle, skin and abdominal organs may affect the normal gait. Brain lesion may cause circling. Cerebellar lesions may cause dysmetria with incordinated gait (goose stepping).

4.6.2 Polyneuritis

It is characterized by disturbances in motor functions or peripheral neuritis that produce sensory disturbances in animals. Deficiency of neurotropic B-vitamins B_1, B_6 and B_{12} are the main attributable factors for polyneuritis. Besides the deficiency of neurotropic B-vitamins, pyemia, septicaemia, meningitis, myelitis that damage the nerves may lead to polyneuritis.

Treatment

1. Drug containing B-vitamins along with anabolic steroid may be tried.
2. Specific cause should be ruled out and treatment should be extended. For infectious etiology, broad spectrum antibiotics (see antibiotics) to be administered.
3. Neurotropic B-vitamins (B_1, B_6, B_{12} formulation) *e.g.* Inj. Tribivet (Intas), Inj. Neuroxin-12 (Sarabhai Zydus), Inj. Neurovet (Alved) @ 5-10 ml IM should be administered.

4.6.3 Motor Disturbances

Disturbances in nervous functions affect the muscles in two ways, *viz.*, (1) Spasm (2) Paralysis and paresis. In muscle spasms there are sudden, violent involuntary contractions which may be continuous called tonic spasms or intermittent called clonic spasms.

If muscle spasms are widespread and involve the whole body including limbs they are called convulsions. In the second form of neuromuscular functional disturbance paralysis and paresis may occur. The underlying cause is the defective innervations of the muscles.

There would be involuntary movement and loss of muscular co-ordination resulting in irregular movement, gait or paralysis.

Types of Paralysis

Hemiplegia – When paralysis is unilateral owing to disturbances in nervous function arising from brain cortex and peripheral nerves.

Paraplegia – A bilateral paralysis of the posterior parts of the body and hind limbs resulting from the injury of spinal cord, called paraplegia.

Quadruplegia – It is a condition where all the fore legs are affected.

Monoplegia – When paralysis is confined to a single organ.

Diplegia – It is a condition in which both sides of the body are involved.

Principle of Treatment

1. Specific treatment for specific diseases showing nervous manifestations as in cases of Trypanosomiasis, Nervous form of Bovine Ketosis, milk fever, Hypomagnesaemia, Listeriosis *etc.*
2. Supportive and symptomatic treatment.
3. Antibiotics for control of infections (the antibiotics which can cross the blood brain barrier – *e.g.* Cefotaxim, Britax, Cefstan *etc.*)
4. Use of hypertonic solutions *e.g.* IV Calcium Borogluconate (Inj. Calgonate, Inj. Mifex, Inj. Intacal *etc.*)
5. Diuretics can be used to relieve intracranial pressure.
6. Application of CNS depressants.
7. Use of CNS stimulants as the case may be.

CNS Stimulants

(*a*) Cerebral stimulants – Caffein, ephedrine, cocaine.

(*b*) Brain stem stimulants – Camphor, Caffein, Nikethamide.

(*c*) Spinal cord stimulants – Strychnine.

Formulations

Atropine – (Inj. Atropin sulphate), Dose: Cattle and Buffalo 15-100 mg SC.

Caffein (Caffein citrate) – Dose: Cattle and Horse – 2-4 mg SC and 2-8 mg orally.

Amphetamine (*e.g.* Methedrine, Dexedrine) – 100-300 mg SC for Cattle and Horse, Dog 1-4 mg/kg.

Leptazol (Cardiazol) – Horse and Cattle 0.5-1 g, Dog 50-100 mg.

Useful to counteract effects of barbiturates.

Strychnine – (Strychnine HCl) Horse and Cattle 15-60 mg, Dog 0.3-1 mg.

It acts as spinal cord stimulant.

Liquour Strychrine HCl – 4-8 ml orally for Horse and Cattle.

Nervine Tonics

Tr. Nux vom – 15 ml

Tr. Gentian – 12 ml

Liq. Arsenicalis – 25 ml

Aqua – Q. S.

Mft. Haust, Adv. one dose orally on 3-6 occasions.

Arsenicalis acts as alterative and tonic, hence combined with nerve tonics.

Phosphorus compound is also useful in stimulating the motor activity (acts as nerve stimulant).

1. Inj. Uremin (Glaxo SmithKline)
2. Inj. Tonophosphan (Intervet) 10-15 ml SC or IV
3. Inj. Alphos-40 (Alved) @ 10-15 ml by IM
4. Inj. Tonoricin (Wockhardt) @ 10-15 ml for large animal and 1-3 ml for small animal.

Calcium preprations act as nerve stimulants. The trade names of such preparations are

1. Inj. Calborol (Novartis)
2. Inj. Calgonate (Indian Immunologicals)
3. Inj. Intacal (Intas)
4. Inj. Calmex (Vetnex)

These can be employed as nervine stimulants in large animal by IV and SC routes.

Neurotropic B-vitamins act as nervine stimulants and tonics. The trade names of such preparations are

1. Inj. Neuroxin 12-V (Sarabhai) – Dose: 5-10 ml IM daily.
2. Inj. Neurovet (Alved) – Dose: 5-10 ml IM daily.
3. Inj. Tribivet (Intas) – Dose: Large animal 4-5 ml, Small animal 0-5-1 ml by IM.
4. Inj. Polyvet (Excell) – Dose: Large animal 10 ml, Small animal 2-3 ml by IM.

CNS Depressants

Indicated in nervous excitement, hyperaesthesia, hyperirritability, titanic convulsion, epilepsy, strychnine poisoning, prolapse of uterus with severe straining, epileptic fits and seizures *etc*.

The drugs are:

Chloral hydras, potassium bromide, sodium bromide *etc*. can be used in cattle, buffalo and horse.

1. Chloral hydras 30 g in 200 ml distilled water can be given by slow IV route.
2. Sodium bromide or Potassium bromide – 4 g as treacle – Q.S., Mft. Haust, Sig. as required.
3. Chloral Hydras – 30 g

   Aqua – 150 ml

   Oil Lini – 400 ml

   Mft. Haust – Sig. Stat.

Common Tranquilisers Used in Veterinary Practice

Triflupromazine HCl and Chlorpromezine HCl can be used in cattle and buffalo.

Inj. Triflupromazine HCl *e.g.* Inj. Siquil (Sarabhai Zydus)

Dose: Cattle and Buffalo 10-20 mg/100 kg body weight IM or IV.

Inj. Chlorpromazine HCl-5 per cent *e.g.* Inj. Largactil

In dogs the commonly used tranquilizers are

Inj. Diazepam, Inj. Calmpose, Inj. Anazepam @ 1-2 ml by IM or IV.

Inj. Largactil 25 per cent solution @ 1-2 ml by IM or IV or Tablets @ 25 mg BID.

Inj. Siquil (Sarabhai Zydus) 20-40 mg SC or IV.

Phenobarbitone *e.g.* Gardenal Tablets 30 mg

Drugs like Epsoline, Mysoline @ 0.25 g/5 kg BID orally, Tab Dilantin @ 1 tab TID orally can be used.

Paralysis

It is a condition where there is complete or incomplete loss of nervous control over any bodily function occurs. This may comprise loss of sensory or motor power both. It is characterized by total inability to perform voluntary movements.

Anatomically paralysis may be of three types. These are (*a*) Cerebral paralysis, (*b*) Spinal paralysis and (*c*) Peripheral paralysis.

Etiology

Paralysis results due to encephalitis, infection of CNS, compression of brain, space occupying lesions in brain (Tumor, cyst, abscess), injury of spinal cord due to trauma, fracture of vertebral column, Myelitis, abscess in spinal cord, ancylosis of vertebrae, injury to the nerve trunk, deficiency of vitamins B_1, B_6 and B_{12}.

Treatment

1. Specific treatment should be given in case of infective etiology.
2. Core and nursing of the animals are essential to restore the paralytic condition.
3. Physiotherapy *e.g.* massaging of the spinal cord and the affected part of the body with liniments, *e.g.* Lint. Terebenthene, Infrared ray, moist hot fomentation with Epsom salt can be tried.
4. The liniments commonly used are
   (*a*) Ammoniated camphor liniment
   (*b*) Oil turpentine liniment
   (*c*) Weak ammonia liniment

Nervine tonics, neurotropic B-vitamins *e.g.* Inj. Tribivet, Inj. Neurovet, Inj. Polyvet *etc.*, anabolic steroids, phosphorus preparations *e.g.* Inj. Uremin, Inj. Tonoricin, Inj T. Phos @ 5-10 ml IM or SC can also be used.

For abscess and tumour *etc.* surgical intervention is advised.

For spinal injury NSAIDs *e.g.* Neoprofen, Inj. Ketop or Inj. Meloxicam *e.g.* Inj. MP3, Inj. A_3vet plus, Inj. Melonex *etc.* @ 10-15 ml by IM route for large animal and 3-5 ml for small animal can be tried.

4.6.4 Epilepsy/Epileptic Seizure

Any thing that alters neuronal function in the brain is potentially seizure producing. The word epilepsy in Greek means "Seizure" characterized by abnormal body movement, profuse salivation, a loss of consciousness, abnormal behavior, involuntary behavior, involuntary urination and defecation. Epilepsy is only a symptom of an underlying neuronal dysfunction occurring primarily within the brain or secondarily caused by toxic substances, or metabolic or electrolyte abnormalities.

Etiology

Seizure disorders constitute about 1 per cent of all canine diseases. It is mainly caused by damage to brain tissue which acts as a focus of seizure.

1. Virus – *e.g.* Distemper virus
2. Protozoa – *e.g.* Toxoplasmosis.
3. Metabolic – *e.g.* Hypoxia (lowered oxygen tension of the blood).

Hypoglycaemia and Hypocalcaemic hepatic encephalopathy and chemical intoxication (*e.g.* Large dose of penicillin, insecticides, pesticides, strychnine, lead, cyanides *etc.*)

4. Cerebral trauma
5. Cerebral neoplasm
6. Mycotic – *e.g.* Cryptococcosis.

Treatment

1. Removal of underlying causes.
2. To control seizures with anticonvulsants. Since hard or continuous seizures are devastating to CNS, anticonvulsants are used to control seizures while the primary disorder is being treated.

Phenothiazine transquilizers should not be given to epileptic patient.

Drugs to be used are:

1. Pheno-barbitone: It is effective in all forms of epilepsy seen in dogs and cats. The recommended dose is 1-5 mg/kg daily in one or two days.
2. Primidone (Mysoline, Mylepsin) – It is effective in all types of seizures, has a rapid action when given orally. The recommended dose is 1.7-7.0 mg/kg daily in three divided doses.
3. Diphenyld hydantoin (Dilantin, Phenytoin) – It is indicated in generalized major motor seizures, focal motor seizures and psychomotor behavioral-hysterical seizures.

   Recommended dose is 20-35 mg/kg at every 8 hours interval.
4. Diazepam (Valium) – It is indicated for status epilepticus. It is the only tranquilizier, which is not epileptogenic. Recommended dose is 1-2 mg/kg body weight.
5. Carbamazepine (Tegretol) – It is also an effective anticonvulsant. Dose is 8-10 mg/kg body weight.
6. Sodium valproate – It is the drug of choice for primary generalized epilepsy or dogs suffering from Idiopathic epilepsy @ 75 mg/kg body weight/day in 3 divided doses.

Biochemic Remedy

Magnesia phosphorica–a biochemic remedy of seizures and epilepsy.

Mag Phos – 6x, 3 tabs placed on tongue once daily for a month gives better response in epilepsy in dogs.

4.6.5 Brain Trauma

Brain trauma in bovines is common in field conditions. It may also occur in other animals too. In animals, brain injury may be caused due to sudden falling, blow, accidental collision, violent stretching of head and neck, in fighting or trauma due to casting.

The direct trauma is an uncommon cause of brain injury in large animals because of the force required to damage the cranium. In bull, cow, calf and buffalo this occurs due to blow, hit by stone over poll, forehead or due to attack by adult cow or sudden falling.

Symptoms

Circling, falling immediately after trauma, recumbancy, dilatation of pupils, slow irregular respiration. Anorexia and cessation of rumination, defaecation and urination. There may be signs of excitement, bellowing, salivation, falling and convulsions. The signs exhibited may be due to concussion or contusion leading to increased intracranial pressure and damage to nervous tissue.

Diagnosis

Based on history of injury, evidence of injury to the skull, symptoms and sudden onset of signs without rise in body temperature.

Treatment

1. Sedatives to be given to prevent and to control nervous excitement.
2. Antibiotics to check secondary bacterial infection – *e.g.* Inj. Enrofloxacin @ 2.5 mg/kg body weight, *e.g.*, Inj. Britax (Brihans), Inj. Intacef (Intas) by IM route for 3-5 days.
3. NSAIDs as anti-inflammatory and analgesic *e.g.* Inj. Melonex, Inj. Proxivet, Inj. Zobid-20, Inj MP_3, Inj. Analgin NP *etc.*
4. Steroids to reduce inflammation and to prevent shock – *e.g.* Inj. Enidex, Inj. Brisone, Inj. Dexona *etc.*
5. IV injection of Manitol to reduce intracranial pressured for its vasoconstrictive and diuretics effect. Mannitol @ 0.5 g/kg body weight by IV.
6. 20 per cent Dextrose IV infusion or Intalyte, Rintose, Wocktrose @ 500-1000 ml can be infused.
7. Neurotropic B-vitamins (B_1, B_6 and B_{12} formulations) *e.g.* Inj. Tribivet (Intas), Inj. Polyvet (Excell), Inj. Neurovet (Alved) @ 5-10 ml by IM daily for 3 to 5 days.
8. Inj. Chloropromazine HCl @ 1 mg/kg body weight by IM or IV can be tried.
9. Osmotic diuretics to be used to reduce intracranial pressure.

4.7 DISEASES OF LOCOMOTOR SYSTEM AND MUSCLES

Skeletal System and its Therapeutic Management

The most common conditions are acute trauma, laminitis, myositis, injuries of ligament, joint or muscles, sprains, sprain of muscle and tendons, paresis, tendonitis, bursitis, muscle contracture, contracted tendons, ligaments and muscles. Besides these affections, large animals those are used for draught or fast work are prone to the orthopedic affections involving joints. Bursitis, synovitis, tendovaginitis, arthritis and osteroarthritis are also the common affection of locomotory system.

For all such conditions excluding fractures some common modes of treatment can be advocated.

1. Physiotherapy – by use of cold therapy, heat therapy (including diathermy and ultrasound therapy), electrical stimulation, laser therapy, magnetic field therapy, massage, acupuncture, controlled exercise *etc.* and other modalities can be tried.

   Example: Cold water application can be advocated for acute trauma, laminitis and ligament joint or muscle injuries or sprains.
2. Local application with Liniment Ammonia in cattle and horse.

   Application of iodex ointment, application of cat gall on yokegall, massage with Rumalaya cream, Briclofen Plus gel (Brihans).
3. Massaging – by stroking, kneading, compression or fiction of the part (*e.g.* Inflamin ointment, Briclofen Plus gel, Iodex ointment, Mastilepgel. Olive oil, mustard oil, coconut oil or a fine grainded talcum powder can be used to reduce friction, to soften skin and avoid pulling of hair. Massage for 10-15 minutes for obtaining good results.
4. Oral or parenteral administration of NSAIDs – 20 ml for large animal, and 5 ml for small animal *viz.* Inj. Boline, or Inj. Artisone (Alved), Inj. Esgipyrin @ 15-25 ml for large animal, or Inj. Meloxicam, Inj. Melonex, Meloxy by deep IM @ 1-2 ml for small animal.

   Inj. Zobid-M, Inj. Proxivet *etc.* or Inj. Ketop, Inj. Ketoprofen (Neoprofen) *etc.* for large animal @ 10-15 ml, and for small animal @ 3-5 ml and for dog and cat 0.5-1 ml by IM route can be administered.

For Arthritis

In addition to above treatment the following may be tried. R-compound (Alarsin) for large animal @ 10 tabs TDS for 15 days. For small animal 2 to 5 tabs TDS for 15 days. Rumalaya (Himalayan Drug) for large animal 10-15 tabs TDS for 15 days, and for small animal 2-3 tabs TDS for 15 days can be administered.

Infra red fomentation can be advocated, Inj. Esgipyrin (Sarabhai Zydus), Inj. Phenyl Butazone, Inj. Artisone(s) (Alved) @ 10-15 ml for large animal by IM route for 2-3 days, and for small animal 2-3 ml by IM route can be administered.

Oral bolus like Oxalgin NP, A_3 vet bolus, Paralgin DP, Melonex Plus bolus along with serratiopeptidase bolus like Seri-D (March India), Inflamin/Inflazyme vet (Excell) can be recommended (which act as a proteolytic enzyme counteracting inflammatory signs and dissolves fibrous tissue).

Anthrocentesis for the treatment of joint diseases it is mandatory to perform arthrocentesis properly. It would not only relieve increased intra articular pressure associated with joint affection but also as an avenue for injection of therapeutic medicament into joint cavity.

The following drugs can be administered – as an intra-articular therapy:

1. *Corticosteroids, viz.*
   (*a*) 9-Fluroprednisolone acetate – 5-20 mg
   e.g. Inj. Prednisolone
   (*b*) Triamcinolone acetonide (Synthetic corticosteroid) *viz.* Inj. Vetalog 5-15 mg
   (*c*) Betamethasone acetate and Betamethsone disodium phosphate – 6-12 mg
   e.g. Inj. Betnesol
   (*d*) Methyl Prednisolone – 40-80 mg
   (*e*) Flumethasone – 1.5-2.5 mg

(Here corticosteroids act as buffer between irritant and susceptible cells, inhibit the release of prostaglandins, collagenase, the leucocytic migration and suppress superoxide formation.)

Antibiotics

For infections arthritis antibiotics alone or in combination with other drugs should be administered. Almost all antibiotics cross the synovial membrane and antibiotics when given intra-articularly are more beneficial due to a rapid therapeutic concentration at the affected site.

The common antibiotics for intra-articular therapy are:

1. Penicillin 40 lakh to 80 lakh, IU/joint.
2. Streptomycin and Rifamycin 0.5-1 g/joint
3. Chloramphenicol and Neomycin 1-2 g/joint
4. Gentamycin 50-150 mg/joint.

Non drug therapy – which includes the use of drainage and lavage of the septic joint using large bore needles in each side of joint capsule and flushing of the joint.

The use of specific antibiotic along with joint drainage hastens the recovery from arthritis or joint affections.

4.7.1 Sprains

Sprains are the painful condition of animals characterized by the injuries in the neighbourhood of joints, tearing of a ligament or tendon. Usually it occurs in the limbs of animals as a result of slipping or stumbling, falling and slipping when muscular effort is more to carry a heavy load or other conditions where the tendons are subjected to severe stress or strain or pull, heavy exercise *etc.*

Treatment

Apply liniment of ammonia. Lint ABC, Relaxyl or Iodex ointment can be locally applied. NSAIDs orally or parenterally can be used. *e.g.* Inj. Esgipyrin (Sarabhai Zydus), Inj. Artisone(s) (Alved), Inj. Ketop, Inj. Neoprofen (Vetnex), Inj. Meloxicam (*e.g.* Inj. Meloxi, Inj. A_3vet, Inj. Zobid-M, Inj. Analgin, Inj. Oxalgin NP by IM route (see NSAIDs in the Drug Index).

Or orally spasmonim bolus (Excell), Inflamin, Oxalgin NP (Sarabhai Zydus), Melonex Plus bolus, A_3 vet, Melonex bolus can also be used.

4.7.2 Myositis

It is a common condition occurring in cattle and buffaloes characterized by the inflammation of the muscle fibres.

Etiology

Traumatic injury of the muscle, tearing of muscle fibres, violent blow *etc.* Infighting injury and tauma forced work and heavy exercise. Some diseases may cause Myositis – *e.g.* BQ, FMD *etc.*

Symptoms

Severe pain in muscles, swelling, lameness, stiffness in gait due to muscular rigidity. In acute myositis, muscles are swollen and painful, crepitating muscles in BQ haematoma may also develop.

Treatment

1. Application of liniment.
2. Cold application initially – followed by moist hot fomentation.
3. Application of Briclofen plus gel, Iodex, *etc.*
4. NSAIDs (*e.g.* Meloxicam, Analgin, Neoprofen *etc.*) should be administered.
5. Specific therapy for specific etiologies, as for example in BQ Inj. Streptopenicillin, Inj. Enrofloxacin can be used.
6. Corticosteroids can be used.
7. Inj. E-care Se (Vetnex) @ 10 ml IM by for large animal 2-3 injections can be administered.

4.7.3 Myopathy

It denotes non-inflammatory degeneration of skeletal muscles.

Etiology

1. Vitamin E and Selenium deficiency.
2. Plant toxins and Mycotoxins.
3. Nerve damage leading to muscular atrophy.
4. Violent trauma, blow and prolong exercise.
5. Prolong use of cortico-steroids.
6. Post parturient paresis
7. Prolong recumbency.

Symptoms

Weakness of muscles, abnormal gait, muscles are swollen, hard and painful, inability to rise and walks, stiffness of joints and lameness. Animal may become paretic or recumbent.

Treatment

1. Inj. Vitamin-E with selenium – *e.g.* Inj. E-Care Se (Vetnex)–@ 10 ml IM daily for 3 to 5 days to cattle.
2. Give comfortable bedding to present sores.
3. Neurotropic B-vitamins *e.g.* Inj. Neurovet, Inj. Tribivet, Inj. Neuroxin-12 @ 5-10 ml by IM route on alternate day for 3 occasions can be administered.
4. Parenteral calcium *e.g.* Inj. Orical (IBC), Inj. Cal BD (Vets Farma), Inj. Brical (Brihans) @ 10-15 ml IM daily for large animals @ 2.5 ml IM daily for small animals can be tried.
5. NSAIDs if necessary can be administered.

4.7.4 Arthritis

Inflammation of the joints is called arthritis. There are inflammatory changes of synovial membranes of multiple joints. Joints may be swollen, thickened, stiff and synovial fluid may become turbid. There may be deposition of fibrin within the synovial membranes. Lameness is the cardinal signs of arthritis.

Etiology

Bacteria, virus, mycoplasma infection (*Mycoplasma mycoides*). Autoimmunity and hypersensitivity have also been incriminated rheumatoid arthritis in dogs. Virus – *e.g.* Bovine viral diarrhoea, Chlamydia – Polyarthritis.

Symptoms

Lameness, hot, swollen and painful joints, deformities of the joint, defect in locomotion (ataxia) difficult movement, painful sitting and rising up Hypophegia to off fed, in long standing cases there may be ankylosis of joint.

Treatment

1. Inj. Phenylbutazone (*e.g.* Esgipyrin), Inj. Artisone (s) (Alved) @ 10 ml IM, Inj. Ketoprofen, Inj. Neoprofen, Inj. Ketop (Alembic) @ 10-15ml IM, Meloxicam *e.g.* Inj. MP_3, Inj. A_3vet, Inj. Zobid-20 @ 10-15 ml by IM route can be administered to relieve pain and inflammation.
2. Moist hot fomentation with Magsulf (Epsom salt) can be done.
3. Hot water and weak liniments can be used for fomentation.
4. In severe cases Inj. Prednisolone, Inj. Vetalog or Inj. Dexamethosone (*e.g.* Dexona, Enidex, Vetcort, Dex-10) *etc.* can be used.
5. Parenteral antibiotics *e.g.* Streptopenicillin, Ampicillin, Ampicillin Cloxacillin, Enrofloxacin, Cephalexin, Cefotaxim, Chloromphenicol (See antibiotics in the Drug Index) can be administered by IM route.
6. Aspiration of fluid from joint capsule with sterile needle may give relief from tenderness.

7. Intraarticular injection of corticosteroid may be tried;
8. Surgical intervention may be required in extreme cases.

4.7.5 Radial Nerve Paralysis

The radial or muscular spiral nerve is the largest branch of the brachial plexus. It supplies the extensors of the fore arm and the extensors and external flexor of the metacarpus and extensor pedis and extrensor Suffraginus. Radial nerve paralysis is frequently observed in animals especially in horse, bullock, ox and dog.

Etiology

Casting of the animals under field conditions on hard ground without proper bedding may lead to radial paralysis, compression of the nerve between shoulder, chest wall, fracture of the first rib and prolonged recumbency on field conditions or under operation, due to fall or kick *etc.*

Symptoms

Non-weight bearing on the forelimbs.

Treatment

The surgical treatment is the only alternative if the nerve is completely severed. The disease is amenable to medical treatment in mild (neuro preaxia) to moderate injury (axonotmesis).

Hot fomentation, massage, anti-inflammatory drugs and neurotropic B-vitamins can improve the condition.

Moist hot fomentation with Epsom salt (Magsulph) on upper fore arm (affected fore limb) twice or thrice daily.

Iodex ointment, Briclofengel can be used for massaging of the upper arm thrice daily.

Neurotropic B-vitamins like Inj. Tribivet (Intas). Inj. Neurovet (Alved), Inj. Pollyvet (Excell) Inj. Neuroxin-12 (Sarabhai) @ 10 ml in Horse, 2 ml in Buck, Ram, Doe and Ewe by IM route daily for 6 days; then alternatively for one week, followed by twice in a week or once in a week for 3 weeks can be recommended (as per need).

Injection Tonoricin (Wockhardt), Inj. Alphos-40 (Alved), Inj. Aciphosh (Excell) @ 10 ml by IM route alternatively for 1-2 weeks for the large animal and 2-3 ml for the small animal. Anti-inflammatory analgesic injection like Melonex (Intas), Inj. Mecloxi (Vets Farma), Inj. Zobid-M (Sarabhai Zydus) @ 10-15 ml daily for 5 days for large animal and 1-2 ml daily for small animal.

4.7.6 Rickets (Infantile Tetany)

Rickets is a disease of bone that occurs in young animals because of phosphorus or vitamin-D deficiency where defective mineralization occurs not only in bone, but also at the cartilaginous portion of the growth plate. A good number of conditions that could give rise to rickets that share a common feature of inadequate intake or endogenous production of cholecalciferol (Vitamin D) in relation to calcium content of the diet. The most common cause of rickets could be the deficient diet in both bio-available calcium and Vitamin D.

Symptoms

It is a chronic disease affecting the pups mainly. Bones remain soft, spongy and swollen. Bowing of radius, focal swelling, hind quarter weakness, pain on palpation of joints may be evident. Shaft of the bones become weak and bending of bones occur (bowed leg condition). Feet may become flat owing to laxity of muscles and ligaments. Pica may develop and the animal may become prone to fracture.

Treatment

1. Ossopan Granules (TTK) or Ossopan liquid 1 tsf orally BID.
2. Inj. Vitamin D_3 (Arachitol) – 3 lakh by IM weekly for 3-5 weeks.
3. Inj. Vitamin A (Arovit Vet-A) – 2 ml IM once in a week.
4. Multivitamin and Multi mineral – like Sypradyn (Piramol Health Care) ½ to 1 tab BID. Becadexamin Cap (GlaxoSmithKline) Ossivite Capsule (Wyeth).
5. Oral Calcium Symp – Calcicare-C, Ostovet fort (GlaxoSmithKline), Intacal Pet liquid (Intas) @ 5 ml BID.

4.7.7 Osteomalacia/Adult Rickets

Osteomalacia is an adult form of rickets affecting bones where endochondral ossification has completed. Etiology and occurrence of osteomalacia are the same as for ricket except that predisposing cause is not the increased requirement on growth but the drain of lactation and pregnancy. In this disease bones are demineralised and become soft.

Symptoms

In adult, milk production declines, bones become fragile and feed intake poor. Lameness, stiffed gait, reduced appetite, anoestrus, low conception, collapsed udder, chewing or licking of inanimate object (Pica) *etc.*

Treatment

1. Parenteral administration of organic or inorganic phosphorus *e.g.* Inj. Tonophosphan (Intervet), Inj. T. Phosh (Sarabhai Zydus), Inj. Uremin (GSK), Inj. Tonoricin (Wockhardt) @ 10 ml IM or IV on alternate day for 3- 5 occasions.
2. Parenteral calcium *e.g.* Inj. Caldee – 12 (Wockhardt), Inj. Orical (IBC), Inj. Brical (Brihans), Inj. Cal BD (Vets Farma) @ 10 ml IM for 3-5 days.
3. Mineral mixtures *e.g.* Ramix (Vetnex), Minfa (Intas), Agrimin Fort (Glaxo) @ 25-30 g for one month.
4. If necessary antibiotic like Alincomycin (Alved) 5-10 ml IM for 3 days can be administered.
5. Oral supplementation of calcium tonics like Capsola, CalShakti, Calcicare, Vitacalci plus, Calcimilk *etc.*

4.7.8 Osteoporosis

It usually occurs in adult animals and the occurrence is high in pregnant and lactating animals just post partum due to heavy drain of calcium leading to calcium depletion from the bones, the calcium reservoir of the body of the mother. It causes disappearance of bone matrix, making the bone porous called osteoporosis. The condition mainly arise due to deficiency of Vit. D and calcium salt in diet.

Treatment

1. Oral supplementation of calcium, mineral mixtures like Calphosh D_3, Ranmix, Grovimin, Supplevite-M, Agrimin Fort, Proteimin Fort @ 25-30 g OD.
2. Parenteral administration of calcium like Inj. Caldee-12, Orical, Brical @ 10-15 ml IM.
3. Oral supplementation of calcium syrup like Capsola, Calshakti, Calcimilk, Ostovet Fort *etc.*
4. Parenteral administration of Inj. Tonophosphan, Inj. Tonoricin, Inj. Aciphosh, Inj. Alphosh-40 *etc.* @ 10 ml twice in a week for 1-2 weeks by the IM route. Parenteral therapy of Calcium gluconate (Calborol, Calgonate, Mifocal, Calmax) IV or SC route and with the use of calcium levulinate therapy with IM route and supplementation of Vitamin D, the deficiency disease of adult can be prevented.

4.8 DISEASES OF THE EYE

4.8.1 Examination of the Eye

Examination of the eye and particular structures are essential before going to treat a patient suffering from ophthalmic disorder or ocular affection.

Ophthalmic Examination Includes

1. Evaluation of vision by noting the hand movements. Bright light application to visual field (Bright light stimulation). Cotton balls tossed into the visual field (Cotton ball testing) and Meance response.
2. *Ocular examination* : (*a*) Examination of orbit and adenexa a for studying deformities or enlargements *etc.* (*b*) Examination of eyelids for abnormalities of position, function structures *e.g.* lagophthalmos, ptosis, trichiasis, ectropion, entropion, blepharitis, neoplasms *etc.* Blink response, its rapidity of completeness should be evaluated.
3. Examination of conjunctiva and Nictitating membrane. This can be done by manual eversion of upper and lower eyelids.
4. *Examination of sclera* – for change in its colour, tear, lacerations, presence of any foreign body, abnormal matter *etc.*
5. *Examination of cornea* – Examine for studying corneal reflex. Examined for loss of transparency (Edema or infiltrates). Examined for opacity, dryness, foreign bodies and lacerations, ulceration *etc.*

6. *Examination of anterior chamber* – Iris is generally examined with a focused beam of light and magnification for color, shape, pupil size, surface and movement.
7. *Examination of cornea* – Examined for studying corneal reflex. Examined for loss of transparency (Edema or infiltrates). Examined for opacity, dryness, foreign bodies lacerations, ulceration etc.
8. *Examination of lense* – It is examined for opacities cataracts, position and presence of cataract and its size.

Examination of Vitreous

It is to be examined by slit lamp bimicroscope with added lenses for studying abnormalities like vitreous strands, asteroid, hyaloids, haemorrhage and inflammation.

Examination of Fundus

It needs direct and or indirect ophthalmoscopy. It is examined for studying or examining the changes of vascular patterns, detachment of retina, congestion, haemorrhage, scars and for foci of inflammation. Swelling and inflammation of the optic disc occurs with optic neuritis and is characterized by blindness.

4.8.2 Conjunctivitis

Inflammation of the conjunctival mucous membrane is called conjunctivitis. In dog, it is called red eye. According to the development of lesions it is of many types which include vesicular conjunctivitis, catarrhal, follicular, dipthetic, granular and purulent type of conjunctivitis. This may be caused by virus, bacteria, fungus, parasites, trauma, chemicals and allergies.

- ☆ *Bacterial conjunctivitis* could be due to *Streptococcus* and *Staphylococcus* species.
- ☆ *Mycoplasma conjunctivitis* is due to *Mycoplasma* species.
- ☆ *Viral conjunctivitis* is due to systemic infection of virus origin (*e.g.* CD, LCH in canines).
- ☆ *Mycotic conjunctivitis* is due to *Candida* and *Aspergillus* sp.
- ☆ *Parasitic conjunctivitis* – Owing to eye worm infesation like *Thelazia* species, *Oxyuris* species, filarial worms *etc.*
- ☆ *Traumaic conjunctivitis* – Owing to trauma, laceration, dusts, dirts, blow, injury, smokes, foregign body, self inflicted trauma *etc.* Lice and ticks infestation on eye lid, eye lashes.
- ☆ *Chemical conjunctivitis* – Owing to accidental access to corrosive agents like acid, alkali, irritant chemicals like soda, phenol, turpentine oil.
- ☆ *Allergic conjunctivitis* is due to various allergens, drugs and foreign proteins may cause sensitization of ophthalmic mucosa leading to allergic conjunctivitis.

Symptoms

Redness and swelling of mucous membrane of eyes, tears (excess lacrimiation) and tendency of animal to keep its eyelid closed.

Treatment

Affected eyes should be washed first with 1 per cent warm boric acid solution. Then broad spectrum antibiotic eye ointment or eye drops to be applied. Ointment like Neosporin eye ointment, Soframycin ophthalmic ointment, Nebasulf eye ointment. Eye drops *e.g.* Genticyn eye drop, Gencyl eye drop (Gentamycin eye drop), Ciplox (Ciprofloxacin eye drop), Ranicol eye drop, Chloramphenicol eye drop *etc.* 1-KUL eye drops (Intas) 10 ml – non-antibiotic preparation containing phenylephrine HCl, Naphazoline HCl, Menthol and camphor ophthalmic solution can also be used. In severe cases some topical antibiotic eye preparations with steroids can also be used *e.g.* Dexacol eye drop, optidex eye drop, Dexacort-N eye drop, Sofracort eye drop, Ranidex eye drop *etc.* Systemic antibiotics should also be recommended in acute cases *e.g.* Inj. Gentamycin, Inj. Oxytetracycline, Inj. Ciprofloxacin, Inj. Enrofloxacin (See antibiotics in the Drug Index). In allergic conjunctivitis steroids *e.g.* Inj. Dexamethasone, Inj. Prednisolone and antihistaminic preparations *e.g.* Inj. Avil, Inj. Antilar, Inj. Anistamin *etc.* (See antihistamines in the Drug Index) are indicated.

In parasitic conjunctivitis parenteral Inj. Ivermectin SC, Inj. Livamisole HCl and topical application of Piperazine compound in normal saline solution may be tried with eye instillation and mechanical removal of worm with forceps can be attempted.

4.8.3 Keratitis and Keratoconjunctivitis

Corneal inflammation is known as Keratitis. Sometimes conjunctiva may also be involved leading to a condition known or Keratoconjunctivitis.

Etiology

Like conjunctivitis it may be due to chemicals, trauma, parasites, fungus, bacteria and virus.

Lesions may be superficial or deep. There may be suppuration (suppurative Keratitis).

Symptoms

Lacrymation, Photophobia, Congestion and changes of cornea. Corneal opacity may develop.

Treatment

Irrigate the eye with antiseptic ophthalmic solutions *e.g.* Boric acid (Boric acid 1 part + Aqua 100 ml), Boro zinc eye lotion (Boric acid 10 g + $ZnSO_4$ 2 g + Aqua up to 1000 ml) 3-8 drops to be instilled in eye TID. Boro alum zinc eye lotion (Boric acid 0.5 g, Alum 0.5 g, $ZnSO_4$/zinc sulphate 0.5 g in 100 ml Aqua, 5-10 drops to be instilled in eye twice daily. Topical antibiotic and steroid preparations *e.g.* Dexacort-N eye drop, Optidex eye drop or Ranidex eye drop *etc.*

Sub-conjunctival injection with Betamethasone or Dexamethasone *e.g.* Dexona, Enidex, Brisone *etc.* can be used.

In severe cases systemic antibiotics *e.g.* Inj. Oxytetracycline, Inj. Ampicillin, Inj. Ciprofloxacin, Inj. Enrofloxacin, Inj. Gentamycin *etc.* can be used for 3-5 days by IM route.

4.8.4 Corneal Opacity

Opacity or cloudiness of cornea is common affection of eyes encountered in cattle. The non-infectious etiology other than trauma, irritant chemicals, and foreign bodies, vitamin-A deficiency may lead to the development of corneal opacity in bovines.

Usually the first signs of vitamin-A deficiency are excessive lacrimation, night blindness, white spot, opacity and cloudiness of cornea develops latter.

Treatment

1. Administration of vitamin A *e.g.* Injection Veta-A (TTK) Inj. Vitamin A (Legend) 6 lakh I.U. @ 5-10ml IM for 3 alternate days or Inj. Vitamin AD_3E *e.g.* Inj. Betade (Bee Tee Pharma), Inj. Intavita (Intas), Inj. Vet ADE (Sarabhai) @ 5-10 ml/animal for 3 alternate days by IM route.
2. Instillation of Boro zinc solution or Boric acid and Calomel one pinch each in equal quantity to be instilled in both eyes mixed in sterile distilled water.
3. Eye drops like Ciplox, Optidex, Ranidex, Dexacort-N can be instilled 3-4 times a day for 5 days.

4.8.5 Otitis

It is an inflammatory condition affecting the ears that may involve external ear causing otitis externa, and inner ear causing otitis interna, and may also affect middle of the ear causing otitis media.

Symptoms

Pain to the affected ear, tilting of head to the affected side, irritation, foul smelling dischargess, bad odour, accumulation of purulent materials (Otorrhoea), pain around ear, inappetance, depression, wheening and crying.

Etiology

Allergies, fungi, parasites, bacteria, yeast, foreign bodies, trauma, hormonal abnormalities, ear mites (Otoacariasis), neoplasm *etc.*

Treatment

The key to healthy ears is to keep the ear clean, periodical cleaning of the ear canal can keep the dog free from ear problems.

1. For parasitic etiology specific acaricide (*e.g.* Benzyl benzoate), oral ivermectin or parenteral Ivermectin (*e.g.* Inj. Parid, Neomec, Ivectin, Hitex, Trumectin @ 1 ml/50 kg body weight by SC route) should be administered.
2. Aural broad spectrum antibiotics with or without steroids can be used to check bacterial infection and in severe cases systemic antibiotic can be administered. Inj. Enrofloxacin, Inj. Gentamycin (Optisol) – Inj. Chloramphenicol *etc.* owing to bacterial etiology can be safely used for ear problem.

3. Analgesics and local anaesthetic drugs may be used while cleaning the ear wax (*e.g.* 0.5 per cent Cetrimide solution, sterile normal saline may be used to clean the ear canal. Cotton applicator swab or ear buds can be used to clean the ear).
4. Ear drops *e.g.* Pomisol ear drops (Intas, 15 ml and 30 ml phyles) – administer liberally 5-10 drops in each affected ear twice daily. Besides, Pomisol Optidex ear drop, Dexacort-N ear drop, Genticyn ear drop, Otek ear drop, Sofra Cort ear drop *etc.* can also used.

4.9 DISEASES OF SKIN

Skin diseases in domestic animals often go unnoticed and even neglected and in long run they account for considerable loss in terms of health and production.

Etiology of Skin Diseases

The etiology of skin diseases is complex. There are several factors that may affect the skin *i.e.* external factors, internal factors and may be both.

External factors – *e.g.* virus, bacteria, fungus, protozoa, helminth, arthropod, mange mites, chemicals, injurious plant materials, radiation *etc.*

Internal factors – *e.g.* genetic, metabolic, hormonal, internal disease, hypersensitivity, allergy *etc.*

Skin Lesions

May be macule, papule, vesicle, pustule, nodule, wheal, scale, crusts, ulcer, scar, leukoderma, excoriation, hyperpigmentation, hypopigmentation etc. lesions of skin disease may be discrete, circumscribed, Patchy or diffuse. Identification of causal agent of skin scrapings examination is must for confirmatory diagnosis. Note whether dermatitis accompanied with itching or pain. Rule out allergic eruptions (Urticaria). Chronic skin disease is an indication of reduced vitality and resistance.

General Principles of Treatment

1. Isolate the animal.
2. Clip the hairs and removes the scales, crusts, flakes or debrises for easy contact and smooth application of medicines (topical preparations).
3. Prevent secondary bacterial invasion.
4. Administration of antihistaminics and central sedatives should be done for control of itching and extensive injuries caused by self inflicted trauma.
5. Ointments containing local anaesthetics may be applied.
6. Avoid use of detergents.
7. Ensure protein rich diet especially provide diets rich in sulphur containing amino acids.
8. The skin should be cleaned and kept dry.

Dermatitis with Bacterial Invasion

Apply any one of the following ointments externally after proper cleaning with antiseptic solution and drying of the dermal lesions.

1. Betadine ointment with Povidine iodine – 5 per cent (Wockhardt)
2. Soframycin vet cream (Roussel)
3. Himax ointment (Indian Herbs)
4. Topicure ointment (Natural Remedies)
5. Betnovate ointment (Glindia)

In large animals parenteral antibiotics in combination with local application of topical gels/ointments hastens the recovery. Antibiotics *e.g.* Inj. Streptopenicillin, Inj. Munonycin Fort (Glaxosmithkin), Inj. Bistrepen (Alembic), Inj. Enrofloxacin (*e.g.* Inj. Enrocin, Inj. Enrored, Inj. Floxidin) (See antibiotics in the Drug Index)

In small animals oral antibiotics can be tried. Herbal capsule – Tee burb (Indian Herbs) one cap daily for small animals, 2 capules BID for large animals can be recommended. Besides ointment – Acriflavin solution, Mercusochrome solution 2 per cent can also be applied locally.

4.9.1 Urticaria

Uniform weals like eruptions on the cutaneous surface is known as urticaria. Urticarial lesions are most common in horse and pig and rarely occurs in cattle, sheep, goat and dog.

Etiology

Insect bites, contact with stinging plants, irritant chemicals *viz.*. turpentine oil, carbolic acid,exposure to scorching sun ray, Penicillin group of drugs, allergic reaction, absorption of toxins from internal organs, intake of unusual foods *etc.*

Symptoms

Lesions appear very rapidly, lesions are elevated, flat, topped and round in outline. They may appear in large numbers on the skin of eyelids, neck regions or other regions of contact. There is oedema and erythema. Itching is less prominent except plant or insect stings cases.

Treatment

1. Local application of Sodi bi-carb solution, white lotion, Lactocalamine lotion is beneficial.
2. Parenteral administration of antihistaminics *e.g.* Inj. Avil, Inj. Antilar, Inj. Anistamin, Inj. Chlorazin, Inj. Chloril, Inj. Zeet *etc.* @ 5-10 ml for large animal and 1-2 ml for small animal by IM route gives prompt result.
3. Adrenaline may be used parenterally in severe cases.
4. Corticosteroids *e.g.* Inj. Prednisolone (@ 5-10 ml IM) Inj. Dexona, Inj. Enidex, Inj. Vetcort *etc.* (2-4 ml for large animal, 1-2 ml for small animal) can be given by IM route.

5. Calcium preparations *e.g.* Inj. Orical, Inj. Sancal, Inj. Brical, Inj. Cal BD, Inj. Calcinet @ 10ml for large animal and 2-3 ml for small animal by IM route can be given.

4.9.2 Eczematous Dermatoses

It is otherwise known as allergic dermatoses. Allergic response involving the skin of domestic animals may be an inflammatory reaction of the epidermis to certain exogenous or endogenous substances against which cells are sensitized. Eczema is always allergic origin. It may be dry or moist.

Etiology

1. Allergens, foreign serum, egg albumin, drugs, antibiotics etc.
2. Physical agents – *e.g.* cold, heat, light, dust etc.
3. Hormonal imbalance
4. Hepatitic disorders
5. Diets – Oats, clover, alfa-alfa, allergic to horse; cow milk, pork *etc.* allergic to cat; excess carbohydrate may be allergic to dog.
6. Rubber metals and dyes, synthetic fibres may be allergic to both small and large animals.

Treatment

1. Avoid allergens.
2. Supression of action of histamines by use of antihistaminics *e.g.* Inj. Zeet, Inj. Cadistin, Inj. Avil, Inj. Allergo, Inj. Anistamin (See antihistaminics in the Drug Index) for cat and dog oral antihistaminic *e.g.* Levocetriz, Cezor, Cetrizine, Xylera *etc.* can be prescribed.
3. Application of Benadryl, Caladryl, Lactocalamin lotion.
4. Inj. Phenergan is the best (it is highly potent and highly sedative).
5. Topical applications are of value in case of insect bites.
6. Systemic corticosteroids may provide adequate relief *e.g.* Inj. Prednisolone, Inj. Dexamethasone sodium – *e.g.* Inj. Enidex, Inj. Vetcort, Inj. Curadex, Inj. Brisone *etc.*
7. Inj. Placentrex (Albert David) @ 2 ml IM for one week may be given for dog patient with eczema.
8. Topical application of Topicure ointment, Himax ointment can be used.

4.9.3 Pyderma

It is a most common clinical condition of the skin originating from invasion of the pyogenic organisms characterized by the accumulation of pus seen in canine species.

Etiology

Streptococcus pyogens, Staphytococcus species, *E. coli, Pseudomonas* sp., *Corynaebacterium* sp.

Symptoms

Vesicular and pustuler lesions are common with exudation of pus and serum. In deep pyoderma there may be micro abscess formation. Alopecia, erythema and scales may be formed. Interdigital pyoderma is painful for dogs.

Treatment

1. Cleaning of the lesion with condys lotion or povidone iodine.
2. Remove dead tissues and exudates properly.
3. Topical antibacterial preparations *e.g.* Soframycin, Furacin, Betadene ointment.
4. Parenteral or oral antibiotics.

Parenteral antibiotics are Inj. Intamox (Intas), Inj. Inclox (Brihans), Inj. Britax (Brihans), Inj. Cefavet *etc.* (see antibiotics in the Drug Index) which can be administered by IM route. Oral antibiotics are Cifran 250-500 mg tab, Sporidex tab *etc.* which can be prescribed.

4.9.4 Photosensitization

It is a kind of dermatitis, otherwise known as slough sickness, commonly seen in cattle, characterized by the inflammation, erytheme as well as sloughing of the affected skin. The lesions are observed mostly on the unpigmented skin. It occurs owing to aberrant pigment metabolism with photosensitizing reactions.

Primary photosensitization occurs due to ingestion of some toxic plants *e.g. Lantana camara* and some photodynamic agents. Hepatogenous photosensitization occurs due to hepatic insufficiency and with the obstruction of bile ducts. As a general rule all the photodynamic agents *e.g.* Phylloerythrin, the end product of chlorophyll are absorbed in the gut, detoxified in the liver and excreted through the bile. But owing to hepatitis or bile duct obstruction the mechanism detoxification and exertion are disturbed, which in turn goes to epidermis and with the exposure to actinic rays of sun it cause photosensitization reaction or slough sickness.

Symptoms

Lesions start with redness followed by oedema of hairless part of the body. In sheep, goat and cattle ears are mostly affected. Ears are dropped and deformed. Necrosis and peeling of skins occur from the perineal region, under surface of belly, inner surface of thigh, ears, muzzle, eyelid etc. There may be rise in temperature and signs of jaundice. Anorexia, pyrexia constipation, dermatitis, dermal sloughings are main symptoms.

Treatment

1. Protect the affected animal from sunlight and avoid grazing.
2. A course of antihistamin *e.g.* Inj. Zeet, Chlorazin, Chloril, Avil, Anistamin @ 5-10 ml by IM route for 5-6 days should be given.
3. A course of antibiotic to check the bacterial infections to be given for 5 to 7 days (See antibiotics in the Drug Index).

4. A course of liver extract with B-complex parenterally should be given (*e.g.* Inj. Levadex, Inj. Stronic, Inj. Belamyl, Inj. Livobex *etc.* @ 5-10 ml for large animal and 2 ml for small animal by IM route for 3-5 occasions.
5. Dextrose (5 to 10 per cent) should be administrered by IV route.
6. Oral administration of Herbal liver tonics *e.g.* Vet liv powder, Livol powder or liquid livertonic *e.g.* Liv-52 vet, Lifer, Livsee, Meboliv, Livonine etc. (See liver tonics in the Drug Index) can also be done to counter hepatotoxic effects.
7. Local treatment with astringent lotions *e.g.* Lotio Calamine, ZIPP, BIPP *etc.* can also be done.

   Calamine – 15 parts

   Zinc oxide – 5 parts

   Glycerine – 5 parts

   Liquid phenol – 0.5 parts
8. Vitamin-A injection *e.g.* Inj. Vita-A (TTK), Inj. Vitacept, Inj. Intavita (Intas) *etc.* @ 5-10 ml at 2-3 days interval is also beneficial.
9. For constipated animals purgatives can also be given.

4.9.5 Ring Worm

It is not a worm or helminthic disease. It is a dermal disease caused by the invasion of keratinized epithelial cells and hair fibres by dermatophytes. Different species of dermatophytes produce ring worm in different animals. They belong to the genus Trichophyton and Microsporum. Trichophyton occurs in all species and Microsporum occurs in small animals, pigs and horses. It has got zoonotic importance too.

Symptoms

Circular, raised, gray or white (asbestors like) lesions are observed in calves. Lesions are commonly seen in head, neck and perineum. In horse lesions are confined to superficial layers. In sheep and goat lesions are seen on face, head, neck and back region characterzed by scales and crusts.

Diagnosis

Examination of skin scrapings and fungal culture.

Treatment

1. Strong Tr. Iodine application to the affected part after proper removal of crusts and scales are found effective.
2. White field's ointment – Salicylic acid-1 part, Benzoic acid-2 parts and Vaseline – Q.S.

   Or Acid Salicyclic – 2 g

   Acid carbolic – 2 g

   Vaseline – 30 g

3. Antifungal ointments available in the market for human use can be used in small animals and dog (*e.g.* Dermoquinol cream, Quadriderm *etc.*)
4. Sodium iodide injection (10 per cent) @ 1 g/14 kg body weight by IV route can be tried.
5. Systemic antifungal preparation *e.g.* Griseofulvin, Grisovin, Fulvin @ 25 mg/Ib body weight daily for 3-4 weeks can be orally administered for small animals.
6. Povidone iodine, Betadine ointment can also be used.
7. If necessary antihistaminics can be used.

4.9.6 Para Keratosis

Parakeratosis in domestic animals is characterized by alopecia and parakeratosis of limbs, muzzle and jaw usually seen 4-8 months after birth. The animals become stunted and if untreated died in about 4-6 months. Parakeratosis may be hereditary and called inherited Parakeratosis or Adema disease. It mainly occurs due to deficiency of zinc.

Symptoms

Exanthema, alopecia and parakeratosis in the form of scales and thick crusts of the head, abdomen, neck and limbs. Nervous signs, retarded growth and alopecia and encrustation of the lesions are usual.

Treatment

1. Zinc oxide @ 0.5 g orally or Zinc sulphate @ 1 g daily for 3-4 weeks.
2. Zinc containing mineral mixture *e.g.* Nutrisacc power pack (Vetcare), Minfa (Intas), Ranmix (Vetnex) *etc.* @ 15-20 g orally daily for one month is recommended.

4.9.7 Hypodermatosis

It is an obligatory myiasis in animals caused by hypoderma larvae. Mainly Hypoderma lineatum cause myiasis or hypodermatosis in animals. Lesions are usually found on the skin with fissures and nodules. Fissures and nodules usually develop in the back area in the muscular tissue surrounding the vertebral column and ribs. The lesions may develop elsewhere on animal's body. Crepitant feeling and excretion of some larvae through the perforated skin may occur on application of moderate pressure on the skin.

Treatment

Inj. Ivermectin *e.g.* Alverin, Trumeetin, Virbamec, Parid,, Neomec *etc.* @ 1 ml/50 kg body weight is highly effective. Ivermectin pour on (*e.g.* Impour, Ranboxy) 1 ml/10 kg body weight along the back line from shoulder to sacrumcan be tried.

4.9.8 Mange

Mange is a contagious disease of animals caused by Parasitic mites and in human it is called as scabies. Mange mites in domestic animals usually belongs to the genera Sarcoptes, Psoroptes, Chorioptes, Notoedres, Psorergrates, Otodectes, Demodex, Cheyletiella and the disease caused by them are called as Sarcoptic mange, psoroptic mange, choioptic mange *etc.* Demodectic mange causes demodecosis.

Table 4.5: Mites of Different Livestock Species

Host/Species	*Species of Mites*
Cattle	*Sarcoptes scabei, Demodex bovis, Chorioptes bovis, Psoroptes bovis.*
Buffalo	*Sarcoptes scabei, Psoroptes bovis, Chorioptes bovis, Demodex bovis.*
Sheep	*Sarcoptes scabei, Psoroptes ovis, Psorptes cuniculi, Chorioptes ovis, Demodex ovis.*
Goat	*Sarcoptes scabei, Psoroptes cuniculi, Psorptes caprae, Demodex species.*
Pig	*Demodex phylloides, Sarcoptes scabei*
Horse	*Sarcoptes scabei, Psoroptes equi, Psoroptes cuniculi, Demodex equi*
Camel	*Scorptes scabei, Psoroptes sp, Chorioptes sp.*
Dog	*Sarcoptes scabei, Demodex canis, Otodectes cynotis*
Cat	*Demodex cati, Cheyletiella blakei, Notoedres cati*

Pathogenesis of Mange Mites

In domestic animals Demodex mites are part of the normal fauna of the skin and when the host parasite equilibrium is disturbed the mites then gain upperhand and produce demodicosis. Sarcoptes mites settle down on the epidermis and avoids areas which are more horny and having a higher fat content.

Sarcoptes feeds on lymph and young epidermal cells. Psoroptes fed on lymph and blood which they suck from the cutis vera (Malpighian layer) through their sharp chelicera. Chorioptes and Otodectes feed on sebacious matter.

The pathogenesis of lesions in sarcoptic mange is due to mechanical damage caused by the parasite during excavation, irritant action on their secretion and allergic reaction to extracellular products. Psoroptic mites do not burrow the skin and they pierce the epidemis and suck tissue fluid and lymph and induce a serous and haemorrhagic exudates.

Demodex mites may live between the hair and root sheath for a long time causing damage to the adjacent tissue. This is called latent phase. But when parasite equilibrium is disturbed, mites move downward and destroy the root sheath and injure the hair bulb. There may be suppurative dermatitis leading to pustulation.

Symptoms

In sarcoptic mange there may be intense itching, papules excoriations, haemorrhagic crusts and alopecia in cattle and buffalo. Due to intense scratching and rubbing, secondary traumatic lesions may appear. In goats and sheep there may be dry scales, later hard crusts and cracks. The skin is thickened and wrinkled. In dogs small papules develop initially, latter converted to vesicles or pustules. There is branny desquamation, formation of crusts., thickening of skin and irregular patches of alopecia, presence of intense prutitus, restlessness, scratching, rubbing and gnawing on the affected part. In prolong illness the animal becomes emaciated and may die due to cachexia.

In goats psorptic mange is also known as ear mange. A brown and hyaline material accumulates in the external auditory meatus, the meator is occluded and the animal goes deaf.

Diagnosis

Symptoms, characteristic lesions and examination of skin scrapings.

Treatment

In sarcoptic, chorioptic and Psoroptic mange, mites – treatment of skin with coumaphos, Amitraz, Trichophoron, Diazinon *etc.* are effective. Ivermectin single subcutaneous injection @ 0.2 mg/kg body weight in cattle, goats, sheep, camels and single subcutaneous injection @ 0.3 mg/kg body weight in produce excellent results *e.g.* Inj. Trumutin (Zydus AHL), Inj. Neomec (Intas), Inj. Hitek (GlaxoSmithKline), Inj. Conmectin (Concept) @ 1 ml/50 kg body weight. In psoroptic mange in sheep, dip with 0.01-0.02 per cent benzene hexachloride, 0.1 per cent caumaphos or 0.05 per cent Amitraz twice at 10 days interval is recommended. Propetamphos at a concentration of 0.005 per cent is claimed to be 100 per cent effective after 2-3 applications at 10 days interval. Inj. Ivermectin @ 0.2 mg/kg body weight is highly effective. Since chemicals cannot penetrate the burrows in sarcoptic mange or the plugs on the hair follicles in demodectic mange, repeated application at weekly interval is necessary. Acaricides *e.g.* Deltamethrin (*e.g.* Butox), Flumethrin, Cypermethrin (*e.g.* Cyprol, Clinar, Ticomax and Tikkil *etc.*) can also be applied externally (see the ectoparasiticides in the Drug Index). In demodicosis the lesion may be washed with soap and lukewarm water to remove the plugs on hair follicles and subsequently with 0.5 per cent Malathion or Amitraz (Taktic 5 per cent) 10 ml/litre, 0.2 per cent Diazinon or 0.1 per cent Asuntol solution should be given 5-6 applications at weekly intervals or 0.5 per cent Carboxyl applied 5 times at weekly intervals claimed to be effective. Subcutaneous injection of Ivermectin (*e.g.* Inj. Trumectin, Inj. Parid, Inj. Conmectin, Inj. Hitek) by single or 2-3 repeated injections at 7-14 days interval has been claimed to be highly effective. Neostomosan pour on, Eprinomectin pour on @ 0.5 mg/kg body weight can also be tried topically. Herbal multipurpose ointment *e.g.* Himax, Charmil etc. or lotion *e.g.* Himex and Charmil can also be applied. This may give some effective result. In all the cases antihistaminic *e.g.* Inj. Chlorpheniramine maleate (Anistamin, Avil, Antilar, Allergo *etc.*) for 2-3 days can also be administered by IM route.

To rejuvenate the body condition good quality vitamin B-complex *e.g.* Inj. Tribivet, Inj. Hivit, Inj. Cociplex, Inj. Pollyvet *etc.* by IM route for 3-5 days can also be administered. For ear mites ear canal should be cleaned with H_2O_2 (Hydrogen Peroxide) and SC injection of Ivermectin @ 1 ml/50 kg body weight at 15-21 days interval give promising response.

Chapter 5

Metabolic Diseases: Their Treatment and Control

5.1 INTRODUCTION

Metabolic diseases or disorders in animals occur mainly due to nutritional disharmony. Metabolic diseases are nothing but the production diseases occurring as a result of higher production as well as nutritional imbalances, deficiencies or erratic feeding management. Milk is synthesized in the mammary gland and the ingredients are drawn from the blood stream. This milk production exerts stress on protein, fat and mineral reservoir of the cow disturbing the systemic homeostasis leading to the development of various metabolic disorders induced due to stress during early lactation.

5.2 IMPACT OF METABOLIC DISORDERS AND NUTRITIONAL DISHARMONY IN ANIMAL PRODUCTION

1. Stress from metabolic problems and or disorders compromise with immune system and invite opportunistic infectious diseases in animals.
2. In effective management problems and ineffective prevention of metabolic diseases leads to very costly consequences in production and reproduction performances of animals.

The most critical time in the life of dairy cow is the first few days post partum. The incidence of metabolic disorders increases in the period commencing at parturition and extending until the peak of lactation *i.e.*, peri-parturient period in dairy animals characterized by dramatic changes in nutrient demand to meet up the requirements for energy, glucose minerals, vitamins, fats and amino acids by the mammary gland following parturition.

5.3 HOW DO THE METABOLIC DISEASES PRECIPITATE?

Insufficient nutrient reserves during peri-parturient period and during the period of high productivity may further reduce below critical levels following parturition and thus precipitates clinical metabolic disease.

The deficiency of various trace minerals leading to reduced performance in reproduction which is further augmented by higher demand for prolific reproduction, and higher lactation and various interaction between the elements should be tackled properly otherwise metabolic diseases and deficiency related disharmony would supervene.

5.4 IMPORTANT METABOLIC DISEASES OF LIVESTOCK

The most important metabolic diseases are parturient paresis (milk fever), bovine ketosis, downy syndrome, hypomagnesaemia, post parturient haemoglobinuria, fatty cow syndrome *etc.*

5.4.1 Parturient Paresis (Milk Fever)

It is an acute to peracute afebrile disease of high yielding cows characterized by flaccid paralysis with the manifestation of generalized paresis and circulatory collapse occurring mostly soon after parturition.

The incidence is recorded immediately after parturition or at or near parturition in cows and to a lesser extent in ewes, sows, bitches and does, characterized by low serum calcium *i.e.*, depression of the level of ionized calcium in serum and tissue fluids.

Etiology

1. Heavy calcium drain through milk.
2. Poor nutritional status during pregnancy.
3. Nutritional imbalance.
4. Oxalate toxicity.
5. Sudden stress of heavy lactation.
6. Hormonal imbalance.
7. Long treatment with antibiotics and diuretics reducing calcium absorption.
8. Renal failure leading to excess elimination of calcium.
9. Impaired absorption of calcium from the intestine.
10. Placental oxidative sweets.
11. Increased alkaline phosphatase.

Symptoms

The disease usually occurs within a week after parturition. The clinical account of the disease is characterized by excitement, loss of appetite and incoordination of gait at initial stage, followed by remor of muscles (mainly head and limbs) and sternal recumbancy. Lateral recumbancy and flacid paralysis are noticed at the terminal stage.

In most of the cases of milk fever cattle and buffaloes –

1. Sits down on sternum or lateral recumbancy.
2. Half conscious and dry muzzle.
3. Head resting on the chest wall towards the flank making 'S' shaped turn to the neck.
4. Shievering and muscle weakness.
5. Inability to stand.
6. Subnormal temperature and cold extremities.
7. Sphincter relaxed.
8. Animal become dyspnoeic.
9. Heart rate feeble but accelerated (tachycardia).
10. Complete anorexia
11. Eyes are dry and staring.
12. Gastrointestinal stasis and bloat
13. Progressive deterioration of condition with weak pulse.
14. Coma and death due to respiratory failure.

Treatment

Since the disease results from an acute calcium deficiency where the serum calcium goes below (< 7 mg/dl), the normal level of 9-12 per cent, therapy to be started instantly with calcium borogluconate by slow IV method. Preparations can be used are –

- ☆ Inj. Calborol (Novartis) – 450 ml bottle
- ☆ Inj. Calgonate (Indian Immunologicals) – 450 ml bottle
- ☆ Inj. Intacal (Intas) – 450 ml bottle
- ☆ Inj. Calcicat (CRIL) – 450 ml bottle

Dose: Cattle and Buffalo @ 200-300 ml by IV; Ewe and Sow @ 30-50 ml by IV.

Dose: 1 g/100 Ib body weight by slow IV or 300-450 ml by IV and SC); most of the preparations contain 8-12 g of elemental calcium per bottle.

Toxicity Hazards of Calcium IV Therapy

Fast IV calcium infusion particularly in debilitated animals leads to heart block (cardiac arrest). Treatment with corticosteroids and antihistamines relieves the toxicity of calcium if used judiciously.

Dose: 300-450 ml by slow IV infusion to be repeated after 12 hours in cattle and buffaloes. Warm the bottle to body temperature and interrupt IV infusion for few seconds at least twice during infusion. The full dose is to be infused very slowly in 20-30 minutes. Monitoring of heart by careful auscultation is mandatory.

Complicated Milk Fever

Low magnesium levels may be associated with non-responding milk fever cases. Where milk fever is complicated with hypomagnasemia and hypocalcaemia in that case magic relief is obtained by slow I/V administration of following I/V calcium and magnesium combine preparations –

- ☆ Inj. Lactomag (Intas) – 450 ml bottle
- ☆ Inj. Calmax M (Vetnex) – 450 ml bottle
- ☆ Inj. Mifex (Novartis) – 450 ml bottle
- ☆ Inj. Calcimag (Cattle remedies) – 450 ml bottle
- ☆ Inj. Miphocal (Indian Immunologicals) – 450 ml bottle

Dose: Cattle and Buffalo 200-300 ml by slow IV

Ewe and Sow – 30-50 ml by slow IV

Injectable calcium preparation used in IM route is useful in reducing the volume of IV calcium infusion and for the maintenance of blood calcium level, *e.g.*

- ☆ Inj. Capsola (Vetnex) – 45 ml.
- ☆ Inj. Orical (IBC) – 30 ml
- ☆ Inj. Brical (Brihans) – 30 ml
- ☆ Inj. Cal BD (Vest Farma) – 30 ml.

@ 10-15 ml by IM route daily for 3-5 days for cattle and buffalo and @ 3-5 ml by IM route daily for 2-3 days for doe, ewe and sow can be administered. Use of calcium levulinate by IM route has got superior bioavailability and is less irritant. Injection Vitamin D_3 should be administered for correcting calcium level in blood.

Supportive Therapy

Injectable Phosphorus

Inj. Uremin (Glaxo), Inj. T-Phos (Zydus Sarabhai), Inj. Tonoricin (Wockhardt), Inj. Alphosh-40 (Alved), Inj. Aciphos (Vets Farma), Inj. Tonophosphan (Intervet) @ 10-15 ml by IM, IV or SC route daily or on alternate day for 3 occasions can be administered in cattle and buffalo and for doe, sow and ewe @ 2-3 ml by IM or IV route for 2-3 occasions.

Injectable Vitamin B-Complex

Inj. Hivit (Vitnex), Inj. Conciplex (Concept), Inj. Beezet (Vets Pharma), Inj. Pinkojet (Alembic), Inj. Vitamyl (Nugen Pharma) @ 10-15 ml to cattle and buffalo and @ 3-5 ml to doe, ewe and sow by IM route daily or on alternate day.

Injectable Neurotropic B-vitamin

Inj. Polyvet (Excell), Inj. Neurovet (Alved), Inj. Tribiivet (Intas), Inj. Neuroxin-12 (Zydus Sarabhai) @ 5-10 ml to large animal and @ 3-5 ml for small animal by IM route on alternate day or daily can be used.

Good quality enriched mineral mixtures to be supplemented with ration.

1. Ranmix Total (Vetnex).
2. Calphos D3 powder
3. Calcistrength powder (Brihans)
4. Minfa (Intas)
5. Metabolite (Glaxo)
6. Agrimin Fort (GSK) @ 25-40 g orally daily for cattle and buffalo and @ 5-10 g OD for sow, ewe and doe.

Ammonium chloride @ 25-30 g orally BID is beneficial for absorption of calcium from the diet.

Inclusion of ammonium chloride and magnesium sulphate along with calcium chloride in the diet in the last month of pregnancy may help in reducing the incidence of the disease. The important determinants of acidity and alkalinity are considered to be (SO_4^+ + Cl^+) and (Na^+ + K^+) respectively.

Preparturient Hypocalcaemia

Preparturient hypocalcaemia may occur when there is insufficient or low plasma calcium level (having calcium less than 8 mg/day) leading to paresis, uterine inertia, dystokia during parturition. Prolapse of the uterus is very common in highly hypoglycaemic and hypocalcaemic cows. Insufficient calcium in heavy animals suffering from preparturient paresis may result in incomplete response and lead to failure of animal to rise. If these animals are not treated soon, ischemic necrosis of muscles will occur leading to permanent recumbency even if the animal is subsequently treated with sufficient calcium.

Treatment

The best treatment is to administer calcium borogluconate solution through IV route without any delay. About 8-12 g of calcium may be required for the desired response. Inj. Calborol (Novartis), Inj. Intacal (Intas), Inj. Calmax (Vetnex), Inj. Mifex (Novartis), Inj. Lactomag (Intas) etc. with the single dose gives clinical recovery and if the cow fails to show clinical recovery within 5-8 hours, the cow should be treated with further calcium through IV route. If repeated calcium therapy fails to elicit response it is declared 'Downers cow'.

Prevention Tips

Inclusion of ammonium and magnesium sulphate along with calcium may help in reducing the incidence.

Administration of Vitamin D_3 (Inj. Arachitol) a week before calving may be helpful in reducing the occurrence of the disease.

5.4.2 Bovine Ketosis

It is a condition characterized by abnormally elevated concentrations of ketone bodies *e.g.* acetoacetate, acetone and 3-hydroxy butyrate in the tissue and fluids. Bovine ketosis is synonymous to Acetonemia, and hypoglycemia. A negative energy balance in early lactation predisposes the dairy cow and buffalo to metabolic imbalances and diseases such as Ketosis and fatty liver. This is due to impaired carbohydrate metabolism.

Clinical ketosis typically occurs between 2nd and 7th week of lactation in high producing dairy cows and buffaloes. It may also occur in Marwari and other high producing goats. Prevalence of subclinical ketosis in lactating dairy cattle is evident during first 60-65 days of lactation. It occurs mainly during winter and spring months in the immediate post parturient period.

Symptoms

Anorexia, inappetances, hypophagia, depression, loss of weight, reduced milk yield, hypocalcaemia, ketonuria, Ketonaemia and low level of hepatic glycogen.

Diagnosis

The examination of milk or urine by Rothera's test can rule out Ketosis. High concentration of Ketone bodies in urine and significant increase of serum ketone bodies and decrease in serum glucose are the indication of Ketosis.

Types of Ketosis

Ketosis has got two major forms. These are (*a*) Wasting form (*b*) Nervous form.

A. Wasting Form of Ketosis

1. Most common form of Ketosis.
2. Hypophagia and decrease in milk yield.
3. Refusal of grain and continue to eat hay
4. Rapid loss of body weight
5. Woody appearance
6. Firm and dry dung
7. Characteristic odour (sweet smell) in milk and breath.

B. Nervous Form of Ketosis

1. Signs are bizarre and begin all on a sudden.
2. Walking in circles and staggering gait
3. Head pushing
4. Apparent blindness
5. Vigorous licking of body
6. Chewing movements
7. Depraved appetite (Pica)

Treatment

Various treatment protocols have been suggested for the disease but the main aim of treatment would be to relieve the need for formation from tissue and allow ketone body utilization to continue normally. Conventional treatment, *e.g.* IV administration of Glucose/Dextrose 40-50 per cent seems to be the ideal approach.

Solution containing 25 per cent glucose and 25 per cent fructose can also give desired result. Injection Rintose (Wockhardt), Inj. Intalyte (Intas) in 2-3 litres for 2-3 days.

Glucose may be continuously administered by IV @ 0.5 g per minute till the milk ketone test gives negative result.

Propylene glycol 225 g twice daily for 2 days followed by 110 g once daily for 2 days and glycerine or 500 g of glycerol BID for 7-10 days should be given to overcome the necessity for repeated injections. Hormonal therapy with Betamethasone, Dexamethasone or Prednisolone is also helpful in curing the disease. Inj. Prednisolone @ 10 ml by IM route is beneficial as it increases the blood glucose level and help in the elimination of ketone bodies from the circulation, Inj. Dexamethasone @ 40 mg IM and 50 per cent glucose solution 500 ml IV is more effective treatment. Inj. Durabolin/ Nadrolone phenyl propionate) @ 25 mg/ml or 4-5 ml injection is very much effective in eliminating ketone bodies from blood.

Oral feeding of jaggery or honey for 7-10 days is beneficial during sufferings from clinical ketosis.

Anabolic steroid like Inj. Trenbolone acetate @ 60 mg to 120 mg are effective or single injection to make reduction in ketone bodies. Stomachic bolus and microflora rejuvenator bolus *e.g.* Provisacc, Yeasacc, Floraboost, Bioboost, Floratone *etc.* 2 boli BID for 3 days, Rumicare powder 125 g orally BID for 3 days can be used. Vitamin B_{12}, Cobalt and Nicotinamide may be used as supportive therapy. Liver extract with B-Complex Inj. *viz.* Inj. Belamyl (Sarabhai), Inj. Livobex (TTK), Inj. Feroliv (Excell) Inj. Levadex (Glaxo SmithKline) or Neurotropic B-vitamins *e.g.* Inj. Tribivet (Intas), Inj. Neurovet (Alved), Inj. XLplex (Vetnex), Inj. Neuroxin-12 (Zydus Sarabhai) @ 5-10 ml IM daily for 3-5 days or on alternate day administration can be advocated.

If hypocalcaemia coexists with ketosis in that case Inj. Mifex (Novartis), Inj. Lactomag (Intas), Inj. Calmax-M (Vetnex) *etc.* can be administered by slow IV @ 250-300 ml up to 450 ml.

Prevention

Hygest bolus (Natural Remedies) 2 boli once daily one week before and 2 weeks after parturition can be used to prevent ketosis.

Rumicare (Intervet) containing calcium propionate, methionine, picrorhiza dry extract, cobalt gluconate, vitamin B_6 and Dextrose anhydrous in prophylactic dosing (½ sachet 62-63 g per day for consecutive days before and after parturition) is also beneficial for preventing bovine ketosis.

5.4.3 Downers Syndrome

Synonyms

Downers cow syndrome, Downers cow complex, Creepers Cows.

What is Downers Cow Syndrome or Downer?

Downer cow is any cow which was down in sternal recumbency for more than 24 hours. According to Blood, the downers cow syndrom can be defined as a condition occurring following parturient paresis characterized clinically by prolonged recumbency even after 2 successive infusions with calcium. The condition may occur both in cattle as well as buffaloes and is restricted to heavy producers (*e.g.* exotic and crossbred Jersey and Holstein Friesian cows). Holstein breed is highly susceptible to this disease.

When Does the Disease Occur?

The disease occurs most commonly after calving in high yielding dairy animals. This may occur in late lactation too. High incidence is noted in winter but the disease may occur through out the year.

Milk fever may turn to downer and about 30 per cent of cows treated for milk fever will not stand for up to 24 hours after treatment and turn to downers animals.

Factors Incriminated as Possible Cause of Downers

1. Milk fever
2. Persistent hypocalcaemia
3. Persistant Hypophosphatemia
4. Hypokalemia
5. Hepatosis (Fatty liver)/Fat cow syndrome
6. Myocardosis
7. Septic mastitis
8. Muscular injuries, rupture of round ligament, Hip dislocation *etc.*
9. Excessive Protein intake
10. Toxic mastitis and Metritis
11. Vitamin E and selenium deficiency
12. Miscellaneous causes *e.g.* management errors.

Pathogenesis

Many different factors could make the animal recumbent. These may include traumatic injury at the time of parturition and parturient paresis.

Animal could not rise up and remain recumbent which causes muscles and nerve damage. Struggling of animal may lead to bruishes, tear and haemorrhage. Compression leads to obstruction of blood supply leading to ischaemic necrosis.

Symptoms

The disease may be of two types, *viz.,* (1) Alert Downers and (2) Non-alert Downers.

Alert Downers

The cow remains alert, bright and maintains proper appetite. Temperature, pulse, respiration, urination and defecation are normal. The affected animals usually crawl around on the forelimbs while the hind limbs remain in a flexed position owing to potassium depletion. Peculiar dog sitting posture may also be seen. This type of stance is ascribed as 'Creeper Cow'. If the cow remains in this condition for more than seven days, the prognosis is grave. The cow generally dies due to septicaemia or myocarditis. Buffaloes are more responsive to external stimuli and assistance in the attempts of rising.

Non-alert Downers

Animals are dull, depressed and unable to attain sternal recumbency despite assistance and remain in lateral recumbency. Complete loss of appetite, elevated cardiac and respiratory rates, decubital ulcers at pressure points, tachycardia and arrhythmia are evident. Development of myocardial lesions hastens death of the animal despite treatment.

Prognosis

Prognosis is favourable if the disease is due to metabolic disorders.

Treatment

First rull out possible fractures, dislocation, sprain by careful examinations. Metritis mastitis spinal injury, malposition and fixing of foetus in advance gestation by rectal examination. Attempt should be made to lift the cow. Adequate bedding should be provided.

Physiotherapy comprised of soft bedding, frequent rolling, sand or paddy straw bedding needs to be provided. Animal needs to be rolled from one side to another side for every 4 hours interval to prevent bed sores.

Animals need to be assisted to stand for at least 30 minutes four times a day using supportive sillings. Massage of hind limbs with liniment camphor, hot water fomentation, Mag Sulph or Epsom salt formentation may be done.

There is no specific treatment for the disease.

Calcium magnesium borogluconate preparation, Vitamin-E and Selenium preparation, use of potassium, Vitamin D, Corticosteroids, Vitamin B_1 (Thiamine) recommended.

For the cases suspected for hypocalcaemia and hypomagnesaemia and hypophosphataemia.

Parenteral administration of Inj. Mifex, Inj. Calmax, Inj. Calcimal, Inj. Miphocal, Inj. Lactomag @ 1 ml/kg body weight to be slowly infused.

Injection Sodium acid phosphate, organic or inorganic phosphorus *viz.*, Inj. Sodaphos (Vetnex), Inj. T. Phos (Sarabhai), Inj. Beetphos (Bee Te Pharma), Inj. Torpophosphan (Intervet), Inj. Uremin (Glaxo), Inj. Alphos-40 (Alved) @ 10-15 ml by IM, IV or SC as per convenience and need to be administered to reduce myotonia.

Good quality potent neurotropic B-vitamins *viz.* Inj. Polyvet (Excell), Inj. Tribivet (Intas), Inj. Neurovet (Alved), Inj. Neuroxin-12 (Sarabhai Zydus) @ 5-10 ml daily or on alternate day by IM route for 3-5 days can be advocated.

Potassium acetate 10 per cent solution 100 ml IV daily for 10 days or Potassium Chloride @ 30 g orally can be prescribed.

Good quality Mineral Mixtures *e.g.* Minfa (Intas), Ranmix Total (Vetnex), Agrimit Fort (Glaxo SmithKline) 25-30 g OD may be given for 10-15 days.

Vitamin-E and selenium preparation *viz.*, Inj. E-Care Se @ 10 ml IM on alternate day for 3 days can be recommended. If Downers due to pelvic muscles and nerve injuries (owing to forced traction), treatment should be Epidural injection of Neurobion, Gentamycin and Dexamethasone @ 2 ml each daily for 7 days. Potassium chloride 30 g orally for 7 days, Inj. Tribivet, Inj. Polyvet, Inj. Nuroxin-12 @ 5-10 ml by IM route on alternate day for 7 days can also be given.

If Downers due to Post Parturient Septic Metritis

- ✰ Inj. Oxytetracycline – 10 mg/kg IV with NS or DNS
- ✰ Povidone iodine 20-40 ml IU.
- ✰ C-Flox TZ (Intas), Enrocin IU (Vetnex)
- ✰ Ladexin IU (Legend), Lixen IU (Glaxo SmithKline) for intrauterine infusion.
- ✰ Inj. Dexamethasone 1 mg/kg body weight
- ✰ Inj. Meloxicam (*viz.* Inj. Zobid-40, Inj. Melonex, Inj. A3 vet, Inj. Meloxy) 10-15 ml IM daily for 3 days or Inj. Ketoprofen/Neoprofen (Vetnex)/Ketop (Alembic) @ 1 ml/33 kg body weight can be administered.

If Downers Due to Fall on Trenches and Slippery Floor Without Fracture/ Dislocation

- ✰ Epidural injection with Neurobion, Gentamycin 2 ml daily for 5 days.
- ✰ Inj. Dexamethasone sodium 1ml diluted in equal amount of distilled water by epidural route can also be adviced.
- ✰ Inj. Meloxicam *e.g.* Inj. A3 Vet, Inj. Zobid-M,
- ✰ Inj. Zobid-20, Inj. Meloxicam) @ 15-30 ml by IM route or Inj. Ketoprofen (*e.g.* Neoprofen or Ketop) @ 1 ml/33 kg body weight by IM route for 3 days.
- ✰ Potassium chloride orally @ 30 g daily may be tried.

If Downers Due to Pelvic Muscles and Nerve Injuries Due to Fixed Traction

Epidural injection of Neurobion, Gentamycin and Dexamethasone 2 ml each daily for 7 days. Inj. Tribivet/Polyvet/Neurovet @ 5-10 ml IM on alternate day IM for 7 days. Pot chloride of orally for 7 days.

5.4.4 Hypomagnesaemia

Synonyms

Grass staggers, Wheat pasture poisoning, Hypomagnesaemic tetany, Grass tetany, Lactation tetany.

Definition

It is a metabolic disease of cattle, buffalo, sheep and goats characterized by hyperaesthesia, incordination, tetany, tonic and clonic spasms and convulsion due to deficiency of magnesium in the body.

In cows lactation or grass tetany said to be due to grazing exclusively on green grasses or luxuriant pasture grown on heavily manured soil and may occur at any stage of lactation.

Symptoms

Hyperaesthesia/excitability, convulsions, muscle trauma (spasm), incordination and tachycardia (100-120 per min).

Twitching of muscles and ears, nystagmus, frothing of mouth, eye and nasal discharge, champing of sows, scanty feaces and hyper asthesia are predominant symptoms.

Diagnosis

Estimation of magnesium in serum and history of grazing or rearing on lush green pasture.

Whole Milk Tetany

In young calves the disease is called whole milk tetany.

Symptoms

Calf became unable to stand and walk, twitching of muscles, nystagmus, signs of hyperaesthesia, convulsions and tachycardia are prominent, champing of jaws, frothing from mouth, scanty defecation may be seen. The calf may die suddenly after bellowing. Concurrent hypocalcemia is commonly recorded with hypomagnesemia.

Treatment

Inj. Lactomag (Intas), Inj. Mifex (Novartis), Inj. Calmex-M (Vetnex), Inj. Mifocal (Indian Immunologicals) 250-350 ml for adult, 50-100 ml for young (calves) to be administered slow IV. Along this Magnesium sulphate salt is recommended to add in drinking water for calves 15 g/litre for 10 days; and for cattle and buffalo 25 g/litre for 10 days.

Magnesium sulphate (sterile) 50 per cent solution @ 100-200 ml SC for adult may be tried.

Magnesium oxide @ 100-200 g orally daily for a week may be fed.

Rubbing of normal salt on the tongue to increase intake of magnesium salt containing water is adviced.

Mineral mixture like Minfa (Intas), Milmur forte (Novartis), Ranmix Total (Vetnex), Agrimin (GSK) may be given. Calf 5-10 g, cattle and Buffalo (adult) 25 g daily.

5.4.5 Post-parturient Haemoglobinuria

Synonyms

Hypophosphatemia, Phosphorus deficiency, haemoglobinuria.

It is a life threatening metabolic disease continuously seen after parturition more in buffaloes than the dairy cattle. Phosphorus (P) deficiency haemoglobinuria, a metabolic disease of high yielding elderly dairy animals is characterized by intravascular haemolysis, anaemia, haemoglobinaemia and haemoglobinuria. Recently calved or advance pregnant cattle and buffaloes maintained on dry roughage are more susceptible to phosphorus deficiency hemoglobinuria.

High yielding buffaloes are more susceptible than the cattle. Fodder grown on phosphorus deficient soil, drought conditions and prolonged housing are considered to be main determinants. Sporadic cases occur in animals usually in post parturient stage. The disease may be caused due to increase intake of cabbage, turnip rales, brassica and rye grass containing haemeolytic factors.

Symptoms

Usually afebrile disease, the most important symptom is passing of red, blackish urine (hemoglobinuria). Reduced appetite, weakness, depression, constipation, suspended rumination, anaemia, and dehydration are common signs of the disease. Dyspnoea, open mouth breathing, Jaundice and tachycardia in advanced stages are noted. There is increase pulse and respiratory rates and animal may develop pica. These may be sloughing and gangrene of the tail tip.

Diagnosis

Rule out Babesiosis (Piroplasmosis) by blood smear examination with high fever and tick infestation, where post parturient haemoglobinuria is usually afebrile and rule out hematuria too.

Estimation of serum inorganic phosphorus, which will definitely fall down in case of hypophosphatemia.

Treatment

Sodium acid phosphate (SAP) @ 60-80 g IV as 20 per cent solution in 5 per cent dextrose for 3 to 5 days. Injection ascorbic acid @ 5 g total dose per animal by IV route for 3-5 days. Adjuvant therapy consisted of Inj. Feritas (Intas)–@ 3-5 ml IM daily for 5 days. Inj. Intavita (Intas), Inj. Vet ADE (Sarabhai Zydas), Inj. Adevet (Excell) @ 10 ml, 3 doses every alternate day.

Mineral supplementation – Minfa (Intas) 30 g daily orally or Ranmix total (Vetnex), Agrimin forte (Agrivet) (GSK) @ 25-30 g orally daily may be done. Dicalcium phosphate may be added in animal ration as preventive measure.

5.4.6 Fatty Cow Syndrome in Cow–Lipid Mobilization Syndrome

Synonyms

Pregnancy toxaemia of cattle, Fatty liver and fatty infiltration of the liver. It is common in high producing dairy cows occurring few weeks before and or after parturition. The disease is associated with several peri-parturient diseases and an increase in the calving to conception interval.

A severe form of fatty infiltration of the liver immediately before or after parturition is known as fatty liver or fat cow syndrome or pregnancy toxaemia of cattle which can be highly fatal.

The cows which have free access to energy rich diet in the early part of pregnancy become obese and such obese cows if remain off-fed for a long time due to disease and stress, there is mobilization of fat to liver.

Symptoms

Marked decrease in milk production, hypophagia to anorexia or partial anorexia, scanty defecation, suspended rumination with ruminal atony. Retention of placenta at the time of parturition. Ketone bodies would be present in urine and tissue fluid. Prognosis of the disease is grave if the cow is recumbent and semi-comatosed.

Treatment

Animal may be treated with 50 per cent Dextrose IV or IV infusion of 20 per cent Dextrose or Intalyte (Intas)/Rintose *etc.* 1-1.5 litre for 2-3 days followed by propylene glycol orally. Inj. Polyvet (Excell), Inj. Neurovet (Alved), Inj. Tibivet (Intas) @ 10 ml on alternate day for 3 occasions.

Propylene glycol – 350 ml daily orally. Rumentas bolus (Intas), Yeasacc bolus (Vetnex), Bioboost bolus 2 boli BID for 3 days.

Mineral mixtures *e.g.*, Minfa (Intas), Agrimin (GSK), Ranmix (Vatnex) 25-30 g orally daily with feed is recommended.

Antibiotic, steroid along with Insulin therapy may also be tried.

Prevention

Obesity should be restricted during pregnancy and late lactation. High quality palatable roughages should be provided.

Chapter 6

Common Poisonings and their Management

6.1 INTRODUCTION

Toxicology is the branch of pharmacology which deals with the study of harmful effects of drugs and other chemicals administered in over recommended doses (toxic doses) on the biological systems (*i.e.* on animals body). Toxicity of a substance is dose related since a substance at low dose is without effect but may produce harmful effects at some higher dose.

And thus 'poison' may be defined as 'any substance which is consumed in a very small dose or applied in any manner to a living system (body) that depraves the health or entirely destroys life (Offila-1821)'.

The incidence of death (un-natural deaths) due to poisoning is increasing day by day. Everything is poisonous if dosage and route of entry into the living organisms are not restricted. Poisoning and or intoxication may be acute or chronic.

Acute Intoxication

It results from a relatively large intake of intoxicant or poison over a short period of time (minutes, hour or few days). Here illness is usually severe, onset of death is rapid. Sometimes death occurs all on a sudden in acute intoxication or poisoning.

Chronic Intoxication

When relatively small quantities of poison are absorbed over a long period of time (slow poisoning-for several days, weeks, months or years), that causes chronic intoxication and onset of illness is slow. In veterinary practice, most poisoning cases are acute.

How Poisoning Occurs?

Accidental access to poisons and its ingestion is the most common route. The administration of poison may occur through inhalation, ingestion, injection and also through mouth, rectum or other natural orifices and also through skin absorption.

Poison become detoxified in liver to a definite extent and then eliminated mainly through urine. Elimination may occur through saliva, stool or vomit.

6.2 COMMON SYMPTOMS OF POISONING

The common symptoms usually are salivation, trembling, incoordination, dry muzzle, twitching, dilated pupils, spasms, ataxia, convulsion, labored breathing, rapid respiration, paddling, clamping of jaws, hyperthermia, abdominal pain, paresis, loose motion, bloat, frothing of mouth, regurgitation, depressed consciousnesses and coma.

6.3 GENERAL PRINCIPLES OF TREATMENT OF POISONING

These are some general principles of treatment or management of poisoning. These are as follows:

1. Stop further ingestion or absorption of poison.
2. Keep the animal away from the source of poison.
3. Remove the residual poison from the alimentary tract by giving emetics, gastric lavage. For poisoning through skin absorption, washing of the skin with plenty of water is suggested.
4. Prevention of absorption of ingested toxins (poisons) – Absorption can be retarded by precipitation, inactivation, neutralization oxidation and chelation.
5. Neutralization of residual poison – For acid or acidic poison use milk of magnesia, lime water, sodium bicarbonate, chalk (0.3-0.5 g), Mag. Carb @ 15-30 mg/kg body weight. For alkalis/alkaline poison use vinegar, lemon juice, weak HCl (0.5-1 per cent), demulcents like egg, milk, castor oil *etc.*
6. *Adsorbents*: They do not detoxify toxicants but prevent absorption. Use of universal sponge – *viz.* activated charcoal, tanic acid and magnesium oxide at 2 : 1 : 1 ratio in drinking water. Activated charcoal for many toxicants like insecticides, herbicides, mercuric chloride, strychnine, morphine, atropine, barbiturate and ethylene glycol.
7. *Antidote* – Substance used to detoxify the poisons.
   (*a*) *Universal antidote*: In most poisoning calcium can be used as universal antidote.
   (b) *Chemical antidote*: Such antidotes render poison insoluble or harmless *viz.* Barbiturates for chlorinated hydrocarbon, sodium nitrite and sodium thiosulphae for cyanide poisoning. Methylene blue for Nitrite/ Nitrate poisoning, 2-PAM or DAM for organophosphate poisoning and Atroprin. Atropin sulphate for carbamate poisoning. Oxidizing

agents can be used for neutralizing residual poison *viz.* tannic acid which precipitates alkaloids.

8. *Cathartics*: Sodium sulphate can be used orally for the evacuation of the bowel to remove some of the toxicants/poisons not absorbed till that time of treatment. Sodium sulphate is more efficient and preferable agent for evaluation of the bowel than Mag. Sulphate with activated charcoal. The dose of sodium or Mag Sulph is 1 g/kg body weight.
9. *Elimination of absorbed toxicants*: Toxicants are excreted through renal elimination. Hydration by Mannitol.

   Use of diuretics like Frusemide @ 2 mg/kg.
10. *Oxidizing agent*: It can be used for neutralizing residual poison *viz.* Tannic acid which precipitates alkaloids.
11. *Supportive therapy:* Fluids in dehydration, sedatives in excitement, stimulants in depression, demulcents in gastroenteritis.

6.4 COMMON POISONINGS AND THEIR MANAGEMENT

6.4.1 Chlorinated Hydrocarbon Poisoning

This includes BHC, DDT, Aldrin, Lindane, gammaxene, Endrine Toxaphene etc. These are commonly used as insecticides and pesticides in agricultural field usually absorbed through skin and by ingestion of sprayed vegetables and grasses. Chlorinated hydrocarbons are excreted by the kidneys.

Symptoms

Excitement, muscle tremors, spasm, convulsion, grinding of teeth, dyspnoea, incordination, hyperthermia, profuse salivation, running circles, violent seizures.

Treatment

Wash the skin thoroughly with soap water if poison absorbed through the skin. If the exposure is oral route, activated charcoal (1-3 g/kg) and sodium or magnesium sulphate 1 mg/kg should be given orally as slurry. Barbiturates, chlorpromazine HCl (0.5 to 2 mg/kg) by IM route, hydration by saline (NS) or DNS is mandatory. Purgatives, IV calcium borogluconate (*viz.* Calgonate, Calborol, Calmax – 250-300 ml for adult cattle and buffalo) can be tried or 10 per cent calcium gluconate sodium @ 2-4 ml/kg can be administered.

For sedation pentobarbital sodium by IV route should be used. Reduce body temperature by cold water packs. Other drugs can be used are Dexamethasone @ 20 mg/kg or mannitol 1 g/kg can also be used. For dogs emetics and gastric lavage should be used.

6.4.2 Organophosphorus Compound Poisoning

Source of poisoning is either by accidental intake or spray etc. Commonly used compounds or insecticides and pesticides are Malathion, Sumithion, Neguvan, Diazinon, Thimet *etc.* These are also used for spraying over the animal body and animal sheds for ectoparasite control. Specific antidotes for organophosphorus poisoning such as 2-PAM (Pralidoxime) and TMB-4 @ 20 mg/kg is highly effective in organophosphorus poisoning.

Symptoms

Profuse salivation, lachrymation, respiratory distress, proturion of tongue, constriction of purpils, muscle stiffness, incordination, abdominal pain, tremors of head, bloat, watery discharge from nose, collapse and death.

Treatment

1. Saline purgative (*viz.* Mag Sulph orally) should be fed to the animal if poisoning occurs due to accidental ingestion.
2. Atropin sulphate injection by IV or IM @ 0.5 mg/kg body weight and inject additional dose of 0.1 mg/kg body weight if necessary. For cattle average total dose is 50 mg and half of the dose by slow IV and ½ dose by IM. Repeat at 4-5 hours interval.
3. For dogs 0.02 mg/lb (average dose – 1 ml) by IV and SC routes. IV infusion of Dextrose is suggested.
4. Sedation with barbiturates if excessive excitement and convulsions persists. Use pentobarbitone or chloral hydrate injection, and Diazepam injection by IM route can also be tried.
5. Injection Pralidoxime by IV route (@ 4-6 mg/kg body weight). Repeat the injection after 30 minutes.
6. Parenteral calcium *viz.* Inj. Orical, Inj. Brical, Inj. Calcivet, Inj. Calde-12 10 ml IM can be administered.
7. 2-PAM or DAM (15-20 mg/kg body weight) by IV and repeat hourly if required. (PAM-2-Pyridine-2 Aldoxime-N-Methyl Iodide).
8. Activated charcoal together with a saline cathartic should be given orally @ 1-3 g/kg of charcoal and 1 g/kg sodium or magnesium sulphate.

6.4.3 Lead Poisoning

Poisoning occurs through licking of oil paints, lead paints, lead pipes, lubricants licking of metallic lead preparations, car batteries etc.

Symptoms

Bellowing, rolling of eyes staggering, incoordination, spasms and convulsive phases there may be blindness, trying to climb the wall, hyperesthesia, mania muscular spasm, tetany, atony of rumen, colic, constipation followed by diarrhoea *etc.*

Treatment

1. Saline pugitives and emetics orally (*e.g.* Magsulph orally) and gastric lavage may be tried.
2. Sodium sulphate, magnesium sulphate, milk and egg white (albumin) or tannic acid can be drenched.

3. Sedative *viz.* Siquil, Largeaetil *etc.* to control excitement (hyperaesthesia) can be used.
4. Calcium versenate, Ca-EDTA @ 75 mg/kg body weight daily for 3-4 days as 12.5 per cent solution with 5 per cent dextrose by IV or 1-2 per cent solution in 5 per cent dextrose for SC, use in divided doses or slow IV administration of a 6.6 per cent (w/v) solution of calcium EDTA @ 1 ml/kg (67 mg/kg).
5. Large amounts of normal saline solution can be infused by IV.
6. Supportive therapy – Forced feeding and oral fluids are important.

6.4.4 Nitrates and Nitrites Poisoning

Accidental ingestion of fertilizers containing nitrates like Ammonium Nitrate, consumption of plants grown on soils heavily fertilized with nitrates cause this poisoning.

Symptoms

Diarrhoea, abdominal pain, anoxia, muscular weakness, staggering, subnormal temperature, dyspnoea, acute gastroenteritis, progressive cyanosis and other symptoms.

Blood becomes dark, discoloured, coffee brown or tary coloured.

Treatment

1. Methylene blue by IV route @ 8.8 mg/kg body weight as 1 per cent solution. (For Cattle average dose – 20-40 ml of 1 per cent solution IV). Treatment should be repeated in severe cases.
2. Ascorbic acid can also be used @ 15-20 mg/kg body weight by IV.
3. Intensive supportive therapy should be given.
4. Mineral oil via stomach tube can be drenched to counter act the caustic action of nitrate salts.
5. Saline cathartics and intraruminal antibiotics and 10-20 litres of cold water may be beneficial.

6.4.5 Mercury Poisoning

Accidental ingestion, licking of mercury may cause this poisoning.

Symptoms

Ataxia, spasms, convulsions, vomiting, diarrhoea, dyspnoea and pulmonary oedema.

Treatment

1. IV infusion of sodium formaldehyde sulphoxinate 100-200 ml.
2. Sodium citrate 1-4 g at 4 hours interval orally.
3. IV administration of calcium gluconate 250-350 ml.
4. Feeding of albumin, magnesium sulphate.
5.

6.4.6 Arsenic Poisoning

Poisoning occurs through arsenic dip or spraying of animals to control ectoparasites, accidental access to arsenical preparations, over dose of arsenical preparations, contamination of herbage with arsenicals, arsenic weed killers, insect killers *etc*.

Symptoms

Intense abdominal pain, grinding of teeth, staggering gait, salivation, thirst, vomiting, foetid diarrhoea, collapse, paralysis *etc*. In dog vomiting has garlic like odour, cyanosis, weak pulse and collapse.

PM indicates intense rose red inflammation of G I tract.

Treatment

1. Use saline purgative (Mag Sulph) for herbivores and gastric lavage with warm water and enema in carnivores.
2. *IV infusion of sodium thiosulphate*: Horse and Cattle – 10 g as 10-20 per cent solution (IV) and 20-30 g orally in 300 ml of water at six hours interval and 8-10 g in 10-20 per cent solution by IV.
3. Dimercaprol (or BAL) @ 3 mg/kg body weight inject by IM route as a 5 per cent solution of benzylbenzoite in peanut oil at every 4 hours interval for first 2 days followed by twice daily for another 7 days. In small animal a 10 per cent solution of BAL (British antic lewisite) is used @ 2.5-5 mg/kg (5 mg/kg for acute cases only for first day), repeated every 4 hours for first 2 days and at every 6 hours on 3rd day.

6.4.7 Urea Poisoning

Common poisoning in herbivores owing to accidental intake of urea fertilizer or feeding of urea, clinical symptoms of urea toxicity differ from animal to animal and depend upon the species of the animal involved, dose of urea and nature of basal diet. The course is short in acute toxicity and death occurs within 1-4 hours.

Symptoms

Severe colic, shivering, staggering (incordination), weakness bloating, tremors, growing, forced rapid breathing, marked jugular pulse, violent struggling and bellowing *etc*. The animals walk with a proppy gait. The animal goes down on its sternum and later rolls over on to its side. Excessive salivation, frothing at mouth, laboured breathing and paralysis are common signs. As death nears, animal becomes cyanotic, dyspnoic, anuric and hyperthermic. Follow drenching of acetic acid with drenching of large volume of water (Cattle 20-30 litres for adults). The rationale is that water lowers the rumen temperature and dilutes the reacting medium, while acetic acid lowers rumen pH preventing ammonia absorption.

Treatment

1. Diluted acetic acid up to 10-12 litres of 6 per cent acetic acid along with 20-40 liters cold water for cattle buffalo. Goat and sheep – 0.5-1 litre of kitchen vinegar or 5 per cent acetic acid. Vinegar orally 2 ml/kg body weight mixed

in 2 to 5 litres of water can be drenched (for cattle and buffalo 2-8 litres, sheep and goat 0.5-1 litre).

2. Electrolyte solution by IV.
3. Injection of adrenergic blocking agents.
4. Parenteral Calcium-Magnesium preparations like Mifex, Calborol, Calgonate 200-300 ml IV to relieve tetanic seizures.
5. Supportive therapy with isotonic saline solutions by IV route to correct dehydration.

6.4.8 Cyanide Poisoning

The most effective antidote for cyanide poisoning is the combination of nitrate and thiosulfate. The recommended therapeutic regimen is the IV administration of a mixture of 1 ml of 20 per cent solution of sodium nitrite and of 3 ml of 20 per cent sodium thiosulfate @ 4 ml/45 kg body weight.

6.4.9 Lantana camera Poisoning

Feeding of the plant or ingestion of Lantana camera cause this poisoning. In the early stages there is severe constipation, haemorrhagic gastroenteritis, incoordination, progressive weakness and latter hepatogenous photosensitization. Jaundice and cholestasis occurs. Animals look dull, anorectic, do not ruminate properly, peeling of skin, necrosis of skin or subcuites, alopecia on thoracic and abdominal walls.

Treatment

1. Removal of the plants from the diet.
2. Keep the animal in dark place (avoid direct sunlight).
3. Give purgatives.
4. Give antihistaminics like Inj. Avil, Antilar, Allergo, Antilar *etc.* @ 5-10 ml by IM route for 3-5 days.
5. Inject Glucose saline – DNS, 5 per cent Dextrose, 10 per cent Dextrose, Rintose, Wocktrose.
6. Inject Antibiotics like Enrofloxacin @ 5 mg/kg body weight. (with Enrocin, Enrovet, Floxidin) for 3-5 days.
7. Inject Liver stimulant (liver extract with B-complex) *viz.* Inj. Belamyl, Stronic, Levadex, Livron, Livobex @ 5-10 ml for 3-5 occasions.
8. Treat the wounds with antiseptic (herbal) ointment like Sorine, Dermanol, Dressol, Himex, Topicure *etc.*
9. Supportive therapy with Inj. Tribivet/Inj. Neuroxin -12, Inj. Polyvet *etc.* @ 5-10 ml daily for 3-5 days by IM can be administered.
10. Calcium borogluconate IV is also effective in treating *Lantana camera* toxicity.

6.4.10 Plant Toxicity

Members of the solanaceae family having active principles like atropine, solanine nicotine, etc. may cause toxicity in herbivores on ingestion. *Cestrum aurantiacum* (*Bhik phul*) having solanaceous alkaloids may cause poisoning in animal on accidental consumption in large doses.

Symptoms

Incordination, dialation of pupil, dyspnoea, recumbency, tremors, rapid breathing and constipation.

Treatment

1. Demulcents – to be used orally *e.g.* egg white or albumin.
2. DNS or Dextrose 5 per cent to be infused by IV route.
3. Liver stimulant in parenteral route *viz.* Inj. Belamyl, Livobex, Livron @ 5-10 ml by IM route.
4. Antihistaminic injection *e.g.* Inj. Antilar, Anistamin, Zeet @ 5-10 ml by IM route for 5 days.
5. Inj. Oxytetracycline, Inj. Intamycin, Inj. Loxy *etc.* by IM route can also be administered.

6.5 MATERIALS TO BE SENT FOR CHEMICAL ANALYSIS IN POISONING CASES

Arsenic poisoning	Hair, liver, kidneys and urine
Carbon Tetrachloride (CTC) poisoning	Liver, blood, serum
Copper poisoning	Liver, blood and serum
Cyanide toxicity	Rumen content (stomach content), Oxalated blood, plant residues
Insecticides poisoning	
(a) Chlorinated hydrocarbon	Liver, tissue fat and stomach content
(b) Organophosphates	Liver, lumen content, plasma, serum
Lead poisoning	Kidney, liver, hair, urine, blood
Nitrate/Nitrite poisoning	Rumen content, urine, blood, plasma, serum, CSF
Strychnine poisoning	Stomach contents, urine, liver, brain, Blood without anticoagulant 20-25 ml, Rumen content – 250 g.
	Brain – whole brain, hair, body fat, kidney, liver.

Chapter 7
Bacterial Diseases: Their Treatment and Control

7.1 INTRODUCTION

Infectious diseases are caused by the organisms which are infective in nature and are capable of being transmitted rapidly from the infected to the healthy animal. Disease is caused when there is breakdown in the defense mechanism of the host. The diseases are caused by the specific organisms like bacteria, virus or mycotic agents. In this chapter bacterial diseases are discussed.

1. Anthrax
2. Black Quarter (BQ)
3. Haemorrhagic Septicaemia (HS)
4. Brucellosis
5. Tuberculosis (TB)
6. Tetanus
7. Actinobacillosis (Wooden tongue)
8. Actinomycosis (Lumpy jaw)
9. Botulism
10. Colibacillosis
11. Contagious Bovine Pleuro Pneumonia (CBPP)
12. Contagious Caprine Pleuro Pneumonia (CCPP)
13. Enterotoxaemia
14. Listeriosis

15. Leptospirosis
16. Paratuberculosis

7.2 ANTHRAX

This disease is caused by bacteria, *Bacillus anthracis*. It is an acute or peracute wide spread infectious as well as septicemic disease of all warm blooded animals, common in cattle. Anthrax bacillus possesses complex antigen components and produce three types of toxins. The toxins are extracellular in nature and are responsible for causing excessive tissue damage, resulting in death of the animal.

Symptoms

The most common symptoms are high temperature, muscular convulsions, bleeding from natural orifices and dyspnoea. The affected animals die abruptly.

The carcass decomposes rapidly with the formation of gas and distension of abdomen. Rigor mortis is absent. The blood is dark red or black in colour and does not clot. Spleen is greatly enlarged (spleenomegaly). Liver and kidneys are very much enlarged. The anthrax infected carcass should not be opened.

Diagnosis

Blood smear stained with polychrome methylene blue and serological tests.

Differential diagnosis should be made from lightning stroke, Black Quarter, Haemorrhagic septicemia, Babesiosis and acute lead poisoning.

Treatment

Crystalline Penicillin 40-80 lakh IU, Procaine Penicillin like Inj. F.P.P. (Alembic) or Inj. Fortified Procaine Penicillin (Sarabhai Zydus), Streptopenicillin like Inj. Biostrep (Vetnex), Inj. Dicrysticin (Zydus AHL), Inj. Bistrepen (Alembic) 2.5 g IM is specific treatment along with anti-anthrax serum.

Prophylaxis

Anthrax spore vaccine, 1 ml SC injection gives 1 year immunity. Vaccination can be done from 6 months of age onwards. Deep burial of carcass and disinfection of cattle shed should be made carefully.

7.3 BLACK QUARTER

Black Quarter (BQ) occurs in a sporadic form and is caused by bacteria, *Clostridium chauvoei*. It is an acute infection of young bovines usually below 2 years of age. Sheep and goats are also affected.

Symptoms

Sudden onset, high fever, painful swelling of affected quarter, complete anorexia, ruminal atony. Animals show lameness due to hot and painful swelling in the upper part of the leg. This disease causes severe toxaemia resulting in high mortality.

Diagnosis

Examination of exudates smear from crepitating swelling.

Treatment

Incise swelling and remove exudates.

Early therapy with antibiotics is effective and beneficial. The affected animals should be immediately treated with Penicillin @ 6,000 IU/kg body weight by IM route for protection against the disease. Penicillin-G is the drug of choice. Inj. Petromox-C (Novartis) 3 g or Inj. Amoxirum (Glaxo Smithkline) can also be used. Long acting oxytetracycline, newer antibiotics like Enrofloxacin, Cefotaxim, Cephaloridine may also be tried.

Antihistaminic injection like Pheniramine maleate or Chlorpheniramine maleate may be administered.

Anti-inflammatory analgesic injection like Meloxicam (Inj. Melonex, Inj. Meloxi, Inj. A_3 Vet, Inj. Proxivet), Ketoprofen injection like Neoprofen, Ketop may be administered.

Prophylaxis

Prevention is possible by routine vaccination once in a year.

Combined HS BQ vaccine @ 2 ml of Intervet and 4 ml of Biomed company per animal by SC route can be given.

Bovilis HS BQ (Intervet) 50 ml (25 dose vial) may be given to cattle and buffalo @ 2 ml SC injection.

7.4 HAEMORRHAGIC SEPTICAEMIA

It is an acute, fatal septicemic disease of cattle and buffalo, also known as shipping fever caused by bacteria, *Pasteurella multocida*. Sheep and goat may also be affected. Outbreak usually occurs in early monsoon, predisposed by stress and inclement weather. Septicemia results in very high mortality (80-100 per cent). Onset and course of the disease is very rapid.

Symptoms

High rise of temperature (with sudden onset), swelling of neck and throat, profuse salivation, swelling of tongue and its protrusion, open mouth breathing, respiratory distress, laboured breathing, pneumonia and acute enteritis characterized by bloody diarrhoea.

Diagnosis

Examination of blood film and smears from oedematous fluid would reveal Gram negative bipolar coccobacillary organisms. The post mortem findings are mainly petechial haemorrhage in trachea and heart, full of froth in trachea, and phenomonic lungs.

Treatment

The disease can be successfully treated with sulphadimidine ($33^1/_3$ per cent) solution. Give any one of the following: Inj. Diadin (Pfizer), Inj. Sulphadimidine (Indian Immunologicals), Inj. Sulphamin, Inj. Brimdine (Brihans), Inj. Vesadin (IU).

The dose of sulphadimidine in case of cattle and buffalo is 100 ml ($33^1/_3$ per cent solution) as initial dose of which ½ the dose by IV and ½ by SC. Repeat ½ the dose after 24 hours.

Injectable Amoxycillin and Cloxacillin like Inj. Intamox (Intas), Inj. Moxcell (Alembic), Inj. Clomoxy (Brihans), Inj. Inimox (Indian Immunologicals), Inj. Petromox (Novartis) may be given by IM route. Inj. Chloracin (Cipla), Inj. C-flox Powder (Intas) or Inj. Enrofloxacin like Inj. Enrocin (Vetnex), Inj. Enrovet (VetsFarma), Inj. Quin intas (Intas) @ 10-15 ml IM daily for 5 days.

Anti inflammatory analgesic like Inj. A_3 Vet, Inj. A_3 Vet plus, Inj. Melonex, Inj. Melonex plus (Intas), Inj. Nulox, Inj. Meloxi (VetsFarma), Inj. Proxivet, Inj. Zobid-M (Sarabhai Zydus), Inj. MP_3 (Vetnex) @ 15-30 ml IM daily for 3 days.

Antihistaminic injection like Inj. CPM Vet (Cipla), Inj. Chloragin (Vetnex), Inj. Zeet (Alembic) @ 5-10 ml IM daily for 3 days. Corticosteroid like Inj. Dexona (Alembic), Inj. Brisone (Brihans), Inj. Curadex (Concept) 2-5 ml locally at the swollen throat or neck give relief to the animal.

Prophylaxis

A vaccine composed of killed organism in an oil adjuvant base is effective. H.S. alum precipitated veccine at the age of basic of 6 months and at the dose of 5 ml and to be repeated every year.

Combined HS BQ vaccine (Intervet) @ 2 ml SC, Bivilis HS and BQ vaccine (Intervet), HSBQ vaccine (Biomed) @ 4 ml SC can be administered. The vaccine confers immunity for 12 months.

7.5 BRUCELLOSIS

It is also known as Bang's disease, caused by *Brucella abortus* and characterized by abortion in cows during last stage of pregnancy. Aborted animals may develop infertility. The organisms invade gravid uterus mammary glands, testis, lymph nodes and joints. The milk from infected udder serves as a potential source of infection to calves and human beings as well. Brucellosis is considered by FAO, WHO and OIE as the most widespread zoonosis all over the world.

Diagnosis

1. Isolation of organism from the infected tissues.
2. Detection of antibodies by tube agglutination test, complement fixation test and ELISA.
3. Milk ring test – Easy, inexpensive and reliable test.

The disease needs to be differentiated from Trichomoniasis, Leptospirosis, Listeriosis, Vibriosis and Mycotic abortion for diagnosis.

Treatment

The disease does not respond to any treatment. Hence only way for control of the disease is removal of Brucella reactors from the herd.

Vaccination

Vaccination with two injections at 6 months interval may be tried.

7.6 TUBERCULOSIS (TB)

It is a serious disease of cattle (mainly of crossbred cattle) caused by the organism *Mycobacterium bovis*. Bovine TB has largest host range and can be transmitted all warm blooded vertebrates including human and buffalo.

The disease is characterized by progressive emaciation, capricious appetite and fluctuating temperature. When the lungs is affected there is broncho-pneumonia and chronic cough.

Tuberculous mastitis is of great public health importance. Human beings may contract the disease through infected milk consumption.

Diagnosis

Tuberculin test is very efficient in identifying the carriers as well as suffers.

Treatment

Long term oral administration of Isoniazid may be done. A combination of Streptomycin and Para aminosalicylic acid is effective in treating tuberculosis.

7.7 TETANUS

All animals except chicken and cat may suffer from tetanus, caused by *Clostridium tetani* releasing a potent neurotoxin in deep infected would under anaerobic conditions. The toxin is absorbed by motor nerves and transported to spinal cord.

Male calves of cattle and buffalo, male kids and lambs are very much prone to tetanus owing to unhygienic castration in village condition. Besides puncture wounds, obstetrical intervention, dehorning, tattooing,hoof trimming, dog bites, tears and cuts *etc.* are common sources of contracting the infection. During manual removal of placenta the post parturient animals may suffer from tetanus owing to unhygienic handling.

Symptoms

Lock jaw (trismus), stiff gait, wooden horse appearance, stiff tail, stiffness of muscles and tremors, anxious and alert expression with erect ears, falling on ground and death owing to respiratory failure.

Treatment

Acetyl promazine or Chlorpromazine is to be administered.

Penicillin-G is the drug of choice as antibiotic along with Tetanus antitoxin. Dose 10,000-15,000 units IV every 12 hours interval. Muscle relaxant like Largactil-5 per cent (@10ml IM) may be used. Magsulf saturated sterile solution 50-100 ml may be administered through SC route to horse, cattle and buffalo, and in case of sheep and goat 15-20 ml SC. In horses Tubocurarine and Succinyl choline have been successfully employed. Midorine (BW) containing succinyl choline chloride can act as the muscle relaxant and can be mixed with Thiopentone sodium or by slow drip for prolong action. Doses: 30-100 mg IV.

Inj Amoxycillin cloxacillin combination in high dose (like Inj. Intamox, Inimox, Lemox, Moxcell) twice daily, and Diazepam Inj. 3-4 times a day along with antitetanus serum diluted in DNS and infused by IV route are also promising treatment.

Prevention

The disease can be prevented by vaccination with T-tox, Tetvac, Tetanus toxoid.

7.8 ACTINOBACILLOSIS

It is the most frequently occurring bacterial disease of bovine and caused by *Actinobacillus lignieresi*, found involving the soft tissue. The tongue is frequently affected due to loss of pliability it is named *'wooden tongue'*. It is found most frequently in soft tissue of head characterized by acute inflammatory swelling of soft tissues of head, lymph glands, tongue followed by abscess formation of lymph glands.

Diagnosis

Examination of pus smear.

Treatment

Treatment may be carried out with a Sodium iodide IV injection @ 700 mg/kg body weight in normal saline solution or by Potassium iodide 2 g in 20 ml distilled water by IV route, repeated 2-5 times at 3 days interval.

Antibiotic mainly Streptopenicillin in high doses like Inj. Munomycin Fort 2.5 g (GSK), Inj. Bistrepen 2.5 g (Alembic), Inj. Biostrep (Vetnex), Inj. Dicrysticin-S 2.5 g (Sarabhai Zydus) daily for 6 days is highly effective. Pain killer like Inj. Meloxicam, Inj. MP_3 15-20 ml IM daily for 3 days, and surgical drainage of abscess and dressing with Povidone iodine, Ranbidone (Vetnex), Metricare (Zydus AHL) are indicated.

7.9 ACTINOMYCOSIS (LUMPY JAW)

As a general rule actinobacilosis is found involving the soft tissue whereas actinomycosis affects the bony tissue and is caused by *Actinomyces bovis*. It is found most frequently in the bony tissue of jaw. It is actually a rarefying osteomyelitis of mandible and maxilla with poor response to treatment. The affected jaw become granulomatous, immobile, lumpy hard swelling of jaw bone with multiple inter communicating abscesses. Yellow gritty pus is oozed from the abscessed jaw and there is difficulty in prehension and mastication owing to jaw involvement. In complicated cases fistula develops which needs surgical intervention. Osteitis is common sequel of the disease.

Diagnosis

Examination of pus smear and yellogritty pus, Bony spicules or spikes from the affected jaw and lump or abscess is characteristic of lumpy jaw. The organisms are seen in the form of granules in the suppurative foci.

Treatment

Inj. Penicillin-G with aluminium (Sarabhai Zydus) along with oral potassium iodide powder is effective treatment. Streptopenicillin preparation in high doses like, Inj. Munomycin Fort (Glaxo), Inj. Biostrep (Vetnex), Inj. D.C. (Sarabhai Zydus) for 5-7 days by IM route and oral administration of potassium iodide @ 10 g for 7 days is recommended.

Potassium iodide is believed to reduce fibrous tissue reaction and iodides are bactericidal. Analgesic like Inj. Ketop, Inj. Neoprofen (containing Ketoprofen, Vetnex) @ 10-15 ml IM daily for 3-5 days or Inj. Meloxicam (like Inj. Melonex, Inj. Meloxi, Inj. Proxivet, Inj. Zobid M, Inj A_3 Vet, Inj A_3 Vet plus (Brihans) @ 15-30 ml IM daily for 3-5 days may be used.

Cryotherapy with liquid nitrogen is promising in curing Actinomycosis. The method of cryotherapy is detailed herewith. After restraining the animal physically, the lesions are to be enlarged and curetted to drain the necrosed tissue and pus with few bone spicules (if it is present at all). Liquid N_2 is poured slowly into the lesion using an applicator (*e.g.* Teflon goblet) till the entire lesion is frozen with ice ball formation. Next day lesions are again curetted and liquid N_2 is poured as on first day and it can be repeated at 7 days interval for one or two more applications depending on the severity of lesions.

During the period of LN_2 application all the necrosed tissue will slough off and fresh granulation tissue will develop from underneath and healing will occur. Local application of antiseptic cream, gels or herbal ointment should be made liberally for speedy recovery or healing.

7.10 BOTULISM

It is a fatal bacterial disease of cattle, horse, sheep, goat and birds, caused by the neurotoxins of *Clostridium botulinum*, produced in decaying animal tissues. Deficiency of proteins and phosphorus are predisposing factors. The disease may occur both peracute and subacute form.

Symptoms

Peracute deaths sometimes occur without premonitory signs. The disease manifested by restlessness, incordination, stumbling, knuckling, ataxia, motor paralysis, sternal recumbancy with head on ground or turned into flank.

Progressive muscular weakness, tremor, prostration and recumbancy are usual signs in cattle and horse. Stiff gait, incoordination, tilted head, terminal paralysis and rapid death occurs in sheep.

Treatment

Specific polyvalent Botulinum antitoxin in early stages needs to be administered. Purgatives like magnesium sulfate to be fed to the animal for the removal of toxins from the GI tract. Inj. Streptopenicillin or Inj. Penicillin-G in high doses dissolved in chlorpheniramine maleate may be tried along with specific antitoxin. Neurotropic B-vitamins, *viz.*, Neurovet (Alved) can be of use while treating neural problems.

7.11 COLIBACILLOSIS

Colibacillosis is one of the important diseases in neonatal calves characterized by profuse diarrhoea, marked prostration and septicemia. *Escherichia coli* (*E. coli*) still continues to be the predominant cause of collibacillosis in bovine neonates.

Colibacillosis is the common enteric disease of mostly calf, lamb and piglet (neonates at early life). *E. coli* produces septicemic colibacillosis with an acute illness in colostrum deprived new borns. The mortality may occur and sometimes exceed 50 per cent death and prognosis of the disease is poor if the colostral immunity is low.

Symptoms

Fever in early stage with depression, anorexia, followed by diarrhoea and dysentery and death within 24-96 hours. *Enterotoxic colibacillosis*, the most common form in young calf and lamb where profuse foul smelling watery diarrhoea streaked with blood, acidosis, weakness and death within 3-5 days occurs. New born calves should drink colostrums at least 50 ml/kg body weight within 10-12 hours after birth.

Treatment

1. *Sulphonamides*: Sufex bolus, S.D. bolus, Sulphabolus (Sarabhai), Lemidine bolus (Legend-5 g bolus, Duaprim (Brihans), Biotrim DS bolus (Vetnex)

   Dose: Calf – ½ bolus, Lamb/Kid/Piglet – ¼ bolus, BD orally.
2. *Broad spectrum antibiotics*: Oral – Neodox bolus (Vetcare), Cyclin DT (Excell), Amoxirum Bolus (GSK), Alcycline bolus (Alembic), Steclin bolus (Sarabhai), 3-Care bolus, Cyclin bolus (Excell) – ½ to 1 bolus BID.

   Injection – Chloramphenicol sodium succinate, *viz.*, Vetampin 500 mg, Chloraxin (Cipla) @ 2-4 mg/kg body weight by IV route; Inj. Amoxycillin Cloxacillin (Intamox 500 mg) can be administered daily.
3. *Chemotherapy* with Furazolidone (Fagil) 60 mg/kg body weight for 5-7 days are also effective. Antibac-C (Oxfendaem) oral suspension @ 5-10 ml BD is found effective.
4. *Electrolyte solution* like Electrocon liquid, ERS liquid, ORS, Remilyte (Legend) must be given to the neonates to check dehydration. In severe cases DNS must be given by IV route.

7.12 CONTAGIOUS BOVINE PLEURO PNEUMONIA (CBPP)

It's an infectious disease of bovines, also affecting sheep and goat, caused by *Mycoplasma mycoides*. The disease spreads by inhalation and results in pneumonia and pleurisy. CCPP is an infection of lungs. In septicaemic form it is characterized by sudden onset of high fever, anorexia, shallow respiration accompanied by expiratory grunt, and typical pneumonia with pleurisy, respiratory distress and death occurs within 1-2 weeks.

Diagnosis

Auscultation findings are diagnostic. For Mycoplasma detection and confirmation CFT may be done.

Treatment

Tylosin is the drug of choice. Sulphadimidine may be tried. Tylosin tartarate – 2-5 mg/lb body weight by IM route. Inj. chloramphenicol like Inj. Neochlor (Vetcare), Inj. Enteromycetin (Deys vet), Inj. Phenivet (PCI), Inj. Ciptec vet (Cipla), Inj. C-flox

Power/C-plox (Intas) @ 10 ml/50 kg body weight; Antihistaminic like Inj. Zeet, Inj. Avil, Inj. Chlorazin, Inj. Anistamin *etc.* @ 5-10 ml and Meloxicam, Inj. A_3 Vet, Inj. MP_3, Inj. Melonex Plus, Inj. Zobid-M @ 10-15 ml by IM route daily for 3-5 days by can be administered.

Repeated vaccination with live attenuated vaccine can be done for control and containment of the disease. Remove positive animals.

7.13 CONTAGIOUS CAPRINE PLEURO PNEUMONIA (CCPP)

It's a specific injections disease of sheep and goat caused by *Mycoplasma mycoides var capri*, spreads mainly by inhalation. Large numbers of deaths occur every year in unprotected flocks.

Symptoms

Fever, anorexia, weakness, respiratory distress, nasal discharge and foetal pneumonia (60-100 per cent mortality).

Treatment

Tylosin is the drug of choice @ 2-5 kg/Ib body weight. Inj. Ciprofloxacin (C-flox/ C-flox power) @ 1-2 ml for 5-6 days by IM route is effective. Tetracycline in high doses in early stage by IV route is also effective treatment. Inj. Alinchomycin (Alved) @ 1 ml/adult goat is also found effective, Inj. Ciprofloxacin, Inj. Ciptec (Cipla), Inj. C-flox (Intas) @ 10 ml 80 kg body weight can also be tried. Antihistaminic injection (Avil, Zeet, Cadistin) and Cox-II inhibitor NSAID-Meloxicam Injection (Dulonex, Melonex plus, Zobid M, MP_3, Proxivet) may be tried @ 2-5 ml through IM route for 3 days.

Prevention

Prevent the disease by vaccination.

7.14 ENTEROTOXAEMIA

Commonly known as pulpy kidney disease of ruminants. Particularly sheep caused by *Clostridium perfringens* type-D. Lamb neonates (3-10 weeks age) are prone to the disease, Adults may also be affected. Disease is peracute in lambs and adult sheep exhibit temors, ataxia, respiratory distress, bloat, convulsion, and diarrhoea.

Treatment

Treatment is not effective. Inj. Intamox, Inj. Britax, Inj. Ciprofloxacin, Inj. Enrofloxacin can be tried.

Prevention

Prevent the disease by annual vaccination with Enterotoxaemia (Biomed) @ 1 ml per animal.

7.15 LISTERIOSIS

It's an infectious disease caused by *Listeria monocytogens*, a gram (+) ve organism, affects all the livestock and poultry. Three common forms of the disease are noted.

1. *Listerial meningo encephalitis* (*Nervous form*): Dullness, circling, head pressing, dropped jaw, lingual protrusion, Glaxia, recumbency and death.
2. *Listerial abortion*: Ewe aborts in last month of pregnancy. In case of cow there is still birth, fever and retention of placenta.
3. *Listerial septicemia* (*Septicemic form*): It occurs usually in monogastric animals and in lambs and calves.

Treatment

Chlortetracycline in high doses (IV) or Streptopenicillin (Inj. Bistrepen, Munonycin Fort, Inj. Dicrysticin *etc.*) with fluid therapy (Inj. Rintose, Inj. Intalyte 10 per cent, Inj. Dextrose, Inj. Woctrose *etc.*) may be done.

Severely affected animals die inspite of therapy.

7.16 LEPTOSPIROSIS

All animals may be infected by this disease. It is zoonotic in nature. The disease is caused by several species of Leptospira. Rodents act as carries. The organisms localize in kidney and liver.

Symptoms

Anorexia, depression, haemolytic anaemia, intermittent fever, jaundice, dyspnoea, haemoglobinuria and abortion. Some animals may show lameness and necrotic dermatitis. Older dogs suffer from intestinal nephritis.

Diagnosis

Differentiate the disease from babesiosis, anaplasmosis and bacillary haemoglobinuria. Microscopic examination of urine sediment under dark ground illumination or Fontana's silver impregnation staining may confirm the disease.

Treatment

Streptomycin, Tetracyclines and Penicillin are highly effective when given continuously for 7 days.

Prevent the disease by vaccination.

For dogs – combined vaccine like Pentadog, Candur DHL *etc.* can be done.

7.17 PARATUBERCULOSIS

It is also known as Johnes Disease (JD). Cattle, sheep and goats are affected. The disease is caused by *Mycobacterium paratuberculosis* and the organisms localize primarily in the mucosa of intestine and associated lymph nodes.

Symptoms

Emaciation, excessive thirst, chronic recurrent diarrhoea, submandibular edema.

Diagnosis

Rule out enteric parasitic infestation, examination of faecal smear, acid fast bacilli in rectal mucosae, Johnin test (single intradermal test) using 0.2 ml Johnin on loose skin of neck. Chronic emaciation and chronic recurrent diarrhoea when do not respond to treatment leads to the diagnosis of JD. JD positive animals must be slaughtered.

Treatment

Inj. Streptomycin @ 25 mg/lb body weight given for a long period may give transient recovery. However, infection is very resistant to treatment.

Chapter 8
Viral Diseases: Their Treatment and Control

8.1 INTRODUCTION

The most important viral diseases of livestock are enlisted below.

1. Foot and Mouth Disease (FMD)
2. Rinderpest (RP)
3. Bovine Ephemeral Fever
4. Blue Tongue
5. Pox
6. *Peste des petits ruminants* (PPR)
7. Contagious Ecthyma
8. Cutaneous Papillomatosis
9. Hydrophobia (Rabies)
10. Hog Cholera (Swine Fever)

8.2 FOOT AND MOUTH DISEASE

It is a highly contagious disease of cloven footed (hoofed) animals and is caused by a small RNA virus (Picorna virus). The disease is not usually fatal although the morbidity is as high as 100 per cent. It is fatal to suckling calves. Exotic and crossbred animals are very much prone to the disease. Four major strains (types) *viz.*, A, O, C and Asia-I, are prevalent in India. In Buffalo the mouth lesions are quite severe as comparable to cattle.

Diagnosis

Clinical symptoms are so characteristic that diagnosis is not a problem at all. FAT, AGPT, CFT and ELISA are the usual diagnostic technique.

Treatment

There is no specific treatment of the disease. Since lesions develop on tongue and inter digital space of the hoof (feet) care to be taken for speedy healing. Boroglycerine, Alum water washing, mouth washing by potassium permanganate solution and foot washing and cleaning with warm potassium permanganate solution, 5 per cent $CuSO_4$ solution is recommended. Multipurpose ayurvedic ointment like Himax, Sorine, Charmil, Lorexene or readymade antiseptic lotion or dressing oils like Dressit, Dressogen, (Nugen), Bacticon, Suffoil (Legend), Dressol (Kapila) or lotion like Charmil lotion, Himax lotion (Indian Herbs) should be applied on foot lesions.

Broad spectrum antibiotic like Oxytetracyclines, Chlortetracyclines to the non-pregnant and dry animals and Enrofloxacin, Streptopenicillin to the lactating and other animals can be given. Supportive therapy like Inj. Hivit, Inj. Coniplex, and immunomodulator like Inj. Lemasol -75 (Vetnex), Inj. Kalmisol has been found very much Inj. Kal antisol (@ 1 ml/30 kg body weight SC) has been found very much effective in the treatment of FMD and hastens recovery.

For lameness and pain striken condition Inj. Analgin, Novalgin, Vetalgin 10-15 ml IM for 3 days or Inj. Neoprofen, Ketoprofen, Ketop @ 10-15 ml IM daily for 3 days or Inj. Meloxicam, Melonex, MP_3, Zobid-M @ 15-30 ml daily for 3 days may be administered.

Prophylaxis and Control

It is very difficult to eradicate the disease because of high price of FMD vaccine, short lived immunity and thick livestock population of India. Vigorous sanitary measures, prompt reporting system, effective quarantine and correct typing of FMD virus may help in control of the disease.

Tissue culture inactivated polyvalent (O, A, C and Asia I) vaccine like Raksha FMD (Indian Immunologicals) may be used @ cattle, buffalo and calf – 3 ml SC, and sheep and goat – 1 ml SC. Polyvalent FMD vaccine (Hoechst/Internet), BAIF FMD vaccine (multi dose vial), IVRI FMD vaccine (Bangalore) and Raksha-OVAC may also be used. Dose of the vaccine should be as per the recommendation of the manufacturing company. FMD vaccination must be done at least twice in a year.

Protection of calf against FMD: Primary vaccination is to be done between 4-8 weeks of age, then at 5 months and 9 months of age and thereafter at every 4 months interval.

Bovilis Clovax (Intervet) – 10 ml and 30 ml vial.

Dose: Cattle and buffalo @ 2 ml by IM, sheep and goat @ 1 ml by IM route.

FMD vaccine (Intervet) – 100 ml vial.

Dose: Cattle and buffalo @ 2 ml by IM route, sheep and goat @ 1 ml by IM route.

8.3 RINDERPEST (RP)

Synonym

Cattle plague.

It is an acute, febrile, highly contagious and fatal disease of cattle where the death toll may be as high as 90 per cent. Exotic and crossbred cattle are highly susceptible and suffer a severe attack. It is caused by a Morbilli virus. Cattle, buffalo, sheep and goat are susceptible to Morbilli virus (RP). The affected animals show high rise of temperature, anorexia, depression in milk yield, inflammation of buccal mucosa and conjunctivae and focal erosion of the G.I. tract mucosa followed by diarrhoea.

Treatment and Control

There is no effective treatment of the disease, but can be controlled by vaccination and elimination of the sources of infection. Sulpha drugs like Duaprim, Biotrim, Sulphadimidin, Brimdine *etc.* and high dose of antibiotics can be used for control of secondary complications. Fluids and electrolytes therapy and symptomatic treatment must be advocated.

Culture attenuated Kabette 'O' strain of RP is extremely safe and used in RP control programme through vaccination. The Govt. of India declared our country as Rinderpest free zone.

Because of similarity of clinical symptoms of RP and *Peste des petits ruminants* (PPR) in sheep and goats, differentiation of the two infections using recombinant antigens is essential.

8.4 BOVINE EPHEMERAL FEVER

Synonym

Three days sickness, Bovine epizootic fever, Dragon boat disease.

Ephemeral fever is commonly known as 'three days sickness'. It is an acute non-contagious, epizootic arboviral disease of cattle and water buffaloes, characterized by sudden onset of fever, depression, stiffness and lameness with high morbidity and extremely low mortality.

Source of Infection

Source of infection is believed to be arthropod vectors/insect bites *i.e.* Culicoides, Culicine and Anophelis mosquitoes.

The virus has been isolated from mosquitoes and midges. The disease is caused by a single stranded RNA virus under Rhabdoviridae.

Symptoms

Pyrexia or fever which is generally biphasic and sometimes triphasic or polyphasic (104 °F – 107 °F) 12-18 hours apart.

The characteristic signs are accelerated heart and respiratory rates, anorexia, ruminal atony, depression, serous or mucoid nasal and ocular discharge, salivation and shievering.

The muscles of the affected limb become stiff, hard and painful. The animal shows lameness akin to acute laminitis leading to shifting lameness and generalized stiffness. Many animals become recumbent for 12-24 hours but are able to rise if sufficiently stumbled.

Differential Diagnosis

Many diseases or disease conditions may be confused with ephemeral fever. These are Rift Valley fever, Blue tongue, Botulism, Babesiosis, Black Quarter (BQ), Laminitis, Milk fever *etc.* The salivation may suggest FMD, however, there is no vesicular lesion in the mouth and feet in Three days sickness or Ephemeral fever.

Treatment

1. Treatment with anti-inflammatory and antipyretic drugs is beneficial.

   Inj. Analgin, Inj. Oxalgin, Inj. Vetalgin, Inj. Dipravet (PCI), Inj. Paramol, Inj. Paracetamol (Cadila), Inj. Dafomol (Dafodillis), Inj. Boline, @ 10-15 ml IM daily for 2-3 days; or Meloxicam preparation with or without Paracetamol *e.g.*, Inj. MP_3 (Vetnex), Inj. Melonex plus (Intas), Inj. Zobid-M (Sarabhai Zydus), Inj. Meloxi (Vets pharma) @ 30 ml/300 kg body weight by IM route daily for 2-3 days. Injectable Ketoprofen like Inj. Ketop, Inj. Neoprofen (Vetnex) @ 10-15 ml daily for 2-3 days by IM route. During fever the paresis or paralysis responds to injectable calcium borogluconate (Inj. Calborol, Inj. Intacal, Inj. Calmax) in the same manner as Parturient paresis (Milk fever).

   Besides injection oral tablet/bolus may be used like Nimulite Plus bolus (Vets Farma), Oxalgin NP bolus (Zydus Sarabhai), Melonex plus bolus (Intas), A_3 vet bolus (Brihans), Paralgin NP bolus @ 1-2 boli orally BID for 3 days.

2. Antibiotics may be given to prevent secondary bacterial infection.

   For pregnant and lactating animals Inj. Enorfloxacin (Inj. Floxidin, Quinintas, Enrodac, Enrovet, Enrocin, Meriquin), Inj. Ciprofloxacin (Inj. C-flox), Inj. Ampicillin (Inj. Acvet, Conampi) *etc.* for 3 days. For dry and other animals Inj. Oxytetracycline, Inj. Chlortetracycline (Inj. Oxy, Loxy, Biroxy, Intamycin, Terramycin), Inj. Streptopenicillin (Inj. D.C., Inj. Bistrepen, Inj. Biostrep, Munonycin Fort) *etc.* 2.5 g for 3 days by I/M route may be given.

3. Stomachic powder

   Himalayan Batisa. Normal Batisa, Herbogastrine *etc.* 20-25 g orally BID may be fed to the animal.

8.5 BLUE TONGUE

Synonyms

Catarrhal fever, Stiff lamb disease, Sore muzzle.

It is an infectious, non-contagious, arthropod borne virus disease of domestic and wild animals. It is principally a disease of sheep and occasionally of cattle. Six different strains of Blue tongue virus are prevalent in India causing great threat for the sheep industry. A homeopathic medicine – Mercsol and 0.5 ml of Ocimum are dissolved in 30 ml of Vimeral liquid shaken thoroughly and @ 0.5 ml in drops administered orally consecutively for 2-3 days found effective.

Mercsol can exert an antiviral and immunostimulant action. *Ocimum sanctum* has antistress, antibacterial immunomodulatary, respiratory stimulant and ulcer healing actions.

Symptoms

Initially high fever (100-105°F), nasal discharge, salivation and lachrymations followed by drooling of saliva, stomatitis, swelling of gum, tongue and lips. These changes may be followed by ulceration of lips, dental pad, gum and tongue which turns purple in colour. Dypsnoea, lameness, coronitis, laminitis, cyanotic and bluish appearance of the tongue, dry muzzle with burnt appearance are characteristic of the disease. In abortive form there is abortion and congenital deformities of new born lambs. Sub acute or sub clinical form is noted in cattle and generally passed unnoticed.

Diagnosis

Differentiate the disease from FMD and Contagious ecthyma, confirm the disease by CFT.

Treatment

There is no specific treatment of this viral disease. Symptomatic treatment and control of secondary bacterial infections with antibiotics should be done.

Affected animal should be kept away from solar radiation.

Localized lesions should be treated with antiseptic solution (Potassium permanganate solution, Boro glycerine *etc*). Parenteral injection for fever and skin inflammation, Inj. Meloxicam *viz.* Inj. Melonex, Melonex Plus, MP_3, A_3 Vet. Melflam vet (Cipla), Inj. Proxyvet, Inj. Nulox (Karnataka Antibiotics) or Ketoprofen like Inj. Ketop, Inj. Neoprofen (2-3 ml) for sheep and goat, Inj. Nimovet (Indian immunologicals) 1ml IM for 3 days. Antihistaminic injection like Avil, Zeet, Chloril, Chlorazin 1-2 ml IM for 2-3 days. Parenteral Antibiotics like Inj. Alinchomycin,@ 1m, Inj. Ciptec (Cipla), Inj. C-flox/C-flox Power @ 1-2 ml daily for 2-3 days, Injection Chloramphenicol like Inj. Neochlor (Vet Care), Inj. Enteromycetin (Days vet) @ 1-2 ml IM daily for 3-5 days, Injection Enrofloxacin (Inj. Enron, Floxidin, Quinintas, Enrovet, Enrocin @ 1-2 ml IM daily for 3-5 days or combined antibiotics like Inj. Intamox 500 mg IM daily for 5-7 days may be given.

As supportive therapy oral multivitamins like Vimeral, Ambiplex, Lysovit, Oraplex, Livolysin @ 5-10 ml orally BID, parenteral multivitamins like Inj. Hivit, Inj. Coniplex, Inj. Pinkojet, Inj. Pinkojet-L @ 1-2 ml daily for 3 days may be administered by IM route.

Prophylaxis

Tissue culture polyvalent live virus vaccine can be used.

8.6 POX

Cattle Pox/Cow Pox

Cow pox is a contagious, benign viral disease of cattle and is transmissible to human beings by direct contact. The disease is caused by a large DNA Orthopox virus, closely related to small pox and horse pox virus.

Symptoms

In cowpox there is some rise in body temperature, development of pinpoint red sports, papules of the size of mustard, which can be felt by hand, the papules transformed into vesicles later on.

Papules occurring on the udder are generally circular but those on the teats are elongated. The lesions heal in the course of 15-20 days. The lesions are clinically similar to pseudo cowpox and bovine ulcerative mammillitis. Sometimes lesions on teats and udder may lead to mastitis. Lesions are usually observed at scab stage in the field when the animal is brought for veterinary aids.

Treatment

Symptomatic and palliative treatments are to be given. The lesions may be cleaned with 1 : 1000 solution of Potassium Permanganate ($KMnO_4$) followed by local application of antiseptic ointment *viz.* Borolene, Sorine, Dressol ointment and Dermanol cream. To check secondary bacterial invasion, Inj. A_3vet, Inj. Vetclox, Inj. Inclox, Inj. Intamox, Inj. Lemox, Inj. Inimox may be given @ 2 g IM daily for 3 days to the lactating and pregnant animals and Inj. Oxytetracycline to the dry animals.

Inj. Novalgin, Analgin, Valginate, or Inj. Neoprofen, Inj. Ketop, or Inj. Melonex, MP_3, Inj. A_3vet, Inj. Nulox, Inj. Proxyvet, Inj. Meloxi @ 10-15 ml IM for 2-3 days may be given if there is much pain and pyrexia.

Topicure spray may be used on skin lesions.

Buffalo Pox

It is a highly contagious Orthopox viral infection characterized by popular localized lesions on the teats and udder of the milking buffaloes along with pock lesions on ears, eyes and brisket. Sometimes generalized pock lesions are also seen.

The disease is caused by buffalo pox virus (a double stranded enveloped DNA virus under Orthopox genus under Poxviridae family.

Diagnosis

It can be easily diagnosed based on the localized pock lesions on the udder of milking buffaloes. Differential diagnosis requires laboratory confirmation by isolation and identification of the pox virus.

Treatment

Washing of the lesions with Potassium permanganate solution followed by antiseptic gel application like Dermanol cream (Indian Herbs), or paste made out of neem and turmeric onto the lesion can be done. Boric acid powder in neem/coconut oil may also be used on pox lesions. To check secondary bacterial infection antibiotics and anti-inflammatory analgesics can be used, same as mentioned in case of cow pox.

Goat Pox

Goat pox is an important viral disease caused by the genus Capri pox virus generally characterized by fever and appearance of pock lesions. All breeds of goat irrespective of sex are affected. Goat pox can also cause more serious lesions in sheep than sheep pox virus. It is a contagious disease and usual mode of transmission is contact. Biting insects may inoculate the virus.

Symptoms

Skin papules appear in 2-5 days following temperature reaction. Pock lesions appear in all parts of the body, *e.g.* lips, cheeks, snout, nostril, face, ear, feet, thigh, abdomen, eyelid, neck, udder and teats. Mucopurulent discharges from eyes and nose, conjunctivitis, respiratory distress (if pneumonia develops). Pox viruses of sheep and goat are antigenitically distinct although transmissible to each other.

Diagnosis

Diagnosis is based on history and clinical signs. Differentiate from Contagious ecthyma and Blue tongue. Confirmatory diagnosis by virus isolation and characterization needs laboratory facilities.

Treatment

Exposed lesions are to be washed with Potassium Permanganate solution (1 : 10,000). Antiseptic ayurvedic ointment like Sorine, Himax, Dermanol, Charmil *etc.* can be applied on lesions.

As a measure to check secondary bacterial complications a course of antibiotic *viz.* Oxytetracycline 50 mg/ml (Inj. Intamycin, Inj. Oxy, Inj. Loxy, Inj. Terramycin), Enrofloxacin (Inj. Enrocin, Inj. Enrox, Inj. Floxidin), Ciprofloxain (Inj. Cflox, Inj. Cflox power. @ 1ml by IM route for 3-5 days. Inj. Ciptec (Cipla) @ 1-2 ml IM daily for 3 days. For cases having respiratory distresses – Chlorpheneramine maleate 10mg/ml @ 2-5 ml daily by IM route. Analgesic antipyretic like Meloxicam *i.e.* Inj. Melonex (Intas), Inj. MP_3 (Vetnex), Inj. Meloxi (Vets Farma), Inj. Nimovet (Indian immunologicals) can be prescribed.

Vaccination

Freeze dried Goat pox vaccine 75 dose ampules (reconstituted in 75 ml diluent) @ 1 ml by SC route to each animal about an inch inside the tip of ear.

Sheep Pox

Sheep pox is a highly contagious and most serious pox virus disease of animals characterized by acute febrile condition and generalized pock lesions, causing high mortality in lambs. The disease is caused by sheep pox virus (SPV) classified in the genus Capripox virus of the family Pox viridae. The sheep are naturally susceptible. Merino breeds are highly susceptible. The sheep rearing prospects are dampened by the occurrence of such dreadful disease.

Symptoms

The incubation period varies from 4 to7 days. The disease usually causes severe systemic reaction with widespread lesions. The pox eruptions are more prominent on the checks, nostrils, lips and wool free skin. The lesions pass through the typical pox stages. The vesicular stage may be haemorrhagic with a tendency to generalize, followed by development of pustules which later turn to scales. Healing is very slow. Lymphadenitis, and focal viral pneumonia with lesions distributed uniformly throughout the lungs are also seen.

Diagnosis

Clinical signs, electron microcopy, cell culture, immunological tests like FAT, AGPT, ELISA, VNT *etc.*

Treatment

There is no effective treatment. Symptomatic and supportive treatment should be done. To alleviate pain, inflammation, pyrexia and pneumonia Meloxicam or Ketoprofen *viz.* Inj. Melonex, Inj. Melonex plus, Inj. Meloxi, Inj. Neoprofen, Inj. Ketop *etc.* @ 3-5 ml IM daily for 3-5 days may be used. Anti-histaminic *e.g.*, Inj. Zeet, Inj. Phenavil, Inj. Avil, Inj. Chloril @1-2 ml IM daily for 5-7 days, oral tonic like Oraplex, Vimeral, Ambiplex, Lysovit *etc.* may be tried. For topical application Charmil, Himax, Sorine ointment or Dermanol, Dressol, Charmil, Himax lotions can be used.

Vaccination

Alive attenuated sheep pox vaccine using SPV-RF strain or SPV tissue culture vaccine should be used. It provides immunity for six months.

8.7 *PESTE DES PETITS RUMINANTS* (PPR)

It is one of the most destructive viral diseases of small ruminant flocks and number one constraint to intensive small ruminant farming (FAO, 1983).

- ☆ Morbidity – 50 per cent to 100 per cent
- ☆ Mortality – 10 per cent to 50 per cent
- ☆ Abortions – 75 per cent to 95 per cent.

It is an acute viral disease of sheep and goats characterized by fever, erosive stomatitis, conjunctivitis, gastroenteritis and pneumonia.

Etiology

Morbilli virus genus – An RNA virus belongs to Paramyxo virus family with close antigenic relationship to the Rinderpest virus of large ruminants.

Routes of Infection

Transmission through close contact, ocular, nasal and oral secretions, feaces, inhalation of aerosoles, fomites such as bedding.

Incubation Period: 4-5 days.

Symptoms

Pyrexia 104-106 °F (40-41°C), temperature is high for 5 to 8 days and slowly returns to normal and drops below normal leading to death. Serous nasal discharge

– turns mucopurulent occluding the nostrils to cause respiratory distress and sneezing in an attempt to clear the nose.

Necrotic stomatitis lending to depressed appetite, profuse non haemorrhagic severe diarrheoa leading to severe dehydration and emaciation. Secondary complications like Bronchopneumonia and abortions are common findings. Pregnant animals usually abort.

Prevention

Prevention is possible by timely vaccination. A live attenuated homologous PPR vaccine like Raksha-PPR (Indian Immunologicals) – 50 doses vial. 1st vaccination at 3 to 4 months of age @ 1 ml SC (To be dissolved in sterile diluents) storage at (+) 20 °C.

A Homologous live attenuated vaccine developed at IVRI (Mukteswar) in freeze dried form; single vial contains 50/100 doses which are very much effective, give life long protective immunity.

Dose: 1 ml SC (reconstituted vaccine).

Treatment

Antibiotics to be administered to the affected animals to check secondary bacterial complications. Enrofloxacin injection, Floxidin, Enrocare, Enrox, Enrocin @ 10 mg/kg body weight or 1 ml/20 kg body weight IM daily for 5 days; Inj. Ciprofloxacin (Ciplox, Cflox power 1-2 ml) IM daily for 5 days, Inj. Intamox, Inj. Britax, Inj. Exact, Inj. Cefavet 250-500 mg, Inj. Amoxirum (375 mg) IM daily for 5-6 days. Antihistaminic injection like Inj. Zeet, Inj. Avil, Inj. Chlorazin @ 1-2 ml IM daily for 3 days; oral or parenteral NSAID like Melonex, Melonex plus, A_3vet, Emcalm, Oxalgin NP, Paralgin NP bolus or Inj. Melonex, Melonex plus, A_3vet, Proxivet, Meloxi @ 3-5 ml IM daily for 3-5 days should be administered. Oral administration of Cyclin DT, Furazolidone (Oriprim bolus), Sulfaguanidine bolus, Sulphadimidin bolus twice daily can be given for enteritis and diarrhoea. Supportive therapy like vitamin B-complex, or liver extract with B-complex injection or oral liver tonic, vitamin syrup, ORS (oral rehydration solution) or electrolytes should also be given to the animals. IV fluid therapy can decrease death due to dehydration and subsequent electrolyte imbalances.

8.8 CONTAGIOUS ECTHYMA

It is a viral disease of sheep and goat caused by epithellotropic para pox virus which is highly contagious and zoonotic in nature. It is characterized by pustular, scabby and proliferative lesions on the muzzle, lips, face, ears, teats or vulva. It is caused by an epitheliotropic virus which enters through skin abrasions. The virus replicates in proliferating keratinocycles in the damaged epidermis.

The disease appears in the form of papules which progress rapidly to vesicles, pustules and scabs. Crusty proliferative lesions typically on the lips but can also affect the face, ears, coronary band, scrotum, ears or vulva. Bronchopneumonia and gastro-enteritis may develop in kids and lambs.

The intense scab like encrustations around the oral cavity are very much characteristic of orf, a viral infection. Localization of the lesions also ruled out the possibility of Goat pox and Sheep pox. Deaths of the animals may occur because of inanition and dehydration induced by intense oral lesions which unable the animals from feeding along with the secondary bacterial complications.

Treatment

1. Supportive therapy with fluid and palliative feeds to be given.
2. Application of neem leaves paste on to the lesions, or antiseptic lesions like Dressol, Dermanol, Charmil or Himax lotion or multipurpose gel/ointment like Dressol, Himax, Sorine ointment, Charmil *etc.* should be done.
3. Treatment with broad spectrum antibiotics to combat secondary bacterial infections. *e.g.* Inj.Enrofloxacin (5 mg/kg body weight), Inj. Oxytetracycline, Inj. Ciprofloxacin, Inj. Gentamycin, Inj. Chloramphenicol (@ 30mg/kg body weight) *etc.*
4. Antiinflammatory analgesics (NSAIDs) *e.g.* Inj. Melonex, Inj. Meloxi, Inj. A3 vet, Inj. MP_3 *etc.* @ 2-3 ml by IM route or Inj. Analgin, Inj. Oxalgin NP @ 3-5 ml by IM route for 2-3 days can also be given.
5. For cases complicated with rhinitis antihistaminic *e.g.* Inj. Avil, Inj. Zeet, Inj. Chloril, Inj. Chlorazin @ 1-2 ml IM daily for 2-3 days.
6. For malnourished kids and lambs DNS should be administered by IV route to check dehydration and to rejuvenate body condition.
7. Exposed lesions should be washed with 1 : 10,000 Potassium permanganate solution for sufficient numbers of times. Wiped with sterile wet cotton swabs. Exposed lesions can be painted with 2 per cent Boroglycerine. Acid salicilate, Dithranol, Derobin skin ointment, Neosporin ointment *etc.* can also be liberally applied to the lesions.

8.9 CUTANEOUS PAPILLOMATOSIS

Cutanous Papilloma or warts are benign and proliferative epithelial neoplasm, caused by the Papilloma viruses of the family Papova viridae. These virus induced papillomas are of two different types. They are squamous papilloma and Fibropapilloma. Intermediate types have also been recorded. The virus type except the bovine papilloma virus are highly host specific and for each species of animals there may be several virus types and these viruses can be distinguished by the endonuclease cleavage of their DNA.

Bovine Papillomatosisis

Bovine papillomatosisis caused by bovine papilloma virus, a papova virus having double stranded DNA in its genome. There are six types of Bovine papilloma virus affecting the cattle. In cattle Bovine papilloma virus type-I produce, fibropapilloma, type 2 and 3 produce cutaneous lesions of squamous papilloma and type-5 produce lesions on the teat (called rice grain papilloma or teat papilloma).

Epidemiology

Papilloma is common in young animals and adult age groups are resistant to infection probably due to acquired immunity derived from apparent infection in the young age. It can spread by direct contact or during tattooing, dehorning *etc.* Persistence of warts for longer periods may be due to immunodeficiency.

Symptoms

Formation of warts are generally seen on skin of face, neck, legs, anteroventral parts of the body and may also at many other parts of the body. The lesions are most typical. Lesions are flat, raised, fissured (spiny) and crusty mats which are attached to skin by a pedicle. The growth may also be sessile. The warts may have the size of a grain to a cauliflower like appearance up to 10-15 cm in diameter. In adult cows multiple sessile and small lesions (1-2 mm in diameter) are observed in teats, during milking. These are elongated up to 1 cm. Fibopapilomatous lesions are usually seen on penis, vulva, anus *etc.* (on its epithelium).

In horses, the warts appear on muzzle, nose and lips and are usually sessile type. In goats the lesions usually appear on teats, in sheep the lesions are common on the face and ears. In dogs oral papilloma are the most common involving muzzle, lips and oral cavity.

Treatment

Warts or papilloma usually regress or resolve spontaneously. However, in most of the cases treatment are required owing to persistent nature of the lesions and also for traumatic wound on papillomas. Injection Antheomaline, Lithiomony etc. (containing antimony or bismuth) by IM route at 3-5 days interval for 3-4 occasions may cause regression of warts. But results are of varying degree of success (dose 10-15 ml IM on young animals up to 150-200 kg body weight). Removal of warts by surgical excision (sometimes aggravates the lesions and cause extensive lesions development). Treatment by autologous vaccine prepared from the wart. (Sometimes such vaccination may increase the size of the warts or prolon the course of disease).

Autohaemotherapy

Blood collecting from the animal (self-blood) suffering from cutaneous papillomatosis to be injected immediately after collection by IM route @ 15-20 ml at weekly interval for 3-4 occasions are also effective in regression or falling of warts.

Cryotherapy

Cryotherapy with liquid nitrogen or solid CO_2 is also very good and effective therapy in wart management. This can be tried easily since liquid N_2 are available in each veterinary centre for preservation of semen for artificial insemination.

In that case area surrounding the wart lesions should be protected with liberal application of vaseline or petroleum jelly to prevent the tissue from cold frosts or burn.

Salicyclic acid 12 per cent daily, salicyclic and lactic acid lotion (Salactol) topically under occlusion after removing surface layer with coarse sand paper.

Homeopathic Therapy

Using Thuja orally (200x) or by injection gives very good results. Mother Tincture of Sulphur (Sulphur Q.S.) @ 2 ml diluted in 2 ml distilled water SC or Mother Tincture of Thuja at the same doses is found to be very much effective.

Treatment with Levamisol

Levamisol HCl in prophylactive dose administered by SC route on 1st, 3rd, 5th, 7th, 9th and 16th day gives very good result in recovery.

8.10 HYDROPHOBIA (RABIES)

Rabies is a highly fatal zoonotic disease of all warm blooded animals involving CNS and is caused by *Rhabdovirus* (Lyssa virus infection). Dog is the principal transmitter of infection to man and animals. Both sylvatic and urban rabies is present in India. Since the virus is present in the saliva, infection by bite is facilitated by dog, wolves, jackals *etc*. The time between the exposure and first appearance of clinical signs of the disease may range from days to years but the majority of incubation periods observed, are between 4 to 6 weeks. This again depends on the proximity of the site of the bite to the brain.

Transmission

Transmission of rabies virus usually begins when infected saliva of a host is passed to an uninfected animal. The most common mode of transmission is through the bite and virus containing saliva of an infected host. Through contamination of mucous membranes (eyes, nose and mouth) aerosol transmission and through corneal transplantation, the disease may also be transmitted.

Pathology

Pathology of rabies infection is typically defined by encephalitis and myelitis frequently showing cytoplasmic eosinophilic inclusion bodies (Negribodies) in neuronal cells, especially pyramidal cells of the hippocampus and purkinjie cell of the cerebellum. The virus replicates in the infected perikarya of neurons and appears as inclusion bodies histologically demonstrable as Negri bodies.

Symptoms

Affected and or infected animals exhibit nervous signs restlessness, excitement, bellowing, salivation, paralysis and death.

Rabies in dogs is manifested in two forms (i) Furious forms and (ii) Dumb form. Both forms terminate in death following paralysis. The first symptoms of Rabies may be non-specific flu like signs. Malaise, fever or headache, which may last for few days progressing within 1-2 days to symptoms of cerebral dysfunction, anxiety, confusion, agitation progressing to delirium, abnormal behaviour, hallucinations and insomania. Once clinical signs of rabies appear, the disease is nearly fatal and treatment is typically supportive.

Furious Form (Violent Form)

The virus reaching the brain, damages the nerve cells and causes the animal oversensitive and over alert. They chase and attack other animal furiously. Animal develops a tendency to attack and lick every moving objects. It chews bricks, stones, mud, wood etc. Hoarse voice in this stage is very typical. This stage is quickly followed by paralytic stage. There is incordination in gait and frequent loud bellowing. The animals collapse in a paralytic state with in 24-48 hours after the onset of symptoms.

Dumb Form

In this form the animal cannot chew its flood and cannot drink water. It can neither bite nor close its mouth. Lower jaw hangs down, saliva dribbled down owing to paralysis of muscles of head, mouth and neck too. Paralysis gradually extends to the limbs. Death occurs within 3-4 days after the onset of symptoms. In the dumb form the animal goes down to paralysis and succumbs with in 48 hours of recumbency. In paralytic form severe depression, recumbency and profuse salivation occur and animal unable to swallow anything. At any rate death occurs within 10 days.

Confirmation

Detection of Rabies inclusion bodies in cells of acetone fixed brain smears by Florescent antibody testing. Impression smears from hippocampus for Negri bodies.

Prevention and Control

For effective control of rabies in livestock and human beings, the population of stray dogs is to be controlled on priority basis.

Disease prevention is entirely prophylactic and includes both passive antibody (Immuneglobulin) and vaccine.

Immunization and Post Bite Prophylaxis

The most effective mechanism of protection against rabies is to wash and flesh wound with soap and water, detergent or plain water, followed by application of ethanol or Tr. iodine.

Active immunization and Post Bite Vaccination against Rabiaes

(i) Raksharab (Indian Immunologicals)

An inactivated tissue culture vaccine (contains tissue culture Rabies virus; CVS strain) produced in BHK-21 cell line and inactivated with a Ziridine compound.

Dosage and Schedule: Dog, cattle, sheep, camel and all other species – 1 ml by SC or IM route on 0-3-7-14-30-90 days as post bite case.

Prophylactic uses: At 3 months of age and above. In case primary vaccination is given below 3 months, a booster dose should be given at 3 months age.

(ii) Defensor® -3 – 1 ml and 10 ml vial (Pfizer Animal Health)

It can be used in dog, cat, cattle, sheep and goat.

Dose and administration: Administer 1 ml SC or IM at 3 months of age followed by annual vaccination.

For post exposure prophylaxis (Post bite vaccination) 1ml on 0-3-7-14-30-90 by SC or IM route.

(iii) Rabdomun (Sarabhai Zydus) – 1 ml and 10 ml vials.

An exceptionally safe, potent and stable inactivated vaccine against fatal Rabies.

Composition: Flurry low egg passage (LEP) strain of rabies virus, propagated in BHK-21 suspended cell culture.

Indication: For the active immunization of dogs, cats, cattle, horses, sheep, goats, pigs and foxes of all ages against rabies.

Dose and administration: All domestic animals 1 ml by IM or SC route.

(iv) Nobivac Rabies (Intervet) – 1 ml and 10 ml vials.

Each dose contains rabies strain Pasteur RIV, grown on BHK-21 clone CT cell line inactivated with β-propiolactone and adsorbed on aluminum phosphate. This vaccine is used for active immunization of animals against rabies.

For livestock: For cattle, horse, sheep and goat, primary vaccination at the age of 6 months and revaccination at 2 years.

For dog and cat: Primary vaccination after 3 months of age and revaccination at 3 years of age. Annual revaccination is recommended in endemic areas.

All domestic dogs should be immunized with prophylactic rabies vaccines. Rabies virus flurry strain attenuated vaccine is maximally used in immunoprophylaxis of dog. Inactivated vaccine of nervous tissue origin is also used. Modified live virus vaccine and inactivated cell culture vaccines, attenuated and inactivated virus vaccines containing rabies virus antigen alone *viz.* Cadur R and vaccines in combination with antigens of other infectious agents (*e.g.* Pentadog and Megavac-6) are also in use.

8.11 HOG CHOLERA (CLASSICAL SWINE FEVER)

It is one of the most important viral disease of pigs and has been occurring as a regular feature in North-Eastern states of India including Assam. No antibiotic or other curable treatment is available to veterinary doctors. It is endemic in West Bengal and Assam along with many other states of India. It is a highly contagious viral disease of pigs caused by a virus belongs to Flaviviridae (Genus-Pestivirus).

Hosts

Pig and wild boar are the natural reservoir.

Transmission

Direct contact between animals, secretions, excretions, serum, blood, transplacental transmission and indirect contact through premises, implements, vehicles and instruments *etc*. The incubation period of the disease is 2-14 days. Clinically the disease has got many forms like (1) acute form, (2) chronic form, (3) mild form and (4) congenital form

Acute Form

High fever (41°C), anorexia, lethargy, haemorrhagic lesions of the skin, conjunctivitis, cyanotic changes of extremities *e.g.* ears, limbs, tails and snout, dyspnoea, coughing and occasional vomiting. Transient constipation followed by diarrhoea, ataxia, paresis and convulsion. Pigs handle together. Seaths occurs 5-15 days after onset of illness. Mortality in young pigs can approach 100 per cent.

Chronic Form

Dullness, capricious appetite pyrexia and diarrhoea up to one month. Apparent recovery with eventual relapse and death.

Milk Form

Transient pyrexia and inappetence, foetal death, resorption, mummification, still birth and in rare case abortion and congenital deformities.

Lesions

Enlarged haemorhogic lymph modes in acute form widespread potechiae and ecchymoss, specially in the skin, lymph nodes, laryax, kidney and ileocaecal junction. Lesions in chronic form are button ulcers in the caecum and large intestine.

Diagnosis

Signs and symptoms, pathognomonic lesions, serological tests like ELISA, Fluorescent antibody technique, Neutralisation, Peroxidase linked assay, direct immunofluorescent test *etc.*

Prophylaxis

Vaccination with modified live virus strains is effective (swine fever vaccine). Protection will be solid after 15-20 days post vaccination.

Treatment

There is no effective treatment of the disease. Only symptomatic treatment can be given. To reduce the temperature (Pyrexia) Inj. Boline, Inj. Melonex plus, Inj. MP3, Inj. A3 vet plus etc. (See NSAID. Antipyretics can be administered by IM route for 3-5 days. To control and combat secondary bacterial infections broad spectrum antibiotics *e.g.* Inj. Enrofloxacin (Enrored, Enrovet, Enrocin, Floxidin), Inj. Fortius (Virbac) @ 2.5-5 mg/kg body weight single injection and repeated after 72 hours. Inj. Ciprofloxacin (*e.g.* C-flox, C-flox power), Ampicillin-Cloxacillin or Amoxycillin- Cloxacillin combination for 5-7 days by IM route should be administered.

To check the diarrhoea anti diarrhoeal preparations *e.g.* Neblon, Diarex, Astrinex powder and other antibiotic and chemotherapeutic preparations like 3-Care bolus, Cyclin DT, Cflox-TZ, Biotrim DS, Pabadene Intrim, Genprim, Sulcoprim bolus *etc.* can be tried. Good quality vitamin B-complex like Inj. Hivit, Inj. Conciplex, Inj. Pinkojet, Inj. Tribivet can be administered (as rejuvenator).

A course of antihistaminic (*e.g.* Inj. Avil, Inj. Zeet, Inj. Chlorazin, Inj. Chloril) @ 3-5 ml IM for 2-3 days can be recommended.

During outbreak thorough disinfection, strict sanitary measures, disposal of carcasses and bedding materials *etc.*, efficient sterilization, prohibition of waste food fed to pigs *etc.* should be adopted.

Chapter 9

Protozoan Diseases: Their Treatment and Control

9.1 INTRODUCTION

The most important protozoan diseases of livestock are enlisted below.

1. Anaplasmosis
2. Babesiosis (Piroplasmosis)
3. Trypanosomiasis (Surra)
4. Coccidiosis

9.2 ANAPLASMOSIS

It is also known as Gall sickness caused by *Anaplasma marginale.* Anaplasmas are the parasites of RBC of sheep, goat and cattle. Based on its structure and behaviour it can also be regarded as Rickettsial group of organism, affects cattle, sheep and goat in which erythrocytes are parasitized. The disease is principally transmitted through tick bites (Ixodes) and also through Tabanus flies. The disease is severe in exotic and crossbreds. Indian breeds of cattle are carriers. The incubation period varies from 20-125 days.

Symptoms

Sudden rise in temperature upto 105°F, soon followed by dullness, anorexia, rough hair coat, cessation of milk yield, dyspnoea, tachycardia, lachrymation constipation followed by diarrhoea, abortion in pregnant animals, jaundice, anaemia (rapid and progressive anaemia) and continuous high fever are the major signs and symptoms of the disease. Animals become weak, tremble and die within 2 days to 3 weeks. Some animals may manifest aggressive symptoms attacking attendants.

Confirmation

1. Examination of blood smear by Giemsa or Leishman's stain.
2. Direct and indirect FAT (Fluorescent antibody technique)
3. CFT (Complement Fixation Test)

Treatment

All tetracyclines are equally effective for this disease. Injection Oxytetracycline HCl (Inj. Terramycin, Inj. Loxy, Inj. Brioxy), Inj. Oxytetracycline dihydrate (Inj. Intamycin), long acting Tetracycline like Oxy LA, Terramycin LA, Intamycin LA (@ 1 ml/10 kg body weight) by deep IM route for 5-7 days; IV administration of Oxytetracycline along with DNS is highly effective in the treatment of this disease.

Supportive Therapy

Oral liver tonic like Ferroliv (Excell), Tefroli (TTK) *etc.* @ 10-15 ml orally BID for sheep and goat, and @ 50 ml orally BID for cattle and buffalo. Ayurvedic liver protective and stimulant powder like Livol, Vetliv @ 50 g orally BID or injectable liver extract with B-complex *viz.* Inj. Belamyl (Sarabhai Zydus), Inj. Stronic (Vetnex), Inj. Pepsid (Concept), Inj. Ferroliv (Excell) @ 5-10 ml thrice in a week by IM route. Oral multivitamin syrup like Vimeral (Glaxo SmithKline) @ 10 ml daily or Ambiplex (Alembic) @ 20-25 ml, Tefroli (TTK), Stressvit (Excel) @ 15 ml BID for 10 days in feed or water should be recommended.

9.3 BABESIOSIS (PIROPLASMOSIS)

It is one of the most important fatal haemoprotozoal diseases of animals where the protozoan parasite inhabits the RBC, producing haemolysis, haemoglobinemia, haemoglobinuria and icterus. The haemoprotozoan parasites or the Piroplasms namely *Babesia bovis, B. argentina, B. bigemina, B. major* are the major pathogenic species of cattle and buffaloes. Main economic loss is caused in cattle and buffaloes by *B. bovis* and *B. bigemina.* The disease is mainly transmitted by cattle tick *Boophilus microplus.*

Disease caused by *Babesia bovis* is very severe and the disease caused by *B. bigemina* is less severe.

Symptoms

Fever higher than 40°C (pyrexia), red urine, haemoglobinuria, in later stages jaundice and anaemia may develop, loss of appetite, depression, weakness and reluctance to move, nervous signs sometimes develop in a condition known as 'Cerebral Babesiosis'.

The symptoms include circling, head pressing, hypersensitivity, aggression, convulsions and paralysis. When nervous symptoms develop, outcome is always fatal.

Confirmation

Simplest method to confirm infection is by laboratory examination of Giemsa stained blood smears from sick animals at the height of fever.

Treatment

Diminazine accturate is the drug of choice. Injection Nilbery (Intas) @ 8-10 mg/kg body weight or 1 ml/10 kg body weight) by deep IM Injection. Protonil (Excell), Inj. Berenil (Intervet) @ 1.5 g for 100 kg body weight (average dose 4-5 g) for adult cattle) by deep IM injection along with Inj. Copper glycinate (Curan-BH 500 mg, Care vet Pharma) in fluid is highly effective.

For equine @ 6 mg/kg body weight, dogs @ 3-4 mg/kg body weight. Berenil is the drug of choice.

If treatment is delayed supportive therapy becomes essential for the survival of animals. (1) Use of blood supplements, (2) Injectable vitamins like Hivit, Pinkojet, Conciplex *etc.*, (3) Liver extract with B-complex like Inj. Stronic, Inj. Livron, Inj. Ferroliv, (4) IV administration of fluids like Inj. Intalyte, Inj. Rintose, 10 per cent Dextrose, (5) Good nutrition and shade, (6) Antioxidants *e.g.* Vitamin E (Inj. E-Care-Se @ 10 ml one or two injections by IM route) and (7) if necessary corticosteroids can be administered.

Prevention and Control

Control of ticks by use of Cypermethrin, Flumethrin, Deltamethrin *etc.*(*e.g.* Clinar, Cyprol, Tick kill, Butox *etc.*) should be used.

9.4 TRYPANOSOMIASIS (SURRA)

Surra is a common and most dreadful haemoprotozoan parasitic disease of cattle and buffaloes. It is also known as *'Makhiki Bimari'* in Punjab. Cattle and buffaloes are considered to be main reservoir of infection due to subclinical infection.

Etiology

The disease is caused by *Trypanosoma evansi*, a monomorphic intercellular parasite, occurring in blood plasma and lymph.

Transmission

Tabanus and other biting flies mechanically transmit the diseases during monsoon and post monsoon season.

Symptoms

Depending upon the intensity of the disease, symptoms vary in peracute, acute, subacute and chronic.

Peracute form: Peracute cases characterized by high fever, abdominal pain, difficulty in breathing and groaning.

Acute form : Animals shows staggering gait, high rise of temperature, starring eyes (wide open eyes), circling movement, nervous excitement, striking the head against hard object, stamping of feet, frequent micturation, salivation, twitching of muscles, shivering of body, followed by coma, collapse and death.

Degree of parasitaemia is directly proportional to degree of fever.

Subacute and Chronic: Animals are dull and sleepy, lacrimation from eyes, emaciation, rapid pulse, intermittent fever, oedema of legs, diarrhoea and death from exhaustion.

Diagnosis

Clinical history, microscopic examination and immunological tests (ELISA, Western blotting, SDG-PAGE). Microscopic examination of lymp node smears, blood smear examination during febrile condition. Thick films stained with Giemsa reveals Trypanosomes, the flagellate extracelluar protozoa.

Treatment

A combination of Quinapyramine SO_4 and chloride is the drug of choice.

Inj.Tvansi (Vetnex) @ 7.4 mg/kg body weight by SC or Triquin Injection (Wockhardt) @ 5 mg/kg body weight by SC route should be administered. (The average dose for adult bovine 2 to 2.5 g suspended in 15 ml distilled water single dose). Besides quinapyramine SO_4 and chloride, Inj. Dimenazene aceturate and Phenazone @ 3.5-7 kg/kg body weight *viz.* Inj. Prozomin (GSK) @ 1 ml/10 kg body weight; Inj. Nilbery (Intas) @ 5 ml/100 kg body weight can be administered. Antihistaminic injection (like Avil, Zeet, Chlorazin) @ 5-10 ml IM for 2-3 days; IV infusion of Rintose, Intalyte or 10-20 per cent. Dextrose or 25 per cent Dextrose solution is recommended as a supportive therapy because Trypanosomes produce hypoglycaemia. Neurotropic B-vitamins like Inj. Polyvet, Inj. Nuroxin-12, Inj. Tribivet @ 5-10 ml by IM route is indicated.

9.5 COCCIDIOSIS

It is not at all a hemoprotozoan disease, but definitely a contagious protozoan (parasitic) disease. It is predominantly a disease of young calves caused by *Eimeria* species (mainly *Eimeria bovis* and *E. zurni*) resulting in contagious enteritis in young calves below 6 months age.

Symptoms

Disease may be acute or chronic. In acute case the calves die without any symptoms. The disease starts with sudden onset of severe diarrhoea, faeces containing mucus and blood. In chronic case the disease may last for weeks together showing anaemia, diarrhoea, dehydration and weakness.

Confirmation

Faecal examination showing oocysts of coccidian (Eimeria).

Treatment

Sulphamezathine, Sulphadiazine, Sulphadimidine, Sulphadoxine and other sulpha drugs (*viz.* Duaprim, Biotrim, Sulfa bolus, SD bolus, Sulcoprim) orally 5 gram bolus for 50 kg body weight for 3 days.

Amprolium, Amprosol (20 per cent) the @ 100mg/kg body weight daily for 5-6 days in water can also be given.

Supportive Therapy

Oral rehydration solution, ERS liquid (Excell) @ 20 ml-25 ml BID, Electrocon, Remilyte @ 2-3 ml daily. Ambiplex 5 ml daily or Lysovit 5-10 ml BID, parenteral Vitamin A Inj. like Vita A @ 2 ml IM, oral liver tonic Livtus, Livsee @ 10 ml, Livonine syrup, or injection Belamyl, Inj. Stronic, Inj. Levadex 2 ml on alternate day by IM route should be administered.

9.6 DRUGS ACTING AGAINST HAEMOPROTOZOAN PARASITES

9.6.1 Diminazine Diaceturate

Indication

Babesiosis, Trypanosomiasis, Theileriosis, mixed infections and pyrexia of unknown orign (PUO), dosages – 3.5-7.0 mg/kg body weight.

Prozomin (PM) Injection (GSK) – 30 ml vial.

Composition: Each ml contains Diminazine Diaceturate, 70 mg, Phenazone 375 mg.

Dose: For large animals (cattle and buffalo) – 30 ml IM (or 1 ml/10-20 kg body weight).

Nilbery injection (Intas) – 30 ml vial.

Composition: Diminazine diaceturate – 70 mg/ml.

Dose: 1 ml/10-20 kg body weight (3.5-7.0 mg/kg body weight) by deep IM injection.

Berenil injection (Intervet) – 20 ml vial.

Composition: Each ml contains 70 mg Diminazine diaceturate.

Dose: 20 ml for adult cattle and buffalo (1 ml/10-20 kg body weight) by deep IM injection. Besides parenteral liquid preprations, injectable powder preparations are also available.

Berenil Injection (Intervet) – 4.5 g, 22.5 g (with plastic measuring spoon).

Dose: For all species of animals 0.8-1.6 g/100 kg body weight (5 ml distilled water is added per 0.8 g/1 measuring spoon). Total dose should never goes beyond 9 g.

Protonil injection (Excell) – 5.6 g/pack.

Composition: Each g contains 4-4 Diamidihodinzo amino benzene Diacetuorate Tetrahydrate/Diminazene Aceturate – 0.444 g.

Dose: 7.37 mg/kg body weight @ 5 per cent solution.

Exotic breeds of cattle (325-350 kg body weight) 5.6 g Protonil (*i.e.* 2.4864 g Diminazine aceturate).

9.6.2 Quinapyramine Sulphate/Chloride

It is used for both curative and prophylaxis against Surra (Trypanosomiasis).

Triquin™ (Wockhardt)–Quinapyramine SO_4 and chloride injection.

Dose: 0.025 mg/kg body weight by SC route.

Triquin™ – *S* (Wockhrdt) – Quinapyramine SO_4.

Dose: 5 mg/kg body weight by SC route.

It is used for curative purpose.

Chapter 10
Parasitic Diseases: Their Treatment and Control

10.1 INTRODUCTION

Invasion of tissues by parasites produces an infection that results in diverse pathologic processes, causes severe structural and biochemical alterations in submucosa and often deeper tissues of respiratory and G.I. tract. These changes lead to further complications of bacterial infection. Chronic debility, rough body coat, indigestion, diarrhoea, retarded growth, anaemia, low milk yield, unthriftiness, convulsion, loss of disease resistance *etc.* are the effects of parasitism on the host.

10.2 INTERNAL PARASITES: THE WORMS

Worms or helminthes which are parasitic to livestock and birds belong to different taxonomic groups and invade various structures of the body and they can be elsewhere in the animal's body.

Three types of worms parasitic to livestock are

1. Nematodes
2. Trematodes and
3. Cestodes.

10.2.1 Nematodes (Round Worms)

1. G. I. Tract–Strongyles and Ascarids
2. Respiratory Tract – Lung worm (Dictyocaulus)
3. Body cavities – Filarids
4. Tumour forming – Spirocercaria.

Pathogenecity

Namatodes cause pathogenecity by making tissue damage. They penetrate and destroy mucosal cells, and severely impair the host's ability to digest (metabolism) *e.g.* strongly larvae, blood sucking (stomach worm – Haemonchus), gastroenteritis, destruction of lung tissue (Dictyocaulus), obstruction, toxic secretions and excretions, gastric and enteric pathology. Visceral larvae migrans (*i.e.* migrating stages affect lung and liver), physically obstruct the gut lumen *e.g.* (Ascarides), block the airways and impair respiratory function *e.g.* Dictyocaulus.

Ascarids

Common round worm in cattle is *Toxocara./Neoascaris vitulorum*. This does not occur in sheep and goat. Calves, pigs and goats are affected with ascarids.

Symptoms

Both adult worms and the migrating larvae can produce tissue damage or injury to host. Migrating larvae may produce cough by damaging lungs. Animals feel exhaustion or tires easily.

Adult worms – Symptoms exhibited are poor growth, pot belly, loss of appetite, loss of weight, low resistance to disease, unthriftiness, a tendency to diarrhoea and colic, diarrhoea with mucous or blood clots, anaemia, and exhaled air will be of garlic odour. The skin is rough and hairs may drop from the body coat (alopecia). Jaundice may occur due to intestinal obstruction. Calves usually suffer from diarrhoea, anaemia, alopecia and stunted growth.

Diagnosis

Examination of faeces for ova (eggs) and larvae in sputum.

Treatment

The following groups of anthelmintics are effective against ascarids as described below.

1. *Piperazine* @ 100 mg/lb body weight (10 g/100 lb body weight)

   The trade names of this group of drug are –

   Knock-45 (Piperazine hydrate) @ 15 ml/25 kg body weight for calf.

   Bripazine (Piperazine hydrate) @ 15-20 ml for calf. It is effective against the larvae and parasites in the gut but not effective against the visceral larvae migrating through the tissues.

   Piperazine hydrate (Glaxo) @ 5 ml/10 kg body weight (45 per cent solution).

   Piperazine adipate powder @ 8-10 g (in solution form) orally, repeat at monthly interval up to six months.

2. *Fenbendazole* (Fentas plus 150 mg, Panacur 150 mg) @ 1 tab/30 kg body weight.

   For adult cattle the dose of fenbendazole should be @ 7.5 mg/kg body weight.

3. *Albendazole* (Wormer, Albomar, Suprazole Suspension) @ 2 ml/kg body weight.

   For adult cattle the dose of albendazole should be @ 7.5 mg/kg body weight.

4. For visceral larvae migrans, *Ivermectin* injection (Inj. Parid, Hitek, Neomec, Virbamec, Conmectin, Vectin) @ 1 ml/50 kg body weight SC is highly effective. Besides oral use, use of Ivermectin pour on drop Ipour (Ranbaxy) @ 1 ml/10 kg body weight poured on the back midline from shoulder to sacrum is effective.

Gastro-intestinal Worms

The followings are common G.I. nematodes of cattle, sheep and goat.

Stomach Worms

- ☆ Mecistorrus species – cattle
- ☆ Haemonchus sp. – More in sheep and goat
- ☆ Medium stomach worm – *Ostertagia* sp.
- ☆ Small stomach worm – *Trichostrongylus* sp.

Intestinal Worms

- ☆ Very small worms – *Cooperia* sp.
- ☆ Hook worms – *Bunostomum* sp.
- ☆ Thread worms – *Strongyloides* sp.
- ☆ Nodular worms – *Oesophagostomum* sp.
- ☆ Large mouthed bowel worms – *Chabertia* sp.

Pathogenesis and Symptom

Stomach Worm

Haemonchus species is known as stomach worm. Food source is blood. Larvae burrow in the abomasum. Young worm sucks blood, and often causes heavy blood loss. Anaemia may be slight or severe especially in terminal stages. Diarrhoea, constipation, anaemia, weakness, weight loss and death may occur.

Ostertagia Species

Food source is tissue and mucus. Larvae may encyst in gastric glands. Encysted larvae emerge and develop to adults. Persistent diarrhoea, anaemia, unthriftiness and weight loss are predominant signs.

Bunostomum Species (Hook worm)

Food source is blood. Larval skin penetration causes local irritation. Diarrhoea, anaemia, weakness and death are predominant signs.

Trichostrongylus Species

Food sources are tissue, mucus and blood. Tissue migration causes many complications. Trichostrongylus causes destruction of abomasal mucosae including gastric pits. Mainly epithelial damage and desquamation, diarrhoea and polycythaemia are seen.

Cooperia Species

Food sources are blood and tissue. Mucosal penetration in small intestine and intestinal mucosa, desquamation of epithelial mucosa and secondary anaemia with heavy infections are seen.

Chabertia Species

They feed on tissue and cause tissue damage on migration. They cause blood loss, anaemia and loss of weight.

Strongyloide Species

Strongyloidosis is a helminthic disease of cattle and sheep caused by *Strongyloids papilosus*. The larva enters the body via skin and through capillaries and carried to the lungs through oesophagus, trachea and cause heavy infection.

Symptoms

Coughing, diarrhoea, entertis, abdominal pain, anorexia and loss of weight.

Diagnosis

Examination of faecal sample (for Gastro Intestinal Nematodiosis).

Treatment

Treatment may be done with various groups of anthelmintics as described below.

1. *Albendazole* @ 5 mg/kg body weight orally to be given to all the animals in case of G.I. nematodes and repeat it after three weeks (Albendazole bolus like Analgon, Wormer, Suprazole, Albidol, Albomar *etc.*, 1.5 g to 3 g bolus for adult cattle and buffalo and for calf, sheep and goat Albendazole tab 150-200 mg or suspension to be fed.
2. *Oxfendazole* (*viz.* Axefendol suspension 2.265 per cent w/v) @ 1 ml for 5 kg body weight for cattle and sheep, 1ml for 2.25 kg body weight for horse, and 1 ml for 3.20 kg body weight for goat can be used.
3. *Ivermectin* injection @ 200 mg (microgram)/kg body weight SC (or 1 ml/50 kg body weight) like Virbamec Alverin, Conmectin, Mectin, Neomec, Parid, Hitek, Trumutin @ 0.2 mg/kg body weight single injection is very much effective against all G.I. nematodes.
4. *Fenbendazole* (Panacur, Allclear, Fenbezole, Fentas) @ 10-15 mg/kg body weight.
5. *Levamisole* (Regain bolus) @ 5 mg/kg body weight can also be used.

Lung Worm

The other major round worm of cattle and sheep is the lung worm (*Dictyocaulus viviparous/D. filariae*). The worms may physically block the airways and impair respiratory function. Dictyocaulus species (Lung worm) feeds on tissue and mucus and causes catarrhal bronchitis, chronic cough and lobular pneumonia. Exudates block the bronchioles, and bronchial rales are audible as such. Verminous pneumonia in sheep and goats are caused by *Dictyocaulus filariae, Mullerius capillaries* and *Protostrongylus rufescens.*

Treatment

Treatment may be done with various groups of anthelminthics as described below.

1. *Albendazole* (Albomar, Analgon, Suprazole, Wormer *etc.*) @ 7.5-10 mg/kg body weight.
2. *Ivermectin* Injection (Parid, Hitek, Neomec, Virbamce, Alverin, Trumectin) @ 1 ml/50 kg body weight or 0.2 mg/kg body weight.
3. *Levamisol* (Lemasol-75, Kalmisol) @ 3.9 mg/kg body weight SC (Average dose is 10 ml SC or Regain bolus 1.5 g orally (5-10 mg/kg body weight) for large animal.
4. Fenbendazole (Panacur, Fentas, Fenbezole) @ 5-7 mg/kg (for adult lung worms only).
5. Oxfendazole suspension (2.265 per cent w/v) (Axefendol) @ 1 ml/5 kg body weight for cattle and sheep and @ 1 ml/3.20 kg for goat can be used.

Nodular Worm

Oesophagostomum species causes helminthic disease in sheep, goat and cattle and is found in colon cause severe persistent diarrhoea, dropping of mucus and blood, loss of body condition, formation of nodules which may be palpated through rectum. Anaemia, emaciation, persistent diarrhoea with mucous and blood clot and straining at defecation are predominant signs of Nodular worm/or Oesophagostomiasis.

Treatment

Like other G.I. Nematodiasis as stated above.

Heart Worm

Dirofilaria immitis is known as heart worm. Dogs usually are the sufferer of Dirofilariasis.

Treatment

Ivermectin injection (Trumectin, Ivermectin, Hitek *etc.*) @ 0.05 to 0.2 ml/10 kg body weight in precardiac stage of Dirofilaria is very much effective.

(Exact dose – 0.2 mg/kg body weight).

Hook Worm

Hook worm in dogs is a common problem, caused by *Anchylstoma caninum.*

Treatment

Treatment may be done with various groups of anthelmintics as described below.

1. *Ivermectin* injection (*e.g.* Trumectin, Hitek, Neomek *etc.*) @ 0.05 to 0.2 ml/10 kg body weight SC.

2. *Levamisol HCl* is also effective @ 8 mg/kg body weight orally. Injection Vemasol-75, Kalskisol *etc.* by SC route @ 1 ml/10 kg body weight can be administered.

10.2.2 Trematodes (Flukes)

Fascioliasis and Distomiasis

Trematodes are commonly known as *flukes* and they are mainly Liver flukes and Rumen flukes, which are common in certain areas where marshy lands, tanks and ponds are more. Intermediate host is small.

Liver flukes are

1. *Fasciola hepatica* (Host – sheep, goat, cattle and most other mammals)
2. *Fasciola gigantica* (Host – sheep, goat and cattle).

Stomach flukes are *Cotylophoron cotylophorum.* They invade rumen and reticulum of ruminants. Infection occurs after grazing on pasture contaminated by infective Metacercariae. The infective form of the flukes is Cercaria that escapes from the snail and encyst on garbage. This is called Metacercaria which are swallowed by the grazing animals. These immature flukes tunnel through liver tissue and feed themselves on liver tissue and damage the blood vessels. Sometimes the extensive damage and bleeding leads to sudden death of the animals which are not commonly diagnosed and treated in the field practice.

Immature flukes are more dangerous and cause great damage while wandering through liver and cause liver cirrhosis, anaemia, and bottle jaw. Among the ruminants cattle and sheep are more susceptible than the goats. Cattle usually suffer with chronic form. Digestive disturbances, diarrhoea with emaciation, anaemia, reduced milk yield, rough coat and loss of appetite are usual symptoms.

In acute form the animal die suddenly with blood discharge from anus. In chronic case liver gets enlarged. There will be marked anaemia, hypoproteinemia, fall of calcium and phosphorus level and metabolic energy, pot belly and submandibular oedema.

Treatment

Flukicides are to be used when they remain in the bile duct. Treatment may be done with various groups of flukicides as described below.

1. The most accepted flukicides when they remain in the bile duct is *Oxyclozanide.*

   Dose – 10-15 mg/kg body weight.

   Zanil (GSK) @ 1 ml Zanil suspension/3 kg body weight. It is very good for Distomiasis.

   Nilzan suspension @ 1 ml/3 kg body weight.

   Distonex (Neospark) suspension @ 1 ml/3 kg body weight.

   Neozide (Intas) @ 90 mg/300 kg body weight for cattle.

Neozide Plus (Intas) @ 1 ml/4 kg body weight for sheep and goat.

Distodin Tab -100 mg @ 1-2 tab once only for sheep and goat.

2. *Rafoxanide* is also a very good flukicidal drug (*viz.* Rafoxin, Ranide–10 g powder suspended in 80 ml water).

   Dose – Young animal 20-50 ml, adult 75-80 ml.
3. *Triclabendazole* is the drug of choice for both mature and immature flukes. It is safer than Oxyclozanide. Fluzic suspension – 90 ml for adult cattle or Helino (Triclabendazole + Levamisol) (Intas) @ 1 ml/5 kg body weight for sheep, goat and cattle. Fluzic Bolus 900 mg (Vetnex) @ 12-15 mg/kg body weight may be used.
4. *Albendazole* (Anlgon, Suprazole, Albidol, Albomar *etc.*) @ 10-15 mg/kg body weight is also effective.
5. *Closantel* (Xycloz) @ 1 ml/10 kg body weight or Zenvet bolus (Intas) @ 15 mg/kg body weight is also effective. Zenvet (Closantel 15 per cent w/v) @ 1-1.5 ml/10-15 kg body weight can also be tried.

Paramphistomiasis

Paramphistomiasis is a serious helminthic problem and livestock industry suffers heavy losses due to this infection. The mature ones in the fore stomach are less harmful, while immature counterparts in the abomasum and small intestine are highly pathogenic causing disease condition known as immature paramphistomiasis. Sheep and goats are most susceptible to this worm infestation. The worms cause patchy haemorrhages at the pyloric part of abomasum, patchy haemorrhages and marked thickening of duodenal mucosa, and thickening of ileum. The symptoms produced by the worms are anaemia, emaciation, debility, submandibular oedema and diarrhoea with blood.

Treatment

Treatment may be done with various groups of anthelmintics as described below.

1. Tolzan-F (Oxyclozanide) @ 10 mg/kg body weight or Distodin (Hexachlorophene) (Pfizer) @ 10-15 mg/kg body weight. In general for sheep and goat – 1-2 tablets only once. Or Hexanide bolus 1000 mg @ 1 bolus/65 kg body weight.
2. Albendazole (Analgin, Wormer, Suprazole, Albomar) @ 10-15 mg/kg body weight is also effective.
3. Rafoxanide 20 per cent water dispersible powder suspended in 80 ml of water. Sheep and Goat – 10-20 ml (@ 7.5 mg/kg body weight).
4. Tolzan plus (Oxyclozanide + Tetramisole compound) (Intervet) @ 10 ml/30 kg body weight. Or 0.33 ml/kg body weight orally or Nilzan suspension (Oxycloxamide + Tetramizole) @ 30 ml/100 kg body weight for cattle and buffalo.

Amphistomes

There are also the flukes mainly found on the wall of rumen and reticulum, causing an important parasitic disease known as Amphistomiasis in cattle, buffalo, sheep and goat caused by Cotylophoron, Gastrothylax, Paramphistomum *etc.* Immature flukes are very pathogenic. Adult parasites are harmless.

Symptoms

The immature flukes cause severe enteritis. Heavy infestation causes even death of the individual. Anaemia, emaciation, diarrhoea with blood and mucous, submandibular oedema (bottle jaw) and general debility are the usual signs. Mortality is very high in small ruminants (sheep and goat).

Treatment and Prophylaxis

Rafoxanide (7.5 mg/kg body weight), Niclosamide, Oxyclozanide (10-15 mg/kg body weight) are the drug of choice. Albendazole and even Closantel are also effective in amphistomiasis.

Line of treatment is same as Fascioliasis.

1. Rafox plus suspension,Vet Alben R, Nilzan are very much effective.
   Dose – 10-15 mg Oxyclozanide per kg body weight.
2. Olgard (Intas) – (Triclabendazole + Ivermectin) @ 1 ml/5 kg body weight can be used in case of sheep and goat.

Nasal Schistosomiasis

It is otherwise known as Nasal Granuloma, caused by blood flukes namely *Schistosoma nasale*. The eggs and parasites give rise to inflammation of nasal mucosa and produce cauliflower like growth.

Symptoms

Granulomatous growth in the nasal chambers causes dyspnoea, sneezing and snoring (stenotic) sounds and respiratory distress. The disease is transmitted through the snail as intermediate host.

Diagnosis

Faecal examination and examination of nasal discharge.

Treatment

The drug of choice is Lithium Antimony Thiomalate.

Anthiomaline or Lithiomony injection (6 per cent) @ 10-15 ml by deep IM 4-6 occasions at an interval of 3-4 days. The injection sites should be changed on alternate occasions. Injection XLT 4 per cent (30 ml vial) (Excell) along with dextrose saline by slow IV has been claimed to be effective too.

10.2.3 Cestodes (Tapeworms)

Tapeworm is common in young calves, sheep, goat and dog. Moniezia are the common tapeworms of sheep, goat and calves. *Avitellina* species are also common.

Calves under six months of age are mostly affected. Worms resides in the gut lumen and absorbing the nutrients from host's food lead to weakness, debility and nutritional deficiency.

Symptoms

Unthriftiness, vague digestive troubles, diarrhoea, pot bellied appearance (ascites), rough body coat and paralysis are recorded. Cucumber seed like segments and even long segments and tape like worms are also voided through faeces. Dog rubs its anus on the ground.

Treatment

Dichlorophene, Niclosamide, Praziquental, Albendazole are the drug of choice.

1. Albendazole (*viz.* Wormer, Albomar, Suprazole, Wormpar, Kalbend, Endoban) @ 10-20 mg/kg body weight orally.
2. Oxfendazole @ 5 mg/kg body weight.
3. Rafoxanide @ 3-7.5 mg/kg body weight. Cestophen (Dichlorophene) @ 0.2 g/kg body weight for cattle and buffalo, and 0.5 g/2.5 kg body weight for sheep and goat.
4. Fenbendazole (Fentas, Fenbezole, Panacur) @ 6 mg/kg body weight. Fentas Plus tablet (Fenbendazole + Praziquintal) 200 mg is also effective in sheep, goat and calf. Fentas Plus suspension @ 1 ml/3 kg body weight can also be drenched.
5. Ayurvedic medicine like Wopell (Indian Herbs) @ 25 g as a single dose and Wormena powder (Bioherbs), Helmex powder (Vetmed) @ 50 g for sheep, goat and calf may be used safely.
6. For dog – Eazypet (Intas) combination of Praziquantel, Pyrantel pamoate and Tenbendazole) @ 1 tab/10 kg body weight is recommended. For the best result two oral treatments two weeks apart are advised. Besides Eazypet,.Prazisom Tablet can also be used. Tablet Plozin @ 1 tab/10 kg body weight or Tab Praziplus @ 1 tab/10 kg body weight.
7. Cestophene suspension 20 per cent w/v (Pearl chemical) @ 30 ml/500 ml bottle.

   Dose – Cattle and Buffalo calf – 0.1 ml/kg body weight.

   Cestophene tab (Dichlorophen 0.5 g tab) @ 0.2 g/kg body weight for dog and cat; and 0.3-0.5 g/kg body weight for cattle, buffalo, sheep and goat.

Supportive therapy with liver extract with B-complex is beneficial to rejuvenate body condition and to boost up liver function. Injection Belamyl, Inj. Stronic, Inj ND Plex-L *etc.* @ 5-10 ml IM twice in a week or ayurvedic liver tonic like Vetliv, Livol, Liv-52 tonic should be fed.

Table 1: Common Internal Parasites in Domestic Animals

Abomasum	:	*Hemonchus contortus, H. bubalis, H. placei, Mecistocirrus digitatus, Ostertagi, Trichostrongylus, Metastrongylus, O. ostertagi* (cattle, buffalo and sheep), *O. lyrata* (sheep, goat and cattle) *O. gruhneri* (sheep and goat), Marshallagia–*M. Marshallia* (sheep and goat), Mecistocirrus–*M. digitatus.*
Intestines	:	Amphistomes (more than 12 species) *Paraamphistomes explanatum*, Nematodirus sp., *Neoascaris vitulorum, Bunostomum phlebotomum, Strongyloides papillosus, Bunostomum trigonocephalum, Gaigeria pachyscelis, Cooperia punctata*, Paracooperiosis (*P. nodulosa*), Visceral schistosomiasis, Oesophagostomum sp., *Taenia pisiformis, Monezia* sp. *Paramphistomum* sp. (Intestinal flukes).
Liver	:	*Fasciola hepatica, F.gigantica* (Snail vector – *Lymnea auricularia*).
Nasal cavity	:	*Schistosoma nasale.*
Blood	:	*Schistosoma* sp. (Blood flukes)
Lungs	:	Lung worms *Dictyocaulus* sp., Mullerius, Protostrongylus, *Paragonimus* sp. (Lung flukes).

Small Intestines

- ✰ *Cooperia oncophora* (cattle)
- ✰ *Cooperia curticei* (sheep and goat)
- ✰ *Cooperia punctata* (cattle)
- ✰ Nematodirus sp.–*N. fillicollis* (sheep and goat)
- ✰ *N. spathigar* (sheep and goat)

Bunostomum

- ✰ *B. trigonocephalum* (sheep and goat)
- ✰ *B. phlebotomum* (cattle)
- ✰ Gaigeria–*G. pachyscelis* (sheep and goat)
- ✰ Strongyloides–*S. papillosus* (sheep, goat, cattle and buffalo)

Chabertia Species

- ✰ Oesophagostomum –

  O. columbianum (sheep and goat)

  O. venulosum (sheep and goat)

  O. radiatum (cattle and buffalo)
- ✰ Toxocara –

  T. vitulorum (cattle and buffalo)

  T. canis (dog)

Gastro Intestinal Tract

G.I. Nematodes – Trichostrongylus sp., *Metastongylus* sp. *Cooperia* sp., *Nematodirus* sp., *Neoascaris vitulorum, Oesophagostomum* sp., *Chabertia* sp., *Bunostomum* sp., *Capillaria* sp., *Trichuris* sp., *Strongyloides* sp., *Hylostrongylus rubidus, Ascaris suum*

G.I. Tapeworm – Moniezia sp.

Heart: Heart worm – *Dirofilaria immitis* (Dog)

Kidney: Kidney worm – *Dioctophyma renale*

Eye: Oxyuris equi (Pin worm), *Thelazia* sp.

Mesenteric Artery: Strongylus vulgaris (larvae)

Stomach worm: Haemonchus contortus (sheep and goat)

Brown stomach worm: Ostertagia circumcincta

Hook worm: Ancylostoma caninum

Whip worm: Trichuris vulpis

Brown stomach worm: *Ostertagia circumcincta*

10.3 DEWORMING SCHEDULE OF ANIMALS

Deworming should be done regularly following a schedule. The deworming schedules of various categories of animals are given in the following sections.

10.3.1 Deworming Schedule for Cattle and Buffalo

Physiological Stages of Cattle and Buffalo	*Deworming Schedule*
Calf	At 15-21 days of age and thereafter every month
Heifer	Once every 2-3 months
Adult Cattle/Buffalo	Once every 3-4 months
Pregnant cow/Pregnant she buffalo	5th month of pregnancy and 2 weeks after calving.
Post parturition cow and she buffalo	2 weeks post calving, to be repeated twice at one month interval.

10.3.2 Deworming Schedule for Sheep and Goat

Physiological Stages of Sheep and Goat	*Deworming Schedule*
Kid/Lamb	4, 8 and 12 weeks.
Adult Sheep and Goat	Once every 2 to 3 months
Pregnant Doe/Ewe	4th month of pregnancy and 2 weeks pre lambing and kidding.
Post kidding/lambing	4 weeks pre-lambing or kidding.

10.3.3 Deworming Schedule for Pig

Physiological Stages of Pig	*Deworming Schedule*
Young	5-6 weeks, repeat after 4 weeks.
Adult pig	Once every 3 to 4 months
Pregnant Sow	1 week pre farrowing
Post farrowing	5-6 weeks post farrowing

10.3.4 Deworming Schedule for Dog

Physiological Stages of Dog	Deworming Schedule
Pup	1st at 2 weeks age, repeat after 2 weeks; 2nd at 2 months age.
Adult dog	Once every 3-4 months.
Pregnant Bitch	2 weeks pre whelping
Post whelping	2 weeks post whelping.

10.4 ECTO PARASITISM (DISEASES CAUSED BY ECTOPARASITES)

Ectoparasites represent one of the most costly nuisances for livestock holders. The common veterinary ectoarasites that cause menace to the livestock industry are the ticks, lice, flies, fleas and mites. These parasites cause constant irritation, itching, alopecia, dermatitis and so many nuisances if not controlled in time. It affects production of the livestock greatly. Flies cause myasis, blood loss, irritation, annoyance and above all disease transmission.

10.4.1 Types of Ectoparasites of Veterinary Importance

1. *Fleas:* These ectoparasites cause irritation, annoyance, allergy and disease transmission (*viz.* Mastitis, Keratoconjunctivitis).
2. *Lice:* These ectoparasites cause annoyance and irritation, hair loss, broken hairs, moth eaten coat.
3. *Ticks:* These ectoparasites cause blood loss, irritation, toxicity, tick paralysis anaemia and disease transmission (Haemoprotozoan infections) *viz.* babesiosis, anaplasmiosis, dermatophilosis, theileriosis and heart water.
4. *Mites:* These ectoparasites cause mange mites cause skin disease, irritation, scab, scaly legs, itching, crusting lesions, loss of hair, debility *etc.*

In general ectoparasitism is basically a flock disease rather than one of the individual animals. External parasites harm (affect) animals in many ways including irritation, blood sucking, destruction of tissues and spread of associated diseases.

Disease Transmission by External Parasites

Disease	Vector	Causal Agent	Species Affected
Babesiasis	Vector is ticks	*Babesia* sp.	Cattle, Sheep, Goat, Horse and Pig.
Analplasmosis	Vector is ticks	*Anaplasma* sp.	Cattle, Sheep, Goat, Horse and Pig
Tick Pyaemia	Ticks	*Staphylococcus aureus*	Lamb
Tuleraemia	Ticks	*Pasteurella tulerense*	Sheep
Brucellosis	Ticks	*Brucella* sp.	Cattle, Goat and Pig

Contd...

Disease	*Vector*	*Causal Agent*	*Species Affected*
Tick Borne fever	Ticks	*Rickettia* sp.	Dog and Cat
Epizootic bovine abortion	Ticks	Virus	Cattle
Oncocercosis	Flies	Filarid worm	Sheep
Blue tongue	Culicoides	Virus	Sheep
Ephemeral fever	Biting midges	Virus	Cattle
Japanese Encephalitis-B	Culicoides mosquitoes	Virus	Pig and Human

10.3.2 Medicines Used for Ectoparasitic Control

External antiparasite drugs are used to control flies, fleas, grubs, ticks and mange mites on livestock. Most of the compounds are toxic to animals, hence these are to be used very carefully.

Insecticides and External Parasite Formulation

Insecticides and anti external parasites are available in many formulations as follows.

Flea products: Collars, Powders, Dips, Aerosol sprays, Pump sprays, Baths, Foggers, Foams, Pourons, Dropons and even Rollons.

Insecticides: Pour-on products, Dips, impregnated ear tags.

Method of Application

Pouring, spraying, dipping, swim bath, hand bath *etc.*

Trade Names

1. *Pestoban* (Indian Herbs): It is a herbal acaricide. It should be diluted in the ratio of 1 : 10 dilution for application on animal body. It is very much effective on *Boophilus micropluse.*
2. *Dicosul Liquid Spray* (Pear chemical) – 30 ml, 50 ml, 100 ml, 500 ml and 1 litre

   It is a liquid combination of Dichlorophen, Coumaphos and Sulphanilamide. Indications are control of ticks, sucking and biting lice, sheep keds, fleas, mange mites, biting and sucking flies, fly larvae in wounds.
3. *Ektomin* (Novartis) – 15 ml, 50 ml and 1 litre bottle

   It should be diluted @1-2 ml per litre of water for application on animal body as topical spray.
4. *Citox Liquid* (Oxen labs) – 15 ml, 50 ml and 1 litre

   It contains Cypermethrin 10 per cent E.C.

   Dose: 1-2 ml/litre of water for spray or bath.
5. *Clinar* (Glaxo Smithkline) – 5 ml, 15 ml and 50 ml

   It contains Cypermethrin 10 per cent E.C. for external use only as spray or dip or bath (hand bath) @ 1-2 ml/litre of water.

6. *TIK-KIL powder* (Indian Immunologicals) – 5 g sachet/pouch to be mixed in water and sprayed on the animal.

   Each gram contains Cypermethrin high cis 10 per cent w/v.

   For external use – Cattle 5 g/litre back line spray per animal.

   Camel – 1 g/litre of water.
7. *Megacide vet* (Venky's) – 15 ml, 50 ml and 1 litre

   For whole body spray/wash in case of sheep and goat.
8. *Butox liquid* (Intervet)

   It is a deltamethrin compound, effective against all kinds of ectoparasites.

Type of Ectoparasites	*Dose for Spray*	*Dose as a Dip*
Ticks and Flies	2 ml/litre of water	3 ml/litre of water
Mites	4 ml/litre of water,	
Repeat after 8 days	6 ml/litre of water,	
Repeat after 8 days		
Lice	1 ml/litre of water	1 ml/litre of water

9. *Ticomax* (Vetnex): It contains fenvalerate 20 per cent EC. It can be used as an acaricide.
9. *Gammaxine*: Application of *Gammaxine* dust 5 per cent combined with hand picking of ticks is the safest method.
10. Other drugs like Malathion, Sumithion and Asuntol can also be used. But all these are deadly poisons, to be applied externally with due precautions and giving mouth tie or net.

    Malathion (Cynamider) 50 per cent w/v

    0.1 per cent solution for spraying over animals body, 2 per cent solution for spraying over cattle shed.

    Sumithion (Tata Fison) 50 per cent w/v

    For spraying 50 ml in 20 litre of water for lice and mites.

    Asuntol (Bayers) and *Neguvon* (Bayers) – 0.15 per cent solution as spraying is effective against ticks and lice.
11. Some safe ectoparasiticide are *Bayticol Pour* on drop (Pfizer), *Poron* (Bayer) for topical use and *Flupor* (Vetnex) pour on the back or for topical drip application.

    Each ml contains Flumethrin – 10 mg.
12. *Ivermectin Injection* (Avermectin, Alverin, Neomec, Clovotin, Virbamec, Alverin Plus, Parid, Hitek, Ivomac, Ivectin) @ 1 ml/50 kg body weight is safe and can be used for control and prevention of ectoparasites including mange and mites.

    (*See the drug index for ectoparasiticides in detail*).

Chapter 11
Nutritional Diseases: Their Treatment and Control

11.1 VITAMINS DEFICIENCY DISEASES

All the vitamins (fat and water soluble vitamins) are essential micronutrient for animals and plays vital role in normal functioning of animal body, for maintenance, growth, health and production performances. In ruminants, fortunately, most of the vitamins are synthesized either by ruminal microbes or by the host animal in sufficient quantities or are present in required amount in the feeds and fodders of livestock. Green forages are rich source of Beta (β) carotene, Pro-vitamin-A, and if available in sufficient amount can met the demand of vitamin A requirement of the animal. Vitamin A may lead to reproductive failure in both male and female due to change in epithelia involved. Ruminants appear to be more sensitive to vitamin B_{12} deficiency than the non-ruminants, largely because of their dependence on gluconeogenesis to meet up the needs of tissue glucose and vitamin B_{12} dependent enzyme is required for this process. Vitamins occupy key and indispensible position in maintenance of normal reproductive system of the animal body. Deficiency of vitamins leads to reproductive disorders like anoestrus, repeat breeding, abortion, delayed puberty, ovarian degeneration.

In this chapter some of the vitamins and their features are presented in tabular form (Table 11.1). Besides, the most important vitamin deficiency diseases are discussed here. The formularies containing different vitamins either oral or parenteral uses have been given in Veterinary Drug Index (Chapter 19).

Table 11.1: Some of the Vitamins and their Important Features

Vitamin	*Physiological Functions*	*Deficiency Disorder and Remedy*
Vitamin A	Maintains the normal structure and function of epithelium of reproductive and other organs of the body.	Infertility in breeding animals Abortion or production of dead, weak or blind calves. Treatment: Inj. Vitamin A (*e.g.* Veta-A, Prepaline Fort), Inj. Vitacept, Inj. Vetade, Inj. Intavita @ 5-10ml I/M twice weekly.
Vitamin E	Supports reproduction and acts as antioxidant	Reproductive failure Inj. E-Care-Se (Vetnex) @ 10 ml intramuscularly twice weekly for 2 weeks; Inj. ADEVET, Inj. Vet ADE, Inj. Intavita @ 5-10 ml intramuscularly twice in a week can also be given.
Vitamin B_2	Plays role in cellular oxidation. It has direct effect on metabolism of carbohydrates and amino acids.	Decreased fertility (good quality product of B-complex) *e.g.* Inj. Hivit, Inj. Coniplex, Inj. Pinrojet @ 10 ml intramuscularly daily or on alternate day can be given.
Vitamin B_{12}	Maintenance of ovum and sperm production	Infertility Inj. Polyvet, Inj. Trinural-H, Inj. Neurovet @ 5-10 ml intramuscularly on alternate day should be given.
Vitamin H (Biotin)	Gluconeogenesis, Fatty acid synthesis activation of enzyme systems involved in amino acid metabolism	Ill hoof health, rough skin and congenital foetal abnormalities. Treatment: Inj. Intavita-H (Intas) @ 5-10 ml at 3 days interval.
Vitamin D_3	Calcium and Phosphorus absorption, better bone growth.	Rickets, predisposing milk fever. Treatment: Inj. Intavita, Inj. ADE Vet, Inj. Vitacept @ 5-10 ml intramuscularly at 2 days interval.

11.1.1 Hypovitaminosis A (Vitamin A Deficiency Disease)

Primary Vitamin-A deficiency is of major economic importance in animals. Animals at pasture or maintained on greens, receive adequate supplies of Vitamin A or its precursors except during prolonged drought when animals confined indoors (zero grazed animals) and stall fed may be deficient if not adequately supplemented. Secondary Vitamin A deficiency may occur in cases of chronic disease of the liver or intestine.

Role of Vitamin A

Vitamin A is functional in almost all tissue cells of the body for different functions and is essential for normal epithelial development. It is essential in muscle cells and other somatic cells for growth and multiplication, reproductive cells of ovary and testicles for reproduction and retina of eye for visual function.

Deficiency Symptoms

Hypovitaminosis is characterized by night blindness, xerophthalmia, retarded growth rates, failures and increased mortality. In new born calves blindness, with dilated pupils, nystagmus, weakness and incordination are characteristic. Other deficiency symptoms are scouring, low resistance to bacterial infection, stiffness of joints and in-coordinated movements (staggering), lesions around the eyes, dull watery eyes followed by night blindness in advanced stages.

Vitamin A Deficiency Disease Recorded in Different Species

1. *Night blindness*: Inability to see in dim light, twilight or moonlight night is the early sign in all species.
2. *Blindness*: The first sign of ocular form of the disease is blindness in both eyes. Both pupils are exophthalmic and excessive lacrimation may be evident.
3. *Xerophthalmia*: Thickening and clouding of the cornea occurs only in calf. In other species a thin, serous mucoid discharge from the eyes occurs followed by ulceration and photophobia.
4. *Parakeratosis*: In cattle, X-disease or hyperkeratosis occurs, characterized by Keratinization of skin affecting the dermis; abnormal epithelial lining with reduced feed intake, slow growth, diarrhoea and disease susceptibility.
5. *Reproductive failure*: Both male and females are affected equally. In male there is degeneration of germinal epithelium causing reduced number of normal motile spermatozoa affecting fertility. A shortened period of gestation, a high incidence of retained placentas, still births and abortions are common in vitamin A deficiency. Often calves born blind and their gaits are uncoordinated.
6. *Paralysis*: The paralytic force is manifested by abnormalities of gait due to weakness and in-coordination. The hind limbs are usually affected first and the forelimbs later. Complete limb paralysis occur terminally.

Long term deficiency of Vitamin A has overriding impact on intra-uterine foetus. Anoestrum, repeat breeding, congenital anomalies, pituitary hyperplasia and still births are certain outcome of prolonged Vitamin A deficiency.

Feeding of balanced ration with supplementation of quality fodder and or greens are imperative for optimum reproduction.

Treatment and Control

Animals should be treated immediately with Vitamin A injection. The proprietary drugs are Vita-A (TTK), Inj. Vitamin A (Legend), or injection Vitamin ADE combination, *e.g.* Inj. Intavita (Intas), Inj. Vitacept (Concept), Inj. Vet ADE (Sarabhai Zydus) *etc.* at a dose rate equivalent to 10-20 times the daily maintenance requirement. A single injection of 6000 IU aqueous Vitamin A solution/kg body weight is suggested to be adequate therapy for two months for a serious deficiency in canines; oral dose should not exceed 400 IU/kg/day for 10 days in dogs. Overdosing and over treatment may produce Vitamin A toxicity.

11.1.2 Polyneuritis

It is a neurological disorder commonly occurs due to thiamine deficiency. It is common in swine, caprine and in poultry.

Symptoms

Sudden onset of anorexia, absence of water intake, stiff gait, upward deviation of neck. Dullness, depression, Gynophobia, buldging of eyes, disinclination to move and stiff gait, typical stargazing attitude (looking to the sky) are usual signs.

Etiology

Thiamine deficiency occurs because of build up bacteria in rumen which produce on enzyme that destroys thiamine in the food before the animal can absorb it. Administration of thiamine antagonist *e.g.* Ampicillin to lambs and calves may be responsible. Thiamine deficiency may result from digestive disturbances which can block either synthesis or absorption of thiamine or by the presence of antimetabolics *viz.* flavour in onion, rice, soyabean, and thiaminase containing plants and weeds may also cause thiamine deficiency and polyneuritis.

Treatment and Control

Neurotropic B vitamins containing thiamine should be administered. *E.g.* Inj. Tribivet (Intas), Inj. Neurovet (Aldved), Inj. Neuroxin-12 (Sarabhai Zydus), Inj. Polyvet (Excel) @ 2-3 ml I/M daily and in severe cases at six hours interval for 2 days followed by @ 2 ml daily for 2-3 days by IM route can be administered. I/V infusion of dextrose 10 per cent once daily for 2-3 days can also be tried.

11.1.3 Polyencephalomalacia

It is a thiamine responsive metabolic disease sometimes occurring in young calves (cattle and buffalo) 2-12 months age group owing to thiamine inadequacy (thiamine deficiency). Both cattle and buffalo calves those are well maintained, stall fed and fed on concentrates with lack of greens are prone to such threatened malady.

Thiamine inadequacy is seldom seen in ruminants in natural condition. Young cattle 6 to 12 months of age including buffalo calves, in well nourished condition are mostly affected. An inadequate amount of roughage and increased amount of concentrate feeding can result in decreased amount of thiamine synthesis. It has a direct metabolic effect on neurons and that results in polioencephalomalacia, softening of grey matter.

Symptoms

Dullness, apparent blindness, weak, unable to bear their weight, swaying from side to side, incordination, falling easily with slight disturbances. Temperature goes down. Salivation, spisthotonus, blindness, nystagmus, aimless walking and occasional clonic convulsions etc. are the usual signs.

Diagnosis

Based on clinical signs and measuring the level of thiamine in blood.

Treatment and Control

The recommended treatment of choice is Thiamine HCl @ 10mg/kg body weight initially followed by similar doses every 3 hours for a total of five treatments. To treat the condition, neurotropic B-vitamins like Inj. Tribivet (Intas), Inj. Murovet (Alved), Inj. Neuroxin-12 (Sarabhai zydus) may be administered, on 1st day @ 10-15 ml (large dose), 2nd day @ 10 ml, 3rd day onwards @ 5 ml by IM route.

Ancillary treatment like I/V administration of DNS, 5 per cent Dextrose, antihistaminic and parenteral administration of Vitamin A, and B Complex *e.g.* Hivit, Conciplex, Hitone, Pinkojet, X-L-plex *etc.* can also be done.

Rumenotonic bolus *e.g.* Rumentus, Rumisac, Anorexon forte, On feed, Insta feed FS, Feedon, Gofeed, Rumen bolus, @ ½ to 1 bolus twice daily can also be given.

11.2 MINERAL DEFICIENCY DISEASES

There are 22 essential mineral elements out of which two macro and six micro minerals are very much important in terms of dietary supplementation for sustenance of optimum productive and reproductive performance due to their role in structural, physiological, catalytic and regulatory activity of the body mineral elements. These two macro minerals are calcium and phosphorus, and the six important micro minerals are zinc, cobalt, copper, iodine, manganese and selenium. Micromineral deficiency disorders may be acute, subacute and marginal. Animals suffering from acute or subacute deficiency may develop clinical signs and pathological changes, while it is difficult to diagnose marginal deficiencies.

11.2.1 Macromineral Deficiency

Macrominearls are required in larger quantities for various functions (Table 11.2). Out of various macro-minerals calcium and phosphorus deficiencies are more pronounced in farm animals. These are described at length in the following section.

Table 11.2: Macromineral Requirements for Cattle

Minerals	*Requirement (% Total Feed)*
Calcium	0.43-0.77
Phosphorus	0.28-0.48
Magnesium	0.20-0.25
Sodium	0.18
Chlorine	0.25
Sulphur	0.20

11.2.1.1 Deficiency of Calcium and Phosphorus

Both the elements are required in large quantity as they are the basic structural material of the skeleton. About 1 per cent of the Ca and 20 per cent of the P that remain in the body fluid and soft tissues control various physiological functions including nerve excitability, blood clotting and some enzymes. Phosphorus is required for energy metabolism as a component of energy rich compound like ADP, ATP and Creatine phosphate. Phosphorus is a component of phospholipids which are important in lipid metabolism and transport and is a constituent of cell membrane.

Deficiency symptoms are decreased growth, unthriftiness, decreased milk production, poor conception and pica in addition to skeletal abnormalities.

Lactational Osteoporosis

Demineralization of bones may occur through the mobilization of about 20 per cent calcium (Ca) and Phosphorus (P) from bones during early lactation. A negative balance of either Ca or P will demineralise bones but with different results. When calcium balance is negative, bone is promptly demineralized and the level of Ca in blood is maintained. In severe cases of calcium deficiency there will be reduced milk production and milk fever. When P is the limiting factor a reduction of inorganic P in plasma occurs and metabolism is severely disturbed.

Treatment and Control

1. Supplementation of calcium and phosphorus with feeds.

   Source: Calcium phosphate and De-fluorinated rock phosphate.

   Ca: Steamed bone meal, ground lime, De-fluorinated rock phosphate, Di-calcium phosphate.
2. Oral supplementation of Calphos D_3 Bolus (Excell).
3. Oral supplementation of calcium tonics/syrups *e.g.* Ostovet, Ostovet fort, Capsola, Calcicare, Calcimilk, Orical, Vita Calciplus *etc.*
4. Parenteral administration of injectable calcium preparation *e.g.* Inj. Orical, Inj. Brical, Inj. Cal BD, Inj. Calcinet, Inj. Synccal, Inj. Caldee-12, Inj. Capsola, Inj. Sancal *etc.* by I/M route.
5. Parenteral administration of inorganic phosphorus *e.g.* Inj. Alphos-40, Inj. Aciphos, Inj. Uremin, Inj. Sodaphos (20 per cent solution), Inj. T-Phos *etc.* by IM route (Large animal 10-15ml, Small animal 1-3ml).
6. In severe cases I/M, I/V and S/C administration of Mifex., Calmax-M, Lactomag, Mifocal *etc.*
7. Multimineral supplements *e.g.* Agrimin fort, Ranmix total, Minerin ERS Powder for 25-30 days.

11.2.2 Micro/Trace Mineral Deficiency

Trace minerals or microminerals play a significant role in animal production and reproduction. These minerals cannot be synthesized by the animal and for what these must be present in appropriate amount in the feed.

The trace minerals are related with the synthesis of vitamins, production of hormones, enzyme activity, collagen formation, tissue synthesis, oxygen transport, energy production and other physiological processes related to growth, reproduction and health.

Subclinical trace mineral deficiencies in cattle may be larger problem than an acute deficiency, because specific clinical symptoms are not evident to allow the producer to recognize the deficiency.

Table 11.3: Micromineral Requirements for Cattle

	(PPM)
Zinc (Zn)	23-63
Cobalt (Co)	0.1
Copper (Cu)	12-16
Iodine (I_2)	17-24
Manganese (Mn)	25
Selenium (Se)	0.30

Table 11.4: Influence of Cu, Zn and Mn on Fertility

Mineral	*Female*	*Male*
Cu	Delayed estrus Embryonic death Decreased conception Delayed puberty Decreased ovulation	Decreased lipids, decreased sperm production.
Zn	Increased dystocia Abnormal estrus Delayed puberty	Impaired growth, decreased libido and decreased testicular size.
Mn	Anoestrus, decreased ovarian activity, decreased conception rates and increased abortion.	Increase in abnormal sperm production.

11.2.2.1 Zinc Deficiency

Zinc is an essential micronutrient and deficiency of zinc in cattle that leads to parakeratosis, alopecia, reduced growth rate, poor hair coat and bilateral skin lesions. Zinc is known to be essential for sexual maturity, onset of oestrus, sperm quality of males and plays role in epithelial integrity, repair of uterine lining following kidding, calving and lambing, return to normal estrus cycle and implantation of embryo etc. Subclinical Zn deficiency cause decreased weight gain, reduced milk production and reduced reproductive performance.

Symptoms

Clinical manifestations may be the alopecia, bilateral wrinkling and crust formation on the skin of ear, neck, hump region, muzzle *etc*. Pathognomonic signs are bilateral symmetrical parakaratosis of skin, keratinization of epidermis and alopecia. Impaired growth, delayed puberty, decreased testicular size, decreased libido, abnormal oestrus, increased dystocia, abortion, foetal in mummification, lower birth weights, prolong labour have also been observed in bovines owing to zinc deficiency. Signs of severe zinc deficiency are listlessness, excessive salivation, swollen feet, loss of hair, failure of wounds to heal, reduced feed intake and lesions with horny growths on legs, neck, head and around nostrils.

Treatment and Control

1. Oral administration of pure zinc sulphate and topical application of zinc oxide ointment once daily can be recommended.
2. Trace minerals bolus *e.g.* Cyclomin-7, Flomine-C, Nutrisacc bolus, Minotus bolus, Minerex bolus @ one bolus daily for 10-15 days.
3. Zinc sulphate @ 250 mg total dose orally daily for 20-25 days for calves and @ 500 mg for cattle daily.
4. Mineral mixture like Minfa, Minerex-L; supplevite-M, Vitaprotein DS, CRC (Vetnex), Minameal, Minerin, Rammix total @ 25-30 g orally once daily.

5. Ancillary treatment like anti-histaminic and B-complex therapy can also be done.
6. Zinc can be supplemented as zinc oxide, zinc carbonate and zinc sulphate.

11.2.2.2 Copper Deficiency

Copper deficiency is also called *hypocuprosis*. Various levels of copper deficiency may become a serious problem for young ruminants and is characterized by multiple clinical and subclinical syndroms such an unthriftiness, coat changes, diarrhoea, lameness. It occurs in cattle and buffaloes as a primary or secondary problem owing to decreased level of copper in the diet or due to failure of copper absorption or utilization caused by an imbalance or excess of other elements in the ration respectively.

Role of Copper

Copper (Cu) has roles in several enzymatic systems and is required for normal red blood cell formation, bone formation and elastin formation in the aorta and cardiovascular system. It is important for normal expression of estrus, maintenance of pregnancy, antioxidant activities and in the formation and functionality of connective tissue such as bones, tendons and ligaments. Flaccid paralysis or progressive ataxia at birth has also been recorded in bovine calves owing to Cu deficiency.

Symptoms

Inappetance to anorexia, discoloration of skin, diarrhea, anaemia and localized alopecia. Achromtrichia (distinct areas of depigmentation), poor performance, slow growth rate, low milk production, delayed puberty, anoestrus, defective keratinization of wools and hairs, graying of black or brown hair are associated with Cu deficiency. In young animals abnormalities in bone development, spontaneous fractures, stiff gait, lameness with marked swelling of distal metatarsal and metacarpal physis, pigeon toed, stiff legged condition are seen.

In young calves ataxia, inability to suckle, in coordination, stiffgait, diarrhoea, opisthotonus *etc.* occurs whose dams are copper deficient.

Anaemia in cattle is of hypochromic and macrocytic type and which could be due to Cu deficiency. Delayed estrus, decreased libido, decreased spermatogenesis, decreased conception, delayed puberty, decreased ovulation, embryonic death *etc.* are associated with Cu deficiency.

Treatment and Control

1. Supplementation of mineral mixtures.
2. Supplementation of copper or copper sulphate (@ 1-2 g of 1 per cent $CuSo_4$ by drenching.
3. Vets cuco tab or Cofecu tab can be tried.
4. Adequate copper has to be provided to pregnant cattle to meet early post natal requirement of calf. Mineral mixtures *viz.* Minerex-L, CRC (Vetnex), Ranmix, Minfa @ 25-30 gram once daily can be tried.
5. By pass bolus (Excell) can be fed orally to the pregnant ones.

11.2.2.3 Iron Deficiency

Iron deficiency seldom occurs in adult cattle and other ruminants unless there is considerable loss of blood due to haemorrhage, blood sucking endoparasitic load and other disease conditions. Iron is abundant in all feeds and green leafy vegetables, fodders and forages. However, some roughages may be deficient or low in iron content. The daily requirement of iron in adult cattle is 20-50 ppm in adult cattle and 100 ppm in calves.

Symptoms

Anaemia, unthriftiness, impaired fertility and delay in conception.

11.2.2.4 Iodine Deficiency

It is an integral component of thyroid hormones that plays important role in the synthesis of thyroxin by the thyroid gland and regulates energy metabolism. The requirement of iodine is 0.1 ppm for ruminants.

Symptoms

Enlargement of thyroid, calves born weak or dead, reduced reproduction with irregular cycling, low conception rate, retained placenta and decreased libido and semen quality in bulls.

Iodine deficiency causes a disease known as Goitre. Anoestrus, irregular oestrus, suppressed oestrus, retention of placenta, extended gestation period, abortion and still births are usual outcome of iodine deficiency of ruminants.

Treatment and Control

1. Iodine deficiency can be checked by providing iodized salt licks.
2. Supplementation of trace mineral bolus *e.g.* Bioplex High Five, Minerex bolus, Cyclomin-7 bolus *etc.*

11.2.2.5 Selenium Deficiency

Selenium (Se) is required for maintaining integrity of cellular membranes, normal pancreatic morphology and is involved in normal absorption of lipids and tocopherols. Its functions are interrelated with Vitamin E, and it is important to the function of immune system of animals. Higher concentration of Selenium in ration (> 5 ppm) may cause chronic selenium toxicity characterized by dullness, emaciation, alopecia, soreness, gangrenous syndrome, overgrown hooves, stiffness of joints, atrophy of heart and cirrhosis of liver *etc.* Dietary requirement of Se is 0-1 ppm.

Symptoms

Selenium deficiency causes stunted growth in calves and reproductive disorder in cows. It also causes white muscle disease in calves. Deficiency symptoms in animals are stiffness, lameness and possible cardiac failure and in older animals are unthriftiness, weight loss, diarrhoea, anaemia, and reduced immune responses. Infertility, early embryonic mortality and high incidence of retained placenta are seen in cattle, which can be reduced by adding proper supplementation of selenium in feed.

Treatment and Control

Inj. E-Care-Se (Vetcare) – by IM route (Large animal @ 10 ml twice a week).

11.2.2.6 Manganese Deficiency

It is an essential trace mineral element require for the synthesis of gonadal hormones. It stimulates and activates a number of enzymes that function in carbohydrate and lipid metabolism, also stimulates a number of other enzymes. It is needed for normal bone structure, reproduction, growth and proper functioning of CNS. The daily requirement of Manganese is 20-40 ppm in the ration.

Symptoms

Impaired growth, disturbed and depressed reproductive function (*e.g.* suspension of estrus, silent heat, defective ovulation delayed ovulation, reduced conception in female and inhibition of male libido), ataxia of the new born, low birth weight, and disturbance in metabolism. There may be still birth, calf mortality and premature birth of the calf with low body weight. In males there may be testicular degeneration.

Treatment and Control

1. Give rice bran and paddy straw to animal as these are rich in manganese.
2. Trace mineral bolus *e.g.* Cyclomin7, Flomin-C, Minotus, Nutrisac bolus, Minerex bolus, Bioplex High Five bolus *etc.* @ 1-2 bolus daily for 10-15 days in cattle.
3. Manganese can be supplemented by providing salt licks containing the mineral in adequate amount.

11.2.2.7 Cobalt Deficiency

Cobalt (Co) is one of the most important micromineral, essential for the synthesis of Vitamin B_{12} in rumen by the microbes. It is also essential for the normal functioning of enzyme systems in energy metabolism. The requirement of cobalt as estimated is 0.1 ppm in the ration.

Symptoms

Loss of appetite, listlessness, loss of body weight, weakness, anaemia, general debility, emaciation, decline in milk production, reduced conception rate *etc.*

Cobalt deficiency produces 'Wasting Diseases' of cattle and sheep, characterized by severe emaciation and anaemia. Animal suffers from cellular energy deficit and become extremely emaciated.

Treatment and Control

1. Cobalt tablets like Vets cuco, Cofecu, Cumin *etc.* orally for 10-15 days.
2. Give trace mineral bolous *e.g.* Bioplex High Five, Cyclomin-7, Minerex bolous, Minotus bolous *etc.*
3. Supplementation of multiminerals preparation *viz.* K-Cmin, Grovimin, CRC (Vetnex), Kalvimin, Minfa, Ranmix, Agrimin fort *etc.* 25-30 g.
4. Cobalt can be supplemented by providing salt licks containing the mineral in adequate amount.

Chapter 12
Common Ailments and their First Aid Treatment

12.1 PNEUMONIA

Any inflammatory disease of the lungs with copious exudates filling the alveoli is called pneumonia. It is a very common disease of animals except the cat. It is the lobular pneumonia which is frequently seen in animals and different grades of pneumonia may occur with the same etiological factors too.

Etiology

Common causes are bacteria, viruses, fungai and parasites. Irritants like dust, pollen, foreign bodies, hot and cold air *etc.* may cause pneumonia in animals. Faulty drenching in cattle, aspiration of gruel, milk *etc.* may also cause pneumonia. Exposure to sudden cold and damp climate are predisposing or attributory factors to pneumonia too.

Symptoms

Dull and depression, anorexia, coughing progressive dyspnoea, moderate fever (Pyrexia), increased respiratory rate, inspiratory and expiratory dyspnoea. Auscultation may reveal moist rales, crepitating rales along the lower border of the lungs. Mucopurulent or purulent nasal discharge is commonly observed in pneumonia.

Prognosis

Prognosis is poor in advanced disease.

Treatment

An antibiotic, sulfonamides and antihistaminics are commonly used. The line of treatment is as follows.

1. Medicated inhalation to relieve expiratory distress, like oil eucalyptus in hot water.
2. Message with liniment of ammonia or camphor liniment.
3. Herbal cough mixtures for relieving pulmonary distress, bronchitis, pain and bronchial spasm.
   (*a*) Biocof (Bioherbs Pharma) – 100 g

   Cattle and Horse – 20-30 g; Sheep and Goat – 10-15 g BID or 4 times a day.

   (*b*) Caflon (Indian Herbs) – 30 g BID for cattle

   (*c*) Bronchopyrin liquid (Vetmed) – 15 ml BID for sheep and goat. Dose – Large animal – 20 ml BID x 5 days.

   (*d*) Bronchopyrin powder (Vetmed) – 25 g BID for cattle; 10 g for sheep and goat orally BID.
4. Antibiotics – namely Inj. Intamox, Inj. Lemox, Inj. Moxcell, Inj. Vetclox, Inj. Inclox, Inj. Intacef, Inj. Wocef, Inj. Alinenomycin, Inj. Enrocin, Inj. Enrovet, Inj. Cflox *etc.* may be used in proper dose and schedule.
5. Sulpha drugs like Inj. Oriprim, Biotrim, Duaprim *etc.* can be used daily for cattle and buffalo @ 15-30 ml daily [Duaprim @ 1 ml/20 kg body weight], Inj. Sulphamezathine (331/3 per cent solution), Brimdin, Diadia *etc.* (as per drug index) can be used.
6. Analgesics and antipyretics in the form of bolus or tablet and or injection should be administered. *viz.* Inj. Analgin, Inj. Valginate, Inj. Melonex, Inj. Melonex Plus, Inj. Meloxi, Inj. Proxivet, Inj. MP3, bolus like Oxalgin NP, Melonex Plus, A3vet bolus *etc.* (See the index-NSAIDS).
7. Antihistamin preparations as indicated for relieving respiratory distress, bronchial spasm *etc.* Inj. Chloril, Inj. Anistamin, Inj. Phenavil, Inj. Zeet *etc.* Corticosteroids like Inj. Dexona, Inj. Dexavet, Inj. Brisone, Curadex, Vetcort, Inj. Vetalog *etc.* (as per drug index) should be used.

12.2 FEVER

Abnormal in temperature (or elevation of body temperature) above the normal range is called fever. Long continued fever is harmful to animal body owing to breakdown and loss of proteins leading to loss in antibody producing tissues. Fever also causes degeneration of heart, liver and kidneys. In any inflammatory disease there is rise in body temperature.

Symptoms

Fever is a syndrome and besides pyrexia these are other signs and symptoms. These could be anorexia, off-fed (Hypophagia), increased pulse rate, nausea, vomiting, constipation, scanty urine, elevated thirst and dehydration.

Etiology

Causes are many and could be the endotoxins produced by Gram (- ve) organisms, Gram (+ ve) bacteria, viruses, protozoa, fungi, rickettsiae, injuries, pyrogens.

Treatment

Treatment should be carried out as per etiology. To subside the temperature antipyretics should be administered orally or parenterally. Paracetamol injection shows analgesic and antipyretic effect like salicylates.

Dose: Large animal – 10-30 ml preferably by deep IM; Small animal – 1-5 ml preferably by deep IM (see the index).

Meloxicam and Paracetamol combination like Inj. A3vet plus, Melonex plus, MP3 *etc*. @ 10-15 ml for large animal and @ 3-5 ml for small animal by deep IM or Nimesulide injection like Nimovet can be administered by IM route.

Or Combipack of Paracetamol + Analgin like Inj. Boline or Inj. Artisone, Inj. Esgipyrin can be administered.

Oral preparations like Boline bolus, Oxalgin NP, Paralgin NP, Melonex plus, A3 vet bolus *etc*. can be used @ 1 bolus per 20 kg body weight.

12.3 DIARRHOEA

Diarrhoea is not a disease. Rather it is an enteric condition or signs of a disease. In other words diarrhoea can be regarded as a natural protective response of body to expel out the toxin, irritant materials *etc*. The consequences of diarrhoea are mainly the dehydration and electrolyte loss which should be prevented while treating diarrheoa.

Etiology

Causes are many. It is invariably a sign of parasitic infections like G.I. nematodes, liver flukes, amphistomes *etc*. Bacterial infections like Pasteurellosis, Salmonellosis, Colibacillosis, *etc*. Viral etiology like B.V.D., mucosal disease, PPR *etc*. Protozoa like coccidian parasites, and irritant chemicals, stale food *etc*.

Treatment

1. *Astringent preparations* like
   - (*a*) Light Kaolin – 15 g, Calcarb – 20 g, Magcarb – 15 g.
     Mft. pulv, prepare 8 such doses (for cow).
   - (*b*) Acid Tanic – 15 g, Kaolin 30 g, Pulv. ginger – 1.5 g with gur or gruel once in 12 hrs for adult.
   - (*c*) Astrinex powder (Vetmed)
     Large animal – 25-30 g orally BID, Small animal 10-15 g orally BID.
   - (*d*) Neblon powder (Indian Herbs)
     Cattle, Buffalo and Horse – 30-50 g; Calf, sheep and Goat – 6 -10 g orally BID.
   - (*e*) Diarex powder (Dabut Ayurvet)
     Calf, Sheep and Goat – 6 -10 orally BID.
   - (*f*) 3-care bolus (Vetcare)
     Large animal 2 boli orally BID.

(*g*) Diarex tablet (Himalayan Drug)
Calf 5 tabs BID for 2-3 days.

(*h*) Fazol bolus, Furovet bolus, 0-prim bolus 1-2 boli/50 kg body weight for 3 days can be given.

2. *Sulpha drugs viz.* sulpha bolus (1-2 boli/50 kg body weight) followed by ½ dose daily, Biotrim DS (Vetnex) may be given.
3. *Broad spectrum antibiotics* like Cyelin bolus (Excell), Steclin bolus (Sarabhai) – 500 mg *etc.* Neodox bolus, Cyclin DT (Vets Farma) *etc.* can be given (as per index).
4. *ORS* or balanced electrolyte solution with potassium supplementation or parentral (IV) fluid therapy with DNS should be done.

Treatment Aspects of Diarrhoea Syndrome in Dogs

Dogs with diarrhoea are routinely seen in veterinary clinics and it is manifested with diversified etiology varying from dietary abnormality to infections and infestations. Specific therapy should be done as per etiology comprising anthelmintics, antimicrobials, antiprotozoals, babesiccidals, antirickettsial, hepatostimulant etc. as per following protocol.

Ascariasis (*Toxocara* and *Toxascaris* sp.)	:	Fenbendazole @ 100 mg/kg PO for neonates and for others @ 50 mg/kg/day for 3 days.
Hook worm (Ancylostoma and *Unicinaria dipylidium*)	:	Albendazole @ 25 mg/kg P.O. BID for 3 days.
Whip worm (*Trichuris vulpis*)	:	Praziquantel @ 10 mg/kg PO for 3 days and 15 mg/kg PO for 3 days for puppies < 6months.
Strongyloidiasis	:	Fenbendazole @ 50 mg/kg PO for 3 days. Fenbendazole @ 50 mg/kg P.O. for 5 days.
Fluke	:	Praziquantel @ 20 mg/kg or Albendazole – 50 mg/kg PO daily till faeces cleared from fluke egg (usually 10-15 days) or Fenbendazole 50 mg/kg/days for 10 days,
Coccidiosis	:	Trimethoprim-sulpha @ 30 mg/kg/days for 10 days.
Giardiasis	:	A combination of Tinidazole and Ciprofloxacin @ 7.5 mg – Tinidazole/kg PO BID for 7 days.
Chronic colitis	:	Sulphasalazine @ 15 mg/kg PO TID for 2-3 weeks
Babesiosis	:	Diminazine aceturate @ 3.5-5.0 mg/kg body weight IM once only and Clindamycin @ 25 mg/kg body weight IM and or PO BID for 4 days initially.
Ehrlichiosis	:	Doxycyclin @ 10 mg/kg PO OD for 14 days.
Hepatobilliary Disease	:	Silymarin 16 mg/kg PO BID for 3-4 weeks. Vitamin-E 400 mg PO OD for 2 weeks.
Dietary Diarrhoea	:	Stop the diet which does not suit. Give Lactobacillus orally (probiotics)
Wheat Sensitive	:	Exclusion of wheat from diet.

Contd...

Table 4.1–Contd...

Enteropathy (Glutum intolerance)	:	Rice and corn included in the diet, Folic acid and Methyleobalam in (B_{12}) are to be added.
Milk Intolerance	:	Exclusion of milks and dairy products from diet. Cereal diet with folic acid and cobalamine should be added.
Antibacterials	:	Metronidazole @ 15 mg/kg IV or PO bid for 3-4 days. Cefotaxime @ 2.5 mg/kg IV or IM BID for 3-4 days. Clindamycin @ 7-10 mg/kg IV or IM BID for 3-4 days.
Garbage Intoxication	:	Diphenhydramine @ 0.5 mg/kg IM to control emesis. Metronidazole @ 15 mg/kg PO BID For 5 days. Lactobacillus 60 X 10^6 PO BID.

12.4 CONSTIPATION

Constipation is infrequent, incomplete or difficult defecation with passage of hard or dry faeces. It is a physiological disorder characterized by the delay in expulsion of the contents of intestine.

Etiology

Change in feed, as in calves from milk to roughage, over age (senility), defective secretion at the intestinal wall, hepatic disorder, less water intake and excess intake of concentrate.

The common causes of constipation in the dog are the presence of any foreign body in colon, excessive fibre in the diet, lack of exercise, especially in older dogs, intra or extraluminal obstruction, abscessed anal glands, neurological disorder. Metabolic and endocrinological diseases, dehydration and certain drugs like diuretics, iron supplement *etc.*

Treatment

Therapy for constipation involves relieving the symptoms, treating the cause where possible. Withdrawal of hard and extremely high fibrous feed. Feeding of laxative diet for cattle.

1. Increase fluid/water intake.
2. Injection Carbacol 2-4 ml IM or SC.
3. Magnessium sulphate – 500 g dissolved in luke worm water. Ayurvedic stomachic powder like Catone, Pachak, Ruhamax, Herbogastrin *etc.* (as per index) and Injection Pepsid, Belamyl, Stronic *etc.* (as per index) can be administered. Dehydrated animals should receive a balanced electrolyte solution with potassium supplementation as needed.

12.5 ANAEMIA

Anaemia can be defined as a decrease in total red blood cell count, haemoglobin concentration and packed cell volume, taking into account variation for the age and breed. Normal range of haemoglobin in cow is 8-14 g/dl. (Brar *et al.*, 2002). There are three (3) types of anaemia. These are (*i*) Haemorrhagic anaemia, (*ii*) Haemolytic anaemia and (*iii*) Anaemia due to decreased production of erythrocytes or haemoglobin.

Haemorrhagic anaemia occurs due to acute haemorrhage or with chronic blood loss owing to coccidiosis (calf), haemonchosis (sheep and goat), strongylosis of cattle, sheep and goat and blood sucking parasites. Haemolytic anaemia occurs in many infectious and non-infectious diseases like piroplasmosis (babesiosis), leptospirosis. Braken fern poisoning, copper poisoning and haemolysis due to toxins. Deficiency of iron, Cu, Co *etc.* are held responsible for causing anaemia which are called nutritional anaemia. Iron deficiency is the major cause of hypochromic, microcytic anaemia, although copper deficiency can produce the same signs and folic acid deficiency also produces anaemia, Defective blood formation causing hypoplastic and or aplastic anaemia are also found in animal kingdom. Haemmorhage, heavy infection of endo and ectoparasites, toxic drugs or chemicals, wasting disease, starvation, *etc.* may result in anaemia.

Symptoms

Common clinical manifestations of anaemia include lethargy, inappetance or anorexia, weakness, exercise intolerance, respiratory distress or occasionally collapse and palor mucous membranes. Haematuria, Haemoglobinuria, muscular weakness and depression may accompany with anaemia owing to Babesiosis, plant toxins (Braken Fern poisoning), Leptospirosis *etc.*

Treatment

Specific treatment for special causes; blood transfusion in acute haemorrhage, supplement mineral mixtures containing copper, cobalt, iron and vitamin B_{12}. Feed hematinic mixtures. Besides treatment nutritional management of anaemia should be done that includes availability of amino acids for synthesis of Haemoglobin (Hb), iron for haemosynthesis and copper for the proper mobilization of iron. Iron is poorly absorbed from the gut (GI tract). Intramuscular injection of iron dextran, Imferon Inj. 6-10 ml or iron solution, citric acid complex, or Inj. Feritas (Intas) @ 1 ml/50 kg body weight by IM route followed by Ferritas bolus orally can be tried. Ferritus bolus containing iron, Vitamin B_{12}, and folic acid @ 1 bolus twice daily for calf, ½ to 1 bolus OD for sheep and goat, 2 boli for large animal for 7 days is highly effective in treating anaemia. The absorption of iron (Fe) is facilitated with a liberal intake of ascorbic acid. Folic acid and Vitamin B_{12} are necessary to support normal cell division.

Liver extracts with Vitamin B-complex injections like Inj. Feroliv (Excell), Inj. Belamyl (Sarabhai), Inj. Stronic (Vetnex), Inj. Bivinal forte (Alembic), Inj. Livobex (TTK) @ 5-10 ml for large animal and @ 2-3 ml for small animal on every alternate day can be administered.

Herbal liver tonic like Livol, Vetliv powder, Haematic powder @ 5-10 g BID Haematol powder @ 30 g BID can also be fed to the animal.

Inj. Polyvet (Excell), Inj. Tribivet (Intas) @ 5-10 ml on alternate day for 3 to 5 occassions can also be administered for better results.

A herbomineral formulation Ferrocom (Indian Herbs) containing 2.76 mg of elemental iron/100 mg powder @ 250 mg/animal/day can also be recommended fo

3 weeks. It is a safe antianaemic herbomineral formulation, can be used in anaemic animals.

If there is endoparasitic (helminthic) loads specific anthelmintic should be prescribed/recommended orally.

12.6 THELITIS

Inflammation of teat with resulting obstruction of the teat canal in animal called thelitis is commonly seen in buffaloes. Varying eatiology are there for such clinical entity; *e.g.* viral, mycotic (*e.g. Candida albicans*). Some unknown etiology causing thelitis has also been reported.

Symptoms

Symptoms of inflammation, pain and swelling, hyperaemic and oedematous swelling of teats. Subsequent cessation of milk from the affected teat.

Treatment

1. Parenteral administration of phenyl butazone and analgin or Meloxicam.
2. A course of antihistaminic *e.g.* Pheniramine maleate.
3. If it is due to cadidiasis local application of Candid ointment to be done.
4. Systemic antibiotic therapy (see antibiotics) *e.g.* Inj. Streptopenicillin, Amoxycillin-Cloxacillin combination, Enrofloxacin *etc.*

12.7 ANOREXIA

Most of the cases of reduced appetite (Hypophagia) and complete loss of appetite (anorexia) generally accompany the fever and the systemic disease. Differentiation should be made between actual loss of appetite and inability to eat.

Inability to eat may be due to some lesions in the mouth (Stomatitis, Sore mouth, FMD *etc.*). Constipation is also associated with loss of appetite. In pepsistent clinical illness nutritional status can be surely compromised by the combined effects of reduced feed intake and tissue catabolism.

Anorexia may arise due to a good number of reasons or factors like liver disease or hepatic disorder, impaction, bloat, constipation, diarrhoea, renal failure, urolithiasis, small intestinal disease (SID), large intestinal disease (LID), colitis, febrile conditions, indigestion, oral or mucosal affection, loosening of teeth, actinomycosis, actinobacillosis *etc.* Low water intake, high ambient temperature, colic *etc.* also may be attributed to anorexia.

Treatment

Nutritional therapy, supportive therapy, stomachic, liver extract with B-complex *etc.* should be tried and treatment should be given as per etiological basis. For febrile condition antipyretic (like Paracetamol, *i.e.* Inj. Dafomol, Inj. Paramol, Inj. Boline *etc.*, Nimesulide *i.e.* Inj. Nimovet, Meloxicam with Paracetamol like Inj. MP3. Melonex Plus etc.), for systemic infection parenteral antibacterial (antibiotics or sulphonamides as per index), to boost up liver functions (liver protectives like liver stimullants like Livol powder, Vetliv powder or liver tonic like Feroliv, Zigbo, Brotone, Lifer) or parenteral liver extract with B-complex (like Inj. Belamyl, Inj. Stronic, Inj. Livron, Inj. Levadex) for indigestion, digestive stimulant and stomachic like Floraboost AD3 powder, Floraboost bolus, Provisac bolus, Yeasac bolus, Floratone bolus *etc.* Stomachic powder like Ruchamax, Herbogastrin, Himalayan Batisa, condition rejuvinants like Inj. Polyvet, Inj. Tribivet, Inj. Conciplex, Inj. Hivit *etc.* can be tried. For gastro intestinal endoparasitism (worm infestation) broad spectrum dewormer should be given. And above all nutritional therapy should be given to all the affected animals where nutritional therapy involves nutrition of clinical cally sick animals, supportive nutrition for the convalescent animals and preventive nutrition to flight against the occurrence of clinical illness and therapeutic diets for different patho or pathophysiological conditions. Establishment of acid base and electrolyte (fluid balance) and stimulation of appetite is the main aim of treatment.

12.8 PICA

It is a condition generally developed in cattle and buffalo and also in dogs when the animals ingest materials other than normal food.

Etiology

When the dog eats non food items, the suggested causes are lack of essential minerals like iron and phosphorus, vitamins, hunger, indigestion, parasitic infestation, teething or rickets. In cattle pica is mainly due to dietary deficiency, specifically for salt, cobalt or phosphorus. It may also be due to indigestion, dietic irregularity, chronic abdominal pain due to peritoritis and nervous acetonaemia, hunger and parasitic infestation too.

Types

1. *Osteophagia* – When the animal will chew the bones.
2. *Geophagia* – when the animals will chew muds or clay.
3. *Urophagia* – When the animals intake urine.
4. *Coprophagia* – When the animal will develop unpleasant habit of eating faeces of other animals.
5. *Salt hunger* – when the animal will lick coat.

Treatment

To correct the dietary aspect of pica the dog's food should contain some common salt, calcium and Vitamin B_1 (yeast). Fresh long bones of healthy carcass can be given. For cattle and buffalo symptomatic treatment should be given.

For salt hunger and urophagia administration of normal salt with feed and drink should be done. Vetlick brick/salt bricks can be supplemented. Of course mineral mixtures like Chelated Agrimin fort (Glaxo), Minfa (Intas) @ 30-40 g for bovines, 10-15 g for sheep and goat should be given.

For cobalt and phosphorous deficiency

1. Ranmix total powder (Vetnex), Proteimin Fort (Oxford), Minerin (Brihans) *etc.* @ 25 g daily for consecutive 15 days should be given.

2. Injection Uremin (Glaxo Smithkline), Inj. Aciphos (Excell), Inj. Alphos-40 (Alved) @ 5-10 ml IM twice in a week for 2-3 weeks can be administered.
3. Proper deworming must be done.
4. Oral formulation of calcium a phosphorous *e.g.* Orcal P granules (TTK) or Ossomin suspension (TTK) @ 20 ml daily for cattle and horse, 10 ml BID for sheep and goat, 5 ml for calf and 10 ml BID for heifer, Large animal 20-30 ml BID.

12.9 SIMPLE INDIGESTION

Simple indigestion is the most commonly encountered problem under field condition occurring due to consumption of indigestible feed material and clinically characterized by inappetance to anorexia, atony of the fore stomach (rumen) and abnormal faeces. Indigestible feed material may comprise excess quantity of roughages. Sudden change in feed or feeding schedule, prolonged or heavy oral or ruminal usage of antibiotics or sulfonamides (anti microbials) and any type of stress most commonly transportation stress may lead to simple indigestion. Sudden introduction of feed containing urea or placentophagia (placenta eating) may also cause simple indigestion.

Pathology

Simple accumulation of indigestible feed in the rumen may physically alter ruminal motility along with the production of toxic amides and amines which ultimately leads to ruminal atony by virtue of the less production of volatile fatty acids and that resulting in depletion in milk production.

Symptoms

Hypophegia, reduction in appetite, depression, depressed ruminal movements, lack of rumination, hard and scanty feaces, decline in milk yield.

Diagnosis

Simple indigestion should be differentiated or differentially diagnosed from vagous indigestion, alkalosis, acidosis, abomasal displacement and traumatic reticulitis.

Treatment

Rumenotorics, liver rejuvenator should be administered. Herbal preparations (stomachic powders) like Herbogastrin powder (Vetmed) Large animal – 25 g orally BID, Small animal 10-15 g orally BID, Himalayan Batisa (Indian Herbs), Natural Batisa, Pachak, Ruchamax, H.B. Strong *etc.* (as per index) should be feed orally BID.

Rumenotoric bolus like Floratone (Concept), Provisac (Vetcare) Yeasac (Vetnex), Rumentas (Intas) one to two boli BID and parenteral preparations as liver function modulator/rejuvenator *viz.* Inj. Ferroliv, Inj. Pollyvet (Excell) Inj. Tribivet (Intas) @ 5-10 ml IM daily or on alternate day may be administered for better result.

12.10 ENTERITIS IN SHEEP AND GOAT

A number of etiologic factors like bacteria, parasite, virus, dietic errors and management practices are responsible for enteritis in kids and lambs.

Enteritis manifests diarrhoea, dehydration, abdominal pain, loss of weight and other evidences of specific deficiency. This complex of symptoms occurs in all ages of sheep and goat but is particularly common and fatal to kids and lambs upto 2-3 months of age. The new born animals deficient in immunoglobulin or having an average low birth weight are much more susceptible to infection as well as diarrhoea.

Etiology

- ☆ *Bacteria* – *e.g. Escherichia coli*, *Proteus* and *Shigella*.
- ☆ *Virus* – Herpes virus, picorna virus, rota virus and PPR virus (Paramyxo).
- ☆ *Coccidia* – *Eimeria* species.
- ☆ *Worms* – Helminthic parasites *e.g. Haemonchous*, *Oestertagia* sp., *Chabertia* sp., *Trichostrongylus* sp. *etc.*
- ☆ *Dietic* error – Scours owing to feeding of excessive amount of milk or change abruptly to milk replacer or if the milk is fed at too high concentration.
- ☆ *Mixed infection* – Mixed infection of *E. coli* with *Proteus* sp., *Klebsiella* sp., *Pseudomonas* sp. and Coccidia are harmful and can produce enteritis.

Symptoms

Mild to severe diarrhoea, dullness, anorexia, subnormal temperature, weakness. coma, tremor and death. It is the common features of coccidiosis in small ruminants. A severe watery, often yellowish or sometimes bloody foetid diarrhoea with passage of mucus are observed with *Salmonella* infection. Gradual loss of body weight, loose faeces, dullness, depression and dehydration in diarrhoeic kids and lambs.

Treatment

For bacterial enteritis Enrofloxacin @ 5 ml/kg body weight and Cephalosporin *etc.*, for Pseudomonas Gentamycin, for *E. coli* Nalidixic acid are highly effective. For parasitic enteritis mainly Haemonchosis, Trichostrongylus *etc.* Closantel (Zycloz), Fentas plus, Rafox plus *etc.* can be administered.

Besides Chloramphenicol, Cephacosporin, Polymyxin and quinolones can also be administered.

Oral antibiotic formulations *e.g.* Cyclin DT (Excell) ½ to 1 h bolus BID, Amoxirum bolus (GlaxoSmithkline) @ 1/3rd bolus OD, Neodox bolus (Vetcare) @ ½ to 1 bolus BID, 3-care bolus ½ to 1 bolus BID. Sulfa drugs like Cobatran bolus, Biotrim DS, SD bolus, Sulfex bolus, Duaprim *etc.* @ ½ to 1 bolus BID can also be tried. Furazolidone @ 60 mg/kg body weight *e.g.* Antibac (c), oral administration of oral electrolyte solution containing glucose and glycine can be made. Remilyte, electral powder, ERS liquid, electrocon *etc.* (as per index) can also be used.

Formulary: Glucose- Glycine-electrolyte solution – Dextrose 11.0 g.

Solution made of NaCl 45 g; Pot. Chloride (KCl) – 3.5 g, Cal. Chloride ($CaCl_2$) – 2.5 g, Magnesium chloride – 3.0 g, Sodium acetate -25 g, Sod. phosphate -2.0 g, Dist. water to make – 10 litres.

Dose: 50-100 ml, 4 times a day orally.

12.11 NEONATAL CALF DIARRHOEA

Diarrhoea in cattle and buffalo calves is quite common and it is one of the most common causes of mortality in calves. Etiological agents are several and the disease is often multifactorial, while an infectious agent may be present in a herd without signs, poor management precipitates clinical diseases. Certain agents such as Rotavirus may predispose for a more serious agents such as *E. coli* infections, other agents could be salmonella, coccidia *etc.*

Etiology

(i) Bacterial

Salmonella and *E. coli* are most common cause of calf mortality. *Providencia, Klebsiella, Serratia* and *Campylobactus etc.* are also involved in neonatal calf diarrhoea.

(ii) Viral

A number of viral agents are involved in calf diarrhoea. The effect of viral invasion is generally seen during first five weeks of life as 'Week calf syndrome'. The majority of the diarrhoea are due to enteric Rota and Corona virus.

(iii) Mycotic

Candid albicans are most common causes of mycotic diarrhoea in calves. Of late many fungi *e.g.* Aspergillus, Mucor, Rhizopus and many mycotoxins *e.g.* Aflatoxin, Zenralenone and T-2 toxins *etc.* have been identified as the contributors to neonatal mortality. Poor management predisposes the animal to fungal infections.

(iv) Parasitic

Helminths and protozoa are responsible for parasitic gastro enteritis. Amongst protozoa, elmeria species are the primary causes whereas Trichostrongylus and cooperia are important helminthes responsible for parasitic gastroenteritis.

Treatment

The faecal loss of large volumes of fluid in the scouring calf results in dehydration that may lead to shock, metabolic acidosis and depletion of Na, K and Cl. When acidosis is severe, a potentially dangerous hyperkalemia develops.

1. Balanced polyionic solutions should be used to correct the multiple deficits and current acidosis *e.g.* Ringer's lactate solution by IV route. Ringer's solution with sodium bicarbonate or commercial preparation containing bicarbonate precursor in the form of acetate alone can be given.
2. Glucose glycine electrolyte solutions for oral use can be safely used (1-2 litres, 2-3 times a day).
3. Commercial preparations like Electrocon, ERS liquid or Remilyte powder 2-3 times a day can be given orally or Remilytic powder 2-3 times a day can be given.

4. Oral antibiotics *e.g.* Amoxirum bolus (½ to 1 bolus OD), Cyclin DT (½ to 1 bolus) BID, Neodox bolus (½ to 1 bolus OD), Steclin 500 mg, Cyclin 500 mg 1 bolus BID, Cephalexin pawder (as per index) can be fed.
5. Sulpha bolus *e.g.* S.D. bolus, Pabadene, Biotrim DS, Duaprim, Intrim, ½–1 bolus BID.
6. Fazol, Fumar, Oriprim orally can be given.
7. Inj. Enteromycetin, Inj. Curacin (Vets Farma), Inj. Amikacin, Inj. Gentamycin can be used. Chloramphenicol @ 25 mg/kg body weight for 3 days and Amprolium HCl @ 25 mg/kg body weight for 5 days is recommended.
8. Other antibiotics *e.g.* Neomycin (Unimycin 140 mg/ml) @ 2.5 mg/kg body weight or Inj. Lincomycin-Specinomycin combination (Lincospectin) @ 15 mg/kg body weight by IM route.
9. For coccidian parasitesSulphadimidin @ 125 mg/kg body weight for 3 days and Amprolium HCl @ 25 mg/kg body weight for 5 days is recommended.

12.12 NEONATAL CALF PNEUMONIA

Pneumonia is the main respiratory disorder responsible for high mortality in calves. Several organisms have been isolated from pneumonic lungs. Apart from neonatal calf diarrhoea (calf enteritis), calf pneumonia is the second major hazard to calf health and may account for 50 per cent of calf mortality.

Etiology

The etiology of calf pneumonia is extremely complex and multifactorial including various infectious agents, environment and managemental practices.

Bacterial cause: Bacteria like *Corynacbacterium pyogenes, Pasteurella multocida, Streptococci, Staphylococci, E. coli, Salmonella, Klebsiella pneumoniae etc.*, and Mycoplasma *Fusiformis necrophorus etc.* are responsible for pneumonia in calves.

Virus: Variety of viruses namely Parainfluenza, Rhinovirus, Adeno virus, Reovirus, and Corona virus are responsible for respiratory disorder and pneumonia in neonatal calves. The pathological changes *e.g.* acute bronchopneumonia, pneumoenteritis, fibropurulent pneumonia and abscess.

Mycotic: Several species of *Aspergillus* and *Candida* are responsible.

Miscellaneous causes: Non-infectious factors *e.g.* nutritional, management practices, and environment.

Symptoms

Pyrexia, coughing, tachypnoea, dyspnoea, adventitious lungs sounds, increased heart rate *etc.*

Treatment

1. *Antibiotic therapy* – Drugs like Ampicillin, combination of Ampicillin and Cloxacillin, Amoxicillin and Cloxacillin combination. Amoxicillin with Clavulanic acid, Cifrofloxacin, Enrofloxacin can be used with better

therapeutic efficacy. Inj. Enrofloxacin @ 5 mg/kg body weight by IM route is the drug of choice.

2. Dexamethasone sodium injection *e.g.* Dexona, Vetcort, Enidex @ 0.5-1ml daily for 3-5 days.
3. Turpentine oil/oil Eucaliptol/Tr. Beazoin inhalation twice daily.
4. Coldex (Oxford Gem), Respigen (Nugen) @ 5-10 ml orally BID can be fed, herbal powder *e.g.* Bronchopyrin, Biocof *etc.* can be fed as electuary.
5. Antihistaminic injection *e.g.* Avil, Antilar, Allergo, Anistamin, Chloril, Chlorazin @ 1-2 ml IM daily for 3-5 days.
6. Meloxicam injection *e.g.* Inj. MP3, Inj. Proxivet, Inj. Melonex, Inj. Melonex Plus 2-3 ml IM daily for 3-5 days.
7. Chemotherapy with Trimethoprime + Sulphametoxazole *e.g.* Robatran 1 bolus BID or antibacterial therapy with Chloramphenicol @ 25 mg/kg body weight may be administered daily for 5-6 days. Ampicillin @ 7-10 mg/kg body weight for 5-7 days may be given orally or parenterally.

12.13 SALMONELLOSIS IN CALVES

It is caused by various species of *Salmonella*. Typically two forms are (*i*) an enteric form in which diarrhoea and vomiting are present and young animals are mainly at risk of dehydration and (*ii*) an invasive form in which the *Salmonella* invade the blood stream and cause septicaemia. It becomes fatal when disease resistance is appeared and late starting of treatment.

Treatment

1. Chloramphenicol is sensitive to this disease @ 25 mg/kg body weight daily IM route for 5-6 days.
2. Supportive therapy as well as fluids for rehydration therapy should be administered.

12.14 MYCOPLASMA IN CALVES

Mycoplasma bovis, bacteria like organism causes a persistent chronic infection in calves and cows. It has been associated with otitis (an infection of the ear), Pneumonia and arthritis in calves. Calves may be infected with *M. bovis* by drinking infected milk (organism causing mastitis in cows) or direct contact with infected calves. In addition to clinical ear infection, numerous calves had a characteristic head tilt and or facial nerve paralysis.

Treatment

Tylosin is the drug of choice (by IM route). Besides Tylosin, Erythromycin, Oxytetracycline and Alincomycin are recommended.

12.15 AGALACTIA

In this condition, the secretory activity of glandular tissue becomes passive and secretory cells become physiologically inactive. Such condition is observed just after parturition and may affect one or more teats. On examination, the gland and teat cistern is found normal and there is no evidence of mastitis.

Treatment

1. Oxytocin injection to be given for let down of milk, as per standard dosing, *e.g.* for sow @ 10 IU/sow twice a day till the restoration of lactation.
2. Quantity of milk to be increased by using different galactogogue *e.g.* Milkotone, Rasol, Galogue powder, Maximilk bolous, Payaprobolous (as per index).
3. Oral supplementation of minerals and vitamin preparations like Prolactic (Nugen), Supplevite-M, Agrimin Fort, Ranmix Total, Minfa *etc.* (as per index).
4. Oral supplementation of calcium tonic *e.g.* Calshakti, Calcimilk, Caldhan, Provical *etc.* (as per index).

12.16 BLOOD IN MILK

The presence of blood in milk is generally seen in high milk yielders. The common cause of this condition can be mechanical trauma to the udder or due to presence of infection in the gland or teat cistern.

Treatment

1. Various types of haemostatics such as Adenochrome (Inj. Dafochrome, Chromostat injection), Inj. Bleed check (BeeTee Pharma) 10-15 ml by IM can be administered.
2. Injection Vitamin-K or oral Vitamin-K preparation can be fed.
3. Parenteral calcium preparation *e.g.* Inj. Mifex, Inj. Calmax-M, Inj. Calborol, Inj. Calgonate, Inj. Lactomag, Inj. Intacal *etc.* by IV followed by SC can be administered.
4. Parenteral administration of Inj. Beet Phos, Inj. Alphos-40, Inj. Uremin, Inj. Tonoricin, Inj. Tonophosphan @ 10-15 ml by IM route twice in a week can be administered.
5. Oral administration of formaldehyde (20 ml in 1 litre water) is also effective.
6. Oral supplementation of calcium tonic *e.g.* Calshakti, Orical oral, Capsola, Calcimilk and multimineral and vitamin formulations *e.g.* Vitromin, Vitaprotein DS, Ranmix total, Calcifort (as per index) @ 25-30 g orally OD for 10-15 days can be fed.

12.17 UDDER OEDEMA

Udder oedema usually occurs in high yielding dairy cows and first calf heifers near parturition and it is characterized by extensive accumulation of fluid in the interstitial space of udder. The exact etiology is not known. However, factors like excessive grain feeding in heifers, high sodium intake in housed cattle and hereditary factors. Persistent and severe udder oedema interferes with suckling and milking. This may lead to common complications like mastitis, haemagalactia and injury to udder and teats and in severe case rupture of ligaments of udder.

Symptoms

Oedematous udder usually becomes pinkish in colour, cold in sensation, pitting on pressure and painful. Oedema may extend the umbilicus and to the base of the teats too.

Treatment

1. Salt restriction.
2. Moist hot fomentation (with Epsom salt/Mag Sulph).
3. Inj. Frusemide, Inj. Lasix, Inj. Redema @ 10-15 ml by IM route for 2 to 3 days.
4. Inj. Dexamthasone (*e.g.* Dexone, Enidex, Vetcort) in severe cases can be administered by IM route under anbitiotic coverage.
5. Inj. Analgin, Inj. Vetalgin, Inj. Melonex, Inj. Meloxicam @ 10-15 ml IM for 2-3 days.

12.18 PARTURIENT PARESIS

Synonyms

Milk fever, Post parturient paresis, Hypocalcaemia.

It is an important production disease and or metabolic disease, mainly seen in high producing animals, occurs due to an imbalance between the rates of input of dietary nutrients and the output of production. The disease occurs at or near parturition, characterized by low serum calcium. Amongst the domestic farm animals, the metabolic diseases achieve their greatest importance in dairy cattle and pregnant ewes.

Etiology

A depression of the levels of ionized calcium in tissue fluids is the basic biochemical defect in milk fever. Nearly all cows experience some degree of hypocalcaemia during the 1st day after calving as the intestine and bone adapt to the Ca demands of lactation.

Predisposing Factors

1. *Age*: Mature dairy cattle at the age of 5-10 years and 3rd to 7th parturition is highly susceptible to milk fever.
2. *Breed*: Jersey and white breeds are highly susceptible.
3. *Dietary calcium*: Manipulation of dietary calcium and phosphorus is known to have dramatic effects on the incidence of milk fever.
4. *Dietary phosphorus*: When prepartum diets are rich in phosphorus ($P > 80$g of P/day), then incidence of milk fever increases.
5. Diets that are high in Na and K increase the susceptibility of cows to milk fever.
6. Starvation, estrogenic hormones, lack of exercise, and stress also plays important role in the occurrence of milk fever in dairy cows.

Clinical Findings

Three stages of milk fever in cattle are usually noted.

Stage – I

Serum calcium level is 6.5-8.0 mg/dl.

There is ataxia, cow is still able to stand but wobbly. There is brief excitement and tetany with hypersensitivity and muscle tremor of the head and limbs. Loss of appetite or hypophagia, alert expression, protrusion of tongue, constipation *etc.* are also usual. Cows may be mildly ataxic, have fine tremors over flanks and triceps.

Stage – II

Serum calcium level is 4.0-6.0 g/dl.

This stage is prolonged and there is sternal recumbency. Depressed consciousness, drowsy appearance and lateral kink in the neck or the head turned into the flank, tetany of limbs, subnormal temperature, ruminal stasis, constipation, bloat, impaction, dry eyes, staring and incomplete light reflex *etc.* are seen.

Stage-III

Serum calcium level is <4.0 mg/dl.

In this stage lateral recumbency occurs. Marked reduction in cardiac output, semi comatose condition, bloat, impalpable pulse and increased heart rate (accelerated heart beat). If the animal is left untreated, the animal dies quickly from shock in a state of complete collapse.

Diagnosis

1. Exclusively on clinical signs.
2. Estimation of serum calcium level.
3. Clinical response to 'Ca' therapy.

Differential Diagnosis

Hypocalcaemia or milk fever may occur as (a) Prepartum or (b) Post partum.

(a) Prepartum

1. Muscles and skeletal injuries – *viz.* luxatious, fractures.
2. Spinal injuries, nerve injuries, spinal compression.
3. Uterine diseases – torsion, emphysematous fetus, hydrops.
4. Dry cow, mastitis, toxic mastitis.
5. Hypomagnesaemia
6. Ketosis (Hepatic lipidosis).

(b) Post Partum

1. Musculo skeletal injuries *viz.* calving paralysis syndrome fractured-pelvis, luxations (Coxo femoral luxation), stifle injury.
2. Septicemia – mastitis, metritis.
3. Haemorrhage – Calving injury, uterine laceration.

4. Peritonitis – hardware, uterine rupture.
5. Ketosis (Hepatic lipidosis).
6. Hypomagnasaemia
7. Chronic disease – lymphoma, pneumonia, aspiration, starvation,
8. Spinal compression.

Treatment

Aim is to restore normal serum calcium level as soon as possible to avoid muscular and nervous damage and recumbency.

Recommended treatment is slow intravenous (IV) injection of calcium gluconate salt @ 1 g/45 kg (100 Ib) body weight. In high yielding cattle, besides intravenous (IV) infusion half of the recommended dose should be administered by SC route to provide a prolonged release of calcium into the circulation.

Inj. Calborol (Provimi), Inj. Intacal (Intas), Inj. Calmax (Vetnex) *etc.* may be used. Many solutions contain phosphorus and magnesium in addition to calcium. Phosphorus and magnesium are not usually necessary in uncomplicated parturient paresis and as such these can safely be used where magnesium could protect myocardial irritation caused by the administration of calcium.

Such preparations are Inj. Calmax-M (Vetnex), Inj. Mifocal (Indian Immunologicals), Inj. Mifex (Provimi), Inj. Lactomag (Intas) *etc.*

12.19 ACUTE PULMONARY EMPHYSEMA

Bovine pulmonary emphysema is caused by pneumotoxic effect of 3-methylindole produced in rumen from bacterial degradation and abundantly present tryptophan in lush green pasture. Dyspnoea after grazing on green lush pasture is indicative of pulmonary emphysema.

Symptoms

Inappetance, dullness, head extended downwards, expiratory dyspnoea with grant on expiration, loud crackling sound on auscultation.

Treatment

1. Antihistaminics *e.g.* Inj. Pheniramine maleate @ 5-10 ml IM daily for 3 days.
2. Antibiotics *e.g.* Inj. Streptopenicillin 2.5 g, Inj. Enrofloxacin 1500 mg IM daily for 3-5 days.
3. Corticosteroids *e.g.* Inj. Dexamethasone sodium or Inj. Prednisolone acetate – 100 mg IM daily for 3 days.
4. Poly ether antibiotic – *e.g.* Monensin (*i.e.* Monensin Sodium/Rumensin-60) orally twice daily @ 200 mg/day for 5 days.
5. Liver extract with B-complex *e.g.* Inj. Stronic, Inj. Livobex, Inj. Belamyl @ 5-10 ml IM on alternate day for 3-5 days.

12.20 RETENTION OF URINE

Retention of urine is common in male animals, although it also occurs in females as a sequale to urogical syndrome. Retention due to urethral calculi and fibroma on the urinary bladder needs surgical intervention. Partial retention of urine is very common; and it is not fatal, however, if urine flow is not restored well in time it may have fatal consequences. Cystitis and urethritis may also cause retention of urine-other than urinary calculi.

Symptoms

Attempting to urinate and maintain a prolonged urination posture with legs wide apart and pumping of the tail. Animals become restless and show straining. There may be colic and grunting, Anorexia suspended rumination. Dribbling of urine occasionally following excessive straining or complete stoppage of urination may be seen.

Treatment

1. IV infusion of normal saline or DNS or Ringer's lactate.
2. Along with the IV fluid antibiotic *e.g.* Tetracycline HCl, Gentamycin, Ciprofloxacin *etc.* can also be administered slowly to control possible bacterial infection of the urinary system.
3. Inj. Spasmoproxivon, Inj. Dicyclomine HCl, Inj. Dextropropoxyphene HCl, Inj. Acetaminophen @ 5-10 ml IM daily can be administered.
4. Cox-II inhibitors, Inj. Meloxicam (*e.g.* Inj. Melonex, Inj. Meloxi, Inj. MP3, Inj. Melobest) @ 10-15 ml for large animal and 3-5 ml for small animal can also be administered IM to relieve pain and colic.
5. If the urine is acidic – systemic alkalizer particularly for pet animals and small ruminant can be used *e.g.* Alkasol, potent urine alkalizer @ 10 ml orally BID for a week can be recommended.
6. Herbal formulations *e.g.* Stonil, Cystone *etc.* can be tried. Dose: Cystone tabs @ 10-15 tabs orally BID for large animal and 5 tabs BID for small animal which acts as a good diuretic and helps in dissolving calculi if any which is usually flushed out with the urine.
7. Ammonium chloride orally @ 20-25 g for 5-7 days can be tried. If antibiotic, analgesic and fluid therapy in the form of normal saline fails to give effective result in urination, pre-scrotal urethrotomy is indicated under local infiltration analgesia using 2 per cent lignocaine HCl.

12.21 TORTICOLIS

Torticolis may be congenital or acquired. Various forms and degrees of torsion of neck (torticolis) have been recorded. The condition is observed in calves, adult cattle and buffaloes. The cause could be otitis media in calves and pigs, involvement of brain in certain diseases such as polio encephalitis, rabies in buffaloes, gid in goats, spasm and paralysis of neck muscles, fracture of articular process of vertebrae, incomplete dislocation of one intervertebral articulation, contracture or spasm of muscles on the convex side of the bent neck in the parturient paretic cow. Pesticide poisoning, hard abscess, intramuscular injection on neck muscle by Berenil, Quinipyramin salts *etc.*

Treatment

Treatment should be given as per etiology.

1. Neurotropic B-vitamins *e.g.* Inj. Tribivet, Neurovet, Polyvet, *etc.* in order to facilitate neuronal transmission and skeletal muscles action @ 5-10 ml by IM route to large animal, and @ 2 ml by IM route to small animal.
2. Mag Sulph (Epsome salt) moist hot fermentation twice daily.
3. Massaging with iodex ointment, cat gall, briclofen plus gel *etc.* can be done.
4. Inj. Prednisolone, Inj. Vetalog, Inj. Dexamethasone *etc.* can be administered by IM route.
5. If there is history of poisoning Inj. Atropin Sulphate 1 per cent (*e.g.* Domesto) @ 5-10 ml IM.
6. IV administration of Ca, Mg, P *e.g.* Inj. Mifex (Novartis), Inj. Calmax M (Vetnex), Inj. Lactomag (Intas) 250-300 ml.
7. IV infusion of Dextrose 5 to 10 per cent. Rintose, Intalyte *etc.* can be tried.
8. Liver extract with B-complex can also be given in case of poisoning.
9. If it is due to hard abscess in neck muscle – surgical intervention should be made.
10. NSAIDS *e.g.* Inj. Analgin, Inj. Boline, Inj. Artisone, Inj. Oxalgin NP, Inj. Nimovet, Inj. MP3, Inj. Melonex Plus, Inj. Melobest *etc.* (any one) can be administered by IM route.

12.22 PAROTITIS

Parotitis is the inflammation of any of the salivary glands. The clinical cases occurs sporadically. It occurs suddenly characterized by the swelling at the mandibular region. Pyrexia, anorexia, tachycardia, rapid and labored respiration, congested mucosae, dullness and depression are the usual signs. The swelling may be unilateral or bilateral. On touch the swelling may be felt warm, hard and painful. There may be difficulty in mastication and deglutination (swallowing).

Treatment

1. Broad spectrum antibiotic coverage for 3-5 days *e.g.* Inj. Oxytetracycline @ 10 mg/kg body weight IV, Inj. Streptopenicillin @ 2.5 g, Inj. Enrofloxacin *etc.*
2. NSAIDS *e.g.* Inj. MP3, Inj. Melonex, Inj. A3vet, Inj. Melonex Plus, Inj. Artisone S, Inj. Oxalgin NP, any one can be administered by IM route for 3-5 days.
3. IV administration of fluid *e.g.* DNS can be done to rejuvenate the body condition in case of anorexia.
4. Good quality vitamin B-complex *e.g.* Inj. Hivit, Inj. Conciplex, Inj. Polyvet, Inj. Tribivet @ 5-10 ml IM for 3-5 days can be given.

5. Potassium iodide @ 5-7 g orally daily for a week.
6. Hot fomentation with Mag Sulph and massage with iodovet ointment, Briclofen plus gel *etc.* can be tried.

12.23 FIRST AID IN BLEEDING

(*a*) External Bleeding

Bleeding or haemorrhage from small wound or surface wounds can be stopped by pressing down hard on the wound with a sterile or clean cloth. If the blood soaks through the cloth, another piece of cloth may be placed on top rather than removing the first one.

When bleeding stops, cleaning and treatment of the wound can be done with antiseptic solution, gels or ointments. Bandage can be applied. However, bleeding from larger or deep wounds cannot be stopped using hard pressure with pieces of cloth. Such bleeding can be managed by using a tourniquet. A tourniquet is a piece of rope or cloth which is tied across a blood vessel. It can only be used for wounds in the appendages or tail but should never be used around the neck.

(*b*) Bleeding from Broken Horn

If the horn of the animal is broken, bleeding may be stopped by putting a pad or clean cloth on it and holding it in place with a bandage. A temporary tourniquet around the base of the horn will stop bleeding. If this does not help, a red hot piece of metal can be placed directly on the bleeding spot for half a minute to cauterize the horn and the blood vessel. Potassium permanganate crystals can also be used with wet cotton pad cauterization. A tourniquet cannot be used for a long time. Tourniquet must be released every 20 minutes after that again tighten the tourniquet in case of bleeding that continues.

(*c*) Internal Bleeding

This type of bleeding is dangerous. It can occur from the lungs and gut after an accident or from the uterus or vagina after giving birth. An animal with internal bleeding should be placed in quiet and warm place and should be given water with a pinch of salt in it. Walking such animal should be prevented, since such act may cause the animal to collapse or die.

Internal bleeding from the vagina can occur after birth. In such cases packing the vagina with a clean cloth or towel which has been boiled and then cooled and leaving the towel in the vagina for a day or two that helps to stop the bleeding.

12.24 CUTS AND WOUNDS

Cuts, wounds and injuries are most common in domestic animals irrespective of their age and sex. Types of wounds in clinical cases varies from clean, contaminated, infected and maggot wounds. The treatment of fresh wounds is comparatively easier if it is attended in time. But healing gets delayed if the wound is attended too late.

The cases of wounds are broadly classified as (*i*) clean or fresh wound and (*ii*) old or contaminated wound.

(*a*) Fresh Wound

Fresh wounds are generally the clean wounds defined to be a fresh breach of the continuity of the soft tissues of the body produced by sharp objects, accidents or due to breaking of the horn etc. this type of wounds should be attended immediately to check the bleeding, to prevent contamination and by further delay to prevent possible maggotization.

Treatment

1. The wound should be cleaned gently with Condy's is solution or Acriflavin solution (1 g Acriflavin in 1000 ml of 90 per cent alcohol).
2. If blood oozes a bandage of Tr. Benzoin, Dettol will help to control bleeding.
3. If there is no bleeding simple dressing with Tr. Iodine is adviced.
4. If the injury or cuts are big in size suturing is advisable.
5. If the wound cannot be bandaged, a dressing with antiseptic ointment *e.g.* Betadine (Povidone iodine 5 per cent), Himax, Charmil, Sorine, Dressol, Dermanol, Lorexene ointment *etc.* is suggested.

(*b*) Old Wounds

Uncovered fresh wound or unattended fresh wounds would turn into unhealthy-old wound. Such wounds are usually contaminated with dung, muds, dusts and bacteria or infective agents (the microbes). It becomes prone to maggots formation and that gives an ugly looking wound emitting putrified smell with oozing of blood and exudates.

Treatment

1. Wounds to be cleaned with 1 per cent potassium permanganate solution.
2. Remove all the dead tissues and debris.
3. If there is maggot formation apply Turpentine oil or Dressing oil (*e.g.* Dressol, Dressogen, Bacticon, Saaf oil *etc.*) soaked cotton to remove the maggots from the wound.
4. For maggot wound a mixture of oil turpentine, camphor and coconut oil or linseed oil in equal parts also gives good result.
5. Then dress the wound with multipurpose herbal gel *e.g.* sorine, charmil, Himax, Dressol, Topicure gel/ointment or with charmil or Himax lotion.
6. Besides such ointment ZIPP, BIPP or zinc oxide ointment can also be used.
7. If necessary a course of antibiotic with Inj. Oxytetracycline or Inj. Streptopenicillin can be done by IM route to combat bacterial contamination and for quick recovery.

(*c*) Wounds in Delicate Parts of the Body

For treating wounds in the delicate parts of the body *e.g.* eye, mammary gland, vagina *etc.*, the above mentioned treatment is contra indicated. Rather, it may lead to serious problem instead of healing of the wound.

Treatment

1. Clean the wound with warm 'sterile normal saline solution (NSS).
2. Mild antiseptics *e.g.* Acriflavin solution, Mercurochrome solution (2 per cent) can be used for cleaning of the wounds. (Acriflavin is very much beneficial for wounds over udder region).
3. Antiseptic ointment – *e.g.* Soframycin, Neosporin *etc.* can be used. Topicure gel, Metrogyl-P ointment, Wisprec gel *etc.* can be used.
4. Systemic antibiotic *e.g.* Inj. Oxytetracycline, Inj. Procaine Penicillin, Inj. Streptopenicillin, Inj. Enrofloxacin can be administered by IM route for 3 days.
5. If necessary anti-inflammatory analgesic *e.g.* Inj. Analgin, Inj. Oxalgin NP, Inj. Neoprofen *etc.* can be administered for 2-3 days by IM route.

Wounds over soft tissues usually take lesser time for healing as compared to hard tissue *e.g.* Horn. The wounds over dorsal part of the body showed greater tendency of healing as compared to ventral side.

12.25 HORN INJURIES

Broken horns or horn injuries are very much common in cattle and buffaloes. It is also seen in goats and sheep.

Etiology

Direct violence, infighting, striking he horn against fixed subject.

Treatment

1. Clean the affected part of the horn with antiseptics.
2. If necessary amputee the horn just below the sheath of fracture and protect the wound with antiseptic and bandage.
3. If there is bleeding, it to be checked with local application of styptics – Tr. Iodine, Tr. Benzoin, Adrenaline swab, Potassium permanganate cauterization. Systemic styptic/haemostats *e.g.* Inj. Bleed check, Inj. Chromostat, Inj. Dafochrome @ 8-10 ml by IM or IV route can be administered.
4. Zinc containing compounds or ZIPP (Zinc oxide-1 part, Iodoform -2 parts and liquid paraffin) are very good for horn injuries.
5. A course of antibiotic preferably Inj. Streptopenicillin *e.g.* Inj. Bistrepen, Dicrysticin, Biostrep, Munomycin fort @ 2.5 g daily for 5-7 days should be administered.
6. Regular dressing with antiseptic ointments or dusting powder *e.g.* Nebasulf, Cebazol, Furacin vet should be done.
7. Application of BIPP (Bismuth subnitrate 1 part, iodoform 2 parts and liquid paraffin QS) is beneficial for horn injury and wound healing.

12.26 BURNS AND SCALDS

The tissue changes brought about on excessive absorption of heat by the skin are called burns. Dry heat causes dessication and charring of the skin while moist heat causes boiling or cooking of tissues resulting in opaque coagulation.

Burns and scalds cause inflammatory or gangrenous lesions on contaminations leading to develop toxic complications and even death of the animal that may happen in course of time.

Epidermis being the first tissue exposed to full intensity of flames or heat, the epidermis is the most severely affected structure and tissues lying dipper are injured less.

Effects of Burns

In severe burn there will be difficulty in respiration, fall in blood pressure, traumatic shock. Edema of lungs and nephritis may occur in milder cases of burns which may cause death after several days. If 1/3rd to 1/4th of body surface is affected, death may result within 24-48 hours. The burn wounds are usually infected by bacteria, so suppuration, toxemia and septicemia may result. This condition may cause death of animals.

Treatment

1. Apply cold water immediately after rescue from burns.
2. Apply lime water and oil mixed in equal parts, use carron oil in case of burn on the body.
3. Tincture of iodine, Mercurochrome 2 per cent lotion, Acriflavin solution may lightly be applied after proper cleaning of the charred surface of the body.
4. Antiseptic powder may be applied or spread over the burnt area by dusting or neem oil sprinkling over the thermal burnarea can be done.
5. Burnol ointment, Silverex ointment can be applied locally.
6. For burns caused by acid, require the application of an alkaly.
7. Ringer's solution @ 50 ml/kg body weight and 5 per cent Dextrose @ 30 ml/kg body weight by IV route until diuresis is evident.
8. Parenteral antibiotics, Inj. Oxytetracycline @ 20 mg/kg body weight, Inj. Enrofloxacin @ 5 mg/kg body weight *etc.* should be used.

12.27 TAIL GANGRENE

This is nothing but the necrosis of tail followed by putrifaction. It usually starts from the tip of the tail. Sometimes necrosis may occur at any part of the tail as a circular ring too. Affected area becomes swollen and putrifaction occurs. Hairs may fall out and emits offensive smell. Latter oozing of pus is noticed and the process leads to necrosis or gangrene formation. Sometimes dry gangrene also occurs.

Tail gangrene is most commonly seen in cattle and buffaloes owing to mycotoxicosis (Fusario toxicosis), known as Degnala. Feeding of mould infested rice straw is responsible for such kind of toxicity resulting in tail gangrene and gangrene of extremities (in gangrenous syndrome).

Treatment

1. The dead portion (necrosed part) needs to be cleaned and amputation of tail is suggested.
2. Apply bandage after amputation.
3. Antibiotic coverage by IM route *e.g.* Enrofloxacin, Streptopenicillin.
4. A course of antihistaminic and regular dressing is advised.
5. Analgesic may be used if necessary.

12.28 FRACTURE

Fracture may be defined as a breach of continuity of a bone and may be classified as incomplete and complete fracture.

Types of Fracture

- *Incomplete fracture:* When only a part of the bone thickness is broken it is termed as incomplete fracture, which is again are of 3 types (a) Fissure fracture (b) Partial fracture and (c) Curvature of bone or green stick fracture.
- *Fissure fracture:* Cracks in a bone without any displacement is called fissure fracture.
- *Partial fracture:* A part or some particles of bone is separated or displaced from the main bone owing to violence is called partial fracture.
- *Green stick fracture:* It is characterized by a bent that may fracture on the waves side after the manner of a green stick. It is commonly seen in young animals owing to trauma and violence. Here one side of the bone is broken while the other is intact as occur when a green stick is bent.
- *Complete fracture:* It may be of different types.
- *Simple fracture:* When the bone is broken without making any breach of continuity of the skin at the seat of fracture.
- *Multiple fracture:* When the bone is broken into multiple pieces.
- *Single fracture:* When the bone is broken at one place only.
- *Compound fracture:* When the continuity of skin is breached forming an open wound along with the fracture of bone.
- *Complicated fracture:* When fracture accompanies rupture of an important blood vessel, or a nerve or joint involvement.

Symptoms

Pain at the site of fracture, swelling, abnormal mobility of the fracture site, inability to bear weight, deformity and crepitation.

Treatment

It depends upon the nature of fracture. The aim of treatment is to establish perfect immobilization and setting or fixation of the fractured part in close apposition, to reduce pain and inflammation and to hasten faster healing of fracture.

1. *Application of Plaster Cast*: Generally done in animals for making external immobilization of the fractured limb. It is to be applied under deep transquilization in large animals and under general anaesthesia in dogs on the fractured site incorporating upper and lower joints in plaster cast. Fragments of the fractured bone are to be reduced in their original position by the use of traction and counter traction. In padded type of plaster cast an even layer of cotton is spiraled along around the leg in order to protect bony prominences. In unpadded type of plaster cast splints are applied directly over the skin after bandaging and slightly padding the pressure points. Splints also needs to be bandaged in pressure points. Splints also needs to be bandaged in place with an even pressure. Plaster of paris bandages are soaked in luke warm water, squeezed and wrapped over the splints starting at the fracture site and continuing up and down including the entire limb except hooves in large animals and toe pads in dogs.

   Toes and hooves needs to be examined daily for any swelling, coldness or constriction and affected area may be massaged to promote circulation. Periosteal callus are formed, organized and the bridging of callus made union of the fracture. In larger animals plaster should be removed after a month.
2. Parenteral administration of NSAID – *e.g.* Inj. Esgipyrin, Inj. Oxalgin, Inj. Zobid 20, Inj. MP3, Inj. A3Vet plus by IM route to reduce pain and swelling.
3. Parenteral calcium *e.g.* Inj. Orical, Inj. Cal BD, Inj. Calcinet, Inj. Capsola *etc.* @ 10 ml IM on alternate day for 3-5 occasions to large animal and @ 2 ml IM on alternate day for 3-5 occasions to small animal.
4. Parenteral broad spectrum antibiotics *e.g.* Inj. Oxytetracycline, Inj. Streptopenicillin, Inj. Ampicillin-Cloxacillin, Inj. Enrofloxacin for 3-5 days by IM route can also be administered to combat bacterial infection.

12.29 YOKEGALL

This is an inflammatory condition of the skin and subcutis of neck affecting the front portion of the hump owing to yoke inflicted trauma, frictional trauma owing to faultyyoke, negligence of cart or plough driver and excessive weights loading.

When young bullocks and buffalo young bullocks are trained for agricultural operation they invariably suffer from yoke gall. It may also arise if two bullocks under the yoke are not of same size and height.

Since, constant friction caused by the yoke, is responsible for causing the development of such inflammatory swelling, it is known as yoke gall. It resembles saddle gall in horses and fara gall in elephants. The occurrence of such hot, painful swelling is sudden and may not be noticed during the course of the work.

A yoke gall may be infected and form an abscess which may be acute (hot) or a chronic (cold) abscess which makes the animal incapable for ploughing or carrying carts. The swelling may persist, become fibrous and appears like a fibrous tumour in the course of time. Gangrene and sloughing of tissues may supervene if the injury is severe.

Treatment

1. Moist hot fermentation with Mag Sulph (Epsom salt) or fomentation with warm water containing common salt is beneficial to reduce the pain.
2. Massage with Catgall, Briclofen Plus gel, Inflagel vet, Iodex Vet ointment, Iodovet ointment on the affected part 10-15 minutes twice in a day for 7-10 days is also found beneficial.
3. Needle aspiration of accumulated tissue fluid from the gall can be made to reduce swelling. Local administration of antibiotics *e.g.* Inj. Gentamycin, Inj. Enrofloxacin along with local administration of corticosteroids *e.g.* Inj. Dexamethasone, Inj. Prednisolone *etc.* is very much effective for the quick reduction of the swelling and to combat secondary bacterial infection.
4. Administration of NSAID by IM route to reduce pain and inflammation.
5. If gangrene, necrosis or suppuration occurs, in that case parenteral broad-spectrum antibiotic therapy with Inj. Oxytetracycline, Inj. Streptopenicillin (see antibiotics) for 3-5 days by IM route should be carried out.
6. In case of sloughing and tissue necrosis local application of multipurpose herbal gel *e.g.* Ectosefoint, Himax, Sorine, Charmil, Topicure gel, Dermocept *etc.* can be applied.
7. In case of hard yoke gall, red ointment (blistering ointment) should be applied after applying petroleum gelly or vaseline on the healthy surrounding area of the gall. This will help in ripening of the hard mass.
8. In case of abscess formation of the gall, surgical intervention to be made to make drainage of the accumulated pus or exudates. Regular dressing with Tr. Iodine or Acriflavin lotion or packing the incised cavity with gauge soaked with Himax lotion or ointment *e.g.* Charmil, Himax, Topicure *etc.* helps in healing and recovery of the incised gall.
9. Systemic antibiotic therapy with Inj. Loxy, Inj. Intamycin or Inj. Biostrep, Inj. Bistripen or Inj. Dicrysticin 2.5 g for 5-7 days by IM route should be carried out for speedy recovery.

12.30 ABSCESS

Abscess may develop at any part of the animal's body and its formation is very common in grazing ruminants, although it occurs in all the animals owing to varying eatiologies. It is characterized by a round cavity filled with localized collection of plus under the skin or in any organ.

Symptoms

Swelling of the affected part with pain sensation.. The swelling may be hot and painful. It may turn red. It may have soft point felt on palpation in case of ripened (matured) abscess.

Abscess may be classified as:

1. Acute abscess (Hot or raw abscess)
2. Cold or chronic abscess.
3. Superficial abscess
4. Deep abscess.

When pyogenic organisms enter an organ, an acute inflammation results with death of cells. These dead (cells) material is liquefied by proteolytic ferments resulting in pus in a cavity or abscess. The discontinuity of the skin or mucous membrane that results by opening of an abscess on to the surface is called an ulcer. Ulcer may also develop due to direct action of irritant on the skin or mucous.

Diagnosis

Exploratory needle puncture will help in diagnosis and will differentiate from hematoma, cyst or hernia. If it is abscess, pus will definitely come out.

Treatment

1. To ripen the abscess moist hot fomentation with Epsom salt (Mag Sulph) should be done.
2. Give incision through the lower most part of abscess for maximum drainage of pus. After cleaning the cavity gauge soaked with Tincture of iodine should be packed and if necessary regular dressing can be done.
3. Local application of multipurpose antiseptic herbal ointment *e.g.* Topicure, Himax, Chormil, Dressol ointment can be done.
4. Systemic antibiotic *e.g.* Inj. Oxytetracyline, Inj. Streptopenicillin (2.5 g) IM daily on 3-5 days can be used.

12.31 BROKEN HORN (HORN FRACTURE)

Direct violence, infighting and striking of the horn against a fixed subject etc. usually cause horn fracture. Fracture may occur at the base of the horn or horn may be broken right through the structure. The fracture may be complete or incomplete and direction of the fracture is usually irregular. Avulsion of horn and subsequent fracture or broken horn may also occur in both cattle and buffalo.

Treatment

1. Amputation of horn just below the sheath of fracture.

2. The horn in large animal to be amputed either by flap or direct amputation method with the help of embryotomy wire or saw immediately below the coronary band. In flap method the two edges of the skin flap are brought together in close composition without tension by cutting the extra bone by chisel and hammer. Haemorrhage should be controlled by ligating the vessels. The skin flap is sutured by interrupted or mattress sutures.

3. A course of antibiotic *e.g.* Inj. Oxytetracycline, Inj. Steptopenicillin *etc.* by IM route should be given for 4-5 days.

4. Fly repellant should be used on the skin.
5. The wound should be treated with antiseptics till healing occurs.
6. Protect the wound with antiseptic pad and bandage.
7. Tetanus toxoid should be administered stat during operation or treating broken horn.

12.32 AVULSION OF HORN

Separation of sheath of horn is known as avulsion of horn. The sheath is separated from the horn core owing to direct violence repeated injury by yoke, fighting, trauma *etc*. Sheath of horns may become loose and easily detached by striking it against a fixed object. Haemorrhage occurs with the avulsion even with the mild touch or friction with the hard object. Hence immediate care should be taken to protect the exposed core with antiseptic pad or bandage application.

Treatment

1. Clean and disinfect the horn core.
2. Check the bleeding with the application of styptics (*e.g.* Tr. of iodine).
3. Apply antiseptic pad and bandage on the exposed horn core.
4. If necessary, a course of antibiotic and NSAID may be administered.

12.33 SNAKE BITE

Snake bite is common in domesticated animals and deaths occur due to the venom or by sepsis of the wound. The venom is injected by fangs during bite. Fang marks on skin are diagnostic in bites by poisonous snakes. These comprise a row of small punctures with 2 large punctures outside them. Non venomous snakes leave two rows of small punctures only.

Two common groups of snakes are viperine and elapine where elapines cause flaccid paralysis, mydriasis and respiratory paresis and viperines produce haemorrhage and arteriolar thrombosis and necrosis. Venoms are most toxic to horses and also fatal to dogs. Coral snakes, cobras, kraits and mombus belonged to elapidae, rattle snakes, pit vipers, water moceasins are very much venomous.

Common Poisonous Snakes of India

1. *Naja naja* – Cobra
2. *Naja hannat* – King cobra.
3. Russell's viper – (*Vipera russelli*)
4. Saw scaled viper – (*Echis carinatus*)
5. Krait – *Bungarus coerulens*

The snakes of the genus viperaine contains: (1) Haemolysin (2) Neurotoxin (3) Coagulin, (4) Cytolycin (5) Necrotising factors.

Cobra venome contains (1) Neurotoxin (2) Nephrotoxic factor and (3) hemolytic factors.

Causes of Death in Snake Bite

1. Respiratory failure
2. Intravascular clotting in vital organs
3. Pulmonary oedema
4. Paralysis of muscles of respiration
5. Cardiac failure
6. Acute renal failure (Coagulative necrosis)

Symptoms

Local effects – oedematous swelling, echymosis and extravassation at the site of bite.

Systemic effect – Cobra snake bite produces respiratory embarrassment, restlessness, salivation, dyspnoea, regurgitation of ingesta, vomiting, ataxia, convulsion and death due to respiratory failure.

In rattle snake bite there is restlessness, grinding of teeth vomiting, salivation, dyspnoea, ataxia, convulsions *etc.*

Adder snake bite causes rapid swelling, pain, excitement, salivation, hyperesthesia, tetany, recumbency, paralysis and death due to asphyxia.

Brown snake bite causes drowsiness, muscle tremors, droping of eyelids and lips, tongue paresis, laboured respiration *etc.* Death occurs due to venom or by sepsis of wound. Treatment includes administration of Antivenom IV, Antibiotics IM and Antitoxin IV.

Treatment

1. Tourniquet 1-2 inches above the bite.
2. Washing of wound or fang marks with 5 per cent Pot. permanganate solution.
3. Give incision to bleed out the venom as soon as possible. No use of incision after 30 minutes.
4. IV administration of antivenom (Antivenin). Polyvalent Anti snake venom-serum (PASVS)/Polyvalent antivenin @ 10-20 ml/animal by IV route.
5. Inj. Neostigmine (*e.g.* Prostigmine) @ 5-7.5 mg/calf IV. (Neostigmine stabilizes acetylcholine).
6. Adrenaline (1 : 1000) 1-2 ml IV or SC (for Cobra bite).
7. Corticosteroids, Glucocorticosteroids, Dexamethasone can be administered to counter the effects of hyaluronidase (*e.g.* in Cobra bite).
8. Tetanus toxoid should be given.
9. Fluids and electrolytes can be infused as per requirement.
10. Check convulsions with parenteral administration of Phenobarbital sodium.
11. Analgesics can be used/administered.
12. Inj. Atropine sulphate can be used to check salivation.
13. For haematuria blood transfusion or blood expander can be used.
14. Keep warmth of the animal.

Chapter 13

Common Control Measures Against Infectious Diseases

13.1 TIPS FOR CONTROLLING INFECTIOUS DISEASES OF ANIMALS

1. Proper maintenance of barn or shed with respect to sanitation and disposal of sewage.
2. Animals should be kept in a clean, well lighted and well ventilated shed (place) with adequate floor space and head space.
3. Avoidance of damp floor and muddy housing system.
4. Provision of adequate clean drinking water.
5. Provision of exercise for animals.
6. Fly repellents may be used to ward off the insect population.
7. Adoption of hygienic measures against ecto-parasites (ticks and lice)
8. Proper disposal of infected litter and carcass.
9. Proper disposal of after birth (placenta/foetal membrane).
10. Regular grooming of animals, cleaning of animal's body to be done.
11. Routine deworming to be carried out.
12. Disinfection of the barn/byre at regular interval with formalin (10 per cent), caustic soda (10 per cent), phenol, lime or bleaching powder.
13. Regular screening of animals against Tuberculosis, Brucellosis and Paratuberculosis.

14. Routine prophylactic vaccination against common bacterial and viral diseases.
15. Isolation of sick animals from apparently healthy animals for treatment.
16. Provision of strict quarantine of newly introduced animals.
17. Movement restriction of animals suffering from contagious diseases.
18. Dead animals (carcass) should be properly disposed off either by deep burial with lime and bleaching or by incineration (burning).
19. Postmortem (autopsy) examination to be carried out by qualified veterinarian for knowing the cause of death.
20. Carcass should not be opened in an open place to avoid contamination of soil.
21. Serological tests to be carried out to ascertain the presence of antigens.
22. Aborted foetus and foetal membrane should be disposed off properly.
23. Proper care should be taken to keep the newborn soon after its birth.
24. Perineum and udder of the cow should be washed with clean water before calving and during milking.
25. The navel region of the calf should be properly disinfected with 2 per cent Tr. Iodine solution soon after birth.
26. Calf should be fed with colostrum @ 1/10th of calf's body weight preferably within the first hour after the birth, and to be continued for 3-5 days. If sufficient colostrum is not available, colostrum substitute should be fed to the newborn calf (Table 13.1).
27. Crow scavenging, and entry of stray dogs to the herd needs to be restricted
28. Insecticides, rodenticides *etc.* to be used with caution for the control of pests, insects, rats and rodents.

Table 13.1: Composition and Dose of Colostrum Substitute for Calf

Ingredients	*Quantity*	*Dose*
Raw egg	1 piece (50-60 g)	Thrice daily for 3-5 days @ 1/10th of calf's body weight
Warm water	275 ml	
Castor oil	5 ml	
Warm whole milk	525 ml	
Aureomycin	80 mg	
Vitamin – A	10,000 IU	

13.2 PROPHYLACTIC VACCINATION SCHEDULE FOR VARIOUS SPECIES OF ANIMALS

The prophylactic vaccination schedules for young calf, cattle and buffalo, goat, sheep, pig, dog, broiler and layer are depicted in Table 13.2 to 13.9.

Table 13.2: Vaccination Schedule for Young Calves

Sl.No.	*Name of the Vaccine*	*Age at Vaccination*	*Booster/Revaccination*
1.	Foot and Mouth Disease (FMD) vaccine	6 to 8 weeks	At 6 month age; then repeat biannually
2.	Black Quarter (BQ) vaccine	6 months	Annually (May/June)
3.	Haemorrhagic Septicaemia (HS) Alum precipitated vaccine	6 months	Annually (May-June)
4.	Anthrax spore vaccine	6 months	Annually
5.	Brucella Cotton strain 19 vaccine	6-9 months	Only once, immediately after calving.

1: Dose should be as per manufacturer's recommendation.

2: HS-BQ combined vaccine and HS, BQ and FMD combined vaccines are available in the market, which may be used instead of individual vaccine.

Table 13.3: Vaccination Schedule for Cattle and Buffalo

Disease	Vaccine	Vaccination Schedule (Age)			Remarks
		Primary/Booster	Revaccination	Dosage and Administration	
Anthrax	Anthrax spore vaccine (Live)	All ages (Preferably above 4 months of age)	Annual	1ml SC	Immunity lasts for 1 year
Black Quarter (BQ)	Polyvalent killed BQ vaccine	Calves – 6 months of age	Annual	5 ml SC	Immunity lasts for 1 year
Haemorrhagic Septicemia (HS)	HS Oil adjuvant vaccine	Calves – 6 months and above	Annual	2-3 ml, IM (Bovilis HS 2 ml SC)	Massage the vaccinated area
	HS alum precipitated broth vaccine	Calves – 6 months and above	Biannual	5 ml SC	Massage the vaccinated area
Brucellosis	Live vaccine *Brucella abortus* Cotton strain – 19 vaccine	Calves between 6-9 months of age	Biannual	5 ml SC	Lactating animals after parturition may also be vaccinated.
HS and BQ	Combined HS and BQ commercial vaccine	Above 4 months	Annual/Biannual	@ 2 ml SC (HS-BQ vaccine, Intervet)	Bovilis HS and BQ (Intervet) Cattle and Buffalo @ 2 ml by SC;
				@ 4 ml SC (HS-BQ vaccine, Biomed)	Raksha HS and BQ (Indian Immunologicals) 3 ml SC, 90 ml bottle/30 doses
Foot and Mouth Disease (FMD)	Polyvalent (0, A_{22}, C and Asia-I) cell culture vaccine	4 months and above	Biannual	@ 5-10 ml SC	
	Raksha -FMD vaccine (Indian Immunologicals)	4 months and above	Biannual	@ 3 ml SC	1st vaccine on 'O' day and revaccinated at 22nd day and then 6 months interval.
	Bovilis FMD V Gel	Cattle and Buffalo–6-8 weeks; then 1-1$^1/_2$ month later.	Biannual	Cattle and Buffalo 2 ml SC	
Theileriosis	Attenuated vaccine	4 months and above	Annual	@ 3ml SC	For exotic and cross bred animals.

Table 13.4: Vaccination Schedule for Goats

Disease	*Name of the Vaccine*	*Age/Schedule of Vaccination*	*Dose and Administration*	*Remarks*
Goat pox	Goat pox vaccine (Tissue culture vaccine, IVRI)	1st vaccine at 3 months; then yearly.	0.3 g to be pulverized and mixed in 30 ml glycerin saline, @ 0.3 ml/goat SC at tip of ear.	It can be stored for 15 days at 20-25°C and 3 months if kept in refrigerator.
Peste des petits ruminants (PPR)	Tissue culture PPR vaccine (IVRI)/ Raksha-PPR (Indian Immunologicals)	1st vaccine at 3 months; immunity lasts for about 3 years.	1 ml/goat SC	Safe vaccine; can be given to pregnant animals also; can be stored in refrigerator at 4°C for 1 year.
Foot and Mouth Disease (FMD)	Polyvalent (A,O, C, Asia-I), *e.g.* Raksha-Ovac (Indian Immunologicals)	1st vaccine at 4 months; booster dose after 9 months; then yearly.	1 ml/goat IM	Clovax FMD Vaccine (Intervet) can be given to goats at 3 weeks of age.
Enterotoxaemia	Multicomponent, *e.g.* Enterotoxaemia vaccine type C and D (Intervet)	1st vaccine at 1-1½ month (if mother doe was vaccinated 1 month prior to kidding) or at 1 week (if mother doe was not vaccinated during pregnancy); then booster dose after 21 days; then at 6 months interval.	5 ml/goat SC	Raksha-ET (Indian immunologicals) can be given first time at 4 months of age, then annually.
Contagious Caprine Pleura Pneumonia (CCPP)	CCPP vaccine (IVRI)	6 months interval	0.2 ml/goat SC at the tip of ear.	Can be preserved for 1month at 2-5°C
Haemorrhagic Septicaemia (HS)	Oil adjuvant vaccine, H S vaccine (Intervet)/Raksha-HS (Indian Immunologicals)	1st vaccine at 6 months of age or more, then annually.	2 ml/goat SC	This vaccine should be given if the disease is prevalent in the goat rearing area.
Black Quarter (BQ)	BQ Vaccine (Intervet)/Raksha-BQ (Indian Immunologicals)	1st vaccine at 6 months of age or more, then annually.	2 ml/goat SC	This vaccine should be given if the disease is prevalent in the goat rearing area.
Anthrax	Anthrax Spore Vaccine, Live (Intervet)	Once in a year	1 ml/goat SC	This vaccine should be given if the disease is prevalent in the goat rearing area.

Table 13.5: Vaccination schedule for sheep

Disease	Vaccine	Vaccination Schedule (Age)			Remarks
		Primary/Booster	Revaccination	Dosage and Administration	
Enterotoxaemia	Enterotoxaemia vaccine (*Clostridium welchii* type-D cell culture puppy kidney vaccine)	Lambs above 3 months of age	Booster after 14 days, then annual.	@ 2.5 ml SC, repeated after 14 days with same quantity, then annual vaccination.	Produced by IVRI, Izatnagar; IAH and VB, Bangalore; IVP, Pune; APVB and R, Hyderabad.
Clostridial Diseases (Pulpy kidney disease, Struck, Lamb dysentery, Black disease and Braxy)	Multicomponent clostridial vaccine	All ages above 3 months; dose is same for lamb and adult.	Booster after 14-21 days; then annual.	@ 5 ml by SC route at an interval of 14-21 days in the first year; later subsequent years (Annual vaccination)	
	Bovilis MCV	4-6 weeks of age in lambs born to vaccinated ewes and 1 week of age in lambs born to unvaccinated ewes.	Booster after 3-6 weeks of primary vaccination	Revaccination at six months. Dose @ 2 ml SC	Vial 50ml (Bovilis MCV – Intervet); Vial 100 ml (50 dose) Inactivated Enterotoxaemia vaccine.
Enterotoxaemia	Bovilis ETV (Toxoid of *Cl. perfringens*)	Do	Do	Revaccination at six months @ 2 ml SC	Inactivated Enterotoxaemia vaccine
Black Quarter	Polyvalent Black quarter vaccine	All ages above 3 months. All seasons preferably May-June	Annual revaccination	Lamb – 2 ml SC Adult – 3 ml SC	Combined HS-BQ vaccine may be used.
Haemorrhagic Septicaemia (HS)	HS Oil adjuvant vaccine	Adult (May-June)	Annual	HS Oil adjuvant vaccine (Intervet) 1ml SC	Combined HS-BQ vaccine may be used.

Contd...

Table 13.5–Contd...

Disease	*Vaccine*	*Vaccination Schedule (Age)*			Remarks
		Primary/Booster	*Revaccination*	*Dosage and Administration*	
Foot and Mouth Disease (FMD)	FMD vaccine	At 3 months and above	Booster after 4-6 weeks of primary vaccination; 2nd booster after 24 weeks	@ 1ml IM	FMD vaccine (adjuvant with mineral oil (Intervet)
Sheep Pox	Sheep pox vaccine	At 3 months and above	Booster after 4-6 weeks of primary vaccination; 2nd booster after 24 weeks. Revaccination every 24-48 weeks.	Lamb – 3 ml SC Sheep – 5 ml SC	Raksha–SP freeze dried vaccine –(50 doses with diluents)
PPR (*Peste des petits ruminants*)	PPR Tissue culture vaccine	At 3 months and above	Primary vaccination	Reconstituted vaccine	Immunity may last for 3 years. Raksha-PPR vaccine (Indian Immunologicals)

Table 13.6: Vaccination Schedule for Pig

Disease	*Name of the Vaccine*	*Age/Schedule of Vaccination*	*Dose and Administration*	*Immunity*
Swine Fever or Hog Cholera	Tissue Culture Vaccine, Swine Fever Vaccine (Intervet)	1st vaccine at 6-8 weeks of age, then annually.	1 ml./pig IM.	1 year
Foot and Mouth Disease (FMD)	Polyvalent (A,O, C, Asia-I), *e.g.* Raksha-Ovac (Indian Immunologicals)	1st vaccine at 2 months; then at an interval of 6 months.	2 ml/pig IM	Clovax FMD Vaccine (Intervet) can be given to pig at 3 weeks of age.

Table 13.7: Vaccination Schedule for Dog

Disease	*Name of the Vaccine*	*Age at Vaccination*	*Booster*	*Revaccination*
Canine Distemper	Modified live virus vaccine against CD	6-8 weeks	12-16 weeks	Annual
Infectious Canine Hepatitis	Modified live virus ICH vaccine (CAV-1 or CAV-2) or Inactivated (CAV-1) vaccine	6-8 weeks	12-16 weeks	Annual
Rabies	Modified Rabies Live virus/ Inactivated Rabies virus vaccine	3-4 months	10 months	Annual or at an interval of 3 years or as per the specific product/recommendation of the manufacturer
Canine Leptospirosis	Killed Leptospira vaccine (Bacteria)	9 weeks	12-16 weeks	Annual
Canine Parvovirus	Inactivated Parvo viral vaccine	6-8 weeks	12 weeks	Annual

Table 13.8: Common Vaccination Schedule for Broiler Chicken

Sl.No.	*Age*	*Disease*	*Vaccine*	*Dose and Route of Administration*	*Remarks*
1.	4-7 days	Ranikhet Disease	RDF_1 or LaSota strain (live)	1 drop, nasal or ocular route; or oral through drinking water.	Booster dose is to be given at 21-23 days of age.
2.	12-14 days	Gumboro Disease (IBD)	IBD/ Gumboro vaccine (live)	Oral through drinking water	May be repeated at 28-30 days of age.
3.	21-23 days	Ranikhet Disease (Booster dose)	LaSota vaccine (live)	1 drop, nasal or ocular route; or oral through drinking water.	–

NB: This is a typical vaccination programme in broiler chicken production areas. Individual programmes are highly variable and reflect local conditions, disease prevalence, severity of challenge, and individual preferences. Some vaccines may be combined in some areas. Vaccination for some diseases depends on local requirements. However, modification of this schedule, if needed, should be done with the help of experienced veterinarians or poultry specialists.

Table 13.9: Common Vaccination Schedule for Layer Chicken

Sl.No.	*Age*	*Disease*	*Vaccine*	*Dose and Route of Administration*	*Remarks*
1.	1 day	Marek's Disease	HVT MD vaccine	0.2 ml/bird, IM injection	Generally it is given at hatchery level; it can be given up to the age of 3 days.
2.	4-7 days	Ranikhet Disease	RDF_1 or LaSota vaccine	1 drop, nasal or ocular route; or through drinking water.	Booster dose to be given at 5-6 weeks of age.
3.	12-14 days	Gumboro Disease (IBD)	IBD/Gumboro vaccine	Oral through drinking water.	Booster may be given at 6-7 weeks of age.
4.	5-6 weeks	Ranikhet Disease (Booster dose)	RDF_1 vaccine	1 drop, nasal or ocular route; or through drinking water.	–
5.	6-7 weeks	Gumboro Disease (Booster dose)	IBD/Gumboro vaccine	Same as Sl.No. 3	–
6.	7-8 weeks	Fowl Pox	Fowl Pox vaccine	0.01 ml/bird, injection at wing web or 1 drop by picking of feathers.	One vaccine is sufficient for bird's life. However, it may be repeated at 14 weeks of age.

Contd...

Table 13.9–Contd...

Sl.No.	*Age*	*Disease*	*Vaccine*	*Dose and Route of Administration*	*Remarks*
7.	8-10 weeks	Ranikhet Disease	RDR_2B or Mukteswar strain vaccine	0.5 ml/bird, SC at wing web.	In endemic area, LaSota vaccine is given at this age followed by R_2B at 13 weeks of age.
8.	15-16 weeks	Infectious Bronchitis	IB vaccine	0.5 ml/bird, SC or I/M at wing web.	Booster dose at 40 weeks of age.
9.	18 weeks	Ranikhet Disease (Booster dose)	RDR_2B vaccine (killed)	0.5 ml/bird, SC at wing web.	Then it is repeated at 35 weeks of age, and then LaSota vaccine at the interval of 8 weeks.

NB: This is a typical vaccination programme in layer chicken production areas. Individual programmes are highly variable and reflect local conditions, disease prevalence, severity of challenge, and individual preferences. Some vaccines may be combined in some areas. Vaccination for some diseases depends on local requirements. However, modification of this schedule, if needed, should be done with the help of experienced veterinarians or poultry specialists.

Part – III
Gynaecology and Obstetrics Section

Chapter 14
Reproductive Characteristics of Animals

14.1 REPRODUCTIVE SYSTEM OF ANIMALS

Reproduction simply means propagation of species through production of young ones. Male and female animals have their specific roles in reproduction, and their reproductive systems are also different. Males have the male reproductive system and females have the female reproductive system.

14.1.1 Male Reproductive System

Male reproductive system of farm animals consists of a pair of testis, epididymis, vas deferens, urethra and penis, and accessory sex glands. Testis is the primary reproductive organ, situated outside the body in the skin pouch like structure called scrotum. In ruminants and dogs, testis is located at inguinal region, and in pigs and cats it is located at subanal region. The reproductive tract is formed with epididymis, vas deferens and urethra. The penis is the copulatory organ of male animals. The accessory sex glands are ampula, seminal vesicles, prostrate gland and cowper's gland or bulbo-urethral gland.

14.1.2 Female Reproductive System

Female reproductive system of farm animals consists of a pair of ovary, fallopian tube, uterus, cervix, vagina and vulva. Ovary is the primary reproductive organ, situated in the pelvic cavity at the side of each uterus in case of cow. Each ovary weighs about 10-12 g in cow. Ovary releases ovum and two important female sex hormones, *viz.*, estrogen and progesterone. Fallopian tube is 20-25 cm in length and divided in to four parts namely uterine, isthmus, ampula and infundibulum. Uterus

Table 14.1: Reproductive Characteristics of Female Farm Animals

Species	*Age at 1st Mating*	*Periodicity of Estrous Cycle*	*Duration of Estrus (Heat)*	*Time of Ovulation*	*Right Time of Mating*	*Gestation Period*	*Time of Post-Parturient Mating*
Cattle	Deshi 24 months; Exotic 18-20 months.	21 days interval	12-18 hrs	12-16 hrs after the end of estrus	10-12 hrs after the 1st appearance of heat signs	280 days	2-3 months
Buffalo	2½ yrs	21 days interval	8 hrs – 3 days (average 32 hrs)	At the end of estrus	At the end of estrus (last 8 hrs)	310 days	2-3 months
Goat	12-15 months (earlier age in small breeds)	18-21 days interval	1-2 days	At the end of estrus	10-12 hrs after the 1st appearance of heat signs	150 days	Next season
Sheep	12-15 months	17 days interval (14-19 days)	30-36 hrs	At the end of estrus (last 12 hrs)	20 hrs after the 1st appearance of heat signs	148 days	Next season
Pig	8 months	21 days interval	2-3 days	36 hrs after the onset of estrus and up to next 12 hrs	12 hrs and 24-26 hrs after the 1st appearance of heat signs– 2 times.	114 days	1st heat after farrowing (2½ months later)
Rabbit	6-7 months	No definite estrous cycle	–	Induced ovulation	Any time – at morning or evening	30 days	After weaning
Horse	12-24 months	14-21 days	2-6 days	24-48 hrs before the end of estrus		336 days	21-28 days

is muscular organ and has two parts – body and horns (two in number). Usually uterus is located in pelvic cavity and during gestation it is located in abdominal cavity. Cervix is actually the neck of the uterus, and it is located in between uterus and vagina. Vagina is the copulatory organ of female. It is about 8-10 inches in length in adult female cattle. Vulva is the terminal opening of female reproductive system and consists of two lateral vulval lips and clitoris.

14.2 REPRODUCTIVE CHARACTERISTICS OF LIVESTOCK

Various reproductive characteristics of livestock are given in Table 14.1.

14.3 FORECASTING OF DATE OF PARTURITION

Knowing the expected date of parturition (delivery) is very important for reducing parturition related hazards and also for providing better management. Forecasting of date of parturition in case of various livestock species are given in Table 14.2.

Table 14.2: Forecasting of Date of Parturition*

Date of Service	*Date of Parturition*				
	Cow	*She Buffalo*	*Doe*	*Ewe*	*Sow*
January 1	October 7	November 6	May 30	May 28	April 24
January 16	October 22	November 21	June 14	June 12	May 9
February 1	November 7	December 7	June 30	June 28	May 25
February 16	November 22	December 22	July 15	July 13	June 9
March 1	December 5	January 4	July 28	July 26	June 22
March 16	December 20	January 19	August 12	August 10	July 7
April 1	January 5	February 4	August 28	August 26	July 23
April 16	January 20	February 19	September 12	September 10	August 7
May 1	February 4	March 6	September 27	September 25	August 22
May 16	February 19	March 21	October 12	October 10	September 6
June 1	March 7	April 6	October 28	October 26	September 22
June 16	March 22	April 21	November 12	November 10	October 7
July 1	April 6	May 6	November 27	November 25	October 22
July 16	April 21	May 21	December 12	December 10	November 6
August 1	May 7	June 6	December 28	December 26	November 22
August 16	May 22	June 21	January 12	January 10	December 7
September 1	June 7	July 7	January 28	January 26	December 23
September 16	June 22	July 22	February 12	February 10	January 7
October 1	July 7	August 6	February 27	February 25	January 22
October 16	July 22	August 21	March 14	March 12	February 6
November 1	August 7	September 6	March 30	March 28	February 22

Contd...

Table 14.2–Contd...

Date of Service	*Date of Parturition*				
	Cow	*She Buffalo*	*Doe*	*Ewe*	*Sow*
November 16	August 22	September 21	April 14	April 12	March 9
December 1	September 6	October 6	April 29	April 27	March 24
December 16	September 21	October 21	May 14	May 12	April 8

* This table indicates the expected date of parturition when the females are served on the 1st or the 16th day of the month. If the date of service is after the indicated date, equal number of date is to be added to the date of parturition given in the table.

Chapter 15
Breeding Policy, Andrological Examination of Bull and Artificial Insemination

15.1 BREEDING POLICIES FOR CATTLE AND BUFFALO IN INDIA

During the pre-independent period, India did not have any specific approved breeding policy for development of dairy cattle and buffalo. After independence, Indian Council of Agricultural Research (ICAR) has made the following recommendations:

1. In non-descript cattle, milch and draught qualities should be combined to produce an average kind of animal.
2. For specific types, selective breeding should be utilized to improve their draft and milch qualities.
3. In well defined breeds, the milk production should be increased as far as possible without seriously impairing the draft capacity of these animals.
4. For well defined milch breeds, selective breeding was recommended to develop their milch capacity to the maximum possible extent. This strategy of selective breeding and upgrading of indigenous breeds continued till 1952.

Breed Improvement and Conservation

1. A separate policy for conservation of indigenous cattle breeds and their germplasm should be drawn up and translated into an implemental programme.

2. Crossbreeding with exotic strains needs to be banned in the home tracts of the important cattle breeds and the ban should be strictly got implemented by the State Governments.
3. A judicious mix of cross breeding with exotic strains and preservation of indigenous germplasms should be maintained, while formulating the policy. Import of germplasm should be allowed only in very specific cases and after taking all the precautions to prevent the ingress of diseases into the country.

Breeding Policies Adopted to Augment Productivity of Cattle and Buffaloes

1. Selective breeding of the pure Indian breeds of cattle and buffalo for milk production.
2. Selective breeding of dual purpose breeds for improving their milk and work output.
3. Upgrading of non-descript Indian cattle and buffaloes with selected Indian improved breeds for productivity of milk and work output.
4. Cross breeding of Indian breeds of cattle and buffalo.
5. Cross breeding of Indian breeds of cattle using exotic breeds.

Technologies Involved in Breeding of Cattle and Buffaloes

1. Genetic evaluation of sires and dams for selection.
2. Artificial insemination for maximum use of superior bulls with improved genes in identified populations.
3. Multiple ovulation and embryotransfer to improve the intensity and accuracy of selection and to reduce the period of evaluation.

Bulls to be used for A.I. are evaluated for their ability to transmit economic traits advantageous to the breeders and the industry, *i.e.* milk yield, fat and protein percentage, fertility and number of allied factors.

Open Nucleus Breeding System (ONBS)

This system envisages formation of a nucleus population of breedable animals of exceptionally high genetic merit. The outstanding breedable males are to be let out from the nucleus herd to the farmers or breeders in the neighbouring areas to bring about genetic improvement of their animals.

The Work Plans to be Adopted for ONBS

1. Screening of the unrecorded base population for identifying some outstanding females.
2. Collection of the outstanding females to form a nucleus herd which could be used as test group of animals.

3. Superovulation of the elite animals from the outstanding animals *in vitro* with semen of superior sires.
4. Transfer of the resulting embryos to the test group in the nucleus herd as well as to the females in the unrecorded base population.
5. The best males are selected on the basis of their own performances as well as on sibling's performance. These are then can be extensively used in the field.
6. The female offspring are next considered as potential elite females to donate embryos by MOET for the following cycle after their appraisal against elite cows already present in the nucleus herd and used upon for MOET.

15.2 ANDROLOGICAL EXAMINATION OF BULL

Bulls should be healthy and free from diseases, especially those which may be transferred through semen. Testing for infectious diseases like Brucellosis, Paratuberculosis, Tuberculosis, Campylobacteriosis, Trichomoniasis, Leptospirosis, Bovine viral diarrhoea (BVD) and Infectious Bovine Rhinotracheitis (IBR) should be done before introducing bull into semen collection.

While selecting the bull for breeding purpose its libido should also be tested and it should have short reaction time so that maximum semen doses can be harvested in short period, semen quality and freezability can be improved if bulls are provided thermal comfort throughout the year. The best age to harvest maximum semen doses of good quality from a breeding bull is between three to eight years. Therefore, proper attention should be paid during this age period for harvesting maximum doses of semen.

Bull Health and Hygiene

To harvest quality semen, the bull should be tested and free from any kind of disease which may get transmitted through semen. In addition, proper washing of bull and teaser bull should be practiced before semen collection for abstaining contamination free semen. The prepucial washing just before collection to avoid transfer of any contamination to semen from the bull should be done. Bull apron can also be used to collect clean semen.

15.3 COLLECTION, PROCESSING, CRYOPRESERVATION AND EVALUATION OF SEMEN

Semen Collection

Tying of aprons (65 x 62 cm with semicircular cut at one end by leaving 12 cm., on either side and fixing slightly heavy 2 to 3 metal pieces on opposite side to keep it straight and to avoid folding apron) to the bulls is very important to protect penis from hind quarter of dummy for proper and clean collection of semen.

Semen collection should be made in dust free environment in a sterilized AV (artificial vagina) and use a separate AV for every ejaculate for hygienic semen collection. While collecting the semen precaution must be taken that penis of the bull does not touch hands, which can cause the contamination of semen. Entry of penis into the AV can be made by made by guiding the penis by holding it through prepuce. Dummy/teaser bull should have lower height than the mounting bull so that the mounting is comfortable. Use of gloves by collectors can make hygienic semen collection.

Semen Evaluation

Immediately after collection semen should be brought to the laboratory. After removing from the AV, semen tube should be put in a water bath at 30° ± 2°C for further evaluation and processing. Semen is routinely evaluated for ejaculate volume, color, mass activity sperm concentration and sperm motility for every ejaculate. Mass activity is observed under the low (x100) power on a warm (37°C) stage microscope. The ejaculate having 3+ or more mass activity should be processed further for freezing, otherwise discarded. Other morphoanatomical attributes of sperm cells such as live dead count, sperm abnormality and acrosomal integrity should be assessed periodically in the fresh, cooled and frozen thawed semen of each level.

In certain situations, a farily large number of bulls produce azospermatic semen and poor quality semen which are very poor freezable in nature. This is a serious problem. But recently Sephadex Filtration Technique is being applied which improve the quality of such ejaculates as well as improve the freezability and storage capability of semen.

Semen Dilution

Dilution of bull's semen is made with the use of specific dilutor to achieve acceptable freezability and dilutor should be prepared in the laminar flow chamber. This buffer with 6-7 per cent glycerol and 10-20 per cent egg yolk is commonly used for dilution of buffalo bull semen and results in acceptable freezability. Dilutor being prepared under laminar flow having a pH of 6.8 is autoclaved before use followed by addition of antibiotics.

Semen dilution is done on the basis of the number of spermatozoa required per inseminating dose. In general a total of 40-50 million sperms are kept per insemination dose, out of which at least 20 million should be forward moving sperms.

Glyceralization should be done at room temperature to avoid cold shock to the spermatozoa during the process of pre-freezing cooling. Use of photometer with auto dilutor and printer makes quick and more precision in concentration measurement and dilutor volume. Schedule pH measurement of all equipments and working solution should be done in each step.

Cooling

After dilution semen should be kept for cooling in a cold cabinet to maintain the semen temperature between 3-5°C for five hours. Cooling should be adjusted in such a way that the cold cabinet temperature reaches 5°C within two hours of putting the semen in the cabinet for cooling. Filling and sealing machine, straws and other utensils which come in contact with semen should be kept in cabinet so that they are isothermal to the semen before its filling into straws. Slight rise in the temperature of cooling cabinet during filling and sealing of straws may cause damage to spermatozoa.

Pre-freeze Evaluation

After cooling, semen should be checked for individual sperm motility. Semen having <55 percent individual motility should not be used or filled into the straws for freezing. Sperm motility is assessed on a warm (37°C) stage microscope under low power (x 200) by putting a drop of semen on a slide and covering it with a cover slip.

Trinocular phase contrast microscope with camera monitor and heating stage can increase the efficacy of primary gross evaluation process over the simple binocular one.

Raw semen or frozen semen samples from each semen donor (bull) is taken for different quality control test depending on the test schedule following minimum standard protocol. These are (1) live dead count (2) acrosomal integrity test (3) morphology test (4) hypo-osmotic swelling test (HOST) (5) post thaw viability test of spermatozoa before or after freezing including concentration in each straw.

Recently computer assisted semen analysis system has been adopted for quick quality evaluation of semen. For microbial contamination study, scheduled aerial count, rinse and working solution test should be done.

Semen Filling and Sealing

Nowadays mini (0.25 ml) straw are used for semen filling as universally accepted standard for the best post thaw sperm motility in almost all the farm animals. Semen straw should be printed with bull number, breed of the bull, date of collections and name of the institution for the identification and proper storage of semen. Semen straws should be kept in UV chamber for 15 minutes for sterilization before cooling in the cold cabinet. After cooling, semen samples selected for filling into straws should be filled with automatic or semi-automatic straw filling and scaling machine in order to get better post thaw motility in comparison to manual system.

Comb filling, manual PVC sealing and putting identification were old techniques. Nowadays automatic ultrasonic semen filling and sealing and printing machine has increased the speed of whole process. Filling and sealing machine should also be kept in the cold cabinet to cool it with semen to 5°C. Use of French Mini straw has decreased the dilutor volume and dilution ratio. Dilution ratio in inversely related with sperm quality. Mini straw is useful for equal thawing, less spacious and low freezing and packing cost. Cold handling cabinet and Biological freezer (computerized semen freezing system) are the latest inclusion in frozen semen processing technology. It has got great impact on maintenance of exact temperature and time of freezing than LN_2 plunging into liquid nitrogen.

Vapour Cooling and Plunging into Liquid Nitrogen

After filling and sealing, the semen are kept for ultra cooling in liquid Nitrogen (LN_2) vapour (-120°C) for 12 minutes. After vapourization, semen straws are plunged into liquid Nitrogen (- 196°C) for permanent storage.

Thawing of Semen

Thawing temperature is most vital as it affects the post thaw quality of the semen and conception rate.

Semen sample having less than 40 per cent post thaw sperm motility should not be stored and used for breeding the animals. Thawing at 40°C for 30 seconds and 37°C for 60 seconds can be practiced for obtaining acceptable (> 40 per cent) *i.e.*, more than forty percent post thaw sperm motility with minimum morphological damage to the sperm. Post-thaw incubation and transportation of semen from laboratory to the animal can be done in warm water (at 37°C temperature), tap water or chilled (4.5°C) water for maintaining acceptable sperm motility for insemination.

Permanent Storage

After post thaw evaluation of semen for sperm motility, it should be stored in the narrow mouth cryocans, filled with liquid nitrogen (LN_2). This type of cryocans has lower evaporation rate and less chances of damage to spermatozoa due to exposure during handling. Level of liquid Nitrogen in cryocans should be maintained above the level of the canister to avoid any damage to semen due to atmospheric exposure.

Handling of Frozen Semen

The basic principle of any cold storage is that the cold chain must not be broken. Even at the frozen state temperature fluctuations adversely affect the semen quality, semen transfer from the cryocan to another or from one goblet to another must be done under LN_2. Little exposure of semen straw to atmosphere will adversely affect the semen quality.

For transferring the semen straws from one goblet to another, both the goblets should be kept in liquid nitrogen (LN_2) container (thermocool box) to avoid atmospheric exposure. Straws should be handled with precooled forceps to avoid any fluctuation in straw or semen temperature, while taking the semen straw out of the cryocan, goblet should not be brought above the neck of the cryocan in order to avoid atmospheric exposure to the semen stored in it.

Sterilization System in Semen Processing Laboratory

Since there are so many events or activities involved in collection, processing, freezing, packaging, distribution, thawing and insemination with frozen semen, it is difficult to ensure good quality of semen up to the stage when it is used for AI, until and unless strict sanitation and perfect sterilization system has been adopted in the laboratory.

Air modular system, laminar air flow unit, air shower or air cartoons, ultraviolet light and hatch window devices etc. are the recent advancement and are being used in semen processing laboratory to decrease the chance of contamination in frozen semen during processing

Use of ethylene dioxide gas sterilizer and fumigator over the usual sterilization processes efficiently increase hygienic and clean frozen semen production.

Laxity in even a single step starting from collection, processing, freezing, packaging, distribution, thawing till insemination with frozen semen, will drastically compromises success rates.

Liquid Nitrogen Containers

In animal husbandry practices, normally two types of liquid nitrogen containers or cryocans are used:

1. Liquid nitrogen storage and transport containers: TA type.
2. Semen storage and semen presentation containers: BA Type.
   (*a*) Field level artificial insemination work: Small LN_2 semen storage capacity.
   (*b*) Laboratory/Semen Banks: Large LN_2 semen storage capacity.

For LN_2 storage, transport and for daily routine use 50 liters capacity containers are used while for daily semen usage and transport purpose, 3 liters capacity semen storage containers are in use.

Management of LN_2 Storage Container

1. Cryocans should be kept in cool, dry, confined and well ventilated place and access of unauthorized persons to the room must be strictly prohibited.
2. Always keep the containers cool and never allow them to get dry and warm. Frequent drying and subsequent cooling always shortens the life of the container.
3. Keep the LN_2 can in upright and not at all one above the other, which may lead to damages.
4. Lift the containers properly with due care and do not roll it on the ground.
5. Use the appropriate Rubber rings bottom pads provided by the company for the containers.
6. Cover the container with appropriate mats or gunny bags while transporting.
7. Containers filled with LN_2 may be lifted with the help of trolley while replacing or refilling LN_2.
8. Always replace the lid or neck plug after using the container.
9. Try to keep the lids dry and ensure no ice formation on it. If there is ice or frosting, keep the lid outside the cryocan for a while but don't scratch the ice with sharp objects. Dry the neck plug with dry napkin.

Management of Field Level LN_2 Containers

Management is same as described in case of liquid Nitrogen storage container. Some cautions are specially to be taken care of:

1. Cover the container with a rubber tube outside and then with quire mat. Place a mat in the truck and keep the containers on it during transportation on roads to avoid violent jerks in the transport.

2. Keep all the canisters at their proper place do not replace cansisters from other containers.
3. Label the canisters properly indicating the name of the bull (sire), no. of the bull, breed, blood percentage *etc.*
4. Never touch the canisters with wet hands; otherwise there may be ice formation on the canisters, which may lead to difficulties in replacing the lid causing neck damage.
5. If the lid is open for longer time, check that the lid is properly dried before replacing it. Otherwise the water drops would be in the canister to form ice droplets in the canister neck plug.

15.4 REPRODUCTIVE BIOTECHNIQUES FOR IMPROVING FERTILITY OF DAIRY CATTLE AND BUFFALOES

Fertility is a complex expression of outcome of both male and female reproduction and the objective of which is to maximize the profitability of animal production through effective management.

Reproductive biotechniques include (1) artificial insemination (2) estrous synchronization, (3) super ovulation (4) embryo transfer (5) *in vitro* fertilization (6) cryopreservation of embryos, (7) sexing, (8) cloning (9) transgenic and (10) stem cell technology. This technological advancement can play important role in the genetic improvement of livestock and their conservation. Although several techniques have been developed for the effective control of animal reproduction, yet artificial insemination with frozen semen has almost become a routine practical breeding program.

Artificial Insemination

It is the single most important reproductive biotechnique which has revolutionized the breeding of animals to produce and transfer superior germplasm for higher productivity and also to minimize the transmissible reproductive (Venereal) diseases.

Cryopreservation of semen now enables a single bull to be used simultaneously in several countries and a very small number of elite bulls can be used to serve a large cattle population. Although, modern animal breeding, by virtue of artificial insemination (AI) has got wide popularity, sometimes reduced fertility and or low conception rate obtained by the biotechnique are found to be the major constrain in breeding of cattle and buffaloes in India. And this could mainly because of failure of accurate detection of estrus in animals and timely insemination too. Recognization of oestrous display and insemination close to ovulation is even more imperative because of limited survival of spermatozoa.

Female Fertility

Control of Estrous Cycle

For achieving better reproductive performance, ovarian cycles of female animals must be controlled and ovulation is induced when needed. Estrogens, progesterone, prostaglandins and GnRH are judiciously used for estrous cycle synchronization and superovulation.

Super Ovulation

Ovulation rate can be increased moderately to improve natural prolificacy or it can also be stimulated significantly *i.e.* superovulation to increase the number of high quality oocytes for embryo transfer program. Various treatments of FSH preparation containing a controlled level of LH, GnRH analogues or bovine follicular fluid have been tested for this purpose.

Induction and Synchronization of Estrous

AI would provide a means for circumventing the problem of estrous detection. Induction and synchronization of estrous can be achieved by two alternate approaches. First is by artificially extending the luteal phase (by using progestatimal compounds) and 2nd by inducing device of corpus luteum (by using prostaglandins and its analogue).

Progesterone with some possible adjustment in PMSG and or FSH can be used for anticipated lower response. $PGF_2\alpha$ is widely used to manipulate the early breeding of post partum animals and heifers.

Time and Site for Insemination

Insemination should be done at mid to end period of heat. Best site for insemination is mid cervix and body of the uterus. Deposition of semen nearer to the site of fertilization would result in higher fertility. Animal should be kept calm and quite at time of insemination. In heifers, leave the first heat to make the animal more receptive.

Heat Detection Technique

Wall charts, breeding wheels, herd monitor and individual animal record are the estrous detection aid. These systems are least expensive key to successful use of these management aids are : accurate recording of every heat beginning with the first after calving, their daily use to identify those animals that are due to return to estrous. Sexually active animals can be used to detect the animals in heat.

Use of milk progesterone assay with the help of Radio Immune Assay (RIA) can also be done in estrous detection as an advanced technique. Milk Progesterone level of < 200 pg/ml indicates an animal is in estrous.

A teaser bull may be paraded twice or thrice in a day in cattle or buffalo herd/ sheds where females (dairy animals) are kept open.

Micturation during estrus in buffaloes is quite frequent. They urinate small quantity every 4 to 6 minutes during the estrus period. This helps as an aid in oestrus detection in buffaloes.

Most of the animals (cattle and buffaloes) show clear and transparent cervical mucous at the onset of estrous which becomes cloudy and turbid to dirty translucent with the advancement of the oestrous.

The genitalia of the animals showing vaginal discharge should be examined through rectal palpation for the tone of uterus and the mature follicle in the ovary which proved helpful in detection of estrus in cattle and buffalo.

Estrous Signs in Buffalo

The heat symptoms are prominent in cattle but it is experienced that the buffaloes are normally seasonal and shy breeders. The buffaloes exhibit weak symptoms of heat. The most important reason that limits the use of A.I. in buffaloes is the accurate detection of oestrous signs which is generally exhibited during the night and early morning hours.

Oestrous signs in buffaloes included bellowing. Vulvar discharge of clear mucus, frequent urination, vulvar oedema and hyperemia, rising up the tail, mounting herd mates, being mounted by other animals and decreased in milk yield. The discharge is usually found hanging from vulva or soiling the tail and perineum area.

Gynaecological Investigation during Artificial Insemination in Buffalo

When a buffalo is brought for AI, information about previous breeding dates must be asked to exclude the pregnancy. Oestrous is confirmed on the basis of uterine tone, clear transparent ropy discharge and softening of cervix (cervical relaxation). Uterine tone in buffaloes is not as marked as in cows. Therefore, cervical relaxation should be considered as the better parameter for oestrous confirmation. AI gun covered with sheath may be introduced into cervix to see the degree of cervical relaxation. This is particularly helpful when one fails to confirm oestrous on the basis of history and rectal examination. This is particularly helpful when one fails to confirm oestrous on the basis of history and rectal examination.

Heat (Estrous) Signs in Cattle

The heat symptoms are more prominent in cattle than the buffaloes. Heat symptoms in general are listed below:

Bellowing and anxious look, uneasiness and wandering in search of a bull, erect ears and active eyes, showing excitement, inflammation and swelling of vulvar lips, redness of vaginal passage, frequent urination due to inflammation of vagina, presence of cervical discharge on vulvar lips (sticky in nature, glassy in appearance, thick in consistency and transparent in normal estrous), less feed intake and loss of milk yield. The cattle and buffalo in heat smells other called and buffaloes. In initial stages (early hours) the animals start mounting on another animals, called as 'mounting heat' or early heat. Normally 10-12 hours after onset of mounting, the cattle, heifer starts standing in front of a bull or any other cow and when a bull or any other cow, mounts or rides on her, she standstill and this is the proper time to accept the bull for natural breeding and called as "Standing Heat". Frequent stretching of back and lifting of tail from base due to inflammation of vulvar lips are other signs of heat (estrus in cattle).

It is a skill, art and matter of experience to diagnose, detect and to find out the cow or buffalo in heat that needs constant observation or monitoring in a breedable herd. The heat detection is helpful if it is done in early hours of morning and late hours in the evening when most of the cows or heifers are calm and quiet except the cows or heifers in heat.

Time of Artificial Insemination in Cattle

It is advisable not to inseminate a cattle or heifer in heat when she is in her early estrus stage or when she is mounting others. The discharge at this stage is normally thin, watery, transparent, copious and less sticky and hanging from vulval lips and sticking to the tail and either side of the thighs.

It is always advisable to inseminate the animal little after her 'standing heat'. Preferably 5-6 hours after onset of "standing heat". The discharge is very thick, little turbid and or yellowish in colour, sticky and hanging (4-5 inches from the vulvar lips). If the discharge is yellow, thick and much sticky, examine the cow carefully.

Post Oestrus Bleeding (Metoestrus Bleeding)

Some times mucus discharge with blood or clots of blood observed the next day to five days after the day of oestrous (or A.I. or natural service). It is mainly seen in well fed cows and heifers but not in buffalo cow or buffalo heifers. This condition is due to sudden withdrawal of estrogens in circulation and is considered to be physiological. Post estrus bleeding is seen after the end of estrus before ovulation. If bleeding occurs after the end of ovulation it will be called as metestrus bleeding.

Frozen Semen and Thawing

After confirmation of oestrus frozen semen straw should be taken out from cryocan (LN_2 container) and immediately dipped in warm water. Post thaw motility of spermatozoa remains poor if frozen semen is thawed either in tap water or between the palms of hand (*i.e.* dry thawing).

Thawing the straw at 37-40°C for 30-60 seconds is considered better as thawing at this temperature for more duration does not cause any adverse effect on spermatozoa. Post thaw motility of buffalo spermatozoa decreased sharply following incubation and conception rate is severally compromised. Hence straw should be used immediately after thawing without any delay.

Insemination

Perineal area must be washed or cleaned using a duster before insemination. One person should assist in opening or washing the vulvar lips while introducing the AI gun into vagina. This helps in preventing the entry of infection into the genital tract. The AI gun must be gently passed through the cervix. AI gun should not be introduced beyond cervix, if the animal is making frequent movement while insemination. This is necessary to prevent any accidental injury to endometrium by the tip of the AI gun. Straw must be checked after each insemination to ensure the proper release of semen into the genital tract.

Management and Therapeutic Tools to Enhance Conception Rate

Precaution should be taken to prevent entry of infection into the genital tract while performing insemination.

Perineal area must be thoroughly cleaned and AI sheath particularly its tip at the straw holding side should not be touched. AI sheath must be of superior quality (fine quality) to prevent leakage of semen into sheath or ejection of whole straw from sheath into genital tract while posting the stiletle during insemination.

There are three sites of semen deposition in genital tract. These are

1. Cervix
2. Uterine bod
3. Uterine horn.

Deep uterine insemination ensures the deposition of spermatozoa nearer to the uterotubal junction, which is considered to be the main sperm reservoir prior to ovulation. Poor quality semen even may result in better conception rate if insemination is done into uterine body or uterine horns as compared to cervical insemination.

Conception rate can be enhanced by use of two straws at 12 hours apart rather than using them at a single time.

Clitoris of the animal in estrous at 12 hours apart rather than using them at a single time.

Clitoris of the animal in estrous can be messaged for 10-20 seconds after insemination as it is found to increase conception rate.

In repeat breeding buffaloes, one dose of GnRH (2.5ml, Receptal, Hoechst) may be administered at the time of AI, on day 6-7 or on day 10-12 after AI. Since incidence of delayed ovulation is high in buffaloes, administration of GnRH at the time of AI is beneficial.

If clinical infection is present, antibiotics (antibacterial) can be infused into uterus and the affected animal should be inseminated in next cycle. However, if subclinical or very mild infection is suspected, animals may be inseminated during estrus and antibiotic solution can be infused into the uterus at 24 hours after AI.

In buffaloes fertility is reduced during summer (owing to heat stress and endocrine imbalance) and provision of proper housing, free shade, low fiber diet and wallowing facility should be arranged.

Regular deworming is also necessary in areas where helminthic parasitic infestations are common in cattle and buffaloes due to grazing propensity.

Mineral supplementation and offering of green fodder during summer enhances conception in animals in estrus.

Precautions Before Artificial Insemination

1. Allow the cow, buffalo and heifer to get calm and quiet. If the animal is brought to the A.I. centre with prolong walking (long distance walking) in that case asks the owner to wait at least half an hour to settle the animal at new place and obviously to take rest. New environment may cause adrenaline secretion and long distance walking would cause lactic acid formation which in turn may affect conception.
2. Secure the animal in heat properly otherwise it may not allow examination and to do insemination properly. Since there is anxiety and irritation in

animal while examination and insemination, the sheath and the gun may cause injury to the vagina, cervix, uterus or uterine horns, proper restraining and careful handling is essential.

3. Try to confirm the "standing heat" as much as possible by asking questions to the farmer and try to observe consistency of discharge if it is there. Bellowing, stretching of back, frequent urination, lifting of tail and anxious look can be observed from long distance.
4. (*a*) Before start of per rectum examination lubricate the palm and the hand with the appropriate lubricant *e.g.* jelly, cream, oil or glycerin *etc.*

   (*b*) Evacuate the bowels delicately from the rectum (back recking) without causing any ballooning, lacerations or any injury of rectal mucus membrane.

   (*c*) Hold the cervix carefully and then proceed to uterus. Check for cervicitis, kinked cervix, if possible.

   (*d*) While doing this examination, discharge may be available for the observation and examination of the colour, consistency, volume *etc.*

   (*e*) Check for uterine tone (flaccidity). In normal, healthy cow during heat, the uterus is turgid and heaviest than normal, called as the tone of uterus. Uterus in proper tone helps in conception.

Preparation of an AI Gun

1. Use the clean scissors for cutting the straw and keep it on clean dry napkin only after drying after each use.
2. Prepare sufficient warm water of 37°C in a thermoflask and see that the straw would be completely dipped in it. Record the temperature of warm water with the help of thermometer.
3. Confirm the bull (sire) to be used or frozen semen straw (FSS) to be used and select the canister in which straw is located. Avoid taking out straw unnecessarily and again dipping it in the LN_2 if found not suitable for the same AI. This certainly affects the conception rates in following artificial inseminations.
4. Take out the lid and put it on proper surface, with steel top down. Don't put it in lying down or horizontal condition. Otherwise sand, dusts or soil particles may stick to it which leads to disposition and ill fitting of the canister inviting damages of container (neck of the container).
5. Pick up the required straw from the canister. Avoid any replacement or changing of straw after the straw is out of canister.
6. Leave the canister delicately and carefully in the container.
7. Put the straw delicately in the warm water at 37°C and avoid throwing it. It may lead to breakage of seals and subsequent entry of water in the straw. This will spoil the semen and semen may spill out of straw.

8. Keep the completely dipped straw in the flask or waterbath for 30 seconds. In the meantime replace the canister at its respective place and replace the lid carefully.
9. Take out little portion of the lower end of the sheath from the packet.
10. Pick up the straw from the thermoflask and dry it thoroughly. If there is any water drop on straw it may contaminate semen.
11. Give delicate jerks to the straw and bring down the air bubble to the laboratory seal. Hold the straw straight in the hand or in the AI gun with support of the first finger.
12. Give a bold cut with sharp scissors to the straw exactly at right angles. If there is a slight gradient in the angle or pinch it may cause semen leakage in the sheath or in the gun itself which may cause decreased conception.
13. Take out the sheath from the packet and insert the straw in sheath or gun.
14. Prepare the A.I. gun by fixing the sheath in the knob/lock.
15. Have a prepared gun in hand and ask assistant to lift wide open the vulvar lips. This helps in easy access of the gun to reach at external os of the cervix.
16. Hold the cervix in hand and when gun's tip reaches to the external os of the cervix, ask the assistant to leave the vulvar lips. By passing the cervix gently, reach to the internal os of the cervix and with the first finger check that the gun tip is not beyond the internal os of the cervix.
17. Check that the uterus is held straight and not tilted to left and hold the cervix with left hand. Because of that more than 60-70 per cent semen enters in left horn while more ovulations occur in right side and thus chances of conceptions are less.
18. Leave the semen little ahead of cervix and not directly in uterine body or horns. Take at least 10 seconds to push the stillate. If stillate is pushed faster, the tip may be smaller to pass the semen in the uterus and may spill in sheath.
19. Take out the hand from the rectum and clean it properly. Write details of AI in AI register immediately on the spot.

15.5 REQUIREMENTS FOR FIELD INSEMINATION UNITS

Considering 300 field insemination units with maximum 4 lakh inseminations, the followings are the requirements.

Sl.No.	Description of Articles	Quantity Required	Remarks
1.	LN_2 Cryocan (Small type, capacity 7-10 litres)	320	1 for each unit, and 20 were kept in reserve.
2.	A I Gun (½ ml or ¼ ml)	320	1 for each unit, and 20 were kept in reserve.
3.	Goblet (Small size)	3000	
4.	A I Sheath (for ½ ml or ¼ ml straw)	4.5 lakh	

15.6 RECORDS TO BE MAINTAINED AT THE ARTIFICIAL INSEMINATION (AI) UNIT

For keeping records and evaluation, the following information should be kept in systematic way at the A I centres.

Date of A I	*Name and Address of Owner*	*Breed of Animal and identification No. of Animal, if any*	*Lactation Number*	*Previous Insemination Details*	*Time of AI*
1	2	3	4	5	6

Stage of Heat	*Type of Straw*	*Number of Straw Used*	*Pregnancy Result (P/NP)*	*Date of Calving*	*Body Weight and Sex of Calf*
7	8	9	10	11	12

Chapter 16

Reproductive Disorders and Post Parturient Diseases: Their Treatment and Control

16.1 REPRODUCTIVE DISORDERS

Reproduction is an important consideration in economics of livestock production. In the absence of regular breeding and calving at appropriate time dairy enterprise will never be profitable. The most important problem in animal reproduction is anoestrus.

16.1.1 Anoestrus

When a cow is not observed in estrus or heat, the condition is known as anoestrus. The cow may not come into estrus (not cycling) or the cow has normal estrus but is not observed in estrus due to weak or absent estrus behaviour or insufficient observation. If estrus has not been observed in a dairy cow by 60 days post partum the condition is defined as post partum anoestrus.

Mainly two forms of anoestrus are seen in animals. These are true anoestrus and apparent anoestrus.

True Anoestrus

It is a period of sexual quietude in which there is complete abscess of sexual cycle with no heat manifestation. It may be due to absence of any structure on the ovaries (follicles *etc.*).

Apparent Anoestrus

It is a pathological anoestrus associated with retention of corpus luteum (CL) and cystic condition. In heifers the anoestrus may result from conditions such as (*i*) free martinism, (*ii*) white heifer disease, (*iii*) bilateral hypoplasia of ovaries, (*iv*) congenitál abnormalities, (*v*) infantile genetalia, (*vi*) hypo-functioning of ovaries, (*vii*) under feeding, faulty feeding, parasitism, climatic and nutritional factors, faulty management *etc.*, (*viii*) sub-optimal hormones or endocrinal disorders (sub-optimal functioning of hypothalamus hypophysio gonadal axis and consequent low circulating hormones), (*ix*) bilateral smooth and quiescent ovaries, ovarian inactivity, (x) thermal stress, (*xi*) protein and vitamin deficiency, (*xii*) mineral deficiency (especially low level of potassium, and (*xiii*) senility, lack of exercise, suckling, obesity *etc.*

Treatment and Control

Ayurvedic Heat Inducer

Prajana capsule (Indian Herbs) or *Sajani capsule* (Zydus Sarabhai) 3 caps daily for 2 days; to be repeated on 11th and 12th day if heat is not manifested. *HIT-O-GEN* one bolus in the morning and one bolus in the evening orally with soft jaggery, *Ovatone* (Legend) capsule BD for a week. *Janova* (Dabur Ayurvet) 2 cap BID for 2 days and *Generin Powder* (Vetmed) – 25-50 g, to be repeated after 7 days orally BID till heat appears. *Gestafort bolus* (TTK) – 2 boli daily for 7 days.

Conventional Treatment

1. Iodine Tamponing – Tamponing with Lugol's iodine.
2. Gentle massaging of ovary and genitalia.
3. Phosphorus administration by I/M route.
4. Vitamin A by I/M route.
5. Trace mineral supplementation.
6. Improved feeding and management practices to be followed.
7. Hormone injection like GnRH, LH and progesterone are recommended for treating anoestrus.
8. Natural $PGF_2\alpha$ or its analogue is indicated in cases where anoestrus is caused by retained corpus luteum (CL).
9. Deworming is must for treating anoestrus if there is worm load in the animals.

Mineral Supplementation

The following mineral mixtures may be used orally once daily or at least on alternate day. Chelated Agrimin Fort (GSK) 25 g, Minfa (Intas) 30-50 g, Rannix (Vetnex) 25 g, Supplivite – M (Zydus Sarabhai) 25 g, Concimin (Concept) 25 g, C Min forte Plus (C-Care) 30 g, Gromin (Sarabhai Zydus) 25 g, Encalmin Fort (Enlag Lab) – 25-30 g, Gynomin (Enlag) 10 g.

- ✰ Trace mineral bolus may be used.
- ✰ Bioplex High Five (Vetnex) 1-2 bolus daily.

- ✰ Cyclomin – 7 bolus (Concept) 1 bolus at 3 days interval.
- ✰ Flomin-C bolus 1 bolus BD.
- ✰ Minotas bolus (Intas) Cattle and buffalo 2 boli daily for 2 weeks.
- ✰ Cu-Co tablets 2 tablets BID.
- ✰ Vets cuco tabs 2 tablets BID.
- ✰ Cofecu tabs 2 tablets BID for 10-15 days.
- ✰ Cocu plus – Cattle 2 tablets BID, Sheep and goat ½ tablet BID for 20 days.
- ✰ Aloes compound – 5 to 10 tablets BID for 10-15 days.
- ✰ Gestaforte bolus – 4 boli daily for 5 days.

Vitamin Supplementation

- ✰ Inj. Vitamin A (Legend) 6 lakh I.U. by IM route at 3-5 days interval.
- ✰ Inj. ADE Vet (Vets Farma), Inj. Vitacept (Concept), Inj. Vet ADE (Sarabhai Zydus),
- ✰ Inj. Intavita (Intas), Inj. Intavita-H (Intas), Inj. Brivit (Brihans)

  Cattle and buffalo – 6-10 ml by deep IM route.

  Small animals – 2-3 ml by deep IM route.

16.2 POST PARTURIENT DISEASES

Diseases associated with parturition are estimated to account for 8 per cent of all diseases in cattle and buffaloes, and the most important diseases associated with parturition are Retention of Placenta, Pyometra, Endometritis, Prolapse of vagina and uterus, Metritis and Mastitis.

16.2.1 Retention of Placenta (RoP)

Retention of foetal membrane (RFM) is a common complication in relation to parturition. Incidence varies from 7-21 per cent. Normally placenta is expelled within 6-7 hours after parturition and retention of placenta is defined where the retention of placenta goes beyond 8-12 hours post parturition. It is usually associated with metritis, reduced milk yield and subsequent poor fertility.

This condition is considered pathological and is primarily either due to uterine inertia or due to pathological condition of the placenta which in turn results in the failure of the foetal villi to detach themselves from the maternal crypts and results into retention of foetal membranes. The etiological factors of RFM are nutritional, managemental, endocrinal and infectious in nature. Normally the membranes should be expelled within 4-5 hours after birth of the calf but owing to intricate cotyledonary attachments these are often retained for long periods finally undergoing decomposition. Hasty manual attempts for its removal are followed by serious consequences.

Detrimental Effects of Retention of Placenta

1. Drop in milk production
2. Delayed uterine involution

3. Chronic endometritis
4. Decreased conception rate
5. Repeat breeding
6. Acute septic endometritis
7. Toxemia, which may be fatal.
8. Metritis and Pyometra terminating in infertility.

The cotyledoneny type of membrane attachments do not yield to ergot or estrogen therapy.

Treatment

Use of Uterine Cleansing Agent

Soon after parturition uterine cleansing agent may be drenched or fed to the animal for expulsion of placenta, helping in involution and preparing healthy uterus for next conception.

Involon (Natural Remedies) – 200 ml on first day followed by 100 ml for 3 days.

Exaper liquid (Excell) – 200 ml BID on first day followed by 100 ml daily for 3 days.

Uterotone (Cattle Remedies) – 100 ml BID can be used to expedite the expulsion of placenta.

Hormotone (Novartis) – 450 ml orally immediately after delivery within 4-5 hours, if RoP persists 2nd dose may be given after 6 hours.

Ayurvedic uterine ecbolic powder like *Replanta* (Indian Herb) 50 g orally BID for 3-4 days helps in expulsion of placenta, cleans up lochial discharge and useful in metritis.

Manual Removal

If the placenta is not expelled in spite of above treatment the placenta should be manually removed. Manual extraction should be done with great care and proper hygienic measure. During separation of the retained placenta, caruncles should not be destroyed.

Antimicrobial Therapy

A wide range of antibiotics can be used locally (I/U) to control possible bacterial infection. Tetracycline may be used @ 2-6 g I/U.

Cephalexin, Metronidazole, and Gentamycin are commonly used. The antibiotic may be used as an infusion in 200 to 500 ml of normal saline depending upon the size of uterus.

Bolus C-flox TZ, I/U (Intas) or C-Flox uterine liquid (Intas) – 50 ml I/U daily.

Ledexin (Legend) or Lexin or Lixen I/U (GSK) may be infused.

Recent study revealed the administration of the *combination of a beta receptor blocker e.g.* Carazolol, Oxytocin hormone and an antibiotic *e.g.* Amoxicillinum Anhydricum + Acidum (clavulanicum) is favourable in terms of the expulsion of foetal membranes in cattle with retained placenta. Doses: Beta receptor blocker *e.g.* Carazolol, Suacron @ 5 mg (by IV), Oxytocin 15 I.U. and Amoxicillin @ 8.75 mg by IM.

Pessaries like Uren vet (Deys vet), Furex (Excell), Utrox bolus, Furan bolus (Himachal), C-flox TZ may be placed in the uterus at least for 3 days after manual extraction of placenta.

Intrauterine and Parenteral Antibiotics

If putrifaction has already started the placenta should be removed using sterile hand gloves. In such case both intrauterine as well as parenteral antibiotics should be used.

Inj. Ciptec (Cipla) or Inj. C-flox (Intas) – 10-15 ml I/M daily for 3-5 days and I/U infusion of C-flox Uterine liquid 50 ml. Inj. Enrofloxacin *viz.* Inj. Quinintas (Intas), Inj. Enrocip (Cipla), Inj. Enrocin (Vetnex) Inj. Enrored (Reedson) @ 1 ml/20 kg body weight for 5-7 days and infusion of Enrofloxacin dissolved in distilled water should be done. Metronidazole injectable solution along with Inj. Gentamycin (like Inj. Gentex/Gentabiotic) may be infused by IU route and Inj. Gentamycin may be used parenterally.

Use of Hormones

Uterokinetic hormone like Oxytocin @ 20 IU by IM route at 3-4 hours interval may be tried but not more than 3 days. Estradiol or Stilbosterol may also be used. To reduce pain, oedema, swelling and inflammation – A_3 Vet bolus (Brihans), Melonex bolus (Intas), Oxalgin NP bolus (Zydus Sarabhai) 1-2 bolus; Inj. Meloxicam, Inj. A_3 Vet (Brihans), Inj. Melonex (Intas) 15-20 ml by IM route may be administered for 2-3 days.

16.2.2 Metritis-Pyometra

An infection that is contained in the uterus can exhibit no visible-clinical signs, yet be a quiet site for future systemic problems. The uterine infection causes fever, inappetance, toxemia, weight loss, debility and decreased milk yield. Repeat breeding is the usual sequele to uterine infection owing to metritis and pyometra. Infection like Vibriosis, Brucellosis, Trichomoniasis are also responsible for such condition. A pyometra alters the synthesis of $PGF_2\alpha$ (prostaglandin) by the endometrium. Animal may suffer from anoestrus. Purulent foul smelling discharge observed particularly when animals sit down. Therefore, treatments with GnRH, Oxytocin or Prostaglandin should be done to return the reproductive tract normal and breed when ready. Inj. Utrodex (Hydroxy Progesterone Ceproate 250 mg/ml), Inj. Vetosterol 10-20 mg SC can be given. Inj. Oxytocin @ 20-40 I.U. IM daily for 3-4 days. Inj. Clostenol (Zydus Sarabhai) 2 ml by IM route, Inj. Vetmet (Vetcare) 2 ml by IM route may be tried. Inj. Diethyl Stilbosterol (Distrol, 10 mg/ml) may be given. IU (Intra uterine) antibiotic therapy using insemination pipette should be done. Ledexin (Legend), Lixen IU (GSF), Inj. C-flox uterine liquid (Intas) @ 50 ml, Lexin IU, C-flox IU liquid *etc.* or injectable Metronidazole solution (100 ml), Inj. Gentamycin, Inj. Enrofloxacin diluted in distilled water can be infused in uterus for 3-5 days. Parenteral antibiotic therapy with Inj. Streptopenicillin (Inj. Biostrep (IBC), Inj. Dicrysticin (Sarabhai), Inj. Bistrepen (Alembic), Inj. Enrofloxacin (like Inj. Eroxin (Oxen lab), Inj. Quin intas, Inj. Enrox, Inj.

Floxidin (Intas), Inj. Enrocin @ 1 ml/20 kg body weight by IM route for 3-5 days should be used. Non antibiotic intrauterine treatment with Povidone iodine, Pivipol, Betadine, Wokadine, Ranbidone IU, Metricare IU may be tried for 3-4 days.

Supportive Treatment

Inj. Calmex (Vetnex), Inj. Calborol, Inj. Intacal (Intas) 100-150 ml on alternate day for 3 occasions. Phosphorus injection like Inj. Alphos 40, Inj. Aciphos, Inj. T. Phos @ 10ml for 3 days may be administered to tone up uterine myometrium and helping in early involution. Oral multiherbal preparation like Exapar (Excell), Involon (Natural Remedies), Hormotone (Novartis) – 150 ml per day for 6 days.

16.2.3 Prolapse of Genetalia

Prolapse of reproductive organs either vagina, cervix or both and uterus is one of the grave obstetrical emergencies which may occur both prepartum and postpartum. It is commonly encountered in bovine at late gestation or after parturition. Usually it occurs in case of retained placenta due to severe irritation and excessive straining.

Faulty management practices, hypocalcaemia, mineral imbalances, phytohormones in feed, hormonal imbalances during pregnancy, relaxation of pelvic ligaments etc. are the predisposing factors for the incidence of prolapse of genitals.

Management of Prolapse

Shift the animal on a clean ground with hind quarters on raised level and rest the prolapsed mass on a soft clean cloth. The prolapsed mass and the surrounding parts are to be cleaned properly with potassium permanganate solution. Prolapsed mass is to be lifted to the level of ischial arch and urine if accumulated needs to be relieved by catheterization.

Cold water irrigation or chilled savlon solution irrigation could also be made. Uterosule spray (Goel Pharma) may be sprayed on the prolapsed uterus. Examine for any tear or injury. Bleeding, if any, is to be checked by topical application of adrenaline. Ice blocks rapped with sterile cotton cloth may be applied over the prolapsed mass to reduce its volume. If straining is violent caudal epidural analgesia should be attained injecting 2 per cent Lignocaine Hydrochloride (Xylocain) 10-15 ml at the epidural space.

Prolapsed mass may be covered by a clean soft cloth and gentle squeezing of cloth to be done. This helps the mass to get smaller in size and helps in easy repositioning.

Use the pressure of palm or fist but never the fingers which may cause tear and injury of uterus. Sedative like Triflupromazine HCl (Inj. Siquil) 3-5 ml by IM route may be used. After repositioning of prolapsed mass purse string suture may be applied. Rope truss may be given after reducing the prolapse.

Antibiotic coverage by broad spectrum antibiotic like Inj. Enrofloxacin, Inj. Amoxycillin-Cloxacillin *etc.*; Antihistaminic injections like Inj. Avil (Intervet), Inj. Chloril (TTK), Inj. Chloragin (Vetnex), Inj. Anistamin (Intas) may be administered to prevent shock.

Supportive treatment with parenteral calcium like Inj. Mifex (Provimi), Inj. Calcimal (Oxen lab), Inj. Calmex-M (Vetnex), Inj. Intacal (Intas), Inj. Lactomag (Intas), Inj. Calborol (Provimi) 150-200 ml for 2-3 days may be done. Inj. E-care Se @ 10 ml daily for 3 days may be administered by IM route.

Stomachic powder like Herbogastrin (Vetmed), Himalayan Batisa, Natural Batisa (Nature Care) 25-50 g orally BID or Floratone bolus (Concept), Bioboost, Rumentas (Intas), Floraboost (Excell) @ 2 boli BID may be fed to the animal.

Anti inflammatory analgesic may be administered *viz.* Inj. Meloxi (Vets Pharma), Inj. Zobid-M (Zydus Sarabhai), Inj. MP_3 (Vetnex) or Inj. A_3 vet (Brihans), Inj. Melonex (Intas) – 15-30 ml for cattle and buffalo, Inj. Melonex-P (TTK) 3-5 ml for sheep and goat or Inj. Melonex Power (Intas) @ 2.5ml/100 kg body weight of cattle and buffalo.

16.2.4 Mastitis

Bovine mastitis is a disease complex caused by infections, chemicals, thermal or traumatic conditions. It indicates diverse disease changes in the udder characterized by discolouration, appearance of milk, clots, flakes, pus, blood, blood clots, watery or blood tinged milk, change in consistency and increased number of leucocytes in milk.

Mastitis is nothing but the inflammation of mammary gland or udder caused by mostly bacteria, and rarely by fungi and algae. *Staphylococcus aureus*, *Streptococcus agalactiae* and other Streptococci are the most common pathogens, Coliform bacteria are the next and Pseudomonas, Mycobacterium and Bacillus are occasional. The disease occurs in cow, buffalo, ewe, doe and sow but rarely in mare.

Signs of clinical mastitis include abnormalities of gland and milk and a systemic reaction. It is of 4 types *viz.*, (*i*) Per acute – severe inflammation with systemic reaction, (*ii*) Acute – severe inflammation without marked systemic reaction, (*iii*) Sub-acute – mild inflammation and abnormality of milk, and (*iv*) Chronic – repeated attacks with little change in milk.

Acute inflammatory swelling (hot and painful with gangrene or abscesses in severe cases), fibrosis (firm feel), atrophy of the gland (chronic), lameness in hind limb and swelling of supramammory lymph nodes are usually noted. The systemic reaction in case of peracute mastitis includes toxaemia, pyrexia, depression and anorexia.

Acute Mastitis

It is usually caused by Staphylococci, Streptococci, Pasteusella, *E. coli*, Klebsiella *etc.* Gland becomes hot, painful, hard and swollen. Milk secretion is scanty and watery at the beginning and latter in becomes purulent. Fever and toxaemia are also common signs.

Treatment

Effective treatment of mastitis is a problem due to development of drug resistance. The successful containment of bovine mastitis involves an early diagnosis and institution of immediate and rational therapy.

Remove secretion from all the affected quarters as much as possible. Sterile milk siphon may be used for painful teats and udder and for obliterated teat canal. Milchey (Herbal preparation, Novartis) @ 15 tablets twice daily for 15 days may be fed orally for easy milk let-down. Cultural examination of milk and antibiotic sensitivity test should be carried out for specific treatment.

Intra Mammary Infusion Tubes

- ☆ Inclox – 5 g disposyringe (Brihans)
- ☆ Floclox – L (Vetnex)
- ☆ Pendistrin SH (Sarabhai Zydus)
- ☆ Cobalactan LC (Intervet)
- ☆ Alciclox (Alembic)
- ☆ Vetclox (Zydus Sarabhai)
- ☆ Mammitel (Intas)
- ☆ Tilox (Wockhardt)
- ☆ Tiamutin intrammary (?)

Besides intramammary infusion tube parenteral antibiotic therapy should be combined and the same antibiotic or its combination should be employed in both modes of treatment. Various antibiotics or its combination can be used for treating mastitis, like injection Ampicillin, Ampicillin + Cloxacillin, Amoxycillin, Penicillin + Streptomycin, Enrofloxacin, Chloramphenicol, Amoxycillin + Clavulanic acid, Gentamycin, Cefotaxim sodium *etc.*

To reduce pain, swelling and pyrexia, Cox-II inhibitor *e.g.* Meloxicam Injection or Inj. Analgin, Inj. Novalgin, Inj. Vetalgin may be used for 2-3 days. Mastileo ointment (Dabur Ayurvet) can be applied externally to give relief from pain and swelling. Antihistaminic injection like Pheneramine maleate can be used as and when required as per urgency but never in case of advance pregnancy.

Vitamin-E and Selenium has been found to be effective in preventing and treating mastitis. Hence Inj. E-care-Se (Vetcare) @ 10ml daily for 3 days by IM route may be tried.

Buffer (Excell) 15 g sachet dailyand Mammadium (Intas) may be given @ 50 g daily for clinical mastitis where Buffer ensures milk pH. Mammadium acts as powerful antioxidant, maintains milk pH and acts as immuno-potentiator. Mammadium may be fed to animals after mixing with jaggery or butter as an electuary.

Supportive therapy with topical application of Inflamin ointment (Himalaya drugs), Mastilep (Dabur Ayurvet) may be tried. Serratio-peptidase 75 mg bolus, Inflamin fort (Excell) are found effective in mastalgia and mastitis. Seri-D bolus (Mare India) is also effective in treating mastalgia and mastitis in connection with pain relief and oedema care. Administration of Inj. Levamisol HCl (Lemasol-75, Kalmisol) @ 10 ml by SC route is beneficial while treating bovine mastitis.

Chronic Mastitis

It is usually caused due to incomplete treatment and resistant bacteria. Repeated attacks with little change in milk. Atrophy of the gland, fibrosis (firm fill of the glands and teats) is very much characteristic. There is little or no local reaction, neither swelling nor pain. Cultural examination of milk and antibiotic test should be done wherever possible.

1. Line of treatment is same as in acute mastitis. It needs prolong treatment.
2. Adjunct to antibiotic therapy, Mammadium (Intas) @ 50 g orally daily for 4 days with jaggery.
3. Fibrosin (Legends) 1st day 2 boli BID, 2nd to 5th day (1 bolus BID).
4. Teatasule No. I and Teatasule No. 2 – 20 g each (Goel Vet Pharma)–½ to 1 tsf. BID for 5 days mixed with soft jaggery.
5. Buffer (Excell-Aahar)–15 g daily dissolved in 250 ml water.
6. Systemic antibiotic therapy as per antibiotic sensitivity test:

Inj. Ampicillin sodium, Inj. Ampicillin + Cloxacillin, Inj. Amoxycillin + Sulbactam, Inj. Cefotaxime sodium for 3-5 days.

16.2.5 Agalactia and Hypogalactia

Agalactia and hypogalactia are common problems of dairy cattle and buffalo and are governed by multiple factors. First, study the underlying reasons and try to solve such problems in a systemic way.

1. Enquire about peri parturient and post parturient complications and disease. If the animal is recently parturited enquire about retained placenta, prolapse, metritis, mode of delivery – normal or assisted, generalized illness before and after parturition if any, and parasitic disease.
2. Examine the udder and udder health status. Rule out mastalgia, mastitis, fibrosis, udder abscess, blind teat, congenial udder and teat anomalies like imperforate teat and treat accordingly.
3. Enquire about feeding and nutritional and other management standards adopted for the animal. Not only feeding at adequate level but also its nutrient quality as well as providing *ad libitum* drinking water to the animal needs to be ensured.
4. Enquire about gestational management and feeding standard to assess any nutritional deficiency.
5. Examine for metabolic disorders like Ketosis, hypocalcaemia, hypophosphataemia *etc.* along with nutritional disharmony.
6. Ensure adequate minerals and salt *etc.* are supplemented to the animal.
7. Enquire if there is letting down problem due to death of suckling calf, or calf mortality during parturition.

Treatment

1. Feeding of Oral Calcium Tonic/Bolus

   Liquid like Calcimilk or Capsola or Capsola Gold or Calshakti – 100 ml orally daily for cattle and buffalo for 10-15 days, and for sheep and goat 20-25 ml orally daily for 10-15 days. Caldhan D or Bovical D_3 or Ostovet/ Ostovet fort or Super care 365 liquid – 50 ml orally BID.

   Bolus like Calphos D_3 bolus – 2 boli orally BID.

   Powder like Calphos D_3 powder – 25 g orally once daily.

   Sheep and Goat – 20-25ml orally daily for 10 days.

2. Mineral Mixtures

   Minfa (Chromium rich mineral mixture) is useful in improving milk production. Dose: Cattle and buffalo – 30-50g daily; Sheep and goat – 5-10 g daily.

   Ranmix and Ranmix total – 25 g orally daily.

   Proteimin Fort – 25-50 g orally daily.

   Complemin Fort – 25-50 g orally daily.

   Alvite-M – 25 g orally daily.

   Agrimin/Agrimin Fort – 25 g orally daily.

   Several other mineral supplements are available which may be used.

3. Ayurvedic Galactogogue may be used.

   Milkogen – 5 tablets BID with jaggery.

   Galog – 25-50 g orally daily for 10-15 days.

   Milkotone powder – 25-50 g orally BID for 10-15 days.

   Milkmax/Milchey – 15 tablets BID for 15 days.

4. For correcting letting down problem and to improve milk yield, Leptaden Vet – 10 tablets BID for 10 days.

5. If case of subclinical hypocalcaemia, parenteral calcium may be given.

   For cattle and buffalo Inj. Capsola 15-20 ml by IM route daily, Inj. Caldee-12, Inj. Orical, Inj. Brical – 10-15 ml by IM route daily for 3-5 occasions. Dose for sheep and goat is 3-5 ml by IM route daily or alternate day.

6. Oral calcium preparation like Encalplus, Calcimilk, Encal-12, Calcicare, Mifex oral, @ 40-50 ml/large animal and 20 ml/small animal orally BID may be given for 5-7 days.

Part – IV
Surgery Section

Chapter 17
Elementary Veterinary Surgery

17.1 SURGICAL PACK FOR VARIOUS OPERATIONS

17.1.1 Common Surgical Pack for Large Animal

The following items constitute a common surgical pack for handling preliminary surgical cases of large animals.

1. B.P. Handle (Bard Parker Handle No. 3, No. 4 *etc.*)
2. B.P. Blades No. 3, No. 4 *etc.*
3. Forceps
    (*a*) Allis Tissue Forceps
    (*b*) Rat Tooth Forceps
    (*c*) Dressing Forceps
    (*d*) Artery Forceps (straight)
    (*e*) Artery Forceps (curved)
    (*f*) Iris Forceps
    (*g*) Mosquito artery forceps
    (*h*) Mayo's Needle Holder
    (*i*) Mosquito curved Haemostats
4. Scissors
    (*a*) Scissors Straight
    (*b*) Scissors Curved
    (*c*) Mayo Scissors

5. Buckhaus Towel clamps/clips
6. Crossbar Towel clamp
7. Groove Director
8. Scalpel
9. Curator (Loop head)/Spoon head
10. Needle Holder
11. Sterilized gauge
12. Absorbable and non-absorbable sterilized cotton.
13. Sutures – absorbable and non-absorbable
14. Suturing needle (straight and curve – half circle)
    (*a*) Traumatic

17.1.2 Surgical Pack for Small Animal

The following items should be there in a common surgical pack for handling common surgical cases of small animals.

1. Scissors: 4 pieces
    (*a*) Straight scissors – 2 pieces (1 small, 1 big)
    (*b*) Curved scissors with blunt points – 2 pieces (1 small, 1 big)
2. B.P. Handle No. 3 and 4 (two each)
3. B.P. Blades for B.P. Handle No. 3 and 4.
4. Artery Forceps – 8 pieces (4 curved and 4 straights, 15 cm each)
5. Groove director – 1 piece
6. Dissecting Forceps (Allis type) – 2 pieces (15 cm)
7. Towel clips – 4 pieces
8. Tissue Forceps (Allis type) – 4 pieces
9. Needle Holders – 2 pieces
10. Suture Needles – 4 pieces
    (*a*) Semi circular – 2 pieces (5 cm with non-cutting edge)
    (*b*) Semi circular – 2 pieces (10-12 cm, traumatic with cutting edge)
    (*c*) Semi circular – 2 pieces (7-8 cm, traumatic with cutting edge)
11. Suturing Threads: (i) Linen 20, 60 (ii) Chromic catgut no. 00, 000
12. Surgical gloves – 2 pieces
11. Surgical gowns – 2 pieces
12. Surgical swabs (gauge) – 1 to 2 dozens
13. Surgical towels – 2 pieces (20 cm X 30 cm)
14. Surgical drapes – 4 pieces
15. Medicine cup for keeping sterile saline solution.

17.2 SUTURE MATERIALS

Suture materials are of two types. They are (a) absorbable sutures and (2) Non absorbable sutures.

Absorbable Sutures

Absorbable sutures are digested by the surrounding. This includes plain or chromic catgut, fascia lata *etc.*

Non Absorbable Sutures

These are not affected by enzymatic digestion or enzymatic action by the body fluids and remain in tissues without causing any foreign body reaction until they are removed.

These are cotton sutures, nylon, silk, vetafil, stainless steel suture (metallic suture).

17.3 SUTURE TECHNIQUE

In order to maintain good healing, close apposition of the incised edges with least number of stitches and good quality sutures are essential.

The commonly used suturing techniques are:

1. Simple continuous
2. Simple interrupted
3. Lock stitch
4. Mattress sutures (Horizontal or vertical)
5. Lambert's or Cushing type of suture technique (for suturing of hollow organs like stomach, intestine, bladder *etc.*)

17.4 SUTURE SIZE

Type of Materials to be Sutured	*For Large Animal*	*For Small Animal*
Subcuticular tissue	2/0-0	3/0 and 2/0
Muscle/Fascia	3	1 and 2
Peritoneum	1 and 2	2/0 and 1/0
Vessel	1 and 2	2/0 and 1/0

17.5 STERILIZATION

The instruments, gauge, sponges, suture materials etc. should be sterilized before surgery. The surgical instruments should be cleaned and washed properly with soap or detergent solution or medicated soap solution rinsed and dried properly. Prior to sterilization they should be free from dust, spots of blood, pus, grease, hairs, drugs *etc.* Instruments, gauge sponges, suture material or general surgical pack is best sterilized with saturated steam under pressure. Ten minutes at 20 psi are sufficient to kill both spore forming and non spore forming bacteria but the time may be doubled after sterilization of large packs.

General surgical packs should be sterilized in autoclave at 6.75 kg pressure at 121°C for 15 minutes. Dry heat method of sterilization may also be used for surgical pack. Ethyl alcohol (70 per cent alcohol) can also be used for 30 minutes for instruments sterilization. The usual method of sterilization is using boiling water 100°C for 30 minutes but this is not truly effective. For enhancing the efficacy of this method 2 per cent sodium bicarbonate or 0.1 per cent NaOH may be added to the water to reduce the boiling time from 30-35 minutes. Chemical sterilization is also effective for instruments provided a proper percentage of germicidal solution is used and instruments are submerged in solution for sufficient period. The best method of sterilization for surgical pack is autoclaving.

17.6 PREPARATION OF SITE FOR OPERATION

- Operation site should be shaved properly.
- The site should be cleaned properly with soap and water to remove all dirt and debris.
- The site should be scrubbed with a piece of gauge dipped in 70 per cent ethyl alcohol and allowed to dry.
- Local antibiotics should be given to minimize the chance of infection.

17.7 ANAESTHESIA

17.7.1 Local Anaesthetic Drugs

These drugs produce loss of sensation of a limited body part or organs.

17.7.1.1 Lignocaine HCl

Trade Names

1. *Injection Xylocaine* (Astra) – 30 ml vial
2. *Gesicain Injection* – 30 ml vial

Composition

Lignocaine HCl–2 per cent and 1 per cent.

Indication

Epidural anaesthesia, infiltration anaesthesia, nerve block, obstetrical correction (dystocia).

Dose

For obstetrical correction: Large animal – 5-10 ml, Small animal – 1-2 ml.

For laparotomy operation: Large animal – 10-15 ml, Small animal – 2-5ml.

17.7.1.2 Procaine HCl

Trade Names

1. *Novocain Injection* – 30 ml vial

Composition

Procaine HCl–2 per cent.

Indication

Production of local, regional and epidural anaesthesia.

Dose

For Caudal epidural anaesthesia

Horse – 10-20 ml, Cattle – 7-10 ml.

For Cranial epidural anaesthesia

Cattle – 40-60 ml, Dog – 2-10 ml.

For Conduction anaesthesia

Horse – 20 ml, Cattle – 7-10 ml, Dog and Cat – 2-3 ml.

17.7.1.3 Hexacycloine (Cyclaine)

Indication

Production of local and regional anaesthesia.

Dose

Infiltration 0.5 per cent, Topical – 2.5-5 per cent, Local and regional – 1-1.5 per cent.

17.7.1.4 Butacaine (Butyne)

Indication

Production of local and regional anaesthesia.

Dose

Infiltration – 1 per cent, Topical – 2 per cent, Local and regional – 1 per cent.

17.7.2 General Anaesthetic Drugs

It is known to complete loss of consciousness on the administration of anaesthetic drugs.

17.7.2.1 Anaesthetic Gases

Nitrous oxide – 50-70 per cent with 30-50 per cent oxygen.

Ethylene – 85 per cent with 15 per cent oxygen

Cyclopropane – 20-50 per cent cyclopropane with oxygen.

17.7.2.2 Anaesthetic Agents

Ketamine HCl – 4-8 mg/kg body weight (small animals)

Chloral Hydrate – 0.22-0.33 g/kg body weight for small animals.

Thialbarbitone sodium – 45 mg/kg body weight, 4.5 per cent solution for small animals.

Thiopentone sodium – 22-25 mg/kg body weight

Barbital sodium – 150-1000 mg (oral sedative dose for dog).

Phenobarbital sodium – 25-30 mg/kg body weight

17.7.2.3 Inhalation Anaesthetics

Chloroform – 1.35 per cent for light anaesthesia, 1.65 per cent for deep anaesthesia.

Trichloro ethane – 0.5-0.75 per cent, Vinyl ether – 4 per cent concentrate in inspired air.

Ethyl chloride – 3-4.5 per cent Ether (Ethyl ether) 3.5 – 4.5 per cent concentrate volume.

17.7.2.4 Xylazine Hydrochloride

It is a sedative, analgesic, anaesthetic and muscle relaxant for large and small animals.

Indication

It is used for inducing sedation and analgesia in various animals for restraining animals for routine examination, minor surgical interventions, dystocia handling and immobilization of animals during transportation and transshipment. It can also be used as preanaesthetic to general anesthesia.

Trade Names

1. *Injection Xylaxin* (Indian Immunologicals) – 2 ml, 10 ml and 30 ml vials. Each ml contains Xylazine HCl 23.32 mg.

Dose

Species	*Dose in mg per kg*	*Average Adult Dose per Animal*
Cattle and Buffalo	0.1-0.2	1.5-3 ml
Horse	1.0-2.0	25-50 ml
Sheep	0.1-0.3	0.1-0.5 ml
Goat	0.05-0.5	0.1-0.75 ml
Dog	1.0-2.0	0.75-1.5 ml
Cat	1.0-2.0	0.1-0.5 ml

This should be administered by IM injection in most of the animals. For horse it should be administered by IV route.

Caution

After administration the animals should be left undistributed. Regurgitation may be seen in cattle. In that case head should be raised.

Trade Names

1. *Injection Xylazil -100* (Helpro Health) – 10 ml and 30ml vials. Each ml contains Xylazine HCl 100 mg.
2. *Injection Izine* (Intas) – 10 ml vial. Each ml contains Xylazine HCl 20 mg.

Dose

Cattle and buffalo: 0.5-1.75 ml/100 kg body weight (IM)

0.25-0.75 ml/100 kg body weight (IV)

Sheep: 0.12-0.3 7 ml/25 kg body weight (IM)

0.06-0.12 ml/25 kg body weight (IV)

Horse: 5-10 ml/100 kg body weight (IM)

2.5-5 ml/100 kg body weight (IV)

Dog: 0.25-0.5 ml/5 kg body weight (IM)

0.12-0.25 ml/5 kg body weight (IV)

17.7.3 Tranquilizer

17.7.3.1 Chlorpromazine

It is a phenothiazine derivative. It produces sedation and marked depressant effect on brain stem.

Indication

Excitation along with anaesthetics, as antiemetic, for restraining of animals, castration, travel sickness, tetanus, stiffness of muscle, vomition and post operative analgesic.

Trade Names

1. *Injection Largactil* (Prima Vetcare) – 2.5 per cent solution (1 ml, 2 ml and 10 ml) and 5 per cent solution (5 ml)

Dose

Cattle – 0.2 mg/kg body weight IM; All species – 1-2 mg/kg body weight IM or IV route.

Action starts 40 minutes post IM injection and 5-10 minutes post IV injection.

Largactil is also available in tablet form (10 mg, 50 mg and 100 mg). In case of dog the oral dose is 5 mg/kg body weight dily.

17.7.3.2 Triflupromazine

Trade Name

1. *Injection Siquil* (Sarabhai zydus) – 5 ml vial

Each ml contains Triflupromazine HCl 20 mg.

Dose

Animals	*IV Route*	*IM Route*
Cattle and Buffalo	10 mg/100 kg body weight	20 mg/100 kg body weight
Horse	20 mg/100 kg body weight	30 mg/100 kg body weight (Max. 100 mg)
Sheep and Goat	10 mg/100 kg body weight (Max. 40 mg)	–
Dog	1-2 mg/kg body weight	2-4 mg/kg body weight
Cat	–	4-8 mg/kg body weight

17.7.3.3 Thiopentone Sodium

1. *Inj Intraval sodium* – 0.5 g and 1g ampules

Indication

I V anaesthesia for short duration in small and large animals.

Dose

Make either 2.5 or 5 per cent aqueous solution.

Dog: 30 mg/kg body weight

Goat: 10 mg/kg body weight

Large animal: 1 g/90 kg body weight (10-15 mg/kg, IV)

17.7.3.4 Pentothal Sodium Injection

0.5 g and 1 g vials. Each vial contains 500 mg and 1 g Thiopentone sodium.

Dose

Same as Intraval sodium.

17.7.3.5 Ketamine HCl Injection/Ketamil Injection (Helpro Health)

Each ml contains Ketamine HCl – 100 mg.

Indication

Pre-medication, sedative and as an analgesic.

Dose

Cats – 44 mg/kg body weight. Duration of anaesthesia 30-45 minutes.

17.7.4 Medicines for Sedation, Analgesia and Restraining Animals

Alpha-2 (α_2) adreno receptor agonists are generally used in anaesthetic protocol. Alpha-2 – agonists *e.g.* Xylazine, detomidine, medetomidine and Romifidine are frequently used in veterinary practice for sedation, analgesia, and to facilitate restraint in many domestic and non-domestic species.

Dose Range of α_2-Agonists (mg/kg)

Species	*Xylazine (μg/kg)*	*Medetomidine (μg/kg)*	*Detomidine (μg/kg)*	*Romifidine (μg/kg)*
Cattle	20-2000	20-50	10-40	NA
Dog	200-2000	5-30	5-20	NA
Cat	200-2000	10-80	NA	NA
Horse	200-2000	10-30	5-20	30-80
Pig	2000-4000	30-80	NA	NA
Sheep	20-200	10-20		
Goat	10-50	10		

These Alpha-2 (α_2) agonists also produce regional analgesia when injected epidurally. Optimal dose of Xylazine for perineal analgesia in cattle is 0.05 mg/kg. Xylazine can be combined with lignocaine to produce epidural analgesia for faster onset and longer duration. For flank surgery in cattle, Inj. of Xylazine in first interlumbar (L_1 to L_2) – epidural space @ 0.025 mg/kg Xylazine and 0.1 mg/kg Lidocaine combination is most effective for laparotomy.

17.7.5 Epidural Anaesthesia

It is performed in all species of domestic animals. It is a most popular method of anaesthesia in veterinary surgery. This anaesthesia is done with the use of local anaesthetics. The local anaesthetic first desensitizes the sensory nerves followed by sacral, parasympathetic, sympathetic and motor nerves.

Types of Epidural Anaesthesia

1. Caudal epidural anaesthesia
2. Lumbo sacral epidural anaesthesia
3. Lumbar segmental epidural anaesthesia

A number of surgical intervention or operations are performed under caudal epidural anesthesia *e.g.* Atresia ani, atresia recti, amputation of tail, urethrotomy, recto vaginal fistula, dystocia, embryotomy/foetotomy operation, genital prolapse, episiotomy *etc.*

Anaesthetic Sites

Cattle and Buffalo – Sacrococygeal or at 1st and 2nd coccygeal space.

Horse – Through 1st intercoccygeal space.

Cat and Dog – Saecrococcygeal. In dog anterior epidural anaesthesia is preferred.

17.8 RESTRAINT OF ANIMALS FOR SURGICAL PROCEDURES

Majority of the surgical procedures in large animals can be done with some physical restraint and regional local anesthesia and for small animals majority of operations require general anesthesia.

Physical restraint includes use of nose twitch, nose lead, use of chute, casting *etc.* in large animals and tape muzzle in small animals. Use of sedatives and tranquilizers are indicated for small animals. Restraint achieved with tranquilizers and sedatives usually minimizes the amount of physical restraint.

17.9 COMMON SURGICAL CASES

Common surgical cases like flank surgery in cattle, castration, *atresia ani*, string halt (medial patellar desmotomy), amputation of tail, surgical management of ranula, caesarean operation, hernia, surgical management of urolithiasis, surgical management of penile retraction, affections of horn and euthanasia. These surgical cases are described below.

17.9.1 Castration (Vasectomy)

Indication

- ✰ To render the animal docile.
- ✰ To make the animal sterile
- ✰ To improve the quality of meat
- ✰ Scrotal hernia, malignant disease.
- ✰ Irresparable injury of testes.

Site of Operation

1. Parallel to median raphae and about 3-4 cm lateral to it on the scrotum.
2. Or circular incision on the tip of the scrotum.
3. Equipment – General surgical pack, local anaesthetic, tranquilizer, general anaesthetic, if necessary.

Structures of Spermatic Cord

1. Internal spermatic artery
2. Internal spermatic vein
3. Lymphatic of the testes and epididymis
4. Internal spermatic plexus of antonomic and visceral sensory nerves
5. The ductus deferens
6. The tunica vaginalis visceralis

Surgical Method

The animal should be restrained and anaesthesized. An incision is to be given parallel to the median raphae down the anterior surface of the serotum and it is extended backwards to open the bottom of the scrotum. The testicle and the cord should be freed from the loose areolar tissue with the help of fingers. Then the testicle is to be removed by traction or the cord to be cut after proper ligation. Likewise another testicle is to be removed by traction or the cord to be cut after proper ligation. Likewise another testicle is to be removed through a separate incision or through the same incision by incising the median septum. The skin incision is sutured with 2 to 3 interrupted sutures of non-absorbable material (silk or nylon threads). The following medicines should be used for prompt recovery.

- ✰ Tetanus toxoid must be administered before or at the time of castration to avoid post surgical Tetanus.
- ✰ Systemic antibiotic *e.g.* Inj. Oxytetracycline, Inj. Intamycin, Inj. Loxy, Inj. Teramycin, Inj. Streptopenicillin by IM route for 3-5 days.
- ✰ Parenteral NSAIDS *e.g.* Inj. Analgin, Inj. Oxalgin NP, Inj. Melonex @ 10-15 ml for large animal for 2-3 days.
- ✰ Antiseptic ointment *e.g.* Himax, Charmil should be applied locally. Topicure gel may also be used.

After 7-10 days post castration the skin sutures can be removed and further advice to be given to apply Himax or Topicure gel for another 2-3 days.

17.9.2 *Atresia Ani*

It is a congenital malformation, commonly seen in calves, lambs and kids. It may be a condition on its own or may be assóciated with the following conditions.

(*a*) Recto-vaginal fistula

(*b*) Atresia rectii

(*c*) Recto-cystic fistula

(*d*) Vagino-urethral agenesis.

There is no medicinal treatment of such cases; surgical intervention is must to save the life of the new born.

Surgical Procedure

The animal need to be secured in lateral recumbency. The perineal area (bulging area) below the tail to be prepared for aseptic surgery. Local infiltration with 20 per cent Lignocaine HCl below the base of the tail should be attained. A circular piece of skin as per normal diameter of anus of animals (*e.g.* lamb and kid 1-2 cm diameter-average 1-5 cm) can be excised over the bulge area about 4-5 cm below the base of the tail. Blunt dissection should be done to reach up to the bulging rectal end, which is to be exteriorized and a circular piece of rectal wall is to be removed. After complete evacuation of rectum, the rectal mucosa anterior to the fistulous opening (in case of *atresia ani* with recto-vaginal fistula) can be pulled gently up to the perineum and the wound is to be closed with simple interrupted sutures. The rectal opening is to be fixed to the skin with horizontal mattress suture or patency of anal opening (reconstituted anus) is to be maintained by the application of interrupted sutures by black braided silk between skin and mucous coat. Painting of the surgical wound can be done with Tr. Iodine.

Post Operative Care and Management

1. Systemic Antibiotic coverage with Inj. Ampicillin and Cloxacillin or Inj. Amoxycillin and Doxacillin @ 250 mg to 500 mg daily by IM route for 5-7 days.
2. NSAIDS *e.g.* Inj. Melonex, Inj. MP3, Inj. Neoprofen etc. 1-2 ml IM daily for 2-3 days.
3. Routine dressing of the surgical wound with Soframycin ointment, Lorexene ointment *etc.*
4. The sutures can be removed on 5th to 10th day post surgical intervention.

17.9.3 String Halt (Medial Pattelar Dysmotomy)

It is characterized by upward fixation of patella with locking of stifle joint and dragging of affected limb. Cattle and buffaloes equally suffer from this ailment which needs surgical intervention.

The animal is controlled in lateral recumbancy with the affected hind limb towards the ground and the unaffected hind limb is drawn forward and tied with the forelimb. The affected hind limb which lies downward is dragged backward and tied with a piece of bamboo in order to expose the tense patellar ligaments. Analgesia is achieved on the medial aspect of the stifle joint where medial patellar ligament inserts into the inner aspect of anterior tuberosity of the tibia.

A skin incision of about 3-4 cm in length is made at the posterior border of the ligament. A blunt forceps or scissors is inserted under the ligament and the ligament is cut over the instrument. Tr. Iodine is sprinkled over the incised area and the skin incision is closed by simple interrupted or mattress sutures. The said operation can also be done in close method with the help of a tenotome or fine pointed scalpel. The sharp end of the instrument inserted directly through the skin and fascia at the anterior border of the ligament and the ligament is severed carefully and the instrument is taken out. Few drops of Lugols iodine are poured at the operation site.

A depression may be palpated at the site after cutting the ligament and periarticular fat may bulge out. In chronic condition even after severing the ligament desired result may not be obtained.

A course of anti-inflammatory and analgesic drugs *e.g.* Inj. Neoprofen, Inj. Oxalgin NP, Inj. Vetalgin, Inj. Artisone (S) *etc.* @ 10-15 ml for 2-3 days and a course of antibiotic to prevent or combat possible bacterial contamination or invasion may be given (*e.g.* Inj. Oxytetracycline, Inj. Streptopenicillin *etc.*). Skin sutures to be removed on 8th to 10th postoperative day. If fluids are accumulated, that should be aspirated for prompt healing. The animal should not be used for hard work at least for a week or more.

17.9.4 Amputation of Tail

Surgical intervention on tail sometimes needed for the neoplastic diseases of tail, tail gangrene, major injuries etc. and in severe cases amputation of tail is done. Amputation of tail is done in case of dogs to improve the appearance of the animal (docking).

Surgical Procedure

Operation site is always at the seat of infection at the intervertebral articulation or above the injury. Large animal is controlled either in standing on in recumbent position and the small animal in recumbent position. Posterior epidural anaesthesia or local infiltration anaesthesia subcutaneously encircling the tail above the site of operation can be done for going to amputation of tail. A tourniquet is applied at the base of the tail and then operation can be started. This operation can be done in 2 different methods of using docking scissors.

Using Docking Scissors Method

Docking scissors is placed at the chosen site at the intervertebral space and the tail is amputated. Sterilized gauge soaked in antiseptic, solution is applied over the tail stump and a bandage is applied tightly to check the bleeding. Tourniquet is released after the operation

Flap Method

Two 'V' shaped skin flaps are made one on the dorsal and the other on the ventral side at the site of operation after palpating the articulation or locating intervertebral space. Major blood vessels at the lateral and ventral aspect of the tail pre-ligated and by blunt dissection the joint is disarticulated with the help of knife. The distal portion of the tail is thus removed. Skin flaps are united by simple interrupted or interrupted mattress sutures.

Post Operative Care

1. In first method tail is dressed with antibiotic ointment *e.g.* Soframycin, Betnovet ointment or multipurpose gel *e.g.* Topicure, Skinoment, Himax. ointment *etc.* till the healing is complete.
2. In the second method (flap method) the applied sutures are removed 8-10 days after surgery or after complete healing.
3. A cause of broad spectrum antibiotic coverage should be given to combat possible microbial infection, *e.g.* Inj. Gentamycin @ 3-6 mg/kg, Inj. Streptopenicillin @ 7.5-12.5 mg/kg by IM route for 3-5 days.
4. Anti-inflammatory analgesic *e.g.* Inj. Meloxicam, Inj. Ketoprofen *etc.* can be administered if required for 2-3 day by IM route to alleviate pain and swelling.

17.9. 5 Surgical Management of Ranula

Ranula is transparent retention cyst formed sometimes at the side of the fraenum lingue, or at the ventral surface of the base of the tongue due to obstruction of a mucous gland or one of the ducts of sublingual salivary glands. It is most commonly seen in dogs as compared to other animals. Cattle and buffalo are next to dog in context to its suffering. The cysts may originate from the ducts of sublingual salivary gland and develop due occlusions and continuous accumulation or stasis of saliva in sensory duct.

Signs and Symptoms

Swelling at or near fraenum linguae or under surface at the base of the tongue *etc.* It is soft and fluctuating or tense. The swelling may develop in the caudal border of the vertical part of the ramus of mandiable. There will be profuse salivation, difficulty in mastication and swallowing.

Diagnosis

Oral examination, exploratory puncture sticky alkine/slimy content.

Surgical Management

The animal is to be restrained on lateral recumbency. Then mouth jag is to be applied to pull the tongue gently outside the buccal cavity for ease in operation. The site of incision may be desensitized by local infiltration of 2 per cent Linnocaine Hcl (2-5 ml). The cyst is then cleaned with antiseptic solution. The cyst is then cleaned with antiseptic solution (*e.g.* potassium permanganate solution). Then an incision 1-2 cm as per requirement to evacuate he accumulated sticky fluid. Cauterization of the exotic cavity can be made with pot. Permanganate crystals or with Tr. Iodine gauge soaked or impregnated with iodine can be kept for 3-5 days following cauterization. Daily cleaning of the incised cavity with antiseptic solution for 10-15 days till recovery should be made. Post operatively broad spectrum antibiotic *e.g.* Inj. Loxy, Inj. Intamycin (Oxytetracycline) or Inj. Ampicillin Cloxacillin combination *e.g.* Inj. Acvet Inj. Vetclox *etc.*, NSAID *e.g.* Inj. Melonex, Inj. Oxalgin NP, Inj. Ketoprofen, IV DNS for 3-4 days can be administered.

17.9.6 Caesarean Operation

Pre Operative Protocol

1. Physical examination of animal.
2. Examine heart rate, pulse, respiration and temperature.
3. Haematological and biochemical screening if possible.
4. Broad spectrum antibiotic (having bactericidal effect) *e.g.* Ampicillin, Cloxacillin, Amoxycillin Cloxacillin combination @ 2 g for large animal and 500 mg – 1 g for small animals and Dexamethasone @ 20 mg for large animal and @ 5-10 mg for small animal should be given IV.
5. Drinking water along with salt and sugar can be offered to every dam before caesarean.
6. IV fluid therapy to be initiated with Ringers Lactate, followed by 100-150 ml calcium boro-gluconate and 50-60 ml of sodium bicarbonate can be done for large animals.
7. Then shaving, scrubbing of the surgical site and local infiltration of anaesthetic to be carried out.
8. An anti-inflammatory, analgesic drug *e.g.* Phenylbutazone, Meloxicam can be given before surgery.
9. Keep the animal in lateral recumbancy on cushion beds. Sterile plastic drape/sheet can be covered over it to prevent bacterial contamination.

Intra Operative Protocol

1. Selection of surgical site – low flank, oblique incision just above the flank.
2. Every attempt is made to exteriorize the uterus outside the surgical incision.
3. Incision on the uterus is to be made from ovarian end and to be extended towards the cervix avoiding the cotyledons.
4. Then the foetus is to be removed carefully changing the dams site from lateral to slight sternal position. The foetus is the exteriorized by grasping both the legs of the foetus and removed gently avoiding uterine tear.
5. The placenta is to be carefully removed.
6. To promote uterine involution oxytocin injection @ 40-50 IU for large animal and @ 5-10 IU to small animals can be made.
7. Uterine closure: The exteriorized part of the uterus is to be cleaned properly with sterile gauze and flushing with N.S.S. and then closed by chromic catgut (No. 2). Single inversion/cushings sutures are preferred.

8. Abdominal closure: The peritoneum, abdominus transversus and internal abdominal oblique muscles are to be closed with simple interrupted sutures using chromic catgut (No. 2). Overlapping sutures can also be employed. In case of extreme paramedian (ventral incisions) simple interrupted sutures can also be given.

   Then the external abdominal muscle is to be sutured as a second layer with interrupted sutures. This is followed with subcuticular suture. Lastly the skin is to be sutured using modified vertical mattress without causing much eversion of the skin.
9. Fluid therapy should be continued during entire operation.

Post Operative Care

1. The position of the animal is to be changed from lateral to sternal.
2. Fluid therapy is to be continued for 2-3 hours more even after operation using 5 per cent Dextrose saline (DNS).
3. The animals are to be kept in warmth and comfortable condition.
4. Systemic antibiotic *e.g.* Intamox, Inimox @ 2 g for 7 days.
5. NSAID *e.g.* Inj. Melonex (Meloxicam) for 3-5 days.
6. Steroids *e.g.* Inj. Dexona for 3 days and to be withdrawn in tapering dose.
7. Skin sutures can be removed 15 days after the surgery.

17.9.7 Hernia

Surgical Management of Ventral Hernia

Protusion of the abdominal viscera through a natural orifice or artificial opening is called ventral hernia. Hernias are generally observed as a result of external injuries either due to thrust of horns or falling on blunt pointed objects. In case of small hernias, simple apposition by sutures is possible but in case of large hernia it becomes imperative to use prosthetic implants.

Various Implants Used in Hernia

Nylon mosquito net, stainless steel, Marlex tentalum, Nylon mesh, cotton mesh and carbon fibres.

Classification of Hernia

Depending upon the location, hernia may be external or internal. Among the external, are ventral hernia, umbilical hernia, inguinal hernia, scrotal hernia are common. External hernia usually consists of a hernial sac, a hernial ring and the hernial contents. When the hernia contents can be returned into the abdominal cavity it is called a reducible hernia but when it could not be returned to the abdominal cavity it is called irreducible. In irreducible hernia there must be the adhesion.

Surgical Procedure for All Kinds of Hernia

Animal needs to be fasted for at least 12-18 hours before surgery and sedated 30 minutes before operation. Sedation can be made with Triflupromazine HCl (for bovines) or under Xylazine (Xylocad). Local infiltration analgesia should be made with the use 2 per cent lignocaine HCl to be given around the hernia swelling. An adequate area over and in the continuity of the swelling is to be prepared for aseptic surgery. An elliptical skin incision is to be given over the centre of the swelling and by blunt dissection the subcutaneous tissue, muscle and hernial ring are to be separated from the skin from the edge of the hernial ring. After reducing the hernial contents, the hernia ring is to be freshened and sutured in an over lapping pattern using Vitafil or by inlay grafts techniques using sterile nylon mesh, marlex *etc*, mattress sutures are to be placed to secure the nylon net with hernial ring. The subcutaneous fascia and skin are to be sutured in a routine manner to cover the mesh using braided silk and Tr. Benzoin can be applied over the size.

Post Operative Treatment

1. An antibiotic coverage, *e.g.* Inj. Streptopenicillin, Inj. Enrofloxacin, Inj. Oxytetracycline *etc.* should be given for 5-7 days by IM route.
2. If fluid accumulates at the operation size post operatively that should be aspirated or drained out.
3. NSAID *e.g.* Inj. Melonex, Inj. Meloxi, Inj. MP_3, Inj. Melobest *etc.* (any one) @ 10-15 ml by IM route for 3 days can be given.
4. Neurotropic B-vitamins *e.g.* Inj. Tribivet, Inj. Polyvet, Inj. Nuroxin-N (any one) can be given @ 5-10 ml by IM route daily or on alternate day for 3-5 occasions.
5. Skin sutures can be removed after 12-15 days post surgery.

17.9.8 Surgical Management of Urolithiasis/Urinary Calculi

Urinary calculi results from a combination of physiologic, nutritional and management factors. Obstructive urolithiasis refers to the formation of calculi in the urinary tract with subsequent urinary blockage by uroliths. This results in stoppage of urination and acute discomfort.

Animal shows unconsciousness and abdominal pain manifested by straining, kicking at the belly, swiching of the tail and twitching of the penis and failure of passing urine. Per rectal examination in case of bovine will reveal distension of urinary bladder. It is a fatal disease condition in a suffering animals and fatality mostly occurs due to rupture of the urethra or urinary bladder. The only remedy of obstructive urolithiasis could be the urethrotomy, cystotomy or urethrostomy.

Surgical Management

After aseptic preparation of the site (usual site is post scrotal urethra), an incision about 10-20 cm long can be made through the skin and subcutis exactly on the midline in the post scrotal region under epidural anaesthesia using 10-15ml of 2 per cent Lignocain HCl. Incision needs to be deepened through the fascia between the two retractor penis muscles and through corpus cavernosum urethrae. Urethra is then needs to be incised just above the seat of obstruction and the (urolith) calculi to be removed. A suitable size sterilized catheter or polythene tube can be passed anteriorly towards the bladder and posteriorly towards the external urethral orifice and to be fixed at the orifice. Polythene tube can be removed 5-6 days post surgery and skin sutures to be removed.

Post operatively an antibiotic coverage with Inj. Ceftriaxone, Inj. Enrofloxacin, Inj. Ampicillin Cloxacillin, and NSAID *e.g.* Inj. Melonex, Inj. MP_3, Inj. Melobest-P *etc.* should be given for 5-7 days. Fluid therapy with Ringers lactate and dextrose, normal saline 3-5 litres per day for 3 days should be administered. Normal flow of the urine is indicative of success in surgery and recovery thereafter.

17.9.9 Penile Retraction (Paraphimosis)

Paraphimosis is a condition in which the extended penis cannot be with drawn into prepuce owing to inflammatory enlargement. Paraphimosis is often encountered in young males *e.g.* bulls, bucks, and rams and is quite difficult to treat especially in neglected cases. Direct trauma leading to haematoma, erection through narrow preputial ring, masturbation and administration of tranquilizers are responsible for penile retraction.

Treatment

Conservative treatments *e.g.* massaging, hydrotherapy, lubrication, administration of diuretics are recommended with repositioning of extended (protruded) penis in its original place.

But in neglected cases the penis may be badly mutilated, in that case amputation of penis is recommended.

Surgical Procedure

Analgesia should be achieved locally using 2 per cent lignocaine hydrochloride.

If deep sedation is required Xylazine can be injected intramuscularly as per requirement. The site should be prepared by cleaning the soiled penis with aeriflavin lotion or potassium permanganate solution (Condy's lotion).

Two circular incisions can be made one at glans penis and another at prepucial ring. These incisions are then joined by a longitudinal incision on the shaft of the protruded penis. If there is dead and devitalized (necrosed tissues) on the penis that should be removed carefully. If there is any adhesion then preputial ring and sheath should be made free by gentle dissection.

Two circular incisions need to be joined together by horizontal mattress sutures using chromic catgut and thus retracting the penis into the prepuce.

If there is any haemorrhage that should be controlled by manual pressure or swabbing with adrenaline or swabbing with Povidone Iodine, Tr. Iodine *etc.* (using styptics).

Post operatively prepucial canal should be smeared with non irritant antiseptic, *e.g.*, Silverex, Soframycin ointment or Topicure gel.

17.9.10 Common Surgical Conditions of Horns

Various affections of horns usually need surgical intervention. These are:

1. Avulsion of horn

2. Fracture of horn at base
3. Fracture of horn at middle or tip of the horn
4. Septic horn
5. Overgrown horn
6. Fissures in horn
7. Horn cancer *etc.*

Avulsion of Horn

Among the horn affections avulsion of the horn is a major problem which might be due to vigorous and infighting nature of animals.

In case of avulsion of horn, the horny covering is separated from the bony core. The exposed bony core should be covered with tincture of bezoin dressing.

Treatment

1. The affected horn should be cleaned properly. The exposed corium should be cleaned with 1 : 1000 potassium permanganate solution.
2. Exposed bony core should be covered with Tr. of Benzoin dressing.
3. Fly repellent to be applied to prevent maggot infestation *e.g.* Neem oil, dressing oil, dressogen, saaf oil *etc.*
4. Herbal lotion like Himax, Charmil can also be used.
5. Horn fractures, septic horn and fissures in horn should be best managed by amputation of horn at its base to avoid further complications.

Amputation of Horn

It is indicated for horn fracture, septic horn, horn cancer and fissures in horn. Before commencement of operation deep sedation to be established with the administration of Xylazine HCl (Xylazin) @ 0.04 mg/kg body weight. at least 15 minutes earlier. The base of the horn is to be prepared for aseptic surgery and about 10-15 ml of Lignocaine HCl for cattle and 15-30 ml of Lignocaine HCl for buffalo (with 2 per cent Xylocaine, Astra) should be infiltrated at the base of the horn to carry ring block anaesthesia. A vertical cutaneous incision from the base of the horn at the frontal crest and a horizontal cutaneous incision towards the nuchal crest are to be made. Then an elliptical incision is to be made to connect the two previous incisions on the dorsal aspect of the horn exactly at the base. The skin over the dorsal wall of the horn needs to be separated as a full thickness graft to expose the bony horn. The exposed bony horn is to be transected with a hack-saw-blade up to the half of the horn diameter without causing damage to the ventral edges of the skin. The remaining horn is to be chiseled from one angle from frontal crest towards nuchal crest. After chiseling the entire transected bone is to be lifted to expose the ventral part of the horn through the transacted edge for a ventral skin flap. A series of horizontal mattress with a thick non-absorbable suture material should be applied to close the skin edges.

Post Operative Treatment

1. A course of broad spectrum antibiotic *e.g.* Inj. Oxytetracycline, Inj. Streptopenicillin by IM route for 5 to 7 days should be given
2. NSAID *e.g.* Inj. Melonex, Inj. Zobid-20 *etc.* @ 15-20 ml through IM route daily for 3-5 days.
3. If necessary corticosteroids *e.g.* Dexamethasone or Prednisolone can be administered.
4. Dressing of the wound around the suture line with Topicure, Himax or Charmil ointment should be done till complete recovery.

Horn Fracture

The treatment option is the application of plaster of Paris bandage with or without splints.

Aluminium wire can also be used. If it is not possible owing to complicated fracture amputation of horn up to its base should be done (same procedure as stated earlier).

Overgrown Horn

The treatment in case of overgrown horns can be practiced by sawing he curved portion (in case of buffaloes) and tip of the horn at its bent without touching the corium in case of cattle. After sawing potassium permanganate cauterization should be done for rapid healing and to avoid chances of bleeding if corium is touched.

17.9.11 Euthanasia

The term 'euthanasia' is derived from the Greek terms '*Eu*' means good and '*thanatos*' means death. So euthanasia means 'Good Death'. It is an act of inducing humane death in an animal with minimal pain and distress. Euthanasia technique should give a rapid loss of consciousness followed by cardiac or respiratory arrest (or cardio respiratory failure) and the ultimate loss of brain function. The technique should minimize distress and anxiety in animals prior to loss of consciousness.

Most methods of euthanasia require physical handling of the animal. Proper handling is vital to minimize pain and distress in animals, to ensure safety of the person performing euthanasia.

Indication

Failure of treatment, suffering from excruciating pain, suffering from incurable diseases like rabies, behaviourable problem, and the owner does not want the animal any more due to some reasons. The owner has to take decision and sole responsibility for death (by euthanasia) of the animal.

Basic Mechanism of Euthanizing Agents

The euthanizing agents cause death by 3 basic mechanisms. These are

1. Direct or indirect hypoxia to cause loss of consciousness prior to loss of motor activity.
2. Direct depression of neurons necessary for life function.

3. Physical disruption of brain activity and destruction of neurons necessary for life.

Euthanizing Agents/Methods

1. *Barbiturates: e.g.* Pentobarbital sodium @ 27 mg/lb body weight IV and 40 mg/kg body weight IP or I/thoracic. It is suitable for small animals.
2. *Chloral hydrate*: At the dose rate of 2 g/10 kg body weight, suitable for cattle, buffalo and horse.
3. *Magnesium sulphate*: Saturated solution (1 : 1) at 40-50°C causes cardiac arrest and death. Inject rapidly by IV or intracardiac route.

   Dose: Large animal – 1 g/kg body weight; Dog – 10-30 ml.
4. *Inhalant anaesthetics*: *e.g.* halothane, enflurane. isoflurane, sevoflurane, methoxyflurane, with or without nitrous oxide. Carbon di-oxide (CO_2) gases can be used to induce enthanasia in gas chamber after sedation. It requires special method and chamber.
5. *Shooting*: The shot should be done from a distance of 5-8 ft at the cross point of the imaginary lines drawn from the base of two ears to the opposite eyes. It causes profuse bleeding.

Species-wise Acceptable Method for Euthanasia

Ruminant

Barbiturates, Potassium chloride in conjugation with general anaesthesia, Penetrating captive bolt.

Pig

Barbiturates, CO_2, Potassium chloride in conjugation with general anaesthesia, (Inhalant anaesthetics, Chloral hydrate after sedation) and electrocution.

Horse

Barbiturates, Potassium chloride in conjugation with general anaesthesia, Penetrating captive bolt (chloral hydrate after sedation).

Cat and Dog

Barbiturates, inhalant anaesthetics, CO_2, CO, Potassium chloride in conjugation with general anaesthetics, Mag sulph ($MgSO_4$) saturated solution (IV), N_2 and Argon gases (Ar) can be used.

Zoo animals

Barbiturates, inhalant anaesthetics, CO_2, CO, Potassium chloride in conjugation with general anaesthetics, N_2 or Argon gas and Gun shot.

Free Ranging Wildlife

Barbiturates IV or intraperitoneal, Inhalant anaesthetics, Potassium chloride in conjugation with general anaesthesia.

Consent Form for Euthanasia

Consent form for euthanasia is given in Part-VI of this book.

N.B. *Proforma for taking surgical risk note is given in Part-VI of this book.*

Part – V
Veterinary Pharmaceuticals

Chapter 18
Veterinary Pharmacy

18.1 COMMON TERMINOLOGIES

18.1.1 Pharmacology

Long, long ago special study of the biological effects of drugs had been regarded as 'Pharmacology' as one of the sub-divisions of Physiology. Now, 'Pharmacology' is a special branch of science which deals with drug, its pharmacodynamics, pharmacokinetics and its therapeutic effect, including prescribing systems, cost benefit analysis and official drug regulation *etc*.

18.1.2 Pharmacodynamics

It means the investigation of how drugs, alone and in combination, affect the body of the animal or individual (young, old, well, sick).

18.1.3 Pharmacokinetics

Absorption, distribution, metabolism, excretion or how the body, well or sick, affects drugs is known as Pharmacokinetics. Pharmacodynamics is what drugs do to the body and pharmacokinetics is what the body does to the drugs.

18.1.4 Drug

According to 'WHO', a drug can be defined as a substance or product that is used or intended to be used to modify or explore physiological systems or pathological states for the benefit of the recipient.

A drug is a single chemical substance that forms the active ingredient of a medicine, which latter may contain many other substances to deliver the drug in a stable form, acceptable and convenient to the sick (patient).

According to Indian Drugs Act 1940, drug includes all medicines irrespective of internal and external use intended to be used for treatment.

18.1.5 Pharmacy

It is the art of preparing drugs or combination of drugs or substances so as to make them fit for administration.

18.1.6 Toxicology

'Drugs are useful poisons' (Williams,1787) *i.e.*, poisons in small doses are the best medicines and 'useful medicines' in too large doses are poisonous. Toxicology deals with the study of the symptomatology, diagnosis and treatment of conditions produced when drugs are used in poisonous doses.

18.1.7 Bacterial Toxins

The simplest of free living organisms produce some lethal poisons to man and animals which are several million times more toxic than a dangerous poison *e.g.* Strychnine.

For example, Botulinum toxin produces respiratory paralysis. Tetanus toxin produces muscular spasm and convulsions. Diphtheria toxin damages heart. Staphylococcal toxin ruptures red blood corpuscles.

Bacteria and fungi often produce substances that are toxic to other microorganisms but not to man and animals and these are called antibiotics – those have been a therapeutic GOLD MINE.

18.2 PHARMACOLOGICAL PREPARATION

18.2.1 Alternative

Drugs which modify tissue changes and improve various nutrition to various organs.

18.2.2 Anodynes

Drugs which relieve pain by diminishing irritability of nerve endings.

18.2.3 Antizymotic

Drugs which act against flatulence and help the expulsion of gases and bowel.

18.2.4 Astringent

Drugs used in loose motion (persistent diarrhoea). They act by precipitating proteins of gut mucosa and the proteins protect it from irritant ingesta.

Example: Catechu, Kaolin *etc.*

18.2.5 Carminative

Drugs which prevent the formation and help the expulsion of gases from the G.I. tract.

18.2.6 Diuretics

Drugs which increase the formation and flow of urine.

Example: Frusemide (Inj. Redema, Lasix *etc.*)

18.2.7 Laxative

Drugs which produce soft stool and prevent constipation, helping in evacuation of normal stool. It usually produces single evacuation.

Example: Liquid paraffin.

18.2.8 Analeptics

The agents that stimulate the respiratory, vasomotor, vagal and vomiting centres located in medulla.

Example: Doxapram, Theophylene.

18.2.9 Ecbolics

The drugs or agents that stimulate uterine contractions and hasten parturition (oxytocin) or cause abortion (abortifacients).

Example: Oxytocin and PGF_2a

18.2.10 Tocolytics

Drugs that suppress the uterine contractions.

Example: Isoxuprine (b_2 adrenergic agonist) indicated for threatened abortion @ 0.5 mg/kg body weight.

18.2.11 Urinary Alkalizers

Drugs or medicines that increase the urinary pH and volume. Alkalinization of urine enhances the antibacterial activity of amino glycosides in urinary tract infections.

Example: Sodium bicarbonate, Alkasol.

18.2.12 Anti Tussives

Drugs or substances that reduce the frequency and intensity of coughing by depressing the medulary cough center or by interfering with the cough reflex at the sensory receptors in pharynx and larynx. These are also known as cough sedatives.

Example: Codein phosphate (Corex), Dexthomethorphan, cough syrup, honey *etc.*

18.2.13 Expectorants

Medicines which increase the volume and fluidity of respiratory secretions and expel bronchial secretions.

Example: Respigen syrup (Nugen), Coldex syrup (Oxford).

Benzoin, eucalyptus oil, turpentine oil are inhaled or vapours with steam act as inhalant expectorants.

18.2.14 Hemostatics

Medicines or substances that promote with blood coagulation or arrest bleeding causing obstruction to blood flow or by precipitation of proteins.

Example: Inj. Vitamin K (@ 0.25-2.5 mg/kg body weight.

18.2.15 Anticoagulants

Drugs which prevent clotting of blood.

Example: Sodium citrate, Heparin.

18.2.16 Hematinics

Drugs which increase red blood cells (RBC) production.

Example: Iron, cobalt, vitamin B_{12}, Folic acid, Dexorange syrup, Haematic.

18.2.17 Anaesthetics

Salts of weak bases which reversibly block nerve conduction in sensory and motor fibres leading to a loss of pain sensation and motor function.

Example: Local anaesthetic, Lignocaine HCl, Xylocaine, Lidocaine, *etc*.

18.2.18 Purgative

Agents or medicines which cause expulsion of intestinal contents by multiple evacuation. Purgatives generally act as laxatives in small doses.

Example: (*i*) EPSOM salt (Magnesium sulfate) – It is a saline purgative. (*ii*) Castor oil – It is an irritant purgative.

18.2.19 Enemas

Warm soapy water, saline, glycerol or docusate sodium solution is often infused per rectum to soften impacted colonic and rectal contents and to stimulate defecation in animals (in dog).

18.2.20 Topicals

Drugs/preparations applied to skin, mucosae and ears are called topical. *viz.* antibacterials, antifungals, ectoparasiticides, corticosteroids, antihistaminics and hemostatics for topical/local use (external use).

18.2.21 Demulcents

Water soluble drugs which soothe and relieve irritation particularly of mucus membranes may be applied to skin also.

Example: Glycerin (used as Suppository).

18.2.22 Emollients

Substance used for its soothing effect called emollient. They comprise of fats and oils applied to skin for soothing effect, may be applied to mucosae too.

Example: Vaseline, vegetable oils (arachis, corn oil, olive oil). They act as emollient on skin and mucosae.

18.2.23 Counter Irritants

These are drugs that are applied to skin by friction to increase vascularity of the area. This relieves underlying integument (skin) pain and promotes healing.

Example: Black mustard, Mercuric iodide, Turpentine oil, Methyl salicylate *etc.*

18.2.24 Lotions

Liquid preparations meant for topical application (external use) without rubbing.

Example: Lactocalamine lotion, Himax lotion, Acriflavin lotion.

18.2.25 Cream

Special medicinal preparation resembling ointments and meant for external application. They mostly contain wax, glycerin or liquid paraffin.

Example: Zinc oxide cream.

18.2.26 Pastes

Special preparations having starch, phenol, glycerol or paraffin base intended for external application in skin affections.

Example: Magnesium sulfate paste (Morison's Paste)

18.2.27 Ointment

These are soft or semisolid preparations of various substances having wax or fat base intended for external application (topical use).

Example: sulphur ointment, zinc oxide ointment, methyl/salicylate ointment, Iodine ointment, sorine ointment, Charmil ointment *etc.*

18.2.28 Liniments

Liniments are preparations meant for external application to the skin by rubbing or friction and are usually oily in nature. For better absorptions of medicaments and rubifacient action, alcohol is usually incorporated. It is indicated for painful conditions and sprains.

Example: Ammoniated Liniment of Camphor, Liniment of ammonia, Liniment of turpentine.

18.2.29 Solutions or Liquors

Solutions or liquors are solutions of different substances in some suitable vehicle like water, alcohol or vegetable oil.

Example: Potassium permanganate solution, Electrolyte solution, Liquor Arsenicalis, Hydrogen peroxide solution.

18.2.30 Poultices

Viscous pasty preparations for external use indicated for pains and inflammatory conditions or swelling.

Example: Kaolin Poultice.

18.2.31 Tinctures

Solutions of various crude vegetable substances in alcohol of different strengths prepared either by maceration or percolation.

Example: Nux Vomica Tr.

18.2.32 Syrups

Sucrose based saturated solutions containing certain drugs chiefly used for sweetening and flavouring purposes.

18.2.33 Pessary

Vaginal suppository is called as Pessary where the medicine or drug is liberated in contact with the mucous-surfaces. They are in oblet forms containing antiseptic elements.

18.2.34 Spirits or Spiritus

Alcoholic solutions of volatile substances giving a stable solution for dispensing purpose.

Example: Spirit Nitrous Ether.

18.2.35 Implants

Implants are sterile cylinders prepared by flussing or heavy compressions, intended for subcutaneous implantation for prolong action and slow release.

18.2.36 Electuary

It is a soft paste made by compounding drugs with treacle, sugar or honey.

Example: Ruchi (Kapila)

18.3 HOW DRUG ACTS?

There was no satisfactory answer regarding the exact mechanism of drug action. An overview of the mechanism of drug action may appear thus:

1. Action on the specific receptors or receptor binding (binding site) – which mediates a biological effect. *viz.*
   (*a*) Agonists and antagonists on adrenoreceptors.
   (*b*) Antihistamine drugs on histamine receptors.
   (*c*) Anticholinergic drugs on acetylcholine receptors.

2. Interaction between drug and enzyme like that of drug and receptors.
3. Selectivity of drug action by selective delivery of the drug to the desired site of action alone.
4. Interaction with cell membrane – *viz.* general and local anaesthetics appear to act on the lipid, protein or water constituents of nerve cell membranes.
5. Metabolic process within the cell by (i) enzyme inhibition (ii) blockage of anion transport/inhibition of transport process. (iii) alteration of metabolic process.
6. Direct chemical interactions – *viz.* chelating agents and Neutralization of gastric juice by use of antacids.
7. Produce effects on physical basis – *viz.* Bismuth salts form a protective coating on the intestinal mucosa and act as intestinal sedative.

Kaolin and Magnesium trisilicate act by absorption.

Drugs produce pharmacological effect by producing nerve block *e.g.* Xylocaine, Novocaine, Gesicaine.

18.4 GENERAL IDEA ABOUT PRESCRIPTION

Generally prescriptions are made by the physicians after examining an animal making proper diagnosis of a disease or ailment, suffered by the animal. It includes drugs or combination of drugs used for the treatment or therapeutic measures, directions to the pharmacist and also to the patient or owner of the patients, regarding its use.

Treatment may be classified as (1) General treatment, (2) Specific treatment, (3) Symptomatic treatment, 4) Palliative treatment, (5) Empirical treatment, (6) Rational treatment, and (7) Prophylactive treatment.

Prescription Writing

Prescription writing is an art which includes (1) the superscription (2) the inscription (3) the subscription (4) the signature (5) prescriber's name and his registration number.

1. The Superscription

It is denoted by a traditional esoteric symbol R_x (for the recipe)

R_x means recipe or take thou! Which is addressed to pharmacist.

Originally it means prayer to Jupiter God.

2. The Inscription

It is the body of the prescription which consists of different drugs or combination of drugs with their doses for treating the ailed animal. It may contain only one chief ingredient or medicine which forces the basis and sometimes another drug is used to assist or as adjuvant. Supportive may be given in the form of prescription. This includes the name and dose of the drug or drugs.

3. The Subscription

It gives direction to the dispenser or pharmacist *i.e.* what is to be done? Number of doses, whether it is a mixture, bolus, tablet, caplet, powder *etc.*

4. The Signatures

It is the direction to the patient or the owner of the patient by the pharmacist about how the medicines to be used, how many times to be used, whether to be taken OD, BID, TID (once, twice or thrice daily), route of administration (*e.g.* oral, parenteral, topical *etc.*) *etc.*

5. Last part of the prescription which includes prescriber's signature, name, registration no. *etc.*

PROFORMA OF A STANDARD PRESCRIPION

Date:...........

Name and Address of Veterinary Doctor

Name and address of Patient/Owner of the patient:

For a Cow

(of Sri ....)

Address of the owner ....

....

Ajwan powder – 15 g

Anisi powder – 15 g

Black pepper – 05g

Black salt – 50 g

Ginger powder – 15 g

Mft. Mist, prepare 6 doses, mix with water.

Sig. To be given drench twice daily.

Signature of Veterinary Doctor

Name

Registration No.

18.5 LATIN PHRASES AND ABBREVIATIONS USED IN PRESCRIPTION WRITING

Latin Abbreviations	*Latin Term*	*Meaning*
a.c.	*Ante cibos*	Before feeding or before meals
Ad. lib	*Ad libitum*	As much as wanted, free access
Aq.	Aqua	Water
Aq. Bull	Aqua bullettins	Boiling water
Aq. Dist	Aqua distillate	Distilled water
b.i.d./BID/BD	Bis in die	Twice daily
C	Cum	With
Caps.	Capsula	A capsule
Collut.	Collutorium	A mouth wash
Collyr.	Collyrium	An eye lotion
Cras vesp.	Cras vespere	Tomorrow night
div.	Divide	Divide
div. in pt.	Dividatur in partes aequales	Divide into equal parts
ft.	Fiat	Let it be made
h.s.	Horra somni	At bed time
Inj.	Injecto	An injection
Liq.	Liquor	A solution
m.	Misce	Mix
m. seq.	Mane sequenti	Tomorrow morning
m.d.	More dicto or Modo dicto	As directed
Mist.	Mistura	A mixture
Od	omni die	Every day
Om	omni mane	Every morning
On	omni nocte	Every night
p.c.	*Post cibos*	After feeding or after meal
p.r.n.	Pro re nata	Occasionally, according to circumstances
Po	Per os	By mouth
Pulv.	Pulvis	Powder
q.i.d./QID/QD	Querter in die	Four times a day
q.s.	Quantum Sufficiat	As much as is sufficient
Rep	Repetatur	Let it be repeated
Rx	Recipe	Take
s. i. d./SID/SD	Semel in die	Once a day
s.o.s.	Si opus sit	If necessary/when required
Sig	Signa/Signatura	Write on label/Let it be labeled
ss	Semis	Half
stat.	Statim	Immediately
t.i.d./TID/TD	Ter in die	Three times a day
Tab.	Tabella	A tablet

18.6 WEIGHTS AND MEASURES IN PRESCRIPTION

Weight/Mass

- ☆ 1 gram (g) = 10^3 miligrams (mg)
- ☆ 1 g = 10^6 micrograms
- ☆ 1 g = 10^9 nanograms
- ☆ 1 g = 10^{12} picograms
- ☆ 1 g = 10^{15} femtograms
- ☆ 1 kg = 1000 g   1 tonne = 1000 kg   1 pound = 453.59 g
- ☆ 1 kg = 2.2 pounds   1 g = 15.4 grains

Volume

- ☆ 1 litre = 1000 cc (1000 ml) = 35.196 ft. Oz. = 1.758 pints
- ☆ 1 pint = 568.25 ml
- ☆ 1 ounce (OZ) = 28.35 g
- ☆ 1 milliliter = 10^3 micro litres
- ☆ 1 litre = 10^3 ml
- ☆ 1 litre = 10^6 ml (micro litres)
- ☆ 1 litre = 10^9 nano litres
- ☆ 1 litre = 10^{12} pico litres
- ☆ 1 litre = 10^{15} femto litres

Metric Imperial Equivalent

- ☆ 1 ounce = 28.4 g   1 gallon = 4.546 litres
- ☆ 1 kg = 2.2 pounds   1 inch = 2.54 cm
- ☆ 1 tonne = 0.98 42 ton   1 foot = 30.48 cm
- ☆ 1 ton = 1.016 tonnes   1 yard = 0.9144 meter
- ☆ 1 pint = 568 ml   1 meter = 39.37 inches
- ☆ 1 quert = 1136 ml

Metric Apothecaries Equivalent

- ☆ 1 g = 15.43 grains
- ☆ 1 grain = 65 mg

Metric Household Equivalent (Approximate)

- ☆ 1 tea spoonful (t.s.f.) = 5 ml
- ☆ 1 desert spoonful = 8 ml
- ☆ 1 table spoonful = 15 ml
- ☆ 15 drops = 1 ml

☆ 1 glass = 250 ml

☆ 1 wine glass (peg) = 60 ml

18.7 COMMONLY USED DRUGS(CHEMICALS/PURE HERBAL PRODUCTS) IN VETERINARY FIRST AID

Sl.No.	Name of the Medicines or Drugs	Colour	Texture	Uses
1.	Tincture Iodine	Bluish black	Liquid	Antiseptic, styptic (Haemostatic) dressing of wound
2	Tincture Benzoin	Grayish brown	Stickly liquid	Antiseptic, Haemostatic, Inhalation in respiratory distress (Rhinitis – mucolytic)
3.	Mercurochrome (2 per cent solution)	Green but in water it is red	Crystal	Antiseptic, Haemostatic
4.	Acriflavin	Red but in water it is yellow	Crystal	Dressing of wounds, abscess, used in burn
5.	Potassium Permanganate ($KMno_4$)	Dark purple, in water it is pink	Crystal	Antiseptic, dressing of wound at bleeding points used for cautorization
6.	Zinc oxide	White or faint yellow	Powder	Antiseptic, Eczema, Ring worm
7.	Sulphanilamide powder	White or pale yellow	Powder	Wound dressing surgical wound, burns, wound ointment
8.	Ammonium carbonate ($NaHCO_3$)	White	Powder	Cough mixture and fever
9.	Magnesium sulphate (Epsom salt)	White	Crystals	Purgative, hot fomentation in swelling, yoke gall, mastitis, sprains
10.	Turpentine oil	Pale yellow	Oily	Dressing of maggot wound, preparation of liniment, counter irritant, anti-zymotic
11.	Carron oil	Milky white	Oily	Burn and eye problem
12.	Castor oil	Colourless	Liquid oily	Purgative at initial stage
13.	Sulphur	Yellow	Powder	Ring worms, eczema, skin ointment
14.	Iodine ointment	(Composition: Iodine – 4 parts, Pot. Iodide – 4 parts, Glycerine – 12 parts, Vaseline – 80 parts)		Abscess and wounds
15.	Camphor	White		Mild carminative, topical antipruritic
16.	Catechu			Astringent
17.	Turmeric	Yellow		Antiseptic/antimicrobial, hepato-protective, aromatic/stimulant carminative
18.	Garlic			Antibacterial, carminative/gastric stimulant, Garlic oil as insecticide

Contd...

Contd...

Sl.No.	Name of the Medicines or Drugs	Colour	Texture	Uses
19.	Neem			Antiviral, antifungal, larvicidal
20.	Ginger			Gastric stimulant, carminative, flavouring agent
21.	Pepper			Carminative, antiseptic, sedative, purgative, cough suppressant
22.	Isabgol			Bulk laxative
23.	Chirata			Bitter sialic, febrifuge, stomachic

18.8 COMMON TOPICAL PREPARATIONS

18.8.1 Ointment

(*i*) White Field's Ointment

Benzoic acid – 6 g

Salicyclic acid – 3 g

Paraffin jelly – 100 g

(*ii*) Iodine Ointment (Weak)

Iodine – 1 part

Pot. Iodide -1 part

Glycerine – 10 ml

Paraffin jelly – 40 parts.

(*iii*) Iodine Ointment (Strong)

Iodine – 1 part

Pot. iodide – 1 part

Glycerine – 10 ml

Paraffin jelly – 20 parts.

(*iv*) Sulphur Ointment (For Mange)

Sulphur Sublime – 100 g

Simple ointment 900 g

(*v*) Salicyclic Ointment (For Ringworm)

Acid salicyclic – 2 g

Acid carbolic – 2 g

Vaseline – 30 g

(*vi*) Zinc Oxide Ointment

Zinc – oxide – 15 parts

Vaseline/Paraffin jelly – 85 parts

(vii) Eye Ointment

Boric acid – 18 g

Soft Paraffin – 30 g

(viii) Ointment for moist eczema

Acid salicyclic – 2 g

Tannic acid – 2 g

Spirit – 30 ml

18.8.2 Paste

(i) Bismuth Iodoform Paraffin Paste (BIPP)

Bismuth subnitrate – 250 g (1 parts)

Iodoform – 50 g (2 parts)

Liquid Paraffin – 25 g (Q.S.)

Use: Sinus and Fistula. It is used for horn injury and contaminated wounds.

(ii) Zinc Oxide Iodoform Paraffin Paste (ZIPP)

Zinc oxide -1 part

Iodoform – 2 parts

Liquid Paraffin – Q.S. to make a paste.

Use: Healing promoter of the wounds. It is contaminated wounds and horn injury.

(iii) Morrison paste

Magnesium Sulphate – 10 g

Glycerine – 10 ml

Water – 40 ml

(iv) Viena paste

Caustic potash – 1 part

Quick lime – 1 part

Alcohol or Glycerine – Q.S. to form a paste.

Use: for application over warts and exuberant granulation.

18.8.3 Lotion

(i) Boric Lotion

Used for eye wash (Ophthalmic use)

Boric acid 1 to 1.5 part in 100 ml purified water.

(ii) Boric Alum Zinc Eye Lotion

Boric acid – 0.5 g

Alum – 0.5 g

Zinc sulphate – 0.5 g

Purified water – 100 ml

(*iii*) Betadine Lotion

Povidone Iodine 5 per cent.

(*iv*) Boric-Zinc Lotion (Boro-zinc Eye Lotion)

Boric acid – 10 g

Zinc sulphate – 2 g

Purified water to make 1000 ml.

(*v*) Silver Nitrate Lotion (Eye Lotion)

Silver Nitrate – 125 mg

Purified water – 30 ml

(*vi*) White Lotion

Lead acetate – 5 parts

Zinc sulphate – 4 parts

Water – 100 parts

(*vii*) Golden Lotion

Use: Used for mange infestation in animals.

Sulphur sublimate – 1 part

Quick lime – 2 parts

Water – 10 parts

(*viii*) Refrigerant Lotion (Cooling Lotion)

Use: For sprained and painful limbs.

Ammonium Chloride – 1 part

Lead acetate – 1 part

Alum – 1 part

Vinegar – 40 part

Water – 20 parts

Soak the bandage and apply on sprained limbs.

18.8.4 Solution for Topical Use

(*i*) Lugol's Solution

Iodum – 5 per cent

Pot. Iodide – 10 per cent

Dist. water – 100 ml

(*ii*) Condy's Solution

Pot. Permanganate – 1 part

Dist. water – 1000 parts

(*iii*) Acriflavin Solution (Spirit Acriflavin)

Acriflavin – 1 g

90 per cent alcohol – 1000 ml

(*iv*) Mercurochrome solution (2 per cent)

Sod. Salt of Dibromohydroxy Mercury fluorescein – 2 g

Dist. Water – 100 ml.

18.8.5 Antiseptic

1. Boric acid – 1-2 per cent
2. Cetavlon – 1 : 500 to 1 : 5000.
3. Silver Nitrate – 1 : 1000
4. Potassium Permanganate – 1 : 1000 to 1 : 3000
5. Acriflavin – 1 : 1000 to 1 : 15000
6. Chlorohexidine solution – 2 per cent
7. Mercurochrome – 0.5-2 per cent solution in water.

18.8.6 Liniment

(*i*) Ammonia Liniment

Use: For sprain.

Liq. Ammon Fortis – 30 ml

Oil turpentine – 30 ml

Aqua – 30 ml

Sweet oil – 250 ml.

(*ii*) Stimulating ammonia liniment (strong)

Strong Ammonia Solution – 1 part

Turpentine oil – 1 part

Linseed oil – 4 parts

(*iii*) Camphor Liniment

Camphor – 1 part

Mustard oil – 4 parts.

(*iv*) Turpentine Liniment

Turpentine oil – 65 ml

Camphor – 5 g

Soft soap – 9 g

Water – 100 ml

(v) Aconite Limment (For Sprains)

Aconite – 50 g

Camphor – 3 g

Alcohol (90 per cent) to make 100 ml.

18.8.7 Dressing Oil

Creosote – 10 ml

Turpentine oil – 125 ml

Lini oil – 500 ml.

18.8.8 Carron oil

Use: For Burn.

Lime Water

(Liquor Calcis) – 1 parts

Linseed oil – 8 parts

(Mix by shaking) and use topically.

18.8.9 Astringent Powder

Boric acid – 2 parts

Iodoform – 1 parts

Zinc oxide -2 parts

Use: For dressing of unhealthy wounds and ulcerated surfaces.

18.9 DRUG DELIVERY SYSTEMS/METHODS OF ADMINISTRATION OF MEDICINES

Common sense considerations of anatomy, physiology, pathology, pharmacology, therapeutics and convenience determine the route by which a drug is administered. Usual routes of drug administrations are given below.

18.9.1 Common Routes of Drug Administration

(1) Enteral Route

By oral route through mouth, by buccal/sublingual absorption or by swallowing for systemic effect, per rectum (rectal administration) for local effect, suppositories or solutions.

(2) Parenteral Route

The most common parenteral routes of drug administration are:

(*a*) Intravenous injection or infusion (IV) (for intra vascular administration) (*b*) Intramuscular injection (IM)

(*c*) Subcutaneous injection (SC)

Different sites for giving above injections in different animals are given below.

Species of Animal	*Intravenous Injection (IV)*	*Intramuscular Injection (IM)*	*Subcutaneous Injection (SC)*
Cattle and Buffalo	Jugular vein	Gluteal muscle	Either side of neck
Sheep and Goat	Jugular vein	Gluteal muscle and thigh muscle	Either side of neck and lower part of abdomen
Pig	Anterior vena cava	Gluteal muscle	Outer and lower part of ear
Horse	Jugular vein	Gluteal muscle	Either side of neck
Dog and Cat	Recurrent tarsal vein (in hind legs) and femoral vein (in fore legs)	Thigh muscle	Lower part of abdomen
Fowl	Wing vein	Thigh muscle	Inner side of wing

(3) Topical Application

Local application to skin, eye, anal canal, rectum, vagina *etc.*

(4) Other Routes

Intratracheal	Intraruminal	Epidural
Intradermal	Intramammary	Intra spiral route
Intranasal	Intrauterine	Intra plural
Intra Peritoneal	Intracardiac route	

(5) Miscellaneous Routes

Foot bath, poultice, fomentation, massages, enema (douching). The common forms of medicines are solid, powder, tablets, mixtures, syrups, linctus, suppository, vapours, injectable solutions, ointments, gels, liniments *etc.*

18.9.2 Various Enteral Dose Forms

The most common enteral dosage forms are tablet, bolus, capsule, mixture, syrup and linctus.

18.9.2.1 Tablet

A solid dose in which the drug is compressed or moulded with pharmacologically inert substances (excipients), variants includes sustained release and coated tablets.

18.9.2.2 Bolus

A large solid dose in which the drug is compressed with inert substances and variants to cause sustained release of medicines for oral medications or administration.

18.9.2.3 Capsule

The drug which is provided in a gelatin shell or container for oral administration.

18.9.2.4 Mixture

A liquid formulation of drug for oral administration.

18.9.2.5 Syrup

The drug is provided in a concentrated sugar fructose or other solutions.

18.9.2.6 Linctus

A viscous liquid formulation.

18.9.3 Oral Route of Drug Administration

The most common oral routes for drug administration are drenching and as electuary.

18.9.3.1 Drenching of Medicine

It is a common method of administration of liquid medicines with the help of drenching bottle/bamboo device where one end remains closed and the other end is open.

Besides liquid medicines, farmers also administer the bolus or tablet by drenching method by pulverizing or grinding the boli or tablets and mixing in sufficient water to dissolve and made ready for drenching.

For oral route of medication securing animal from the left side holding the drenching bottle on the right hand, slowly insert the fingers of the left hand in the inter-dental space and the animal will automatically open the mouth. Now hold the lower jaw along with tongue by keeping the animal's head high and then introduce the drenching bamboo funnel or bottle through the mouth and pour the medicine. While pouring the medicine care should be taken to let loose the tongue for easy swallowing by the animal so that the liquid medicine must pass through the oesophagus to the stomach. Otherwise faulty drenching may cause mechanical pneumonia and even death of the animal if liquid medicines pass to lungs in excessive quantity.

18.9.3.2 Electuary

It is a convenient method of applying or administering drugs to the throat and pharynx of the animals. Soft paste or *chatni* is usually made by compounding drugs with treacle; sugar or honey. In pigs, forced drug administration by oral route is very difficult and dangerous. The electuary is applied by means of flat stick (bamboo stick) and is smeared upon the back of tongue and teeth.

18.9.4 Other Routes of Drug Administration

18.9.4.1 Inhalation of Vapours

As a gas (*e.g.* volatile as on aerosol (*e.g.* b_2 – adrenoceptor against bronchodilators).

In this method volatile medicines *e.g.* Tincture Benzoin, eucalyptus oil are introduced through medicated vapours into the nostrils of animals effective in treating in respiratory tract disease. Example of inhalation of vapours – *e.g.* Vix Vaporab nasal inhaler in human being.

18.9.4.2 Suppository

A solid dose form moulded of insertion into rectum or vagina, it may be designed to dissolve or it may melt at body temperature (in which case there is a storage problem when environmental temperature exceeds 37°C), the vehicle in which the drug is carried may be fat, glycerol with gelatin or macrogols with gelatin. For anal and rectal diseases suppositions that are astringent anti-inflammatory or local anaesthesia (lignocaine) can be used.

Example: Vaginal passerines.

18.9.4.3 Foot Bath

This is a very popular method of foot care in farm animals for the treatment and prevention of foot affections like foot rot (*Fusiformis necrophorus* infection) FMD etc. Animals are allowed to pass through a cemented pit containing antiseptic and or disinfectant solution *viz.* 3 per cent Copper sulphate solution, 10 per cent solution of formalin, Potassium permanganate solution *etc.* The bath should have a stopping on entry and at the exit.

18.9.4.4 Poultice

It is indicated for treating local inflammatory swelling in animals to reduce the swelling and pain. In usual practice bran meal, linseed meal or oat meal is added in boiling water and heated to give a pasty consistency. This paste material is known as poultice and is applied to the affected part *viz.* in the treatment of yokegall.

18.9.4.5 Douching

It is other wise known as enema. Enema produces defecation by softening faeces and distending the bowel. Enema is liquid medicinal preparation in lukewarm water, introduced through rectum for local systemic action. For livestock it is indicated for constipation, impaction or bloat. For cattle and buffalo 5-10 liters of luke warm water with soap (soap water enema) is administered with the help of douche can and tube through anus.

18.9.4.6 Fomentation

It is of two types (1) moist hot fomentation by Mag Sulph or Epsom salt (2) dry hot fomentation is commonly used in animal practice and for both types of fomentation which increase the circulation of blood to the affected part to help in healing process, to reduce the swelling and to alleviate pain.

Moist Hot Fomentation

The technique consists of soaking the towel or cloth piece in hot medicated water, then partly squeezing the water out of the cloth and application of warm cloth on the affected part. The temperature of water should not be too high. Temperature should be about 110°F. *viz.* Mag Sulph moist hot fomentation applied on abscess to ripe up. Hematoma, Sprain, Yokegall *etc.*

Dry Hot Fomentation

For this technique rubber bag (Hot water bag) or bottle containing hot water should be applied on the affected part. This will increase the circulation of blood to the affected part which will help in the process of healing.

18.9.4.7 Massaging

This is a very popular method or technique of drug application locally indicated for sprain, muscular pain, trauma etc. It is the method applying medicine to the affected part by rubbing with ointments, liniments *etc., viz.* Briclofen gel, Iodex ointment, Briclofen plus Gel, Mastilep ointment.

18.9.4.8 Liniment

It is prepared for external application only usually oily in nature and indicated for relieving painful inflammatory conditions like sprains and sprains.

18.9.4.9 Eyes and Ears Instillation

Application of medicine in eye and ears are usually made in the form of drops, powder and ointment. But instillation of eye drops and ear drops are most convenient and worthy practice where medicines work locally in very low concentration.

Before applying medicines to ear, ear canal should be cleaned by hydrogen peroxide or by sterile ear buds.

Example of eye and ear drops:

1. Optidex eye drop – 15 ml/30 ml
   To administer 5-6 drops in each eye 3-4 times daily.
2. Pomisol ear drop (Intas) – 15 ml/30 ml
   To administer liberally 8-10 days in each affected ear twice daily.

Chapter 19
Veterinary Drug Index

This index is prepared as per generic names of the drugs/medicines followed by their trade names available in the markets. Pack or presentation of the drugs, indication, dose, and route and frequency of administration in various livestock species are indicated. The trade names indicated in this chapter may not be exhaustive, however, care is taken to include as many names as possible within the purview of this book.

19.1 THERAPEUTIC/PHARMACOLOGICAL LIST OF DRUGS/MEDICINES USED IN VETERINARY PRACTICE

19.1.1 Antimicrobials

Ampicillin, Amoxycillin, Oxytetracycline, Ampicillin + Cloxacillin, Enrofloxacin, Ciprofloxacin, Cephalexin, Pefloxacin, Ceftriaxone, Ceftiofur, Penicillin, Streptopenicillin, Cefotaxime, Chloramphenicol, Neomycin, Amoxycillin + Cloxacillin, Ofloxacin, Gentamicin, Amikacin, Lincomycin, Sulfonamides, Co-trimoxazole/potentiated sulphonamide (Sulphonamide + Trimethoprim).

19.1.2 Antifungal

Amphotericin, Clotrimazole, Griseofulvin, Ketokonazole, Miconazole.

19.1.3 Antiprotozoal

Metronidazole, Tinidazole, Ornidazole.

19.1.4 Antihaemoprotozoans

For Babesiosis: Diminazine, Trypan blue, Diamidine derivatives (Amicarbalide), Acridine derivatives, Quinolone derivatives (Quinuronium), Imidocarb.

For Theileriasis: Buparvaquone, Oxytetracycline (Long acting).

For Trypanosomiasis: Quinapyramine prosalt, Diminazene aceturate, Suramin, Sodium or Potassium Antimony tartarate.

19.1.5 Anthelmintics

Albendazole, Fenbendazole, Mebendazole, Levamisole, Closantel (Ectendoparasiticidal), Ivermectin, Triclabendazole (Flukicide), Oxyclozanide (Flukicide), Dichlorophen, Piperazine, Ayurvedic anthelmintics.

19.1.6 NSAID (Non Steroidal Antiinflammatory Drugs)

Paracetamol, Analgin/Metamizole, Meloxicam, Nimesulide, Phenylebutazone, Ketoprofen.

19.1.7 Steroids

Dexamethasone, Prednisolne, Triamcenolone.

19.1.8 Drugs Acting on Digestive System

Antiemetic: Domperidone, Metaclopramide, Ondansetron, Procloperazine, Promethazine, Triflupromazine.

Antacid: Ranitidine, Cimetidine, Sucralfate.

Anti-diarrhoel: Furazolidone, Diphenoxylate, Loperamide, Halquinol.

Laxative: Bisacodyl, Lactulose.

Appetizer: Cyproheptadane, Fungaldiastage + Pepsine, Pancreatin + Bile salts + Vegetable enzymes, Digyton, Zigup.

19.1.9 Drugs Acting on Respiratory System

Respiratory Stimulant: Doxapram, Nikethamide.

Bronchodilator: Aminophyllin, Atropin sulphate, Theophyllin, Terbutalin.

19.1.10 Drugs Acting on Reproductive System

Estrous inducer: Clomiphene (Fertivet), Indigenous preparations (Projana HS, Sajani, Janova).

Anoestrus, Delayed ovulation, Cystic ovary, Repeat breeding etc: FSH, LH, HCG, PMSG, Buserelin, Gonadorelin, Hydroxy progesterone caproate, Medroxy progesterone acetate, Dinoprost (PGF_2*alpha* analogue), Tiaprost (PGF_2*alpha* analogue), Conjugated oestrogen, Oestrogen, Oxytocin, Valethamate.

Intra-uterine preparations: Povidone iodine, Povidone iodine + Metronidazole, Co-trimoxazole, Nitrofurazone + Urea, Nitrofurazone + Urea + Metronidazole, Cephalexine, Tetracycline.

For Male genital system: Testosteron preparation (Testoviron depot), HCG, PMSG, Oestrogen, Indigenous preparations (Tentexfort vet).

19.1.11 Drugs Acting on Musculo-skeletal System

Succinyl choline, Tubocurarin chloride.

19.1.12 Anti-Neoplastic Drugs

Bleomycin, Busulfan, Cyclophosphamide, Doxorubicin, Fluorouracil, Methotrexate, Vincristine.

19.1.13 Pre-Anaesthetic Drugs

Atropine sulphate, Chlorpromazine, Diazepum, Triflupromazine, Xylazine.

19.1.14 Local Anaesthetic Drugs

Lignocaine, Bupivocaine.

19.1.14 General Anaesthetic Drugs

Halothane, Ketamine, Propofol, Thiopentone sodium.

19.2 ANTIBIOTICS

The most common antibiotics used in veterinary practice are ampicillin, amoxycillin, ampicillin + cloxacillin, amoxycillin + cloxacillin, penicillin, strepto-penicillin, oxytetracycline, Enrofloxacin, cephalexin, pefloxacin, ceftriaxone, cefotaxime, chloramphenicol, neomycin, gentamycin, amikacin and lincomycin.

19.2.1 Ampicillin

It belongs to amino penicillin class. It is a broad spectrum bactericidal antibiotic. It inhibits synthesis of bacterial cell wall, thus effecting bactericidal action.

Indication

Anthrax, BQ, HS, Pneumonia, Nephritis, Metritis, Mastitis, Enteritis, Septicaemia, Foot rot, Synovitis, Wooden tongue, Lumpy jaw, Abscess, Dermatitis, all infections of respiratory, urinary and gastro intestinal tract associated with *Streptococci, Staphylococci, Corynebacterium, Clostridrum fusiform, E. coli* (Colibacilosis), *Klebsiella, Shigella, Salmonella proteus, Brucella, Pasteurella* species and many infections sensitive to ampicillin.

Dose

Cattle, Buffalo, Sheep, Goat, Pig and Horse – 5-10 mg/kg body weight QID by oral, IM, IV, SC route.

Dog and Cat – 20 mg/kg body weight QID by oral route, 10 mg/kg body weight QID by IM, IV, SC route.

Trade Names

1. *Ampixel Injection* (Excell) – 2 g and 2.5 g vials
2. *Oxillin Injection* (Oxen Labs) – 2 g and 2.5 g vials
3. *Solampi Injection* (Brihans) – 1 g, 2 g and 3 g vials
4. *Conampi Injection* (Concept) – 1 g and 2 g vials
5. *Brandocillin Injection* (Intas) – 2.5 g vial
6. *Catcillin Injection* (CRIL) – 2.5 g vial
7. *Kampibiotic Injection* (Karnataka antibiotic) – 1 g, 2 g and 2.5 g vials

8. *Ampicillin injection* (Modern Lab) – 1 g and 2 g vials
9. *Vetampin Injection* (Wockhardt) – 1 g and 2 g vials

19.2.2 Amoxycillin

It belongs to amino penicillin class. It is a broad spectrum water soluble antibiotic having wide range of bactericidal property. It inhibits synthesis of bacterial cell wall, thus effecting bactericidal action. It penetrates well into the fluids of respiratory tract in both mucoid and purulent infections. It should not be given to small herbivores such as rabbits and guineapigs.

Indication

Calf scours, calf enteritis, pneumonia, Mastitis, Metritis, respiratory tract infections, skin and soft tissue infection, HS, BQ, FMD *etc.*

Dose

Cattle, Buffalo, Sheep, Goat, Pig and Horse – 10 mg/kg body weight BID.

Dog and Cat – 10-20 mg/kg body weight BID.

Administration by IM, IV and oral route.

Trade Names

1. *Amoxirum Forte injection* (Agrivet Farm Care) – 300 mg vial

   Composition: Each vial contains Amoxycillin Sodium equivallent to Amoxycillin 200 mg + Sulbactam sodium 100 mg.

   Dose: 7-10 mg/kg body weight by IM or IV and intramammary.
2. *Amoxirum Forte 3000 mg Injection* (Agrivet Farm Care) – 3 g vial

   Composition: It contains Amoxycillin 2000 mg + Sulbactam 1000 mg.

   Dose: 7-10 mg/kg body weight IM or IV.

19.2.3 Oxytetracycline

It is a tetracycline congener. It inhibits bacterial protein systhesis, thus effecting bacteriostatic action. It is a broad spectrum and cheapest antibiotic.

Indication

It is effective against wide varieties of Gram (+ ve) and Gram (- ve) bacteria, Spirochaetes, Anaplasma, Theileria, Diphtheria, Pneumonia, HS, BQ, Bovine Rickettsiae, *E. coli*, Staphylococcus, Streotococcus, *Bacillus anthracis*, Actinomyces, Corynebacterium *etc.* It is effective in the infections of digestive, respiratory and urogenital tracts of livestock.

Dose

Cattle, Buffalo, Sheep, Goat, Pig and Horse – 5-10 mg/kg body weight/day.

Dog and Cat – 10-20 mg/kg body weight/day.

Administration by IM or IV.

Trade Names

1. *Utrox-LA injection* (Neospark) – 30 ml vial

   Composition: Superior long acting Oxytetracycline injectable solution 200 mg/ml provides prolong and sustained antibiotic therapy and prophylactic activity in both livestock and poultry.

   Dose: Large animal 1-2 ml/25 kg body weight; Small animal 1 ml/10 kg body weight IM.

2. *Utrox DS Injection* (Neospark) – 30 ml vial

   Compositi on: Veterinary Oxytetracycline injectable solution double strength 100 mg/ml.

3. *Oxytetracycline dihydrate injection-LA* (Pfizer) – 30 ml and 50 ml vials

   It is a lon g acting injection for the treatment of bacterial infections including Endometritis, Pyometra.

   Composition: Each ml contains 200 mg of Oxytetracycline dihydrate in 2-Pyrrolidone vehicle system.

   Dose: Cattle and Buffalo 1 ml/10 kg body weight by deep IM injection, in divided doses, and administer at 2-3 sites.

4. *Oxyvet-LA injection* (Sarabhai Zydus) – 30 ml vial

   Composition: Oxytetracycline 200 mg/ml.

   Dose: Cattle, Buffalo, Sheep and Goat 1 ml/10 kg body weight. Repeat 96 hours later by deep IM.

5. *Intamycin-LA* (Intas) – 30 ml and 50 ml vials

   Composition: Each ml contains Oxytetracycline dihydrate 200 mg.

   Dose: Livestock 1 ml/10 kg body weight (single shot therapy) by deep IM.

6. *Intamycin* (Intas) – 30 ml and 100 ml vials

   Composition: Each ml contains Oxytetracycline dihydrate 50 mg.

   Dose: Livestock – 1 ml/10 kg body weight by IM and IV route.

7. *Loxy injection* (Legend) – 30 ml, 50 ml and 100 ml vials

   Composition: Oxytetracycline 50 mg/ml.

   Dose: Cattle and Buffalo 2 ml/25 kg body weight; Calf, Sheep, Goat and Pig 1-2 ml/25 kg body weight.

8. *Wolicyclin injection* (Wockhardt) – 30 ml, 50 ml and 100 ml vials

   Composition: Each ml contains Oxytetracycline 50 mg.

   Dose: Cattle, Buffalo Sheep and Goat 5-10 mg/kg body weight; Horse, Dog, Cat and Pig 5-7 mg/kg body weight; In severe cases 10 mg/kg body weight.

9. *Terramycine injection* (Pfizer) – 30 ml and 100 ml vials

   Composition: 50 mg Oxytetracycline/ml, IM, IV and SC routes.

   Dose: Poultry and Rabbit – 1 ml/4 kg body weight SC

   Livestock – 2-4 mg/kg body weight, or 1-2 ml/25 kg body weight.

In young animal – 10 mg/kg body weight

Small animal – 1 ml/5 kg body weight

10. *Oxaclin-LA* (Intervet) – 30 ml and 50 ml vials

    Composition: Each ml contains Oxytetracycline dihydrate 200 mg.

    Dose: Cattle, Buffalo, Sheep, Goat and Pig 1ml/10kg body weight by IM in divided doses at 2-3 sites.

11. *Oxyvet injection* (Oxen Lab) – 30 ml, 50 ml and 100 ml vials

    Dose: Cattle, Buffalo, Sheep and Goat 1 ml/10 kg body weight by IM route daily for 3-5 days.

12. *Oxyvet bolus* (Oxen Lab) – Oxytetracycline 500 mg bolus

    Dose: Cattle and Buffalo 4-6 boli/day; Calf, Sheep and Goat 1-2 boli orally BID.

13. *Steclin bolus* (Sarabhai Zydus) – Strip of 4 boli.

    Composition: Each bolus contains 500 mg Tetracycline HCl.

    Dose: Cattle, Buffalo and Horse for prevention – 1-2 boli/day, and for treatment 4-6 boli/day.

    Calf, Sheep and Goat ½ bolus/day for prevention; and 1 bolus daily for treatment for 3-4 days.

    Ewe and Sow ½ to 1 bolus for treatment.

14. *Loxy bolus* (Legend)

    Composition: Each bolus contains Oxytetracycline 500 mg.

    Dose: Cattle, Buffalo, Calf, Sheep and Goat 1 bolus for 50-80 kg body weight.

15. *Neocyclin bolus* (Intas) – 4 boli strip

    Composition: Each bolus contains Tetracycline hydrochloride 500 mg.

    Dose: Livestock Oral – 4-6 boli daily.

    I/U – 2 boli daily (as passery).

16. *Tetravet bolus* (Marion VCL) – 4 boli strip

    Composition: Each bolus contains Tetracycline HCl – 500 mg.

    Dose: Cattle and Buffalo – 4-6 boli daily.

    Calf, Sheep and Goat – 1-2 boli daily.

17. *Tetracycline WSP Vet* (Intervet) – 100 g sachet

    Composition: Each g contains Tetracycline HCl 500 mg.

    Dose: Sheep and Goat 5 g/15 kg body weight for 5 days; Cattle: 2.5 g -5 g/15 kg body weight for 5 days.

19.2.4 Ampicillin + Cloxacillin Combipack

This is a synergistic combination of powerful antibiotics. Bactericidal and most effective in following indications having broad spectrum antibiotic action, highly effective against penicillin and ampicillin resistant organisms.

Indication

Anthrax, BQ, HS, Pneumonia, Bronchitis, Nephritis, Enteritis, Enterocolitis, Cystitis, Foot Rot, Navel ill, wound, abscess, teat and udder lesions, skin and soft tissue infections, wing rot, secondary bacterial infection in Canine Distemper (CD), Post surgery and other mixed infections of almost all gram negative nature and diseases of penicillinase producing organisms.

Dose

General dose for livestock 6-10 mg/kg body weight daily for 3 to 5 days by IM or IV route.

Trade Names

(*List of Ampicillin and Cloxacillin combipack*)

1. *Injection AC-Vet* (Intas) – 2 g vial (with WFI)
2. *Injection AC-Vet Forte* (Intas) – 3 g vial (with WFI)
3. *Injection AC-VET Max* (Intas) – 4 g vial (with WFI)
   Dose: 6-10 mg/kg body weight for 3-5 day by IM or IV.
4. *Cillox Injection* (Excell) – 500 mg, 2000 mg and 3000 mg vials
   Dose: 6-8 mg/kg body weight for 3-5 days by IM or IV route.
5. *Klox amp Injection* (KAP) – 2 g
   Dose: Cattle, Buffalo and Horse – 2 g to 2.5 g daily for 4 to 5 days by IM or IV route.
6. *Inclox Injection* (Brihans) – 2 g and 2.5 g vials
   Dose: Cattle, Buffalo and Horse – 2 g to 2.5 g daily for 4 to 5 days by IM or IV route.
7. *Injection Vet Clox* (Sarabhai Zydus)–1 g and 2 g vials
8. *Arimox Injection* (Daffodils) – 2 g vial
   Dose: 6-10 mg/kg body weight by IM route.
9. *R.C. Forte Injection* (Vetnex) – 4 g vial
10. *Bothcillin injection* (Oxen Labs) – 2 g, 3 g and 4 g vials
11. *Orlox Injection* (Medivet) – 2 g vial
    Dose: 6-8 mg/kg body weight IM
12. *Cloxillin Injection* (Reedson) – 500 mg, 1 g and 2 g vials
    Dose: Cattle and Buffalo – 2-2.5 g.
    (Recommended dose – 6-10 mg/kg body weight twice daily 3-5 days).
13. *Catlox Injection Vet* (Cattle Remedies) – 2 g vial
    Dose: 5-10 mg/kg body weight daily.
    But may be given twice daily depending upon the severity of infection by IM or IV route.

14. *Maclox Injection* (Marion Pharma) – 2 g and 250 mg vials (with free water for injection)

    Broad spectrum bactericidal agent with synergestic combination.

    Dose: 5-10 mg/kg body weight by IM and IV route for 3-5 days.

15. *Nepoclox Vet* (TTK) – 4 g vial (with 20 ml water for injection)

    Composition: Each 4 g vial contains Ampicillin 2 g and Cloxacillin 2 g.

    Dose: 7-10 mg/kg body weight IM or IV or Dissolve Nepoclox Vet in 15 ml distilled water and administer @ 1ml for 25-30 kg body weight for intramammary or I/U use, dilute 2 ml to 2.5 ml reconstituted solution in 8 ml water for injection and infuse into the affected part.

19.2.5 Enrofloxacin

It is a fluoroquinolone antibiotic. It inhibits the enzyme DNA gyrase responsible for coiling and super coiling of DNA which carries vital information for bacterial metabolism, thus produces bactericidal action. It is a broad spectrum antibiotic.

Indication

It is indicated for high fever, fever due to mixed bacterial infections. Reproductive tract infections, retained placenta, wooden tongue, lumpy jaw, mastitis, metritis, wound infections, HS, Pneumonia, pyometra, Pseudo-rinderpest, Pleuropneumonia, Salmonellosis, Colibacillosis, Pneumoenteritis, CBPP, CCPP. Effective against *E. coli, Salmonella, Pasteurella* sp., *Klebsiella* sp., *Moraxella bovis, Campylobacter* sp., *Haemophilus* sp., *Pseudomonas, Erysipelothrix, Mycoplasma* and *Leptospira* species.

Dose

General dose for livestock is 2.5-5 mg/kg body weight.

Administration by IM, IV or oral route.

Enrofloxacin is not recommended for horse. It is contra-indicated in young animals below 1 year of age, as it may cause arthropathic effect. Sometimes gastro-intestinal and central nervous system disturbances and rashes may be seen.

Trade Names

1. *Menroflox -100 Injection, 10 per cent w/v* (Modern Lab) – 15 ml vial

   Composition: Each ml contains Enrofloxacin 100 mg.

   Dose: 1 ml/20 kg body weight daily for 3-5 days by IM route only (5 mg/kg body weight).

2. *Quin Intas* (Intas) – 15 ml, 50 ml and 100 ml vials

   Composition: Each ml contains Enrofloxacin 100 mg.

   Dose: 1 ml/20 kg body weight daily for 3-5 days (5 mg/kg body weight) by IM or IV route.

3. *K-Flox Injection, Vet* (KAP) – 15 ml and 50 ml vials

   Composition: Each ml contains Enrofloxacin 100 mg.

   Dose: Cattle, Buffalo, Sheep, Goat, Camel, Pig – 5 mg/kg body weight for 3-

5 days by deep IM injection daily.

In poultry 1 ml to be diluted with 9 ml distilled water and 0.5 ml/kg body weight to be administered.

(Indication in poultry: Colisepticaemia, Mycoplasmosis, CRD, Coryza, Fowl cholera, Salmonellosis, Erysipelas, Staphylococcosis also in mixed infections and secondary bacterial complications in GI tract. respiratory tract, urinary tract, skin infections *etc.*)

4. *Enrocin* (Vetnex) – 15 ml, 50 ml and 100 ml vials

   Composition: Each ml contains Enrofloxacin 100 mg.

   Dose: 7.5-12.5 mg/kg body weight IM or SC route, to be repeated after 45 hours.
5. *Enrocip Injection* (Cipla) – 15 ml, 30 ml and 100 ml vials

   Dose: For all animals 1 ml/20 kg body weight.
6. *Fortius injection* (Virbac) – 30 ml vial

   Dose: 3 ml/40 kg body weight by IM, IV and SC route.
7. *Enrobest Injection* (TTK) – 15 ml and 100 ml vials
8. *Enrovet Injection* (Vets Farma) – 15 ml, 30 ml and 50 ml vials
9. *Enrored Injection* (Reedson) – 15 ml vial
10. *Enrobact Injection* (Martin and Brown) – 30 ml and 50 ml vials.
11. *Enrox Injection* (Alembic)– 15 ml vials

    Dose: 1 ml/20-30 kg body weight by IM daily.
12. *Floxidin Injection* (Intervet) – 15 ml and 50 ml vials.

    Dose: Cattle and Buffalo 2.5-5 mg/kg body weight IM;

    Sheep and Goat 2.5-5 mg/kg body weight IM, Dog 5 kg/mg body weight IM.
13. *Meriquin Injection* (Merind)– 15 ml and 50 ml vials

    Composition : Enrofloxacin 10 per cent w/v, *i.e.* 100 mg/ml.
14. *Enrodac-10 Injection* (Sarabhai Zydus) – 15 ml vial

    Dose: 5 mg/kg body weight in all animals.
15. *L-En-RO Injection 10 per cent w/v* (Legend) –15 ml and 50 ml vials

    Dose: Large animal 15 ml daily for 3-5 days.

    Small animal 5 ml daily for 3-5 days by IM route.
16. *Quinrocin injection* (Neospark) – 15 ml and 30 ml vials

    Dose: 1 ml/20 kg body weight (2.5-5 mg/kg body weight) IM.

19.2.6 Ciprofloxacin

It is a fluoroquinolone antibiotic. It inhibits supercoiling of DNA in the bacteria producing bactericidal action.

Indication

Acute infections like HS, BQ, Pneumonia, CBPP, CCPP, Mastitis, Metritis, Pyometra, repeat breeding problem, respiratory tract infections, urogenital infection, pyrexia of unknown origin, in FMD control of secondary invaders.

Dose

Large animal – 5 mg/kg body weight.

Dog and Cat – 5-15 mg/kg body weight BID.

Administration: By oral, IM, IV or I/U route.

Trade Names

1. *Ciptec-Vet Injection* (Cipla) – 30 ml and 50 ml vials

   Composition: Each ml contains Ciprofloxacin lactate equivalent to Ciprofloxacin 40 mg.

   Dose: 10 ml/80 kg body weight for 3 to 5 days.
2. *Cflox Injection* (Intas) – 50 ml vial

   Composition: Each ml contains Ciprofloxacin 40 mg.

   Dose: 10 ml/80 kg body weight daily for 3-5 days by IM or IV.
3. *C-flox Power Injection* (Intas) – 15 ml vial

   Composition: Ciprofloxacin – 40 mg/ml.

   Dose: Cattle and Buffalo – 15 ml/300 kg body weight daily for 3-5 days IM or IV route.
4. *Cipoxin Injection* (Oxen Labs) – 30 ml vial

   Composition: Ciprofloxacin – 40 mg/ml.

   Dose: Cattle and Buffalo – 10 ml/80 kg body weight
5. *Cefloxen-Vet Injection* (Tarun Pharmaceuticals) – 30 ml vial

   Composition: Ciprofloxacin 40 mg/ml.

   Dose: Large animal 10-30 ml by IM route; Small animal 1-3 ml by IM route.

19.2.7 Cephalexin

It is a first generaion cephalosporin. It interferes with bacterial cell wall synthesis by inactivating transpeptidase enzyme, thus producing bactericidal effect.

Indication

Urogenital tract, respiratory tract, soft tissue infection, intrauterine infections like pyometra, endometritis, retention of placenta, cervicitis, repeat breeding, high speed therapy for infected wounds, and prevention of poultry diseases like BWD, fowl cholera, *E. coli*, Fowl typhoid, and early chick mortality *etc*.

Dose

Cattle and Buffalo – 5-10 mg/kg body weight orally BID.

Dog and Cat – 10-30 mg/kg body weight orally TID.

Trade Names

1. *Malexin Powder* (Marion Pharma) – 20 g pack.

   Dose: For livestock 20 g Malexin/300 kg body weight (10 mg/kg body weight twice daily). For poultry, Prevention dose – 5 g daily for 750 chicks for first 5 days, in drinking water; Curative dose – 5 g/375 chicks daily, 65 growers or 25 layers for 3 to 5 days.
2. *Lixen Bolus* (GSK) – Blister of 2 boli

   Composition: Each bolous contains Anhydrous Cephalexin – 1.5 g.

   Dose: 1 bolus/150 kg body weight.
3. *Lixen Powder* (GSK) – 20 g sachet

   Composition: Each 20 g sachet contains Cephalexin – 7.5 per cent w/w.

   Dose: Large animal 20 g BID orally for 3-5 days.

   Poultry 20 g/1500 chicks or 250 growers or 100 layers for therapeutic purpose for 3-5 days and 20 g/3000 chicks for prophylactic purpose for 3-5 days.
4. *Ceflax powder* (Neospark) – 20 g pack

   Composition: Cephalexin 7.5 per cent w/w.

   Dose: Poultry 20 g/1500 chicks or 250 growers or 100 layers for therapeutic purpose for 3-5 days and 20 g/3000 chicks for prophylactic purpose for 3-5 days.

19.2.8 Pefloxacin

It is the latest generation fluoroquinolone having mega spectrum antimicrobial agent, used in livestock and poultry. It inhibits he enzyme gyrase responsible for coiling and super coiling of DNA, which carries vital information for bacterial metabolism, thus produce bactericidal effect.

Indication

Mastitis, Colisepticaemia, Pasteurellosis, Salmonellosis, Mycoplasmosis, secondary bacterial infections, respiratory tract and GI tract infections *etc.*

Dose

Cattle, Buffalo, Sheep and Goat – 10 mg/kg body weight BID orally and 5 mg/kg body weight BID IV.

Dog – 10-40 mg/kg body weight BID orally or IV.

Trade Names

1. *Peflacin bolus* (Neospark) – 1 g bolus

   Dose: 1-2 boli BID for cattle and buffalo.
2. *Peflacin powder* (Neospark) – 100 g and 250 g pack.

   Composition: Pefloxacin soluble powder 10 per cent w/w

   Dose: Poultry 1 g/litre of drinking water for curative purpose; and 1 g/2-4 litres of drinking water for prophylactic purpose.

3. *Pelwin tablet* (Wockhardt) – 4 tablets pack.

   Composition: Eaxh tablet contains 400 mg Pefloxacin.

4. *Pelox tablet* (Wockhardt) – 6 tablets pack

   Composition: Each tablet contains 200 mg Pefloxacin.

19.2.9 Ceftriaxone

Ceftriaxone: It is a third generation cephalosporin, and the most potent bactericidal antibiotic. Sometimes it is combined with Sulbactam.

Sulbactam: It is an irreversible inhibitor of β-lactamase, which binds with β-lactamase enzyme and does not allow interacting with the antibiotic.

Indication

Effective against both Gram positive (+ ve) and Gram (- ve) organisms and some anaerobes, *viz. Streptococcus, Staphylococcus, Clostridium, E. coli, Pseudomonas, Klebsiella, Hemophilus, Enterobacter, Pasteurella, Proteus, Morexella etc.* It is useful in life threatening infections like bacteraemia, septicaemia, CNS infection, per acute and acute Mastitis, Metritis, HS, BQ, RTI, UTI, infection of unknown etiology, mixed bacterial infections, wound infections, osteoarthritis, bacterial nephritis, cystitis, and post operative treatment *etc.*

Dose

5-10 mg/kg body weight for ruminants, dogs and cats.

Trade Names

1. *Cipla Ceft Vet Injection* (Cipla) – 3 g vial

   Dose: Large animals – 5-10 mg/kg body weight; Calf/Sheep/Goat – 10-15 mg/kg body weight; Dogs – 15-25 mg/kg body weight.

   Administration by IM or IV route daily for 3-5 days.

2. *Intacef Injection* (Intas) – 500 mg, 2 g and 3 g vials (combipack)

   Dose: Large animal 5-10 mg/kg body weight; Calf, Sheep and Goat 10-15 mg/kg body weight; Dog 15-25 mg/kg body weight.

   Administration by IM or IV route daily for 3 to 5 days.

3. *Exact Injection* (Excell) – 375 mg, 2.25 g and 3 g vials

   Composition: Ceftriaxone + Sulbactam in 2 : 1 ratio.

4. *Oxcef Injection* (Oxen Labs) – 2 g and 3 g vials

   Dose: Large animals – 5-10 mg/kg body weight. Calf, Sheep and Goat 10-15 mg/kg body weight.

5. *Vetaceph Injection* (Vetcare) – 1 g, 3 g and 4 g vials

   It controls multiple bacterial infection, treats resistant strains of bacteria and achieves peak plasma concentration within 0.5-1 hr. and has got wide spectrum bactericidal property.

   Dose: Cattle and Buffalo 3 g for above 400 kg body weight; 1 g for 200 kg body weight; 2 g for 400 kg body weight by IM or IV route.

6. *Macef Injection* (Marion Pharma) – 250 mg, 500 mg and 2 g vials

   Dose: 5-10 mg/kg body weight by IM, IV route for 3 to 5 days.
7. *T-T-Cef Vet Injection* (TTK) – 0.5 g and 3 g vials

   The top therapeutic Ceftriaxone with water for injection combipack.

   Dose: 5-10 mg/kg body weight by IM or IV.
8. *Vetaceph Plus Injection* (Vetcare) – 3 g and 4.5 g vials

   Combination of Ceftriaxone and Sulbactam.

   Dose: 10 mg/kg body weight by IM and IV for 3 to 5 days.
9. *M-Ceft Injection* (Alembic) 1.5 g vial with 10 ml WFI (water for injection)

   Dose: 5 mg/kg body weight by IV route only that provides optimum bactericidal concentration for 5 days.
10. *Vetaceph-TAZO Injection* (Vetcare) – 3.375 g vial

    A powerful combination of Ceftriaxone with Tazobactam. Best incidated for mastitis and infections of respiratory and genito-urinary tracts.

    Dose: 5-10 mg/kg body weight.

19.2.10 Ceftiofur

One of the latest and most powerful broadspectrum bactericidal third generation cephalosporin antibiotics.

Indication

It is indicated for the treatment of acute and peracute Mastitis, Respiratory tract infections, Reproductive tract infections, Foot rot *etc.*

Dose

Cattle, Sheep and Goat 1.1-2.2 mg/kg body weight by IM route OD for 3 to 5 days; Buffalo 2.2-4 mg/kg body weight by IM OD for 5 days

Horse 2.2 to 4.4 mg/kg body weight by IM route OD only for 3 to 5 days;

Dog 2.2 mg/kg body weight by SC OD for 5-14 days.

Trade Names

1. *Ceftivet Injection* (Vetnex) – 1 g vial

   Dose: Cattle, Sheep and Goat – 1-1-2.2 mg/kg body weight for IM use only OD for 5 days; Buffalo – 2-2.4 kg/mg; Horse – 2.2-4.4 mg/kg body weight OD.
2. *Xnel injection* (Pfizer) – 1 g vial

   Highly effective in post partum metritis, pyometra, respiratory tract infection *etc.*

   Reconstitute with 20 ml sterile water for injection.

   Repeat once daily for 3 to 5 days.

3. *X-Ceft Injection* (Alembic) – 500 mg and 1 g vial

   Benefit: Once daily dose regime, low dose, less antibiotic stress on animals, Maintains 3 times higher MIC, no rumen microbial damage. No antibiotic residue in milk, milk safe for human consumption during treatment.

   Dose: Cattle, Sheep and Goat 1.1-2.2 mg/kg body weight by IM OD for 5 days; Buffalo 2.2-4 mg/kg body weight by IM OD for 5 days; Dog 2.2 mg/kg body weight by SC OD for 5-14 days.

19.2.11 Penicillin

It inhibits the bacterial cell wall synthesis, thus producing bactericidal effect. It is mainly effective against Gram (+ve) bacteria.

Indication

In the treatment of injections caused by Penicillin sensitive organisms such as *Streptococci, Clostridia, Corynebacteria, Bacillus anthracis* and *Actinomyces bovis*. Pneumonia, Anthrax, BQ, calf diphtheria, foot rot, acute mastitis, UTI, leptospirosis, tetanus, wound infections, post castration infection *etc.*

Trade Names

1. *Inj. F.P.P.* (Alembic) – 20 lacs and 40 lacs
2. *Inj. F.P.P.* (Sarabhai Zydus) – 20 lacs and 40 lacs

   Composition: Sterile powder of Procaine Penicillin-A fortified with Penicillin-G sodium.

   Dose: Add 4 ml distilled water to 20 lacs vial and 8 ml to 40 lacs vial. Large animal 4,000 units/kg body weight at 24 hours interval; Small animal 2,00,000 to 4,00,000 units at 24 hours interval.

19.2.12 Streptopenicillin

It is bactericidal in action. Unique and most synergistic antibiotic combination.

Indication

Effective against both Gram positive and gram negative organisms, and indicated for the treatment of systemic infections like Pneumonia, Cystitis, Mastitis, HS, BQ, Anthrax, secondary bacterial infections associated with FMD, retained placenta and metritis.

Dose

10-30 mg/kg body weight for ruminants.

Trade Names

1. *Munomycin forte injection* (Glaxo SmithKline) AFC – 2.5 g vial

   Composition: Each vial contains Procaine Penicillin – 15,00,000 IU, Beazylpenicillin – 5,00,000 IU, Streptomycin sulphate – 2.5 g.

   Dose: Large animal 1-2 vials daily by IM route.
2. *Bistrepen Injection* (Alembic) – 2.5 g vial

3. *Biostrep Injection* (Vetnex) – 2.5 ml vial
4. *Dicrystición-S Large dose Injection* (Sarabhai Zydus) – 2.5 g and 5 g large vials.

   Dose: To each vial (2.5 g) 7.5 ml sterile distilled water to make 10 ml suspension. Large animal 2 ml/50 kg body weight by IM route; Small animal 1 ml/50 kg body weight.

19.2.13 Cefotaxime Sodium

Cefotaxime sodium is the most advanced third generation cephalosporin having broad spectrum bactericidal property and can penetrate into C.S.F., acts even in acidic media and effective against all bacterial infections including anaerobic bacteria like pseudomonas. It has got synergistic action with Gentamycin and Metronidazole. This antibiotic interferes with bacterial cell wall synthesis by inactivating transpeptidase enzyme, thus producing bactericidal effect.

Indication

Septicaemia, HS, BQ, Mastitis, Metritis, Meningitis, acute bacterial Peritonitis, Bone and Joint infections, Cystitis, Urethritis, Dermatitis, Septicaemia, Prostatitis, Seminal vesiculitis, Intra uterine infections and post surgical treatment.

Dose

Cattle and Buffalo – 5-10 mg/kg body weight BID.

Dog and Cat – 10-30 mg/kg body weight TID.

Trade Names

1. *Britax Injection* (Brihans) – 500 mg, 1000 mg, 2000 mg and 3000 mg

   Dose: 10-20 mg/kg body weight.

   Cattle, Buffalo and Horse – 2-3 g; Calf, Sheep, Goat and Foal – 1 g; Cat and Dog – 500g by IM or IV route.
2. *Cefavet Injection* (Excell) – 500 mg and 3 g vials

   Dose: 10-20 mg/kg body weight daily in divided dose through IM or IV route for 3-4 days. Cattle, Buffalo and Horse – 2-3 g/day.
3. *Omitax Injection* (Daffodils) – 500 mg vial

   Dose: 10-20 mg/kg body weight daily by I/M or I/V route.
4. *Toxen Injection* (Oxen Labs) – 2 g and 3 g vials

   Dose: Large animals 10-20 mg/kg body weight (2 g to 3 g); Small animals – 500 mg to 1 g by IM or IV route.
5. *Vetaxim Injection* (Cattle Remedies) – 500 mg, 1 g and 2 g vials

   Dose: Large animal 15-24 mg/kg body weight by IV route; Small animals 20-40 mg/kg body weight by IM or IV route.

19.2.14 Chloramphenicol

It is a potent antibiotic having broad spectrum activity and has got bactericidal/ bacteriostatic action by inhibition of protein synthesis. It readily crosses the blood-brain, pleural and placental barriers.

Indication

Anthrax, BQ, HS, Salmonellosis, Colibacillosis, Nephritis, Cystitis, Enteritis, Metritis, Mastitis, infections of Chlamydiae, Rickettsia *etc*

Dose

Large animal (Cattle and Buffalo) – 2-4 mg/kg body weight BID IV

20-30 mg/kg body weight IM

Small animal (Sheep and Goat) – 10 mg/kg body weight BID IV

30-40 mg/kg body weight IM

Dog – 25-50 mg kg body weight BID IV

It should not be used for prolonged period. It is better not to use in pups.

Trade Names

1. *Neochlor Injection* (Vetcare) – 10 ml and 30 ml vials

   Each ml contains 100 mg chloramphenicol.
2. *Enteromycetin Injection* (Deys Vet) – 10 ml and 30 ml vials
3. *Chloramphenicol Sod. Succinate Injection* (KAP) – 1 g vial

   Dose: For large animals 4 to 11mg/kg body weight; for small animals 20 to 30 mg/kg body weight by IM route.

   For IV route dose is 2 to 4 mg/kg body weight.
4. *Chloraxin Injection* (Cipla) – 3 g vial

   Dose: Cattle and Buffalo 2 to 4 mg/kg body weight by IV route, and 20-30 mg/kg body weigt by IM route.
5. *Chloramphenicol Injection* (Nandini Med. Lab) – 10 ml vial

   Dose: Cattle and Buffalo 20 to 30 mg/kg body weight by IM route.
6. *Chloramphenicol Injection* (Modern Labs) – 30 ml vial
7. *Chlorovet Injection* (G. Loucatos) – 30 ml vial

19.2.15 Neomycin

Neomycin sulphate is an aminoglycoside anti bacterial. It inhibits bacterial protein synthesis, thus producing bactericidal action. It is a broad spectrum bactericidal antibiotic and very stable in organic matter like blood, pus, tissue fluid and secretions. It has unaltered efficacy in a wide range of pH.

Dose

Livestock – 2.5-5 mg/kg body weight BID IM, IV; and 10 mg/kg body weight in divided doses oral.

Dog and Cat – 20 mg/kg body weight oral; and 11 mg/kg body weight TID IM, IV.

Trade Names

1. *Unimycin Injection* (Unichem) – 10 ml and 30 ml vials

   Composition: 140 mg/ml injection.

2. *Unimycin bolus* (Unichem) – Strip of 4 boli
   Composition: 500 mg/bolus.
3. *Neocare Forte powder* (Vetcare) – 50 g and 250 g pack
   Composition: 25 per cent w/w
   Dose: Livestock 50 mg/kg body weight oral.

19.2.16 Amoxycillin + Cloxacillin

It is a unique combination of two modern semi synthetic penicillins. It is the most powerful broad spectrum, synergistic antibacterial formulation.

Indication

HS, BQ, Calf scours, Mastitis, Metritis, Pyometra, *E. coli* infections, Leptospirosis, Listeriosis and other bacterial infections, Pneumonia, Respiratory tract infections, Pyelonephritis, Salmonellosis *etc.* In canines, Bacterial Gastro-enteritis, Otitis, Bronchitis, Pneumonia, External and Internal abscesses *etc.*

Dose

Large animals 6-10 mg/kg body weight daily for 3-5 days by IM or IV route.

Small animals including dog 15-25 mg/kg body weight daily for 3-5 days by IM or IV route.

Trade Names

1. *Intamox* (Intas) – 500 mg, 2 g, 2.5 g and 4g vials in combipack
   Dose: Large animal 6-10 mg/kg body weight by IM or IV for 3 to 5 days.
   Dog 15-25 mg/kg body weight by IM or IV route for 3-5 days.
2. *Inimox Injection* (Indian Immunologicals) – 2 g, 3 g and 4 g vials
   Dose: 10 mg/kg body weight by IM or IV route after dissolving with sterile water for injection.
3. *Megaclox Vet Injection* (Cipla) – 3 g and 4 g vials
   Dose: 6-10 mg/kg body weight for large animals by IM or IV route for 3 to 5 days. Dog: 15-25 mg/kg body weight by IM or IV route for 3 to 5 days.
4. *Clomoxy Injection* (Brihans) – 2 g, 3 g and 4 g vials
   Dose: 7-10 mg/kg body weight.
   Cattle, Buffalo and Horse – 2 g to 3 g; for heavy animals 4 g daily for 4 to 5 days through IM or IV route.
5. *Damox Injection* (Daffodils) – 500 mg and 2 g vials
   Dose: 7-10 mg/kg body weight for IM or IV use only.
6. *Clox Mox Injection* (Daffodils) – 2 g vial
   Dose: 7-10 mg/kg body weight by IM or IV route.
7. *Omoxin Injection* (Oxen Labs) – 2 g, 3 g and 4 g vials
   Dose: 7-10 mg/kg body weight by IM or IV for large animnals. Dog 15 mg/kg body weight by IM or IV.

8. *Emoxel Injection* (Excell-R) – 3 g vial

   Dose: Cattle, Buffalo and Horse 2-3 g daily for 3 to 5 days by IM or IV route.
9. *Moxcell Injection* (Alembic) – 2 g and 3 g vials
10. *Mastox Injection* (Jeps Pharma) – 2 g vial

    Dose: 6-10 mg/kg body weight twice daily for 3-5 days by IM or IV route.
11. *Conmox Injection* (Concept) – 2 g and 3 g vials

    Dose: 6-10 mg/kg body weight by IM or IV.

19.2.17 Gentamicin

Highly effective aminoglycoside antibiotic, effective bactericidal action to treat urogenital, respiratory, G.I. tract infections and mastitis in livestock and can be safely used in poultry. It inhibits bacterial protein synthesis, thus producing bactericidal action.

Indication

Enteritis, Colibacillosis, Mastitis, Metritis, Nephritis, Urethritis, Dermatitis, Respiratory tract infections, Urinary tract infections, Skin and soft tissue infections, Gastrointestinal infections, Otitis externa in canines and felines, secondary bacterial infections specially female genital tract infections.

Dose

Cattle, Buffalo, Sheep, Goat, Pig, Dog and Cat – 4 mg/kg body weight BID IM, IV.

Poultry – 3-5 mg/kg body weight.

Trade Names

1. *Gentamycin Injection* (Vetcare) – 30 ml and 100 ml vials

   Coposition: Each ml contains 40 mg Gentamicin sulphate.

   Dose: Cattle and Buffalo 1 to 2 mg/kg body weight. Dog, Sheep, Goat and Pig 2 to 4 mg/kg body weight. Poultry 0.5 ml/bird IM. For Intra Uterine use 2 ml in 20 ml distilled water (I/U).
2. *Genta Biotic Injection* (KAP) – 10 ml, 30 ml and 100 ml vials

   Composition: Each ml contains 40 mg Gentamicin sulphate.

   Dose: Large animals 1 to 2 mg/kg body weight by IM. Small animals 2 to 4 mg/kg body weight by IM. Poultry 0.5 ml/bird by IM.. For I/U use 2 ml in 20 ml distilled water (I/U infusion).
3. *Gentax Injection* (DPL, Daffodills) – 30 ml vial

   Composition: Each ml contains Gentamicin sulphate 40 mg.

   Dose: Cattle and Buffalo 1 to 2 mg/kg body weight by IM or IV. Sheep, Goat and Pig 2 to 4 mg/kg body weight by IM or IV.
4. *Gentavet Injection* (Oxen Labs) – 10 ml, 30 ml and 100 ml vials
5. *Catlo Genta* (CRIL) – 30 ml and 100 ml vials
6. *Ranbamicin Injection* (Vetnex) – 30 ml and 100 ml vials

7. *Legenta Injection* (Legend) – 10 ml and 30 ml vials

   Composition: Each ml contains Gentamycin sulphate 40 mg.

   Dose: Large animal 2-5 mg/kg body weight.

   1st dose is administered 2 times on 1st day followed by once daily for succeeding days.
8. *Aminocin Injection* (Neo spark) – 30 ml vial
9. *Gentamicin Injection* (TTK) – 30 ml and 100 ml vials

   Dose: Cattle and Buffalo 2.5 ml to 5 ml/50 kg body weight. Calf 0.5 ml/10 kg body weight. Dog and Cat 1 ml/10 kg body weight through IM, IV or I/U.

19.2.18 Amikacin

A narrow spectrum new generation aminoglycoside, effective against Gram positive organisms. It exerts bactericidal action by inhibition of bacterial protein synthesis.

Indication

Urogenital tract, respiratory tract infections, and also infections caused by bacteria resistant to Streptomycin, Neomycin and Gentamycin.

Dose

5-12 mg/kg body weight by SC, IM and IV route.

It is better not to use any aminoglycoside in cows prone to milk fever.

Trade Names

1. *Akayci Injection* (Brihans) – 2 ml, 10 ml and 30 ml vials

   Each ml contains Amikacin sulphate 250 mg.

   Dose: Calf, Sheep and Goat 4-5 ml. Dog and Cat 1-2ml. Cattle and Horse 8-10 ml.

   Or 5-12 mg/kg body weight weigt by IM, SC and IV routes.
2. *Amikox Injection* (Oxen Labs) – 10 ml vial

   It contains Amikacin sulphate 100 mg/500 mg.

   Dose: 5-12 mg/kg body weight by SC, IM and IV routes.
3. *Amix-250 Injection* (Daffodils) – 10 ml vial

   It contains Amikacin sulphate – 250 mg/ml.

   Dose: 5-10 mg/kg body weight by IM, IV or SC route.

19.2.19 Lincomycin

It is a lincosamide antibacterial, producing bactericidal action by inhibiting bacterial protein synthesis. It is a highly potent antimicrobial agent having a good penetrating property. It is a very good antibiotic used for the treatment of livestock diseases.

Indication

It is indicated for Fever, Enteritis, Arthritis, Otitis, Respiratory and Urogenital tract infections, Skin and soft tissue infections, pyoderma of both deep and superficial nature.

Dose

Cattle, Buffalo, Sheep and Goat – 10 mg/kg body weight BID IM, IV, oral.

100-200 mg intra mammary/intra uterine.

Pig – 11 mg/kg body weight BID.

Dog – 15-25 mg/kg body weight BID.

Sometimes this antibiotic may reduce milk yield, and show inappetance, diarrhea and ketosis in case of prolonged therapy. IM use may produce pain and irritation.

Trade Names

1. *Alincomycin Vet* (Alved) – 5 ml vial

   Composition: Each ml contains Lincomycin HCl 300 mg.

   Dose: Livestock 1ml/30-60 kg body weight by IM or slow IV.

   Poultry 10-20 mg/kg body weight by IM or in drinking water 3-5 days.

19.3 SULPHONAMIDES

19.3.1 Sulphadimidin

It is a dependable wide spectrum antibacterial agent. It is a sulphapyrimidine, rapidly absorbed from the gut.

Indication

It is indicated for HS, bovine coccidiosis, Enteritis, Foot rot, pneumonia, Gastro intestinal tract infections, Metritis,and other bacterial infections.

Trade Names

A. Injectable Preparations

1. *Brimdin Injection* (Brihans) – 100 ml vial

   Dose: 30-40 ml/100 kg body weight per day by IM or SC route. For critical cases initial dose may be doubled and to be followed by maintenance dose for 4-5 days. Also suitable for oral route after dilution.

2. *Sulfamin Injection* (Indian Immunologicals) – 100 ml vial

   Composition: Each ml contains Sulfadimidin sodium 333 mg.

   Dose : 30-40 ml/100 kg body weight/day by SC or IM. Dose may be doubled in severe infections.

3. *Sulphadimidine Sodium Injection* (Novartis) – 100 ml vial

   Composition : Sulphadimidine sodium $33^1/_3$ per cent w/v.

   Dose: (IV, IM, SC, IP) – 6 ml/9 kg body weight initially or 30 ml/50 kg body weight initially followed by half of this dose once daily.

4. *Baifidine* (BAIF) – 100 ml

   Composition: Sulphadiazine sodium – 33.3 per cent.

   Dose : All animals 0.2 g/kg body weight IV, SC or intraperitoneally as initial size followed by 0.1 g/kg body weight as maintenance dose.

B. Oral Preparations

Indication

Infections caused by Gram (+ ve) and Gram (- ve) bacteria and certain protozoan diseases of livestock.

Trade Names

1. *Sulphadimidine bolus, 5 g* – Pouch of 2 boli

   Dose: Ruminant 1 bolus/50 kg body weight orally.

19.3.2 Gut Acting Sulphonamides

Oral Sulpha Drugs-Sulphametoxazole and Trimethoprim Combination

Indication

Actinobacillosis, Actinomycosis, Coilbacillosis, Mastitis, Strangles, Salmonellois, Infections keratitis, Infectious polyarthritis, Foot rot, Necrotic rhinitis, Toxoplasmosis, Coccidiosis, respiratory tract infections, urogenital tract infections, G I tract infection *etc.*

Trade Names

1. *Cotrimal Bolus* (Alembic) – 4 boli strip
2. *Oriprim Bolus* (Sarabhai Zydus) – Blisters of 2 boli

   Dose: Large animal – 4 boli daily.

   Small animal – ½-1 bolus daily.

19.3.3 Oral Sulphonamide Bolus

Indication

Different Gram (+ ve) and Gram (– ve) bacterial infections, certain protozoal infections specially in diarrhoea.

Trade Names

1. *Sulphaguanidine Bolus*

   Dose: 100-200 mg/kg body weight.

2. *Guanidin Bolus* (Oxen Lab) – 10 x 4 blister box

   Composition: Sulphaguanidine – 5 g.

   Dose: Cattle and Buffalo – 1-2 boli orally BID.

   Calf, Sheep and Goat – ½ to 1 bolus orally BID.

3. *Lemidine Bolus* (Legend) – 2 boli strip.

   Composition: Sulphadimidine – 5 g bolus.

Dose: Large animal 100-200 mg/kg body weight followed by half dose daily.

Small animal 1 g/5 kg body weight followed by 0.5 g/5 kg body weight daily BID.

4. *Pabadene Bolus* (Intas) – 5 g bolus

   Composition: Each bolus contains sulphadimidine 5 g.

   Dose: Large animal – 1-2 boli/50 kg body weight followed by half dose.

19.3.4 Sulphonamide Combination (Co-Trimoxazole)

Sulphonamide and Trimethoprim combination produces synergistic action against a wide range of bacteria. Common injectable combinations are (*i*) Sulphadiazine and Trimethoprim, (*ii*) Sulphadoxine and Trimethoprim, and (*iii*) Sulphamethoxazole and Trimethoprim.

Indication

Mixed bacterial infections affecting respiratory tract, G.I. tract, urinary and genital tract, HS, BQ, Mastitis, Skin and soft tissue infections and other bacterial infections.

Trade Names

A. Injectable Co-Trimoxazole Preparations

1. *Biotrim Injection* (Vetnex) – 30 ml vial

   Composition: Each ml contains Sulphadiazine 400 mg and Trimethoprim 80 mg.

   Dose: 25 mg/kg body weight (or 1ml/20 kg body weight) only by IM route for 3-5 days.

2. *Duaprim Injection* (Brihans) – 30 ml vial

   Composition: Each ml contains Sulphadiazine 200 mg and Trimethoprim 40 mg.

   Dose: 1 ml/15 kg body weight by IM or IV route daily for 3-5 days.

3. *Sulphatrim Injection* (Vets Farma) – 10 ml and 30 ml vials

   Dose: 3 ml/64 kg body weight.

4. *Injection Oxiprim* (Oxen Lab) – 30 ml and 50 ml vials

   Composition: Trimethoprim + Sulphamethoxazole.

   Dose: 1 ml/15 kg body weight by IM route daily for 3 days.

5. *Oriprim Injection* (Sarabhai Zydus) – 30 ml

   Composition: Trimethoprim + Sulphamethoxazole

   Dose: 1 ml/20 kg body weight. Small animal – 2.5 ml daily. Large animal 15-50 ml daily. It is used through IM or IV route.

6. *Bacterisol Injection* (Alved) – 10 ml and 30 ml vials

   Each ml contains Sulphadiazine 100 mg + Trimethaprim 80 mg.

   Dose: 1 ml/10 kg body weight

7. *Bacteridox Injection* (Alved) – 30 ml vial

   Composition: Each ml contains Sulphadoxin 62.5 mg + Trimethoprim 125 mg

   Dose: 1 ml/5 kg body weight IM or IV route.

B. Oral Co-trimoxazole Preparations

1. *Bactrisol bolus* (Alved) – Strips of 4 boli and 10 boli

   Composition: Sulphadiazine 1 g + Trimethoprim 0.2 g.

   Dose: Cattle and Buffalo 2 boli orally BID; Sheep and Goat 1 bolus BID.
2. *Woktrin tablet* (Wockhardt) –12 tablets pack

   Composition: Sulphadiazine 1 g + Trimethiprim 200 mg.

   Dose: All animals 15 mg/kg body weight. Cattle and Buffalo 4-6 boli daily. Ewe, Sow, Calf 1-2 boli daily.
3. *Atrima Bolus* (Prima Vet Care) – Strip of 4 boli

   Composition: Sulphadiazine 1 g + Trimethoprim 0.2 g/bolus.

   Sulphadiazine 2 g + Trimethoprim 0.4 g/bolus.

   Dose: Large animal 30 mg/kg body weight daily for 2 days. Mare and Cow 2.4-4.8 g. Ewe and Doe 1.2-2.4 g.

   Large animal 2-4 boli/uterine horn; Small animal 1-2 boli/uterine horn.
4. *Oriprim Bolus* (Sarabhai Zydus) – Strip of 2 boli

   Composition: Sulphamethoxazole 2 g + Trimethoprim 400 mg/bolus.

   Dose: Large animal 4 boli daily; Small animal ½-1 bolus daily.
5. *Robatran Vet Bolus* (TTK) – Strip of 4 boli

   Composition: Sulphamethoxazole 1 g + Trimethoprin 0.2g.

   Dose: Large animal 2 boli orally BID. Small animal 1-2 boli orally BID.
6. *Sulcoprim Bolus/Powder* (Concept) – Strip of 10 boli/100 g and 500 g pack

   Composition: Each bolus contains Sulphadiazine 1 g and Trimethoprim 0.2 g.

   Each 5 g powder contains Sulphamethoxazole 2 g and Trimethoprim 400 mg.

   Dose: Cattle, Buffalo and Horse 2-4 boli/2-4 tsf powder orally BID daily.

   Calf, Sheep, Goat and Pig 1-2 boli/½-2 tsf powder orally daily.
7. *Trizol Bolus* (Jeps) – 4 boli strip

   Composition: Sulphamethoxazole 2 g + Trimethoprim 400 mg/bolus.

   Dose: Large animal 2 boli twice daily for 3-5 days; Small animal ½-1 bolus twice daily for 3-5 days.
8. *Oxiprim Forte Bolus* (Oxen Lab) – 10 x 4 boli box

   Composition: Each bolus contains Trimethoprim 0.4 g + Sulphamethoxazole 2 g.

Dose: Cattle, Buffalo and Horse 2 to 4 boli orally daily BID. Calf, Sheep and Goat 1 to 2 boli orally daily.

9. *Intrim Bolus* (Intas) – 1.5 g bolus

   Composition: Each bolus contains Trimethoprim 250 g + Sulphamethoxazole 250 mg

   Dose: Livestock 1 bolus/80 kg body weight oral and I/U route.

10. *Intrim Forte Bolus* (Intas) – 2.4 g bolus

    Dose : Livestock 1 bolus/50 kg body weight oral and I/U route.

11. *Duaprim Bolus* (Brihans) – Strip of 4 boli

    Composition: Trimethoprim 400 mg + Sulphamethoxazole 2000 mg.

    Dose : Large animals 2 boli twice daily; Small animals 1 bolus twice daily.

12. *Biotrim DS* (Vetnex) – 30 boli pack

    Composition: Sulphadiazine – 200 mg + Trimethoprim – 400 mg.

    Dose: Calf scour – 1 bol B.I.D. for 3 days

    Diarrhoea of Bacterial and Coccidial origin – 1 bolus/100 kg body weight

    Or 2-4 boli BID for 2 days.

13. *Genprim Bolus* (Legend) – 4 boli strip

    Composition : Sulphametoxazole 2000 mg + Trimethoprim 400 mg.

    Dose: 4 boli at 12 hours interval for 3-5 days (for large animals).

14. *Trisa-VL* (Pearl Chemicals) – 4 boli strip

    Composition: Trimethoprim 400 mg + Sulphamethoxazole 2000 mg.

    Dose: Cattle and Buffalo – 2 boli BID daily for 3-5 days.

    Calf, Sheep and Goat – 1 bolus orally BID for 3 days.

19.3.5 Oral Broad Spectrum Antidiarrhoeals for Calf, Sheep and Goat

Indication

Broad spectrum antidiarrhoeal covers wide range of mixed infections caused by Gram (+ ve) and Gram (- ve) bacteria (both aerobic and anaerobic). It is indicated in the treatment of diarrhoea, dysentery due to mixed infections like amebiosis, trichomoniasis and giardiasis.

Trade Names

1. *Ciptas-TZ Suspension* (Intas) – 75 ml and 150 ml

   Composition: Each 5 ml suspension contains Ciprofloxacin 125 mg and Tinidazole 150 mg.

   Dose : Calf, Sheep and Goat – 5 ml/20 kg body weight to be repeated for 2-3 days oral route.

2. *Diagen* (Nugen Pharma) – 100 ml, 200 ml and 500 ml bottle

   Dose: Calf, sheep and goat – 10-15ml daily for 2-3 days orally.

3. *Antibac-C* (Oxford Gem) – 100 ml and 500 ml

   Dose: Sheep and Goat 5 ml orally BID for 3-5 days. Calf 10-15 ml orally BID for 3-5 days.

4. *Neodox Bolus* (Vetcare) – Strip of 6 boli

   Composition: Each bolus conatains Neomycin 400 mg + Doxycycline 160 mg.

   Dose: Cattle and Buffalo 4-5 boli per cattle per day.

5. *Fumar Bolus* (Legend) – 4 boli strip

   Composition: Each bolus conatains Metronidazole 1g + Furazolidone 200 mg.

   Dose: Sheep, Goat and Pig (upto 40 kg body weight) ½ bolus twice daily. Calf, Heifer Cattle and Buffalo @ 1 bolus/50 kg body weight in two divided doses for 3-5 days.

6. *BT Flox-TZ Tablet* (Bee Tee Pharma)

   BT FLOX-TZ Bolus (Bee Tee Pharma)

   Composition Each tablet contains Norfloxacin 400 mg + Tinidazole 600 mg.

   Each bolus contains Norfloxacin 1200 mg + Tinidazole 1800 mg.

   Dose: Large animal – 1-2 bolus for 3-5 days. Small animal – 1-2 tab for 3-5 days.

7. *Dydistop Forte* (Oxen Labs) – 4 boli blister

   Composition: Metronidazole 2-0 gram + Furazolidone – 0.5 gram

   Dose: Cattle and Buffalo 2 boli BID for 3-5 days. Calf, Sheep and Goat 1 bolus BID for 3-5 days.

8. *Otrim Bolus* (Excell) – 4 boli strip

   Composition: Metronidazole 1g + Furazolidone 200 mg.

9. *Curacin-O Bolus* (Vets Farma) – 4 boli strip

   Composition: Ofloxacin + Tinidazole.

   Dose: Cattle and Buffalo 1-2 boli BID for 3 days.

10. *Fazole Bolus* (Unichem) – Strip of 4 boli

    Composition: Metronidazole 1 g + Furazolidone 0.2 g/bolus

    Dose: 1 bolus/50 kg body weight orally.

    Calf, Sheep and Goat ½ to 1 bolus BID for 3-5 days.

11. *Cyclin DT Bolus* (Excell)

    Composition: Doxycycline 300 mg + Tinidazole 1500 mg.

    Dose: Cattle and Buffalo 1-2 bolus on 1st day, 2nd day onwards 1 bolus OD.

    Calf, Sheep and Goat ½ to 1 bolus OD. It is once a day oral antibiotic.

19.3.6 Herbal Antidiarrhoeals

Indication

Non specific diarrhoea and dysentry.

Trade Names

1. *Neblon Powder* (Indian Herbs) – 100 g cartoon and 1 kg poly bag

   Dose: Cow, Buffalo and Horss 30-50 g twice or thrice daily. Calf, Sheep, Goat, Pig 8-10 g twice daily. Dog and Piglet 2-3 g twice or thrice daily.

   (to be administered orally with curd or rice gruel)
   In severe cases, the dose may be repeated six hourly.

2. *Diarok* (Ayurvet) – 30 g and 1 kg pack

   It is a protective, adsorbent, antidiarrhoea used for the treatment of diarrhoea of variable eatiology.

   Dose: Cattle and Buffalo – 30 g twice daily orally. Calf, Sheep and Goat – 15 g twice daily orally. In severe cases the dose may be repeated at six hours interval.

3. *Astrinex* (Vetmed) – 100 g, 200 g and 1 kg packet.

   Dose: Cattle and buffalo 40-50 g orally BID for 2-3 days. Calf, Sheep and Goat 20-25 g orally twice daily for 2-3 days.

4. *Becknor Bolus* (Natural Remedies) – 6 boli pack

   A unique polyherbal extract formulation with effective antidiarrhoeal properties.

   Dose: Cattle and Buffalo 1-2 boli orally BID for 3-5 days. Calf, Sheep and Goat ½ to 1 bolus orally BID for 3-8 days.

5. *Diadisco* (Bhartiya Bootee Bhawan) – 100 g and 1kg

   For diarrhoea and dysentery.

   Dose: Cattle, Buffalo and Horse 25-35 g. Calf and Foal 10-15 g. Sheep and Goat 5-10 g. Dog 2-5 g twice daily.

   It should be given with rice gruel or as electuary thrice daily in chronic cases.

6. *Diarex Tablet* (Himalaya) – 100 tablets pack

   Antidiarrhoeal and antibiotic.

   Dose: Cattle, Buffalo and Horse 16-20 tablets daily. Calf and Foal 4-6 tablets. Sheep, Goat and Pig 2-4 tablets twice daily. Dog 1-2 tablets orally thrice daily.

7. *Diardon Powder* (Vets Farma) – 150 g and 1 kg pack

   Herbal product, indicated for non specific diarrhoea and dysentery.

   Dose: Small animal 6-10 g orally TID or BID.

   Large animal 30-50 g orally BID.

   Calf, Sheep and Goat ½ to 1 bolus BID for 3-5 days.

19.4 ELECTROLYTES/ORAL REHYDRATION SOLUTION (ORS)

Indication

Electrolyte imbalance, readymade energy during summer and sickness. Salmonelosis, coli bacillosis and coccidiosis in cattle, stress conditions.

Trade Names

1. *Lemilyte* (Legend) – 25 g and 200 g pouch

   Dose: Large animal 50 g twice daily for 4 days. Small animal 25 g twice daily for 4 days.
2. *Electra-C* (Jeps) – 50 g, 250 g and 1 kg bag

   Dose: Cattle, Buffalo, Camel and Horse 100 g per day. Sheep, Goat and Pig 30-50 g per day. Dog and Cat 10-20 g per day.
3. *E.R.S. Liquid* (Excell) – 200 ml, 500 ml, 1 litre and 5 litres

   Dose: Large animal 50-100 ml daily. Small animal 20-25 ml daily. Chick 100 ml/litre of water, Grower and Broiler 20 ml/litre of water.
4. *Electra* (Sprindles Formulations) – 250 g and 1 kg

   Composition: Sodium, Potassium, Magnessium, Calcium and Vitamin C.

   Dose: Cattle, Buffalo and Horse 25-50 g orally BID. Calf, Sheep and Goat 20-25 g orally BID.
5. *Dextrolyte* (Enlag Lab) – 200 g pouch

   Dose: Cattle 200 g/day; Calf, Sheep and Goat 20 g/day and Dog 10-20 g/day.
6. *Electrocon* (Pharmacon)- 100 ml, 450 ml and 5 litres

   Unique physiological rehydration solution for poultry and livestock.

   Dose: Cow, Buffalo and Horse 500 ml daily for 5 days. Calf, Sheep and Goat 100 ml daily for 5 days. Dog and Cat 50-100 ml daily for 5 days.
7. *Grow-UP* (Vetcon) – 100 ml and 450 ml bottle

   Oral rehydration solution indicated for diarrhoea, dehydration, fluid and electrolyte imbalance, heat stress *etc.*
8. *ROS* (RS Pharmaceuticals) – 200 ml and 450 ml bottle

   Dose: Large animals 100 ml daily for 5 days. Small animals 50 ml daily for 5 days. Poultry 30 ml/100 birds daily for 3-5 days.
9. *Electro Gen* (Nugen Pharma) – 200 ml, 450 ml and 5 litres

   It is an oral liquid rehydration solution and stress eliminator.

   Dose: Large animals 50-100 ml daily for 3-5 days. Small animals 25-50 ml daily for 3-5 days.

9\. *Electrovet* (Marion Pharma) – 200 ml, 450 ml and 1 litre.

   Oral rehydration solution for the replacement of fluid and electrolytes.

19.5 ANTHELMINTICS (DEWORMERS)

19.5.1 Albendazole

Albendazole is a broad spectrum anthelmintic. It inhibits the glycogen metabolism of worms by interfering with fumarase reductase enzyme mechanism, thus worms die of starvation.

Indication

It is used for the treatment and control of parasitic infestations caused by round worms, tape worms and liver flukes.

Dose

For round worms – 7.5 mg/kg body weight.

For tape worms and flukes – 15 mg/kg body weight.

Availability : Suspension, bolus and tablet forms.

Trade Names

A) Albendazole Oral Suspension

1. *Albomar Suspension* (GSK) – 30 ml, 60 ml, 90 ml and 500 ml

   Composition: Albendazole 2.5 per cent suspension (w/v).

   Dose : Large animal – 60-90 ml; Small animal – 5-10 ml; Calf – 15-30 ml.

   Cattle, Calf, Sheep and Goat – 4 ml/kg body weight; Dog – 5-10 ml BID for 3 days.
2. *Albopa Suspension* (Pear Chemicals) – 30 ml and 100 ml bottles.
3. *Expell Suspension* (Excell) – 30 ml, 60 ml, 90 ml and 5 litres

   Composition: Each ml contains Albendazole 25mg.

   Dose : Cow/Buffalo – 60 ml single dose.

   Calf, Sheep and Goat – 10-15 ml single dose depending on body weight.

   Dog – 5-10 ml twice daily for 3 days.
4. *Velminth Suspension, 2.5 per cent w/v* (IBC) – 1 litre jar
5. *Wormer Vet Suspension, 2.5 per cent w/v* (Legend) – 30 ml, 60 ml, 90 ml and 1 litre

   Dose: Cattle and Buffalo – 1 ml/5 kg body weight single dose.
6. *Briben Suspension 2.5 per cent w/v* (Brihans) – 30 ml, 120 ml and 1 litre

   Dose: Cattle, Buffalo and Horse – 60-120 ml. Calf, Sheep and Goat – 10-30 ml. Dog : 3-5 ml twice daily for 3 days.
7. *Endoban Suspension* (TTK) – 30 ml, 60 ml, 500 ml and 1 litre

   Dose: Cattle and Buffalo – 4 ml/kg body weight. Sheep and Goat – 6 ml/kg body weight.
8. *Suprazole Suspension* (Vetnex) – 30 ml and 90 ml
9. *Alben Suspension 2.5 per cent w/v* (Jeps) – 30 ml, 60 ml and 100 ml

10. *Albovet Liquid 2.5 per cent w/v* (Marion Pharma) – 30 ml, 60 ml, 90 ml and 1 litre
11. *Analgon Suspension 2.5 per cent* (Wockhardt) – 70 ml and 1 litre

    Dose: For round worms: Cattle, Buffalo and Horse – 20 ml/100 kg body weight; Pig, Sheep and Goat – 5 ml/25 kg body weight; Dog and Cat – 10-12 mg/kg body weight orally.

    For liver flukes : Cattle and Buffalo – 40 ml/100 kg body weight. Sheep and Goat – 7.5 ml/25 kg body weight orally.

B) Albendazole Bolus

1. *Albicon Bolus* (Pharmacon) – 150 mg, 600 mg, 1500 mg and 3 g

   Dose: 5-7.5 mg/kg body weight.
2. *Albomar Bolus* (GSK) – 1.5 g and 3 g

   Dose : 1.5 g bolus for 150-200 kg body weight; 3 g bolus for above 200 kg to 300 kg body weight. For flukes 1 bolus (1.5 g) for 100 kg body weight.
3. *Albogen Bolus* (Nugen) – 250 mg, 600 mg, 1.5 g and 3 g
4. *Albopa Bolus* (Alembic) – 600 mg and 1.5 g and 3g
5. *Minthal Bolus* (Alembic) – 600 mg and 1.5 g
6. *Valvagen Bolus* (Pfizer) – 600 mg
7. *Wormer Bolus* (IBC) – 150 mg, 600 mg, 1.5g and 3 g
8. *Velminth Bolus* (IBC) – 400 mg and 1200 mg
9. *Briben Bolus* (Brihans) – 1500 mg

   Dose: 5-10 mg/kg body weight orally.

   Large animal – 1-2 bolus ; Medium size animal – ½–1 bolus; Small animals – 1/4 – ½ bolus.

   For flukes and severe worm infestation the dose may be increased.
10. *Kalbend Bolus* (KAP) – 150 mg, 600 mg, 1.5 g and 3 g
11. *Suprazole Bolus* (Vetnex) – 1.5 g and 3 g bolus

    Dose: For round worm Large animal 7.5 mg/kg body weight.

    Or 1.5 g -3 g bolus/animal depending up on size.
12. *Wormpar* (Oxen Lab) – 1.5 g bolus
13. *Endoben Bolus* (TTK) – 4 boli strip

    Composition : Albendazole – 750 mg.

    Dose: Cattle ½–2 bolus (75-150 kg body weight) or 2 boli for 300 kg body weight.
14. *Wormpar DS* (Oxen Lab) – 3 g bolus

15. *Benvet Bolus* (Cipla) – 3000 mg bolus

    Dose: For liver flukes Large animal – 10 mg/kg body weight; Sheep and Goat – 7.5 mg/kg body weight.

    For lung worm and tape worm – 5 mg/kg body weight.

C) Albendazole Tablets

1. *Albogen Tablet* (Nugen) – 150 mg
2. *Albomr Micronised Tablet* (GSK) – 150 mg, 10 tablets strip

   Dose: 5 mg/kg body weight.

   Sheep, Goat and Pig – 1-2 tabs single dose.

   Dog and Cat – 1 tab BID for 5 days.
3. *Wormer Tab* (Legend) – 150 mg
4. *Albicon Tab* (Pharmacon) -150 mg
5. *Kalbend Tab* (Karnataka Antibiotics) – 150 mg
6. *Tablet Albonil* (ACW)–150 mg
7. *Albopa Tab* (Pearl Chemicals) – 200 mg
8. *Alzonex Tablet/Bolus* (Neospark) – 150 mg tablet and 600 mg bolus

D) Albendazole and Ivermectin Combined Bolus

1. *Bandykind plus* (Vetkind)

   Effective against all endoparasites and ectoparasites.

   Composition : Albendazole – 3000 mg + Ivermectin – 100 mg.

   Dose: Cattle and Buffalo – 1 bolus/300 kg body weight.

19.5.2 Fenbendazole

It is a broad spectrum anthelmintic for the treatment and control of round worms, tape worms and lung worms of cattle, buffalo, sheep and goat. It kills all stages of worms (mature and immature), and highly safe and non-teragogenic.

Indication

Round worms, lung worms, tape worms (in ruminants and pigs). Treatment and control of Haemonchus, Ostertagia, Tichostrongylus, Cooperia, Nematodirus, Neoascaris vitulorum, Oesophagostomum, Bunostomum, Trichuris, Strongyloides, Dictyocaulus, Moneizia sp. *etc.*

Dose

5 mg/kg body weight.

Trade Names

1. *Fentas Bolus* (Intas) – 1.5 g and 3 g bolus

   Dose: Large animal 1 bolus (1.5 g)/200-300 kg body weight; 2 boli for above 300 kg body weight.

2. *Fenzole Bolus/Tablet* (Jeps) – 150 mg tablet and 1.5 g bolus

   Dose : One tablet (150 mg) for 30 kg body weight.

   One bolus (1.5 g) for 300 kg body weight.
3. *Panacur Tablet/Bolus* (Intervet) – 150 mg tablet, and 1.5 g and 3 g bolus

   For all animals (except in dog and cat) one tablet for 30 kg body weight; 1.5 g bolus/300 kg body weight.
4. *All Clear Bolus* (Vetcare) – 1.5 g

   Dose: 5 mg/kg body weight
5. *Vet Fen-T/Vet Fen-B* (Indian Immunologicals) – 150 mg tablet and 1.5 g bolus

   Dose: 1 tab (150 mg) for 30 kg body weight; 1 bolus (1.5 g) for 300 kg body weight.
6. *Kira Kill* (Oxen Labs) – 1.5 g bolus

   Dose: 5 mg/kg body weight. 1 bolus for 200 kg body weight (for cattle and buffalo).
7. *Kira Kill-DS* (Oxen Lab) – 60 ml bottle

   Composition: Fenbendazole – 25 mg/ml.

19.5.3 Mebendazole

It is a unique broad spectrum safest dewormer.

Indication

For complete deworming of round worms, tape worms and other worm infestations in all age groups.

Trade Names

1. *Banif Bolus* (Brihans) – Strip of 4 boli

   Composition: 1500 mg Mebandazole.

   Dose: Cattle, Buffalo and Horse – 1-2 boli orally. Calf, Sheep and Goat – ½ to 1 bolus. Dog – 1/4 to ½ bolus (in severe infestation higher dose may be given for 2 to 3 days).
2. *Zodex Bolus* (Concept) – 500 mg bolus

   Dose: 10 mg/kg body weight

   Cattle, Buffalo and Horse – 4-8 boli. Calf, Sheep and Goat – 2-4 boli.
3. *Wormin Tab,* 100 mg (Cadila)– 10 tablets strip

   Composition: Mebendazole – 100 mg.

   Dose: 5-10 mg/kg body weight
4. *Wormin Powder* (Cadila)– 50 g packet

   Dose: Poultry 100 g/100 kg of feed.

19.5.4 Oxfendazole

This is one of the latest Benzimidazole with broad spectrum antihelminthic activity. It has got ovicidal, larvicidal and wormicidal properties. It can eliminate Gastro-intestinal nematodes, lung worms and tape worms.

Dose

5 mg/kg body weight.

Trade Names

1. *Btoxfen Bolus* (Bee Tee Pharma) – 1.5 g bolus

   Dose: Cattle and buffalo – 4.5 mg/kg body weight. Sheep and Goat – 7 mg/kg body weight. Pig – 3 mg/kg body weight.

2. *Axefendol Suspension* (Alved)

   Composition: Oxfendazol – 2.265 per cent w/v.

   Dose: For Sheep and Goat 1 ml/5 kg body weight. For Cattle and buffalo 5 mg/kg body weight or 1 ml for 2.25 kg body weight. Horse 1 ml for 3.20 kg body weight.

3. *Oxyfen Suspension* (Arigo Pharma) – 100 ml bottle

   Composition: Oxfendazole oral liquid 2.265 per cent w/v.

   Dose: Sheep and Goat – 1 ml/5 kg body weight

   Cattle and Buffalo – 5 mg/kg body weight

19.5.5 Levamisole

Levamisole HCl is a broad spectrum anthelmintic and immunomodulator. It inhibits fumarate reductase and ganglion stimulant (Chollinomimetic) and paralyses the nematodes due to sustained muscle contractions. It modulates immune system by modifying activity of T-lymphocytes and phagocytes.

Indication

Nematodes in abomasum, small intestine, large intestine, lungs and eyes like Haemonchus, Ostertagia, Trichostrongylus, Oesophagostomum, Dictyocaulus, Thelazia *etc*.

Trade Names

1. *Regain Bolus* (Excell) – 1.5 g bolus

   Dose: Cattle, Sheep, Goat and Pig – 7.5 mg/kg body weight.

   In eye worm 5 mg/kg body weight. As immunomodulator dose should be divided equally in 3 days.

2. *Noworm Bolus* (Vets Farma) – 1.5 g bolus

   Dose: Cattle, Sheep and Goat – 7.5 mg/kg body weight

3. *Helmonil Powder* (Alved) – 10 g sachet

   Each gram contains Lemamisole HCl – 300 mg.

   Dose: 7.5 mg/kg body weight (or 1 g/40 kg body weight) of all animals orally.

4. *Helmonil Tablet* (Alved) – 150 mg

   Dose: Calf 1 tablet/20 kg body weight.

5. *Ivmasol-75 Injection* (Vetnex) – 30 ml vial

   Dose: 1 ml/10 kg body weight by SC route.

6. *Helmonil Injection* (Alved) – 10 ml and 30 ml vial

   Each ml contains Levamisole 82 mg. This should not be given to dogs.

   Dose: 1 ml/30 kg body weight by IM.

7. *Nemasol Injection* – 30 ml vial

   Each ml contains 300 mg Levamisole HCl.

   Dose: 1 ml/30 kg body weight by deep IM injection.

8. *Kalmisol Injection* (Karnataka Antibiotic) – 30 ml vial

   Each ml contains Levamisole HCl 75 mg.

   Dose: 1 ml/10 kg body weight SC.

19.5.6 Closantel (Ectendoparasiticidal)

A new generation ecto and endoparasiticide.

Indication

It is effective against round worms, liver flukes and tapeworms, and ectoparasites like ticks and lice. It is a safe anthelmintic, useful in both lactating and pregnant animals.

Trade Names

1. *Zycloz Bolus* – Strip of 4 boli

   Dose: 10-15 mg/kg body weight orally.

   For round worm and tape worm, 1 bolus/100 kg body weight. For liver flukes and ectoparasites 1 bolus/66 kg body weight.

2. *Zycloz Oral Solution* (Sarabhai Zydus) – 30 ml and 500 ml

   Composition: Closantel 15 per cent oral solution. Each ml contains Closantel 150 mg.

   Dose: For Cattle, Buffalo, Sheep and Goat

   Fasciola species and Ectoparasites – 1 ml/10 kg body weight or 15 mg/kg body weight. For other endoparasites 1 ml/15 kg body weight (10 mg/kg body weight)

3. *Zenvet* (Intas) – 30 ml, 100 ml and 500 ml

   Composition : Closantel – 15 per cent w/v.

   Dose: As nematicidal 1 to 1.5 ml for 15-20 kg body weight; as a flukicide 1 to 1.5 ml for 10-15 kg body weight.

19.5.7 Ivermectin Oral

It is a new generation endectocide which kills endoparasites and ectoparasites.

It interferes with the transmission of nerve impulses in parasites, paralyzing and killing them.

Indication

It kills external parasites like ticks, lice and mites, and it also kills internal parasites like Dictyocaulus, eye worms (Thelazia) G I nematodes (Haemonchus, Bunostomum, Trichuris *etc.*), skin and muscle worms (Stephanofilaria, Parafilaria), Onchocerca.

Trade Names

1. *Hitek Oral Solution* (GSK) – 100 ml, 500 ml and 1000 ml

   Composition : Hitek 0.08 per cent w/v.

   Dose: 2.5 ml for 10 kg body weight orally (200 microgram/kg body weight)
2. *Endectin Tab* (Excell) – 10 mg and 25 mg

   Dose: 1 tab/50 kg body weight.
3. *Endectin Bolus* (Excell) – 100 mg

   Dose: Cattle and Buffalo 1 bolus for 200-250 kg body weight.
4. *Ivectin Tablet* (Indian Immunologicals) – 10 mg

   Dose: Dog 1 tab/40 kg body weight;

   Other animals 1 tab/50 kg body weight.
5. *Fasimec Suspension* (Novartis) – 100 ml and 500 ml

   Composition: Ivermectin 0.1 per cent + Triclabendazole – 5 per cent.

   Dose: Sheep and Goat – 1 ml/5 kg body weight.

19.5.8 Parenteral Ivermectin (A friendly dewormer of animals) – Ivermectin Injection (1 per cent w/v)

The most powerful broadspectrum anthelmentic and ectoendicide, completely safe in breeding and pregnant animals. Not active against flukes and tape worms.

Indication

Infestation with major endoparasites like G.I. nematodes, lung and heart worms, other endoparasites like eye worms, skin and muscle worms (Stephanofilaria, Parafilaria), Onchocerea *etc.* Also ectoparasites like mange mites, ticks and lice.

Dose

Livestock (Cattle, Buffalo, Sheep, Goat, Pig, Horse and Dog) – 0.2 mg/kg body weight SC.

Trade Names

1. *Neomec Injection* (Intas) – 1 ml, 7 ml, 10 ml and 20 ml vials

   Composition: Each ml contains Ivermectin 10 mg.

   Dose: Cattle and Buffalo – 1 ml/50 kg body weight.

   Sheep and Goat – 1 ml/50 kg body weight.

Dog – 0.05-0.1 mg/kg body weight. (For *Toxocara canis* – 0.4 mg/kg body weight)

Horse and Swine – 0.2 mg/kg body weight.

2. *Vectin Injection* (IBC) – 1 ml and 7 ml vials

   Composition: Each ml contains 10 mg Ivermectin.

   Dose: Cattle, Buffalo and Sheep – 1 ml/50 kg body weight.

   Dog – 0.05-0.1 mg/kg body weight (0.4 mg/kg body weight for *Toxocara canis*)

3. *Ivectin Injection* (Indian Immunologicals) – 1 ml, 7 ml and 50 ml vials

   Composition: Each ml contains Ivermectin 10 mg (1 per cent w/v) and Ethanol 10 per cent w/v.

   Dose: Cattle, Buffalo and Sheep – 1 ml/50 kg body weight.

   Dog – 0.2 ml/33 kg body weight by SC.

   Sheep and Goat – 0.5 ml/25 kg body weight SC.

4. *Alverin Injection* (Alved) – 1 ml, 7 ml, 10 ml, 20 ml and 50 ml vials

   Composition: Each ml contains Ivermectin 10 mg.

   Dose: Cattle, Horse and Camel – 1 ml/50 kg body weight SC.

   Dog and Cat – 0.2 ml to 0.6 ml/10 kg body weight

   Sheep and Goat – 0.5 ml/25 kg body weight SC.

5. *Conmectin Injection* (Concept) – 2 ml, 7 ml and 10ml vials

   Composition: Each ml contains Ivermectin 10 mg.

6. *Parid Injection* (Vets Farma) – 1 ml, 7 ml, 10 ml, 30 ml and 50 ml vials

   Composition: Each ml contains Ivermectin 10 mg.

   Dose: 1 ml/50 kg body weight SC.

7. *Avermac Injection* (Oxen Lab) – 1 ml, 10 ml and 20 ml vials

   Composition: Each ml contains Ivermectin 10 mg.

   Dose: 1 ml/50 kg body weight SC.

8. *Hitek Injection* (GSK) – 1 ml and 10 ml vials

   Composition: Ivermectin 1 per cent w/v.

   Dose: 1 ml/50 kg body weight by SC route.

9. *Alverin Plus Injection* (Alved) – 5 ml and 10ml vials

   Composition: Each ml contains Ivermectin 1 per cent w/v (10 mg/ml) and Clorsulon 10 per cent w/v (100 mg/ml)

   Dose: Cattle – 1 ml/50 kg body weight.

   Sheep and Goat – 0.5 ml/25 kg body weight SC.

10. *Mectin Injection* (Alembic) – 1 ml, 7 ml, 10 ml and 20 ml vials

    Composition: It contains Ivermectin 10 mg/ml.

    Dose: 1 ml/50 kg body weight SC.

19.5.9 Triclabendazole (Flukicide)

The latest new generation flukicide, effective against both mature and immature flukes. It is safer than any other flukicides.

Indication

For complete elimination of mature and immature flukes.

Trade Names

1. *Fluzic Bolus* (Vetnex) – 900 mg
   Dose: Cattle and Buffalo – 12-15 mg/kg body weight
2. *Fluzic Suspension* (Vetnex) – 90 ml plastic bottle
   Dose: Cattle and buffalo – 12-15 mg/kg body weight
3. *Fasinex Bolus* (Novartis) – 900 mg
   Composition: Triclabendazole – 900 mg/bolus.
   Dose: Cattle and Buffalo – 1 bolus/75 kg body weight.
4. *Fasinex Suspension* (Novartis) – 250 ml, 500 ml and 1 litre
   Composition : Triclabendazole 5 per cent w/v
   Dose : Sheep and Goat – 1 ml/5 kg body weight
   Cattle and Buffalo – 90 ml per animal (adult dose).

19.5.10 Oxyclozanide (Flukicide)

It is commonly used as fasciolicide. The mode of action is an uncoupler of oxidative phosphorylation. It has poor activity against the rumen flukes.

Indication

Liver flukes, Amphistomes, Moniezia and N.G.

Dose

Cattle 10-15 mg/kg body weight.

Sheep and Goat 15 mg/kg body weight.

Trade Names

1. *Neozide Bolus* (Intas) – 1 g
   Each bolus contains 1 g.
2. *Oxaclon-200* (Arlgo Pharma) – 10 tablets strip
   Composition: Oxyclozanide 200 mg.
   Dose: Sheep and Goat 1 tablet.
3. *Distonex Bolus* (Neosprak)
   Composition: Oxyclozanide 1000 mg.
   Dose: For Cattle and Buffalo 1 bolus/100 kg body weight.
4. *Zanil Suspension* (Intervet) – 100 ml and 1 litre
   Composition : Suspension containing 3.4 per cent w/v Oxyclozanide.

Dose: Cattle 1 ml /3 kg body weight or 30 ml/100 kg body weight, maximum 100 ml orally.

Sheep and Goat 15 mg/kg body weight.

Do not use in severe liver damage and dehydration condition. The animal may suffer from loose motion and inappetance.

5. *Hexanide Bolus* (Zydus AHL) – 1 g

   Composition: Oxyclozanide – 1 g.

   Dose : 1 bolus/65-100 kg body weight.

6. *Tolzan F* (HPL) – 1 litre and 5 litres

   Composition: Oxyclozonide 3.4 per cent w/v.

   Dose: 10 mg/kg body weight.

Cattle and Buffalo	Sheep and Goat
50 kg – 15 ml	Upto 15 kg – 5 ml
100 kg – 30 ml	15-30 kg – 10 ml
200 kg – 60 ml	30-45 kg – 15 ml
300 kg – 90 ml	

7. *Distonex Suspension* (Neospark)

   Composition: Oxyclozanide – 3.4 per cent suspension.

   Excellent fasciolicide and flukicides for cattle, buffalo, sheep and goat.

8. *Zoonic* (Oxen Labs) – 100 ml, 1 litre and 5 litres

   Composition: Oxyclozamide 3.4 per cent w/v

   Dose: Sheep and Goat – 15 mg/kg body weight

   Cattle and Buffalo – 10 mg/kg body weight

9. *Tolzan-F Suspension* (Intervet) – 90 ml plastic bottle and 1 litre jar

   Each ml contain Oxyclozonide – 34 mg.

   Dose: Cattle and Buffalo – 10 mg/kg body weight.

   Sheep and Goat – 15 mg/kg body weight.

10. *Okazan* (WPL) – Bolus and Suspension (90 ml and 1 litre)

    Composition: Suspension Oxyclozonide – 3.4 per cent w/v; Bolus Oxyclozanide 1 bolus.

    Dose:

    Bolus – Cattle and Buffalo 1 bolus/100 kg body weight.

    Suspension –

Sheep and Goat	Cattle and Buffalo
Upto 15 kg – 5 ml	50 kg – 15 ml
15-30 kg – 10 ml	100 kg – 30 ml
30-45 kg – 20 ml	200 kg – 60 ml
45 and above – 20 ml	300 kg – 90 ml

11. *Neozide Suspension* (Intas) – 90 ml and 1 litre bottle

    Composition: Oxyclozanide 3.4 per cent w/v.

    Dose: Large animal 90 ml/300 kg body weight.

    Sheep and Goat – 5 ml/15 kg body weight.

12. *Clozan Tablet* (200 mg)/*Bolus* (1 g)/*Suspension* 3.4 per cent w/v (Jeps Pharma) – 100 ml bottle/1 litre Jar

    Dose: Suspension 0.33 ml/kg body weight as oral drench.

    Tablet 1 tablet/20 kg body weight.

    Bolus 1 bolus/100 kg body weight.

13. *Distonex Tab* (Neospark) – 200 mg

    Dose: 10 mg/kg body weight. Sheep and Goat -1 tab for an adult sheep/goat.

14. *Zanide Bolus* (Legend) – 1 g

15. *Zanide Tablet* (Legend) – 200 mg

    Dose : 1 tab/14 kg body weight.

16. *Fluknide Suspension/Bolus* (Excell) – 90 ml and 1 litre; strip of 4 boli.

    Composition: Each ml suspension contains Oxyclozanide 3.4 per cent w/v.

    Each bolus contains Oxyclozanide 1.5 g.

    Dose: Suspension 0.33 ml/kg body weight as oral drench.

    Tablet 1 tablet/20 kg body weight.

    Bolus 1 bolus/100 kg body weight.

17. *Trimafen Suspension* (Pearls Chemical) – 90 ml, 120 ml and 1 litre

    Composition : Oxyclozanide 3.4 per cent w/v.

    Dose: Cattle and Buffalo 90 ml/300 kg body weight or 30 ml/100 kg body weight

18. *Tablet Trimafen* (Pearls Chemical) – 200 mg

    Dose: Sheep and Goat – 1 tab/15 kg body weight.

19. *Trimafen Bolus* (Pearls Chemical) – 1 g

    Dose: Cattle and Buffalo – 1 bolus/100 kg body weight.

19.5.11 Dichlorophen

This compound is highly effective against all types of tape worms in livestock.

Trade Names

1. *Cestophen Tablet* (Pearls Chemical) – 10 x 10 strips box.

   Composition : Dichlorophen 500 mg.

   Dose : Calf 0.2 g/kg body weight.

   Sheep and Goat 0.5 g/2.5 kg body weight.

2. *Cestophen Suspension* (Pearls Chemical) – 30 ml and 500 ml bottle
   Composition: Dichlorophen 20 per cent w/v.
   Dose: Cattle and Buffalo – 0.1 ml/kg body weight.

19.5.12 Piperazine Hexahydrate Solution

This is a safe, potent and stable dewormer.

Indication

Ascarid infection (Ascariasis in calves, especially buffalo calves).

Trade Names

1. *Piperazine Hexahydrate* (TTK) – 30 ml
   Composition: Piperazine Hexahydrate – 45 per cent w/v.
   Dose: 100-150 mg/kg body weight.
2. *Piperazine Liquid* (GlaxoSmithKline)
   Composition: Piperazine Hexahydrate 45 per cent w/v.
   Dose: Calf – 4 ml/10 kg body weight.
   Dog – 1 ml/5 kg body weight.
3. *Piperazine Adepate Powder* (KAP) – 450 g
   Composition: Piperazine adepate oral powder – 44.4 per cent w/w.
   Dose: Cattle, Horse, Sheep, Goat, Dog, Pig – 5 g/24 kg body weight.
4. *Piperazine Hydrate Liquid* (Karnataka Antibiotics) – 500 ml
   Composition: Each 5 ml contains Piperazine hydrate – 2.25 g.
   Dose: Calf, Sheep, Goat, Foal, Pig, and Dog – 15 to 30 ml/30 kg body weight.

19.5.13 Levamisole (Parenteral preparation as Immunomodulator and broad spectrum worm eradicator)

It acts as an immunomodulator in addition to its anthelmentic action. It potentiates the natural body defence mechanism against clinical and subclinical disease conditions.

Indication

Prevention and treatment of round worm infestation. In case of canine Ancylostomiasisa and to build up immunity boost up against bacterial and viral attacks. Besides, in all types of viral, bacterial and fungal infections it may be used with the following objectives.

1. To reduce severity, duration and frequency of infection.
2. To help in quick recovery.
3. To reduce chances of relapse.
4. To prevent escalation of outbreaks.
5. In case of Viral papillomatosis.

6. In case of Stephanofilarial worm infestation (Hump sore).
7. Adjunct to antibiotic therapy in Mastitis.

Trade Names

1. *Lemasol-75 Injection* (Vetnex) – 10 ml and 30 ml vials

   Composition: Each ml contains Levamisole HCl – 75 mg.

   Dose: 2.5 mg/kg body weight by SC (or 1 ml/30 kg body weight), to be repeated after 48 hours in cattle, buffalo, sheep and goat.
2. *Kalmisole Injection* (Karnataka Antibiotics) – 30 ml vial

   Composition: Each ml contains Levamisole HCl – 7.5 mg.

   Dose: 1 ml/30 kg body weight in all animals. Administration by SC route. Forty eight hours post vaccination administration is recommendation for immunity boost up.
3. *Helmonil-C Injection* (Alved) – 5 ml vial

   Dose: 1 ml/3 kg body weight by IM route.
4. *Nemasol Injection* (Jeps Pharma) – 10 ml and 30 ml vials

   Composition: Each ml contains Levamisole HCl – 75 mg.

   Dose: 1 ml/10 kg body weight by SC route.
5. *Citarin-L* (Bayer) – 30 ml

   Composition: Levamisol HCl – 10 per cent Injection.

19.5.14 Combined Broad Spectrum Dewormer for the Treatment of Mixed Worm Infestation/Dual Power Anthelmintic

Indication

Treatment and control of mixed worm infestations against mature and immature blood sucking nematodes, lung woıms and adult and young liver flukes.

Trade Names

1. *Rafox Plus* (Alved) – 100 ml and 1 litre

   Composition: Rafoxanide – 1.5 per cent w/v + Levamisol HCl – 1.5 per cent w/v.

   Dose: 1 ml/2 kg body weight orally; can be repeated 4-6 weeks interval if fluke infestation is high.
2. *Nilzan Suspension/Bolus* (GSK) – 100 ml, 500 ml, 1000 ml suspension/10 x 2 bolus

   Composition: Each 5 ml suspension contains Oxyclozanide – 150 mg + Tetramisole – 150 mg. Each bolus contains Oxyclozanide 1.5 g + Tetramisole – 1.5 g.

   Dose: 1 ml Nilzan suspension for 3 kg body weight.

   Cattle and Buffalo 2 boli or 30 ml suspension/100 kg body weight.

   Sheep and Goat – 1 ml/3 kg body weight.

3. *Tetzan Suspension/Bolus* (Jeps Pharma) – 100 ml and 1000 ml

   Composition:

   Suspension: Oxyclozanide – 3 per cent w/v + Tetramisole HCl – 3 per cent w/v.

   Bolus: Oxyclozamide – 1 g + Tetramisole – 1 g.

4. *Fascon Bolus* (Pharmacon) – 5 x 4 boli pack.

   Composition: Oxyclozanide – 1.0 g + Levamisole HCl – 0.5 g

   Dose: Large animal – 1-2 boli/66.6 kg body weight; Small animal – ½–1 bolus/33.3 kg body weight.

5. *Neozide Plus Suspension* (Intas) – 90 ml, 500 ml and 1000 ml

   Composition: Suspension contains Oxyclozanide – 6 per cent + Levamisole – 3 per cent.

   Dose: Sheep and Goat – 1 ml/4 kg body weight orally; Cattle and Buffalo – 90 ml/300 kg body weight.

6. *Helind Suspension* (Intas) – 250 ml and 500 ml

   Composition: Suspension contains Triclabendazole – 5 per cent + Levamisol – 3.75 per cent.

   Dose: Cattle and Buffalo – 90 ml/300 kg body weight; Sheep and Goat 1ml/5 kg body weight.

7. *Olgard Suspension* (Intas) – 500 ml

   Composition : Suspension contains Ivermectin 0.1 per cent + Triclabendazole 5 per cent.

   Dose: Sheep and Goat 1 ml/5 kg body weight; Cattle and Buffalo 60-90 ml/250-300 kg body weight through oral route.

8. *Fentas Plus Suspension* (Intas) – 100 ml, 500 ml and 1000 ml

   Composition: Suspension contains Febendazole 1.5 per cent + Praziquantel 0.5 per cent.

   Dose: Calf, Sheep and Goat – 1 ml/3 kg body weight.

9. *Flukodin-DS* (Arosol Pharma) – 60 ml, 100 ml, 500 ml, 1 ltr.

   Composition: Levamisole 300 mg + oxyclozanide 600 mg per 10 ml.

   Dose: 15 ml/100 kg body weight.

10. *Tolzan Plus* (Intervet) – 1 litre jerry can

    Composition: Each ml suspension contains Tetramisole HCl 30 mg + Oxyclozanide 30 mg.

    Dose: Large animal @ 10 ml/30 kg body weight.

11. *Endex Bolus* (Novartis) – Strip of 4 boli

    Composition: Each bolus contains Triclabendazole – 900 mg + Levamisole – 562.5 mg.

    Dose: 1 bolus/75 kg body weight for cattle and buffalo.

12. *Endex Suspension* (Novartis) – 250 ml jar

    Composition: Suspension – Triclabendazole 0 5 per cent + Levamisore 3.75 per cent.

    Dose: Sheep and Goat – 1 ml of suspension per 5 kg body weight.

13. *Fasimec Suspension* (Novartis) – 100 ml and 500 ml

    Composition: Triclabendazole – 5 per cent + Ivermectin – 0.1 per cent w/v.

    It is effective for all the three stages of liver flukes, major GIT round worms, lung worms, nasal bot and itch mite.

    Dose: Sheep and Goat – 1 ml/5 kg body weight.

14. *Klozanide-L Bolus/Suspension* (KAP) – 90 ml bottle and 1 litre HDPE jar

    Composition: Each bolus contains Oxyclozanide – 1000 mg + Levamisol – 500 mg.

    Suspension contains Oxyclozanide – 3 per cent w/v + Levamisol – 1.5 per cent w/v.

    Dose: 10-15 mg/kg body weight (1 bolus/100 kg body weight) OR 90-100 ml Suspension/300 kg body weight.

15. *Pyramectin* (Bee Tee Pharma)

    Composition: Pyrantel pamoate – 200 mg + Ivermectin – 100 mg.

    It is effective for hook worms, lung worms, heart worms, thread worms, Trichuris, Ostertagia, Toxocara and tape worms.

    Dose: Cattle, Buffalo, Horse, Goat and Sheep – ½ tablet up to 20 kg body weight

    1 tablet above 20 kg (up to 50 kg) body weight.

    Dog and Cat – ½ tablet up to 10 kg body weight

    1 tablet above 10 kg body weight.

    Repeat after 7 days and 21 days.

16. *Levoxy Bolus* (Cattle Remedies) – strips of 4 boli

    Composition: Broad spectrum anthelmintic and flukicide contains Oxyclozanide and Levamisole.

    Dose: Cattle and Buffalo – 1 bolus/100 kg body weight.

17. *Levoxy Suspension* (Cattle Remedies) – 90 ml and 1 litre bottles

    Composition: Oxyclozanide 3 per cent w/v + Levamisole 1.5 per cent w/v

    Dose: 10-15 mg/kg body weight

    Sheep and Goat – 5-10 ml.

    Cattle and Buffalo – 90-100 ml/300 kg body weight.

19.5.15 Ayurvedic Anthelmintic

Safe dewormer, composed of herbal ingredients and can be prescribed during lactation and pregnancy. Broad spectrum dewormer with laxative and stomachic action too.

Trade Names

1. *Helmax* (Vetmed) – 50 g and 100 g pack
   Dose: Large animal 50 g once daily for 2 days.
   Small animal 15g once daily for 2 days.
2. *Wopell* (Indian Herbs) – 100 g and 1 kg
   Dose: Cow, Buffalo, Horse and Mule 50-75 g once daily for 2-3 days.
   Colt and Calf (1-3 months) – 10-12 g for 2-3 days OD.
   Colt and Calf (3-6months) – 15-20 g for 2-3 days OD.
   Sheep, Goats and Piglet – 12-15 g for 2-3 days OD.
   Adult Pig – 20-25 g for 2-3 days OD.
   The dose may be repeated after 4 weeks.
3. *Taenil* (Indian Herbs) – 100 g cartoon and 1 kg poly bag
   It is indicated for complete eradication of tape worm.
   Dose: Sheep and Goat – 12-15 g
   Dog and Piglet (up to 2 months) – 4-6 g
   Adult pig – 20-25 g.
4. *Worm Herb* (Kapila) – 50 g and 100 g
   It contains the best of herbal ingredients and wormherb is completely safe.
   Dose: Cattle and Buffalo – 25 g daily for 2-3 days.
   Calf, Sheep, Goat and Pig – 10-15 g daily for 2 days.
5. *Ascaper* (Angels Group) –120 ml bottle
   Dose: Small animal – 20-30 ml.
   Large animal – 40-60 ml to be given in empty stomach for 4 days and repeat after 15 days.
6. *Kriminth* (Bootees) – 120 ml bottle
   Dose: Small animal – 15-30 ml daily in empty stomach for 2 days.
   Large animal – 50-60 ml in empty stomach orally for 2 days.

19.6 NON STEROIDAL ANTI-INFLAMMATORY AND ANALGESIC DRUGS (NSAID)

(*i*) Parenteral Formulations of NSAID

19.6.1 Paracetamol

Indication

It has got analgesic and antipyretic effect like salicylates. It reduces fever by inhibiting the action of endogenous pyrogens. Pyrexia, Ephemeral fever, pyrexia of unknown origin, as adjuvant with antibacterial therapy.

Trade Names

1. *Dafomol Injection* (Daffodills) – 30 ml vial

   Composition: Injection Paracetamol 150 mg/ml.
2. *Paramol Injection* (Modern Lab) – 30 ml vial

   Composition: Each ml contains Paracetamol 150 mg.
3. *Paracetol Injection* (Sarabhai Zydus) – 30 ml vial

   Composition: Paracetamol 150 mg/ml.

   Dose : Large animal 10 to 30 ml preferably by deep IM route.

   Small animal 1 ml to 5 ml by deep IM route.

19.6.2 Meloxicam

An oxicum group of drug. Most powerful NSAID, selective inhibitor of cox-2, non-mutagenic, non teratogenic, non-carcinogenic, having anti exudative, analgesic and antipyretic activity.

Indication

Acute and chronic inflammatory conditions, colic, soft tissue injuries, lameness, trauma, myositis, mammillitis, laminitis, osteoarthritis, sprain, traumatic and surgical pain, general oedema, bursitis, fibrositis, mastitis, pneumonia, bronchopneumonia, inflammatory condition with arthritis, otitis, renal, intestinal and other visceral colic, fever and at supportive therapy or adjunct to antimicrobials (antibiotic) and surgical interventions.

Trade Names

1. *Melflam Vet Injection* (Cipla) – 15 ml, 30 ml and 100 ml

   Composition: Each ml contains Meloxicam 5 mg.

   Dose: Cattle, Sheep and Goat – Single dose of 30 ml/300 kg body weight in pneumonia and prolapse of uterus. 15 ml/575 kg body weight in other indications daily or 1 ml/10 kg body weight.
2. *A3 Vet Injection* (Brihans) – 30 ml and 100 ml vials

   Composition: Each ml contains Meloxicam – 5 mg.

   Dose: Large animal – 15-30 ml/day. Small animal 10-15 ml/day. Administration by IM, IV or SC route.
3. *Melonex Injection* (Intas) – 2 ml, 15 ml, 30 ml and 100 ml vials

   Dose: Cattle, Buffalo and Horse – 30 ml/300 kg body weight

   Swine – 2 ml/25 kg body weight

   Sheep and Goat – 2 ml/33 kg body weight.
4. *Meloxi Injection* (Vets Farma) – 15 ml, 30 ml and 100 ml vials

   Composition: Each ml contains Meloxicam 5 mg.

   Dose: Cattle, Buffalo and Horse – 1 ml/10 kg body weight.

   Swine – 2 ml/25 kg body weight

   Sheep and Goat – 2 ml/33 kg body weight by IM, IV, SC route.

5. *Nulox Vet Injection* (KAP) – 15 ml, 30 ml and 100 ml vials

   Composition: Each ml contains Meloxicam – 5 mg.

   Dose: Cattle, Sheep and Goat – Single dose of 30 ml/300 kg body weight in pneumonia and genital prolapse.

   For other indications 15 ml/375 kg body weight (or 1 ml/10 kg body weight)

6. *Melonex Power Injection* (Intas) – 10 ml and 30 ml vials

   Composition: Each ml contains Meloxicam 20 mg + Lignocaine HCl 1 per cent w/v.

   Dose: For visceral organ affections, colic, mastitis, pneumonia, bronchopneumonia, uterine prolapse – 2.5 ml/100 kg body weight.

   For musculo skeletal disorders and other conditions –

   Horse : 3 ml/100 kg body weight. Pig 2 ml/100 kg body weight by IM route only.

7. *Zobid-M Injection* (Sarabhati Zydus) – 15 ml and 30 ml

   Composition:Eeach ml contains Meloxicam 5 mg.

8. *Disovet-M Injection* (IBC) – 15 ml and 30 ml

   Composition: Each ml contains Meloxicam 5 mg.

   Dose: Small animal – 1 ml/10 kg body weight

   Large animal – 15-30 ml by IM or I/V.

9. *Xyclofen Injection* (Excell) – 30 ml vial

   Composition: Each ml contains Meloxicam 5 mg.

   Dose: Cattle and Buffalo – 30 ml/300 kg body weight

   Sheep and Goat – 1 ml/10 kg body weight IM and IV route.

19.6.3 Meloxicam with Paracetamol Combination (Injectable Preparations)

Indication

Pain and fever associated with inflammation, Post operative pain, pyrexia of unknown origin (PUO), 3 days fever or Ephemeral fever, any bacterial or viral infection accompanied by fever (Pyrexia). Arthritis, Myositis, Laminitis, Bursitis, Fibrositis. In renal, intestinal and other visceral colic and in any inflammatory conditions. Also to be used as supportive therapy with antimicrobial.

1. *A3 Vet Plus Injection* (Brihans) – 30 ml and 100 ml vials

   Composition: Each ml contains Meloxicam 5 mg, Paracetamol 150 mg and Lignocaine HCl 1 per cent.

   Dose: Large animal – 15-30 ml/day

   Small animal – 10-15 ml/day (1 ml/10 kg body weight) – By deep IM route.

2. *MP3 Injection* (Vetnex) – 30 ml and 100 ml vials

   Composition: Each ml contains Meloxicam 5 mg, Paracetamol 150 mg, Lignocaine HCl 1 per cent w/v, Benzylalcohol 1 per cent w/v.

Dose: 1 ml/10 kg body weight by deep IM route for all animals.

3. *Melonex Plus Injection* (Intas) – 30 ml and 100 ml vials

   Composition: Each ml contains Meloxicam 5 mg, Paracetamol 150 mg and Lignocaine 1 per cent w/v.

   Dose: Large animal – 15-20 ml/300 kg body weight.

   Calf, Sheep and Goat – 1 ml/10 kg body weight.

   Administration by IM route only.

4. *Proxivet Injection* (Wockhardt) – 30 ml and 100 ml vials

   Composition: Each ml contains Meloxicam 5 mg + Paracetamol 150 mg.

   Dose: Large animal – 20-25 ml/300 kg body weight

5. *Melobest-P Injection* (TTK) – 15 ml, 30 ml and 100 ml vials

   Composition: Each ml contains Meloxicam 5 mg and Paracetamol 150 mg.

   Dose: Large animal – 1 ml/150 kg body weight IM for all animals.

   Small animal – 3 ml per animal/day.

19.6.4 Ketoprofen (Safe and Effective NSAID)

It is recommended for both IM and IV use having analgesic, anti-inflammatory and antipyretic action. It rapidly reduces inflammation and mammary oedema. It has got potent antipyretic action, abolishes fever within 3 to 4 hours. It is safe for use in both lactating and pregnant animals. Indications are pyrexia, clinical and subclinical mastitis, udder oedema, lameness, all types of inflammation along with antimicrobial therapy.

Trade Names

1. *Neoprofen Injection* (Vetnex) – 15 ml and 100 ml vials

   Dose: Cattle, Buffalo, Camel, Pig, Sheep and Goat – 3 mg/kg body weight (1 ml/33 kg body weight) by IM/IV for 3-5 days.

   Horse – 2.2 mg/kg body weight (1 ml/45 kg body weight) by IM, IV or SC route for 3-4 days.

2. *Ketop Injection* (Alembic)

   Composition: Each ml contains Ketoprofen 100 mg.

3. *Butagesic-K* (Concept) – 30 ml and 100 ml vials

   Dose: Cattle, Buffalo, Camel, Pig, Sheep and Goat – 2-4 mg/kg body weight IM, IV once daily for 3 to 5 days.

   Dog and Cat – 2 mg/kg body weight by SC for 3-5 days.

   Horse – 2.2 mg/kg body weight by IV once daily for 3-5 days.

19.6.5 Nimesulide Injection

It is a NSAID with selective cox-2 inhibition resulting in decreased gastric irritation and decreased physiological disturbances. It blocks histamine release and reduces the inflammatory pain much faster.

Indication

Pyrexia, musculo skeletal affections, lameness, joint affections, trauma, sprain, wound, arthritis, Bursitis, Sinuvitis, ENT affections (Rhinitis, Otitis, Pharyngitis *etc.*), URT, LLT infections, FMD, Contagious ecthyma, Mastitis, Post operative and surgical inflammatory conditions.

Trade Names

1. *Nimovet Injection* (Indian Immunologicals) – 1 ml, 15 ml and 50 ml

   Composition: Each ml contains Nimesulide – 100 mg.

   Dose: Cattle, Buffalo, Sheep and Goat – 2-4 mg/kg body weight.

   Dog – 3-5 mg/kg body weight at 24 hours interval.
2. *Injection Nimodex* (Oxen Labs) – 30 ml and 100 ml vials

   Composition: Each ml contains Nimesulide 100 mg.

   Dose: Cattle and Buffalo – 2-4 mg/kg body weight

   Sheep and Goat – 2-4 mg/kg body weight

   Dog – 3-5 mg/kg body weight.
3. *Nimesulide Injection* (Daffodills) – 15 ml vial

   Dose: Sheep and Goat – 2-4 mg/kg body weight

   Cattle and Buffalo – 2.4 mg/kg body weight
   Administration by deep I/M injection, daily for 2-3 days.
4. *Oxalgin-Np Injection* (Zydus AHL) – 15 ml vial

   Composition: Nimesulide injection 100 per cent w/v, *i.e.*, each ml contains Nimesulide 100 mg.

   Dose: Cattle and Buffalo – 4 mg/kg body weight

   Sheep and Goat – 2 mg/kg body weight.

19.6.6 Analgin

It is also known as Metamizole or Phenyl dimethyl Pyrazolone. It has got potent analgesic and antipyretic effects.

Indication

Colic and other spasmodic conditions of visceral organs, Neuritis, Neuralgia, Rheumatic conditions of muscles and joints. Post operative pains, injuries, gastritis, chocking *etc.*

Trade Names

1. *Vetalgin Vet Injection* (Intervet) – 30 ml vial

   Composition: Each ml contains 0.5 g analgin.

   Dose: 8 ml/100 kg body weight IM.

Horse 20-50 ml IM; Cattle and Buffalo – 20-40 ml; Foal, Calf, Pig – 5-15 ml IM; Sheep and Goat – 2-5 ml IM; Dog and Cat – 1.5 ml IM.

2. *Analgin Injection* (Oxen Labs) – 30 ml

   Composition: Each ml contains 500 mg.

   Dose: Cattle, Buffalo and Horse – 15-20 ml IM.

   Sheep and Goat – 2-3 ml IM.

   Foal, Calf and Pig – 5 ml IM.

   Dog – 1-2 ml IM.

3. *Bolin Injection* (Merind) – 30 ml vial

   Composition: Each ml contains Analgin 150 mg + Paracetamol 150 mg.

   Dose: Cattle and Buffalo – 25-50ml IM

   Foal and Calf – 8-20 ml IM.

   Sheep and Goat – 3-10 ml IM.

   Horse – 25-30 ml IM.

   Dog and Cat – 2-5 ml IM.

(*ii*) Oral Preparations of NSAID

19.6.7 Meloxicam Group (with or without Paracetamol)

Indication

Pain, inflammation and fever.

Trade Names

1. *Melonex Bolus* (Intas)

   Composition: Each bolus contains Meloxicam 100 mg.

   Dose: Large animal – 2 boli/400 kg body weight daily.

   Small animal – 1/4th to ½ bolus daily orally.

2. *A3 Vet Bolus* (Brihans)

   Composition: Each bolus contains Meloxicam 100 mg + Paracetamol 1500 mg.

   Dose: Large animal – 1-2 bolus/day.

   Small animal – ½–1 bolus/day.

3. *M.P. Con Bolus* (Pharmacon Vet)

   Composition: Each bolus contains Meloxicam 100 mg and Paracetamol 1500 mg.

   Dose: Large animal – 1-2 bolus twice daily.

   Small animal – ½ to 1 bolus daily.

4. *Lofac-M. Bolus* (Legend) – 4 boli blister strip

   Dose: Large animal – 1-2 boli daily.

   Small animal: ½ bolus daily.

19.6.8 Nimesulide + Paracetamol Combination (NSAID)

Indication

Inflammation, pain and fever, Osteoarthritis, Myositis, Barsitis, Fibrositis, Tenosynovitis, Metritis, Mastitis, Prolapse, Pyrexia of unknown origin, post operative therapy, Respiratory tract inflammation *etc.*

Trade Names

1. *Oxalgin-NP* (Zydus AHL) – Blisters of 4 boli.

   Composition: Each bolus contains Nimesulide 400 mg + Paracetamol 1500 mg.

   Dose: Large animal – 1 to 2 boli

   Small animal – ½ to 1 bolus.
2. *Nimulite Plus* (Vets Farma) – 4 boli Strip

   Composition: Nimesulide and Paracetamol bolus.

   Dose: Large animal – 1-2 boli

   Small animal – ½ to 1 bolus orally.
3. *Arogesic-P Bolus* (Anol)

   Dose: Large animal – 1-2 boli BID.

   Small animal – ½-1 bolus BID.

19.6.9 Phenyl Butazone and Analgin Combination

Indication

Fever, pyrexia, pain, rheumatism, arthritis, myositis and neuritis.

Trade Names

1. *Esgipyrin-N Injection* (Sarabhai Zydus) – 5 ml ampoules

   Composition: Each ml contains Phenylbutazone 750 mg, Analgin 750 mg and Lignocaine HCl 50 mg.

   Dose: Cattle, Buffalo and Horse – 2.2 – 4.4 mg/kg body weight.

   Dog – 2.2 mg/kg body weight, maximum 5 ml/day by deep IM route.

   In general for large animal 5-15 ml IM and for small animal1-5 ml IM.

19.7 ANTISPASMODIC DRUG (FOR COLIC)

19.7.1 Dicyclomine HCl

An anticholinergic, antispasmodic drug indicated for G.I. colic and other visceral organ pain – like renal colic, biliary colic, intestinal colic, abdominal pain due to diarrhoea, spasms of uterus and ureters, prolapse of vagina and uterus, irritable bowel syndrome. Reducing pain after manual removal of retained placenta and post dystocia.

Trade Names

1. *Spasmovet Injection* (Wockhardt) – 30 ml vial
   Composition: Dicyclomine HCl
2. *Spasgan Injection* (Oxen Labs) – 30 ml vial
   Composition: Dicyclomine HCl
3. *Spasmonim Bolus* (Excel) – Strip of 6 boli
   Composition: Dicyclomine HCl 60 mg + Nimesulide 300 mg.
   Dose: Large animal 1-2 bolus, may be repeated after 12 hours.
   Small animal ½–1 bolus, may be repeated after 12 hours.

19.7.2 Valthamate Bromide

It is a potent and safe antispasmodic indicated for colic/visceral pains of abdominal origin. It has dual mode of activity, both musculotropic and Neurotropic.

Indication

Intestinal spasms, diarrhoea, renal colic, prolapse of uterus and during AI, all types of visceral pain of abdominal origin (intestinal spasms, uterine pain *etc.*)

Trade Names

1. *Epidosin Injection* (TTK) – 10 ml and 30 ml RC vials
   Composition: It contains Valthamate bromide 1 per cent.
   Dose: Cattle and Horse 8-10 ml
   Sheep and Goat 2-5 ml
   Dog 1-2 ml.

19.8 CORTICOSTEROIDS

The important corticosteroids used in veterinary practice are:

1. Prednisolone
2. Dexamethasone
3. Triamcenolone
4. Betamethasone

19.8.1 Prednisolone

It is a synthetic, dehydrogenated analogue of hydrocortisone. Contraindicated in pregnancy if used in large doses. It is 3-5 times more active than hydrocortisone and does not affect mineral balance.

Indication

Shock, Ketosis (Acetonemia in cattle), Arthrtitis, Allergy, Hypersensitivity, Rheumatoid arthritis, Bursitis, inflammatory and allergic conditions in large and small animals in conjunction with appropriate antibiotic or chemotherapeutic agent when indicated.

Trade Names

1. *Prednisolone Acetate Injection* (Intervet) – 10 ml vial

   Composition: It is an injectable suspension where each ml contains Prednisolone acetate 10 mg.

   Dose: Cattle – 50-200 mg IM.

2. *Predox Injection* (Oxen Lab) – 10 ml vial

   Composition: Each ml contains Prednisolone acetate 10 mg.

   Dose: Cattle – 50-200 mg, Calf – 25-50 mg, Piglet, Dog and Cat – 10-30 mg. Administration by IM route at an interval of 24 hours or 2-4 times if necessary.

   Injection into Bursae – 10-50 mg.

   Injection into joints – Large animal 25-75 mg; Dog and Cat 5-20 mg.

19.8.2 Dexamethasone

Basically it resembles prednisolone. It has no electrolyte retaining property. It is a highly effective glucocorticoid with powerful anti inflammatory and Ketogenic action.

Indication

Ketosis (Acetonaemia), pregnancy toxaemia, induction of parturition, arthritis, synovitis, tendonitis, pruritis, eczema, otitis, inflammation of respiratory tract, urogenital tract, toxaemia, acute and peracute mastitis, dystocia, shocks (*viz.* anaphylactic, traumatic, haemorrhagic, surgical, septic, obstetrical shock), all inflammatory conditions, dermatological disorders *etc.*

Administration : By IM or IV route.

Trade Names

1. *Brisone Injection* (Brihans) – 5 ml vial

   Composition: Each ml contains Dexamethasone Phosphate 4 mg.

   Dose: Cattle, Buffalo and Horse 2-5 ml/day in divided doses.

   Calf, Sheep, Goat and Pig 0.5-1 ml/day.

   Dog 0.2-0.5 ml/day.

2. *Enidex Injection* (Excel) – 5 ml and 10 ml vials

   Dose: Cattle, Buffalo and Horse – 2-6 ml IM or IV.

   Calf, Sheep and Goat – 1-2 ml IM or IV.

   Dog and Cat – 0.2-1 ml IM or IV.

   Intra articular Injection for large animal – 0.5-2 ml.

   Peri articular Injection for small animal – 0.1-1 ml.

3. *Cadex Injection* (Cril) – 5 ml vial
4. *Dexona Injection* (Sarabhai Zydus) – 5 ml vial
5. *Curadex Vet Injection* (Concept) – 5 ml vial

6. *Dexonil Injection* (Reedson) – 5 ml and 10 ml vials
7. *Vetocort Injection* (Alembic) – 5 ml and 10 ml vials

   Dose: Cattle and Horse – 4-20 mg (1-5 ml) daily.

   Calf, Pig, Sheep and Goat – 2-4 mg (0.5-1 ml) daily.

   Dog and Cat – 0.5-2 mg daily.
8. *Dexo Injection* (Daffodil) – 5 ml and 10 ml vials

   Having 100 per cent anti-inflammatory and gluconeogenic activity (anti Ketotic effects).
9. *Anicort Injection* (IBC) – 5 ml vial

   Composition: It is a powerful corticosteroid. Each ml contains Dexamethasone Sodium Phosphate equivalent to 4 mg of Dexamethasone Phosphate.

   Dose: Cattle and Horse – 4-20 mg daily or 1-5 ml daily

   Calf, Sheep, Goat and Pig – 2-4 mg daily *i.e.* 0.5-1 ml daily.

   Dog and Cat – 0.5-2 mg daily *i.e.* 0.25-0.5 ml daily.

19.8.3 Triamcenolone

It is a highly potent synthetic glucocorticoid and anti-inflammatory agent for parenteral administration in the treatment of bovine ketosis and various arthritis and dermatoses in animals.

Indication

Acetonemia (Bovine Ketosis), arthritic disorders (arthritis, tendosynovitis), dermatologic disorders, eczema, dermatitis, frictional allergic reactions like pruritus, conjunctivitis, reaction to insect bites, allergic dermatitis, pain, oedema and inflammation.

Trade Names

1. *Vetalog Injection* (Sarabhai Zydus) – 5 ml vial

   Composition: Each ml contains 6 mg Triamcinolone.

   Dose: 2.5-10 mg to be given in a single IM injection for Bovine Ketosis.

   Horse and Cattle – In intra articular/intrasynovial 6-18 mg IM, SC; in arthritic and allergic condition – 10-20 mg.

   Dog and Cat – 1-3 mg (Intra articular injection) or 0.1-0.2 mg/kg body weight IM or SC.

   Vetalog injection should not be used in pregnant and neonates.

19.9 PARENTERAL ANTIHISTAMINIC

Blocks the histamine effect at receptor sites, thus antagonize the stimulant action of histamine on the smooth muscle of G.I. tract, uterus and blood vessels. This compound has moderate sedation action.

Indication

Allergy, Anaphylactic shock, Dermatitis, Itching, Rhinitis, Pruritus, Urticaria, Laminitis, Eczema, Drug allergy, insect bites, pulmonary oedema, Burns, pregnancy toxaemia, Puerperal toxemia. Bloat, pulmonary emphysema (in horses). Photodermatitis, Retained Placenta.

Trade Names

1. *Inj. Antilar* (Reedson) – 30 ml vial

   Composition: Each ml contains Chlorpheniramine maleate 10 mg.

   Dose: Large animal – 5-10 ml, Small animal – 0.5-2 ml IM.

2. *Inj. Anistamin* (Intas) – 30 ml, 50 ml and 100 ml vials

   Composition: Each ml contains Chlorpheniramine maleate 10 mg.

   Dose: Large animal 5-10 ml

   Small animal – 1-2 ml.

   Dog – 0.5-10 ml IM.

3. *Inj. Cpm Vet* (Cipla) – 30 ml and 100 ml vials

   Composition: Each ml contains Chlorpheniramine maleate 10 mg.

   Dose: Large animals 3-5 ml, Small animal 1-2 ml, Dog – 0.5-1 ml IM only.

4. *Alergo Injection* (Jeps) – 10 ml, 30 ml and 100 ml vials

   Composition: Each ml contains Chlorpheniramine maleate 10 mg/ml.

   Dose: Small animal – 0.5-1 ml.

   Large animal – 3-5 ml IM only.

5. *Chlorazin Injection (CRIL)* – 10 ml and 30 ml vials

   Dose: Cattle and Horse – 3-5 ml

   Sheep, Goat and Pig – 1-2 ml,

   Dog and Cat – 0.5 ml.

6. *Chloril Vet Injection* (TTK) – 30 ml and 100 ml vials

7. *Biostamin Inj.* (IBC) – 10 ml and 30 ml vials

   Dose: Large animal 3-5ml IM. Small animal 0.5-2 ml IM.

8. *Pheniramine Maleate Injection* (Intervet) – 30 ml vial

   Composition: Each ml contains 22.75 mg.

   Dose: Large animal – 5-10 ml.

   Small animal – 2-3 ml by IM route only.

9. *Phenimal Injection* (Oxen Lab) – 30 ml and 100 ml vials

   Composition: Chlorpheniramine maleate – 10 mg/ml.

11. *Phenimal-DS Injection* (Oxen Lab) – 30 ml and 100 ml vials

    Composition: Each ml contains Chlorpheniramine maleate – 20 mg/ml.

12. *Zeet Injection* (Alembic) – 10 ml and 30 ml vials
    Composition: Chlorpheniramine maleate.
    Dose: Large animal – 10-15 ml IM. Small animal – 0.5-2 ml IM.
13. *Avil Injection* (Intervet) – 10 ml vial
    Composition: Pheniramine maleate.
    Chemically it is 1-phenyl 1-pyridyl 2,3-Dimethyl aminopropane maleate (Pheniramine Maleate)
    Dose: Large animal – 5-10 ml or more IM
    Small animal – 0.5 ml or more IM.

19.10 HAEMOSTAT

19.10.1 Ethamsylate/Adenochrome Monosemicarbazone

Most effective for prevention and treatment of capillary haemorrhages associated with haematemesis, haematuria, haemagalactia, malena, epistaxis, post partum haemorrhage, prevention and treatment of pre-operative bleeding in all procedures in highly vascular tissues.

It acts on the first step of haemostasis by improving platelet-adhesiveness and restoring capillary resistance, maintains the fibrinogen level unchanged, inhibits prostacycline synthetase enzyme, helps in the formation of platelet plug, helps in formation of a blood clot. It has no impairment of gestation. Foetal development is normal. It has no malformation or macroscopic abnormality apparent in the embryo or new born.

Dose

Basic dose is 7.5 mg/kg body weight by IM or IV.

Trade Names

1. *Bleed Check Injection* (Bee Tee Pharmaceuticals) – 2 ml x 5 in a box
   Composition: Each ml contains 125 mg Ethamsylate.
2. *Chromostat Injection* – 2 ml and10 ml vials
3. *Botropase Injection* (Juggat) – 1 ml/2 ml amp
4. *Dafochrome Vet Injection* (Daffodills) – 10 ml vial
   Composition: Adenochrome Monosemicarbazone – 0-75 mg/ml.
   Dose : Large animal – 10 ml IM or IV.
   Small animal – 2-3 ml IM or IV.
5. *Sirochrome Injection* (Albert David) – 2 ml amp
   Composition: Each ml containing 0.75 mg Adenochrome Monosemicarbazone.
6. *Styptocid Injection* (Stadmid) – 2 ml amp

19.11 PARENTERAL VITAMINS AND MINERALS

19.11.1 Vitamin-A

Vitamin-A has got most potent epithelial regenerating property, maintains normal activity of osteoblasts and osteoclasts. It crosses placental barrier unlike β-carotene from green grasses. It is an essential vitamin for higher productivity, better eye sight, foetal development and udder immunity.

Indication

Anoestrum, delayed ovulation, repeat breeder, premature still birth, retention of placenta, maintaining healthy epithelial structures and to improve immunity, skin disorders, night blindness, diarrhoea cases to heal the epithelial discontinuity of GI tract, surgical cases for faster wound healing, optimum spermatogenesis in breeding bull, also in Mastitis.

Trade Names

1. *Veta-A Injection* (TTK) – 2 ml ampoules

   Composition: Vitamin-A 6 lakh I.U./2 ml.

   Dose: Repeat breeder (Cattle and Buffalo) – 2-3 ampoules on 1st and 3rd days.

   Pregnant animals (Cattle and Buffalo) – 2-3 ampoules 45 days before parturition.

   Hypovitaminosis-A –

   Large animal 6 ampoules/week.

   Small animal 3-5 ampoules/week.

   Dog and Cat 1-3 ampoules/week.

   (In divided doses by deep IM route).

2. *Vitamin-A Injection* (IBC) – 2 ml amp

   Dose: Large animal 12 ml/week. Small animal 6-12 ml/week.

   Dog and Cat 2-6 ml/week.

   By deep IM route only.

   In infertility condition of females and breeding bulls 6 ml on 1st and 3rd day.

3 *Vitamin A Injection* (Legend) – 2 ml amp

4. *Vitamin A Injection* (GSK) – 2 ml amp

   High potency Vitamin A injection.

   Dose: For treating infertility – Large animal 6 ml on 1st and 3rd day by IM route.

   Small animal 2 ml on 1st and 3rd day by IM route.

   For Hypovitaminosis-A Large animal 12 ml per week.

   In pregnancy 12 ml each month for large animal and 2-6 ml for small animal per week.

19.11.2 Vitamin-AD_3 Injection

Indication

First line therapy in deficient fertility.

Anoestrus, infertility in animals (both males and females), prevention of early abortion, healthy foetal growth, night blindness, rickets and osteomalacia, muscular degeneration, xeropthalmia, keratomalacia, epilepsy, stunted growth, supportive treatment in respiratory, GI and urogenital tract infections.

Trade Names

1. *Vitacept Injection* (Concept) – 5 ml and 10 ml vials

   Composition: Each ml provides Vitamin A 25,000 I.U., Vitamin D_3 25000 I.U. and Vitamin E 100 mg.

   Dose:

   Cattle and Horse – 10 ml/week (5 ml twice in a week)

   Calf, Sheep and Goat – 5 ml/week by IM route.

   Dog – 1-2 ml.

2. *Intavita Injection* (Intas) – 10 ml vial

   Dose: Calf – 2-4 ml.

   Cow, Buffalo, Bull – 6-10 ml.

   Horse – 4 ml.

   Ewe, Ram and Colt – 2 ml.

   Swine – 1ml by deep IM injection.

3. *Betade Injection* (Bee Tee Pharma) – 5 ml vial

   Dose: Convenient weekly dose.

   Cattle, Buffalo and Horse – 5 ml x 2/week

   Dog – 1-2 ml/week.

   Calf, Sheep and Goat – 5 ml/week.

4. *Brivit Injection* (Brihans) – 10 ml and 30 ml vials

   It is a powerful injection of Vitamin A D_3 and E indicated for infertility, repeat breeding, grass tetany, prophylaxis to hypovitaminosis.

   Dose: Large animal – 6-10 ml twice in a week.

   Small animal – 2-3 ml twice in a week.

5. *Vitade Injection* (Sarabhai Zydus) – 10 ml and 30 ml vials

   Dose: Cattle and Buffalo – For prevention 4-6 ml; For treatment 6-10 ml by deep IM route.

   Calf – For prevention 1-2 ml; For treatment 2-4 ml.

   Sheep and Goat – For prevention 1-2 ml; For treatment 2-4 ml.

6. *Adcelin Injection* (Virbac) – 5 ml vial

   Dose: For treating infertility

Large animal – 5 ml on 1st and 3rd day by IM route.

Small animal – 2 ml on 1st day and 3rd day by IM route.

For Hypovitaminosis

Large animal – 10 ml per week.

Small animal – 2-5 ml per week.

In pregnancy for large animal – 10 ml each month.

7. *Lavitone-H Injection* (TTK) – 5 ml vial

   Composition: Vitamin A, D_3, E and Biotin.

   Dose: 5 ml/250-300 kg body weight by IM route.

19.11.3 Injectable Vitamin B-Complex

Vitamin B-Complex are responsible for the biosynthesis of various metabolic enzymes of the body and plays role in protein, fat and carbohydrate metabolism. Choline chloride synthesizes acetylcholine which in turn mobilises fat from the fatty liver thus prevents fatty change in liver. Improves immunity, stimulates nerve and liver function, debility, stunted growth, systemic acidosis, anaemia, nervous disorders, ataxia, paraplegia neuritis, epileptic form of seizures, muscular weakness, rough skin, alopecia, as a co-therapy with antibiotics for fast recovery. The common indications are reproductive disorders, repeat breeding, anoestrous, silent heat, for improving conception rate and improving performance of weak, anaemic and debilitated animals.

Trade Names

1. *Feroliv Injection* (Excell) – 50 ml vial

   Dose: Large animal – 5-10 ml daily for 5-7 days by IM route.

   Small animal – 2.5-5 ml daily for 5-7 days by IM route.

2. *Conciplex Injection* (Concept) – 10 ml and 30 ml vials

   A high potency Vitamin B-Complex for parenteral use.

   Dose: Large animal – 5 ml for 3 to 5 days.

   Small animal – 2 ml for 3 to 5 days by IM injection.

3. *Cavit Injection* (Brihans) – 30 ml and 100 ml vials

   Dose: Large animal – 10 ml/day.

   Small animal – 2.5 ml/day by IM, SC and slow IV route.

4. *Hivit Injection* (Vetnex) – 30 ml and 50 ml vials

   Dose: 1 ml/10-15 kg body weight by IM or slow IV or SC route.

5. *Pinkojet Injection* (Brihans) – 10 ml and 30 ml vials

   Dose:

   Large animal – 6-10 ml

   Small animal – 2.5 ml.

   Daily for 4-5 days through IM or IV route after dilution.

6. *X-L Pex Forte Injection* (Alved) – 10 ml and 30 ml vials
   Dose: Large animal – 10 ml IM.
   Small animal – 3-5 ml IM
7. *Btplex-C Injection* (Bee Tee Pharma) – 10 ml and 30 ml vials
   Composition: B-complex with choline chloride and amino acid.
   Dose:
   Large animal – 10 ml IM
   Small animal – 3-5 ml IM.
8. *Beejet Injection* (Vets Farma) – 30 ml
   Composition: A metabolic stimulant Vitamin B_1, B_2, B_3, B_5, B_6 and B_{12}.
9. *X-L Pex Injection* (Alved) – 30 ml vial
10. *Toxol Injection* (Vesper) – 30 ml vial
11. *Vesplex Forte* (Vesper Pharmaceuticals) – 30 ml vial.
12. *Pepsid-C* (Concept) – 10 ml and 30 ml vials
    Composition: Vitamin B-Complex + Choline.
    Dose: Large animal – 10 ml IM daily.
    Small animal – 0.5 – 1 ml IM daily.

19.11.4 Neurotropic B-Vitamins (B_1, B_6, B_{12})

Composition

Vitamin B_1 (Thiamine HCl), Vitamin B_6 (Pyridoxine HCl) and Vitamin B_{12} (Cyanocobalamin). Vitamin B_1 is needed for energy metabolism, Vitamin B_6 for amino acid metabolism and B_{12} for synthesis of nucleic acid and to maintain metabolic factor.

Indication

Nervine disorders, debility, anaemia, anorexia, liver distress, poor growth, pregnancy, convalescence, adjunct to antibiotic and anthelmintic therapy.

Trade Names

1. *Pyri. B Forte* (Phonex) – 10 ml vial
   Dose: Cattle and Buffalo – 10 ml IM on alternate day by IM or IV route.
   Small animal – 3 ml IM on alternate day by IM or IV.
2. *Tribivet Injection* (Intas) – 2 ml, 10 ml, 30 ml and 50 ml vials
   Dose: Dog and Cat – 0.5-2 ml on alternate day IM or IV.
   Large animal – 5-10 ml.
   Sheep and Goat – 1-2 ml on alternate day by IM or IV route.
3. *Neurovet Injection* (Alved) – 10 ml and 30 ml vials
   Dose: Horse, Cattle and Buffalo – 5-10 ml IM daily.
   Small animal – 1-2 ml IM daily.

4. *Neuroxin-12 Injection* (Sarabhai Zydus)

   Composition : Each ml contains Vitamin B_1-30 mg, B_6 – 13.75 mg and B_{12} – 500 mg.

   Dose: Horse, Cattle and Buffalo – 5-10 ml IM daily for 3-5 days.

   Dog – 2-3 ml IM daily for 3-5 days.

   Sheep and Goat – 2-3 ml IM on alternate day.

5. *Polyvet-B Injection* (Excell) – 30 ml vial

   Dose: Cattle, Buffalo and Horse – 10-15 ml IM or IV.

   Colt, Calf, Sheep, Goat and Pig – 5 ml IM or IV.

   Dog – 2-3 ml IM.

6. *Bion-12 Vet Injection* (Morvel) – 10 ml vial

   Dose: Cattle and Buffalo – 10 ml IM.

   Calf, Sheep and Goat – 2-5 ml IM.

7. *Vitamyl Injection* (Cipla) – 30 ml and 50 ml vials

   Dose: Large animal – 10 ml/day by IM route.

   Calf and Foal – 5 ml/day by IM route.

   Sheep and Goat – 1-3 ml/day by IM route.

   Cat and Dog – 0.25-1 ml/day by IM route.

19.11.5 Vitamin-E Injectable Preparation

Vitamin-E is essential for anti-oxidation, better immune system function and udder immunity.

Indication

Clinical and subclinical mastitis, preventing retention of placenta (ROP) and mastitis in early lactation, muscular dystrophy.

Trade Names

1. *E-Care-Se Injection* (Vetcare) – 10 ml vial

   Composition: Vitamin E + Selenium.

   Dose: Clinical mastitis – 10 ml at 3 days interval 2-3 doses.

   Sub-clinical mastitis – 10 ml at weekly interval.

   Muscular dystrophy – 1 ml/50 kg body weight single dose.

   ROP (retention of placenta) and mastitis in early lactation – 3 injections at weekly intervals, 3 weeks prior to calving.

19.11.6 Liver Extract with Vitamin B-Complex Injection

The parenteral preparations are processed and prepared from detoxified crude liver extract having higher strength of Niacinamide, Decarboxylation, demethylation and deamination properties (metabolic activities) and revitalizing the nerve tissues.

Indication

Supportive therapy in liver disorders (Hepatitis, Jaundice), indigestion, diarrhoea and other G.I. disorders, non-specific anorexia and off fed conditions, debility and general weakness, blood protozoan diseases, skin and neurological disorders, neuropathy, recumbency and downers cow syndrome, anaemia, alopecia, ruminal and intestinal atony, post-insemination vitamin therapy, Vitamin B-complex deficiency and neuralgic convulsions.

Trade Names

1. *Biomex Forte Injection* (IBC) – 10 ml and 30 ml vials

   Dose: 1 ml/30 kg body weight daily or on alternate day for 3-5 days by deep IM route.
2. *Livobex Injection* (TTK) – 10 ml and 30 ml vials

   Dose: Cattle, Buffalo and Horse – 10 ml.

   Sheep, Goat and Pig – 5 ml.

   Dog – 2 ml

   Cat -1 ml.

   By IM route only and for 3-5 days daily or on alternate day.
3. *Nutriliv Injection* (Vet Care) – 10 ml and 30 ml vials

   Dose: Large animal 5-10 ml daily by IM.

   Small animal 0.5-2 ml twice daily by IM.
4. *Stronic Injection* (Vetnex) – 30 ml and 100 ml vials

   Dose: 1 ml/30 kg body weight daily as IM injection for 3-5 days.
5. *Pinkojet-L* (Brihans) – 10 ml, 30 ml and 50 ml vials

   Composition: Liver extract, Vitamin B-complex and Vitamin B_{12}.

   Dose: Large animal – 5-10 ml/day by deep IM injection for 3-5 days.

   Small animal – 1-2 ml/day by deep IM injection for 3-5 days.
6. *Hepatogen Injection* (Jeps) – 10 ml and 30 ml vials

   Dose: Large animal – 5-10 ml on alternate day for 7-10 days.

   Small animal – 1-2 ml on alternate day for 7-10 days by deep IM injection.
7. *Livodex Injection* (Oxen Lab) – 30 ml and 50 ml vials

   Composition: Liver extract with vitamin B-complex and B_{12}.

   Dose: Cattle, Buffalo and Horse – 5-10 ml IM on alternate day.

   Calf, Sheep, Goat and Pig – 3-5 ml IM on alternate day.
8. *Belamyl Injection* (Sarabhai Zydus) – 10 ml, 30 ml and 50 ml vials

   Dose: Large animal – 4-5 ml IM followed by 3 ml after 72 hours.

   Small animal – 0.25-0.5 ml IM followed by 0.5 ml after 72 hours.
9. *Levadex Injection* (GSK) – 30 ml vial
10. *Livron Injection* (Vets Farma) – 30 ml vial and 50 ml vials

11. *Livo-Bee Injection* (Marion Pharma) – 30 ml and 50 ml vials
12. *B-Com-L Injection* (Wockhardt) – 30 ml vial
13. *N-D Plex Forte-L Injection* (Nandini Lab) – 30 ml vials
14. *Bovoplex-C Injection* (Indian Immunologicals) – 30 ml vial

    Composition: B-complex vitamins + Liver extract + Choline chloride.

    Dose: Cattle, Buffalo and Horse – 10 ml daily for 3 or more days.

    Calf, Sheep, Goat and Pig – 5 ml daily for 3 or more days.

    Dog and Cat – 2 ml daily for 3 or more days.

    By deep IM injection.
15. *Zenliv-Fort Injection* (Tanen Pharmaceuticals) – 10 ml and 30 ml vials

    Dose: Large animal 5-10 ml IM daily for 3 days.

    Small animal 1-2 ml IM daily for 3 days.

19.11.7 Power Packed Injection of Calcium, Vitamin D_3 and B_{12} (Injectable Calcium for IM use)

1. Calcium Glucono Lactobionate with Vitamin D_3 and B_{12}.
2. Calcium Levulinate with Vitamin D_3 and B_{12}.

Indication

Prevention and treatment of hypocaecalmia in cows and buffaloes particularly during pre and post calving period, debility and weakness, for early expulsion of placenta and uterine involution, for prevention of ketosis and dystocia, maintaining steady milk production, treating anorexia, to meet up negative calcium balance. both prophylactic and curative purposes in deficiency conditions, stunted growth, stress of various etiology, dermatological disorders, for better health performance and production, weak body skeleton *etc.*

Trade Names

19.11.7.1 Preparations Containing Calcium Levulinate

1. *Brical Injection* (Brihans) – 30 ml vial

   Composition: Power packed injection of Calcium levulinate with Vitamin D_3 and Vitamin B_{12}.

   Dose: Cattle and Buffalo – 10-15 ml thrice in a week by IM route.

   Small animal – 2-3 ml thrice in a week by IM route.
2. *Orical Injection* (IBC) – 30 ml vial

   Composition: A power packed injection of Calcium levulinate with Vitamin D_3 and Vitamin B_{12}.

   Dose: Large animal – 10-15 ml 3 times a week for 1-2 weeks during last trimester of pregnancy; 15 ml 6-8 hours before and after parturition and 20-30 ml immediately after parturition for prevention of milk fever, expulsion of placenta and uterine involution.

   Small animal – 2-3 ml twice a week for 1-2 weeks by IM route.

3. *Hylactin Injection* (Jeps) – 10 ml and 30 ml vials

   Composition: Each ml contains Calcium levulinate 76.4 mg with Cholecalciferol (Vitamin D_3) and Cyanocobalamin (Vitamin B_{12}).

   Dose: Large animal 10-15 ml on alternate day for 10-15 days.

   Small animal 0.5-1 ml on alternate day for 10-15 days by IM injection.

4. *Calcimal Injection* (Oxen Lab) – 30 ml and 50 ml vials

   Composition: Calcium with Vitamin D_3 and B_{12}.

   Dose: Large animal 10-15 ml on alternate day or twice a week for 1-2 weeks.

   Small animal: 2-3 ml twice a week for 1-2 weeks.

   By IM route.

19.11.7.2 Preparations containing Calcium Gluconolactobionate with Vitamin D_3 E B_{12}

1. *Calcinet Injection* (Excell) – 30 ml vial

   Composition: Each ml contains Calcium gluconolactobionate 137.5 mg with vitamin D_3 and B_{12}.

   Dose: For preparturition Cattle and Buffalo 10-15 ml IM thrice a week for 1-2 weeks.

   For post parturition Cattle and Buffalo 15-20 ml IM thrice a week for 2 weeks.

   For Lactating Cattle and Buffalo 10-15 ml thrice a week for 1-2 weeks.

   By IM route.

2. *Sancal Vet Injection* (Novartis) – 15 ml and 45 ml vials

   Composition: Each ml contains Calcium gluconolactobionate – 137.5 mg, Vitamin D_3 – 5000 I.U. and Vitamin B_{12} – 50 mg.

   Dose: Cattle and Buffalo

   To prevent onset of milk fever – 15 ml 6-8 hours before and after parturition, 20-30 ml immediately after calving, by IM route.

   To maintain steady milk production – 10-15 ml thrice a week for 1-2 weeks a month, by IM route.

3. *Capsola Vet Injection* (Vetnex) – 45 ml vial

   Composition: Calcium gluconolactobionate and Vitamin B_{12}.

   Dose: Cattle and Buffalo

   For preparturition 15-20 ml IM twice in a week for 2 weeks.

   For post parturition 15-20 ml IM thrice in a week for 2 weeks.

   For dry Cattle and Buffalo 15 ml IM on alternate day for 2-3 weeks.

19.11.7.3 Parenteral Calcium (IV and SC Use)

Indicated for milk fever complex, downers cow syndrome, metabolic diseases of old cow, hypocalcaemia, post parturient paresis, uterine involution, rumen atony *etc.*

Two types of formulations are available. These are (i) Calcium Boro-gluconate Injection and (ii) Calcium, Magnessium and Dextrose Injection. Before administration of these hypertonic solutions, the solutions should be warmed to body temperature. It is to be administered by slow IV route.

A) Calcium Boro-gluconate: The Leader in Intra Venous Calcium Infusion

1. *Calborol Injection* (Novartis) – 450 ml bottle

   Dose: Large animal 200-350 ml IV.

2. *Intacal Injection* (Intas) – 450 ml bottle

   Composition: Calcium gluconate equivalent to 1.86 per cent w/v of calcium, Boric acid and Calcium ratio 2.26 : 1.

   Dose: Heavy animal – 450 ml.

   Cow, Mare, She buffalo – 200-350 ml.

   Ewe, Doe, Sow – 60 ml slow IV and SC route.

3. *Calvib Injection* (GSK) – 450 ml bottle

   Composition: Calcium borogluconate for IV infusion.

   Dose : Heavy animal – 450 ml IV and SC route.

   Mare, Cow, She buffalo – 200-350 ml IV and SC route.

4. *Calgonate Injection* (Indian Immunologicals) – 450 ml bottle

   Composition: Calcium borogluconate injection for IV infusion.

   Dose: Cow and She buffalo – 200-300 ml.

   Sow, Ewe and Doe – 30-50 ml by IV and SC routes.

5. *Calmax Injection* (Vetnex) – 450 ml bottle

   Dose: Heavy animal 450 ml by slow IV and SC injection.

   Cow, She buffalo and Mare – 200-350 ml by slow IV and SC routes.

   Sow, Ewe and Doe – 30-50 ml by slow IV and SC route.

6. *Calcicat Injection* (Cattle Remedies) – 450 ml bottle

   Dose: Cattle and She buffalo – 200-350 ml by slow IV and SC route.

7. *Thiacal Injection* (Wockhardt) – 450 ml bottles

   Dose: Cow and She buffalo – 250-350 ml by slow IV and SC route.

8. *Calcimal-CBG* (Oxen Lab) – 450 ml bottle

   Dose: Cattle and Buffalo – 200-300 ml IV and SC.

   Ewe and Doe – 25-50 ml IV and SC.

B) Calcium, Magnessium and Dextrose Injection

1. *Lactomag injection* (intas) – 450 ml bottle

   Composition: Each ml contains Calcium gluconate equivalent to 1.86 per cent w/v of calcium, Magnesium hypophosphite – 5 per cent w/v, Anhydrous dextrose – 20 per cent w/v.

   Dose: Heavy animal – 450 ml slow IV infusion.

Cow, Mare and She buffalo – 200-350 ml by slow IV.

Ewe, Doe and Sow – 60 ml by slow IV and SC.

2. *Mifex Injection* (Novartis) – 450 ml bottle

   The most ideal preparation for milk fever complex and associated syndromes.

   Composition: Calcium Borogluconate, Magnesium hypophosphite and Dextrose.

   Dose: 200-350 ml for large animal IV.

3. *Calbim Injection* (GSK) – 450 ml bottle

   Dose: Heavy animal – 450 ml IV and SC route.

   Doe, Ewe and Sow – 60 ml by slow IV and SC route.

4. *Miphocal Injection* (Indian Immunologicals) – 450 ml bottle

   Dose: Cows and Buffalo 200-300 ml by slow IV infusion and SC.

   Ewe, Doe and Sow 30-50 ml by slow IV and SC routes.

5. *Calmax-M* (Vetnex) – 450 ml bottle

   Dose: Heavy animal – 450ml by slow IV and SC routes.

   Cattle and Buffalo – 300-350 ml by slow IV and SC routes.

   Doe, Sow and Ewe – 25-50 ml by slow IV and SC routes.

6. *Calcimag Injection* (Cattle Remedies) – 450 ml bottle

   Dose: Cattle and Buffalo – 300-350 ml by slow IV and SC routes.

19.11.8 Phosphorus

Phosphorus is available in the following forms.

1. Sdium acid phosphate
2. Toldimphos sodium trihydrate
3. Sodium salt of 4-diethylamine 2-methylphenyl phosphoric acid (organic phosphorus).

Indication

It is used for reproductive and metabolic disorders.

Reproductive disorder: Low conception rate, irregular oestrous cycle, anoestrous condition, delayed puberty, underdeveloped genital organs, post parturient haemoglobinuria.

Metabolic disorders: Pica, rickets, milk fever, osteomalacia, downers cow syndrome, Hypophophatemia, Lactation tetany, kidney and heart disorder.

Trade Names

1. *Aciphos Injection* (Excell) – 10 ml and 30 ml vials

   Composition: Sodium acid phosphate – 40 per cent w/v.

Dose: Cattle 8-10 ml on alternate day for 7 days.

Small animal – 2-5 ml on alternate day for 3 days by IM or IV route.

2. *Tonophosphan Injection* (Intervet) – 10 ml and 30 ml vial

   Composition: Each ml contains Sodium salt of 4-diethylamine 2-methylphenyl phosphoric acid – 0.2 g (20 per cent solution). It is an organic phosphorus compound indicated for improving metabolism, production and fertility.

   Dose: Cattle and buffalo – 10-15 ml on alternate day for 5-7 day.

   Sheep and Goat – 2 ml on alternate day.

3. *T-Phos Injection* (Intervet) – 10 ml and 30 ml vial

   Composition : Toldimphos Sodium Trihydrate (20 per cent solution).

   Dose:

   Large animal – 15-25 ml

   Small animal–1-3 ml.

   Half dose by IV and rest by SC or IM divide and give in several sites.

4. *Alphos – 40 Injection* (Alved) – 10 ml and 30 ml vials

   Composition: Sodium acid phosphate – 40 per cent w/v. It is an inorganic phosphorus.

   Dose: Cattle and Buffalo – 10 ml on alternate day for 3 days.

   Small animal – 2-3 ml on alternate day IM.

5. *Urimin Injection* (GSK) – 10 ml and 30 ml vials

   Composition: It contains Acid sodium phosphate 40 per cent and inorganic phosphorus preparation.

   Dose: Cattle and Horse 5-10 ml, Foal and Calf – 1-2 ml, Dog 1-2 ml.

   For infertility Cattle 15 ml on 1st and 3rd day by IM, IV or SC route.

6. *Betphos Injection* (Bee Tee Pharma) – 10 ml and 30 ml vials

   Composition: It is an organic phosphorus, composed of Sodium salt of 4-dimethylamino 2-methylphenyl phosphoric acid – 20 per cent.

   Dose: Large animal 5-20 ml by SC, IM or IV route on alternated day for 5-7 days.

7. *Fertophos* (Glaxo SmithKline) – 30 ml vial

   Composition: Sodium salt of 4-dimethyl amino 2-methylphenyl phosphoric acid trihydrate.

   Dose: Cattle and Buffalo – 10-25 ml every alternate day for 1-2 weeks IM, IV or SC.

   Sheep and Goat – 2 ml IM on alternate day IM, IV or SC.

8. *Ves Phos Injection* (Vesper) – 5 ml ampoules.

   Composition: It contains Sodium acid phosphorus vet equal to elemental phosphorous – 79.4 mg.

   Dose: Cattle and Buffalo – 5-10 ml every alternate day for 1-2 weeks.

9. *Soda Phos Injection* (Vetnex) – 30 ml vial

   Composition: Each ml contains Sodium salt of 4-dimethylamino 2-methyl phenyl phosphoric acid–200 mg.

   Dose: Large animal – 5-15 ml according to body size.

   Small animal – 1-3 ml by IM or SC route on alternate day.

19.12 HORMONES FOR FERTILITY MANAGEMENT

The common hormones used for fertility management are

1. Hydroxy Progesterone Caproate
2. Cloprostenol (PGF2α) – Synthetic Analogue of Prostaglandin F2α
3. Diethyl Stilbosterol
4. Chorionic Gonadotrophin (HCG) – A glycoprotein with Luteinising Hormone activity
5. Dinoprost Trimethiamine
6. Synthetic GnRH Analogue (GnRH) *e.g.* Receptal (Intervet)
7. Pregnant Mare Serum Gonadotrophin (PMSG) *e.g.* Folligon (Intervet).

19.12.1 Diethyl Stilbosterol

Indication

Anoestrous, Mummified foetus, Retention of Placenta, Metritis, Pyometra.

Trade Names

1. *Distrol Injection* (Oxen Lab) – 10 ml vial

   Composition: Each ml contains Diethylstilbosterol -10 mg, for IM use only.

   Dose: For all animals – 20-40 mg/kg body weight SC or IM route.

   For cattle – 50 mg by intra uterine route can be administered.

19.12.2 Hydroxy Progesterone

Indication

Habitual abortion, threatened abortion, corpus luteum insufficiency, for safe pregnancy.

Dose: Cow – 100 mg daily IM or SC; Mare – 100-300 mg daily; Ewe – 10-20 mg daily IM or SC; Dog – 25-50 mg IM or SC.

Trade Names

1. *Fertitone Injection* (Bee Tee Pharma) – 2 ml amp

   Dose : For cow and buffalo

   In habitual abortion 2 ml after 45 days of pregnancy. Repeat the dose after every 10 days for 4-5 times.

   In Repeat Breeders 2 ml/week for 3 weeks.

In Genital prolapses 2 ml/day for 2 days.

Repeat 2 ml after 10 days if required in case of anoestrous.

2. *Duraprogen* (Vet Care) – 2 ml ampoules (250 mg/ml)

   Dose: For threatened and habitual abortion – 500 mg/week.

3. *Utrodex Injection* (Oxen Lab) – 2 ml and 3 ml vials

   Composition: Each ml contains Hydroxy progesterone caproate 250 mg/ml.

   Dose: Cow and She Buffalo – 2-3 ml IM.

4. *Hyprogen Injection* (Reedson) – 2 ml vial

5. *DP-Loton Injection* (Vest Farma) – 2 ml ampoules

   Composition: Injection Hydroxy Progesterone Caproate – 250 mg/ml.

6. *P-Depot Injection* (Sarabhai Zydus) – 2 ml (500 mg) and 3 ml (750 mg) vials

   Composition: A long acting depot progesterone containing Hydroxy progesterone caproate.

   Dose: Early habitual abortion – 2 ml after $1^1/_2$ month pregnancy. Repeat 4-5 times every 10 days interval at late pregnancy. Habitual abortion – 2 ml for 3 days every week for 3 weeks. Repeat breeding – 1-2 ml after A.I. Prolapse of uterus – 2 ml at day 1.

19.12.3 LH Preparation

Indication

Cystic ovaries, repeat breeding.

Trade Names

1. *Lutropin-V* (Vets Farma) – 25 mg/vial + 5 ml diluents

   Dose : 250 mg, repeat in 1-4 week.

2. *Epidosin Vet Injection* (TTK) – 5 ml vial

   Composition: 10 mg/ml.

   Dose: 10 ml IM and repeat if necessary.

19.12.4 Chorionic Gonadotrophin

Indication

Anoestrum, prolonged oestrous, delayed ovulation, nymphomania, cystic ovaries.

Trade Names

1. *Chorulon Injection* (Intervet)

   Composition: Each ml contains Luteinizing hormone (Chorionic gonadotrophin 1500 IU).

   Dose: For Anoestrous Cow 1000-2000 I.U. IM or SC.

   Mare 1500-3000 I.U. IM or SC on the day of service for anovulatory estrous IM or IV or SC.

For Cystic ovaries Rupture manually and then 3000 I.U. IV. May be repeated in 3 weeks cycle.

For Nymphomania with cystic ovaries

Mare – 1800-5000 I.U. IV.

Cow – 1000-3000 I.U. IV.

Combined with rupture or draining of cyst.

19.12.5 Synthetic Analogue to GnRH

Indication

Infertility of ovarian origin, induction of ovulation and improvement of conception.

Trade Names

1. *Receptal Injection* (Intervet) – 10 ml vial

   Composition: 0.0042 mg GnRH equivalent to 0.004 mg Busereline acetate.

   Dose: 5 ml single dose in crossbred animal (As prophylaxis of fertility disorders).

   Cattle and Buffalo for increasing conception rate – 2.5 ml after A.I.

   Follicular cysts – 5 ml. Atresia of follicles – 2.5 ml.

   Fertility disorders of Cattle and Buffalo – 5 ml Im or IV.

   If no estrus occurs within 10-12 days of treatment, treatment should be repeated. Estrus occurs maximally 10-12 days later.

19.12.6 Pregnant Mare Serum Gonadotrophin (PMSG)

PMSG is a gonadotrophin with high follicle stimulating hormone (FSH) and low luteinizing hormone (LH) activity. In males PMSG stimulates spermatogenesis. In females (cow, she buffalo, doe and ewe) PMSG stimulates the growth and maturation of the dominant follicle.

Indication

Anoestrous, estrous induction to increase fertility rate after progesterome pretreatment and superovulation.

Trade Names

1. *Folligon* (Intervet) –1000 IU vial with 5 ml solvent

   Composition: Each vial of contains 1000 IU of PMSG.

   Dose: Cow and Buffalo – 500-1000 IU IM.

   Bull – 1000-3000 IU IM.

   Ewe and Doe – 400-600 IU IM during progesterome based oestrus synchronization.

   Bitch – 20 IU/kg body weight IM daily for 10 days for anoestrus and also at day 10 inject 500 IU Chorulon (HCG).

19.12.7 Cloprostenol (Synthetic PG $F_2\alpha$) as Fertility Solution

It is a synthetic prostaglandin. It is highly safe and does not impair fertility. It is used for synchronized breeding. Owing to its potent luteolytic action it brings about regression of corpus luteum (CL).

Indication

Synchronised breeding, suboestrus (non detected oestrus), removal of mummified foetus, pyometra, chronic endometritis, induction of parturition, ovarian luteal cyst, persistent CL and silent heat.

Trade Names

1. *Cyclix* (Intervet) – 2 ml and 20 ml vials

   Composition: Synthetic analogue of prostaglandin F2α.

   Dose: Cattle and Buffalo – 2 ml IM, Sow – 1 ml IM.

   Goat and Sheep – 1 ml IM.

2. *Juramate Injection* (Vetcare) – 20 ml vial

   Composition: Each ml contains 263 mcg Cloprostenol sodium equivalent to 250 mcg Cloprostenol.

   Dose: 2 ml (500mcg) Cloprostenol per animal by IM injection.

   For pyometra, endometritis and persistent corpus luteum dose 2 ml IM.

   Anoestrus/silent heat – 2 ml IM.

   Cystic ovaries – 2 ml IM.

3. *Vetmate Injection* (Vetcare) – 2ml vial.

   It is a synthetic PG $F_2\alpha$ specially used for fertility solutions. Specially indicated for pyometra, mummified and macerated foetus.

   Dose: 2 ml by IM route.

4. *Clostenol Injection* (Sarabhai Zydus) – 2 ml vial

   Composition: Each ml contains Cloprostenol 263 mcg. It is a most powerful heat inducer, correct metritis and pyometra, terminate pathologic pregnancy.

   Dose: To treat metritis and pyometra Cow and Buffalo – 2 ml, Mare-1-2 ml, Sheep, Goat and Pig – 0.5-1 ml.

   For induction of estrus, for luteolysis – Cow and Buffalo – 2 ml, Mare. 1-2 ml, Sheep, Goat and Pig – 0.5 ml.

4. *Synchromate Injection* (Primavet) – 4 ml and 10 ml vials

   Composition: It is a prostaglandin F_2 analysis. It contains Cloprostenol sodium 263 mg.

   Dose: 2-3 ml IM route.

5. *Iliren Injection* (Intervet) – 10 ml vial

   Composition: It is a prostaglandin $F_2\alpha$ analogue (0.196 mg/ml).

   Dose: Cow and Buffalo – 3.5 ml IV or 5 ml IM.

Sow – 2-4 ml IM.

Mare – 3 ml IM.

19.12.8 Dinoprost Tromethiamine

Indication

It is inidicated for cystic ovarian disease and postpartum fertility. It is used for improvement of conception rate at AI, in anovulation and delayed ovulation, true anoestrus, silent heat, ovarian cyst (follicular), irregular estrus, nymphomenia and anoestrous.

Trade Names

1. *Lutalyse Injection* (Novartis) – 10 ml vial

   Composition: 5 mg/ml.

   Dose: 5 ml IM.

2. *Fertizyl* (Intervet) – 1 ml amp, 2 ml and 10 ml vials

   Composition: 0.1 mg/ml amp and 50 mg/ml vial.

   Dose : 100 mg IM or IV.

3. *Cystorolin* (B & AHP)

   Dose: 250 mg IM or IV.

4. *Hormo P_2 alpha* (BCAHP) – 5 ml vial

   Composition: 5 mg/ml

   Dose: Bovine 5 ml IM.

   Equine 1 ml IM.

19.13 NON-STEROIDAL (NON HORMONAL) SYNTHETIC CHEMICAL FOR SUBFERTILITY/INFERTILITY MANAGEMENT

19.13.1 Clomifene Citrate

It stimulates hypothalamus pituitary axis to release GnRH. It induces ovulatory heat in heifers to make it productive earlier. It acts through stimulating the secretion of pituitary gonadotrophin hormones, particularly leutanising hormone (LH) and inhibits the regulating effect of estrogen on the pituitary.

Indication

Treatment of subfertility due to inactive gonads. Prolonged post partum anoestrous, repeat breeding as a result of anovulatory estrus, nymphomanic symptom and follicular cyst.

Trade Names

1. *Oestrovet* (Excell) – 5 tablets strip

   Composition : Clomifene citrate

Dose: For Anoestrous condition – 1.5 mg Clomifene citrate/kg body weight (Cattle and Buffalo weighting 350-500 kg) daily for 5 days.

For super ovulation in sheep – 10 mg/kg body weight for 3 days (sheep weighing 30-35 kg)

Oestrovet tab. should be given to cows and buffaloes after watering 100 ml of 1 per cent copper sulphate solution.

19.13.2 Valethamate Bromide

Special features of this group of medicine are cervix specific action, neurotropic and musculotropic action, smooth muscle relaxant and anti spasmodic.

Indication

A.I. facilitator. It may be used to facilitate easy delivery and for complete dilation of cervix in dystocia.

1. *Epidosin Vet Injection* (TTK) – 10 ml and 30 ml vials

   Composition : Valethemate bromide 10 mg/ml.

   Dose: Cattle and Horse – 10-15 ml

   Sheep, Goat and Pig – 5 ml

   Dog and Cat – 5 ml

   Administration by IM route only.

19.14 UTERINE TONIC AND ECBOLIC

Indication

Non-hormonal, non-antibiotic herbal medicine for breeding disorders like retention of placenta, endometritis, pyometra, insufficient discharge of lochial and foetal membrane, timely involution of uterus, and uterine tonic and cleansing agent to facilitate easy expulsion of retained placenta, pus, tissue debris and to assist manual removal.

Trade Names

1. *Exapar Liquid* (Ayurvet) – 500 ml bottle

   Dose: Large animal – 100 ml twice on 1st day followed by 50 ml twice daily for next 3 days.

   Small animal – 50 ml twice on 1st day followed by 25 ml BID for next 3 days.

2. *Utro-On* (Natural Herbs) – 500 ml and 1 litre

   Dose: Cow, Buffalo and Mare – 100 ml

   Sheep and Goat – 50 ml.

   Administer one double dose soon after parturition, repeat the single dose twice daily for 3-6 days.

3. *Utrina Liquid* (Kumaon Herbs) – 500 ml bottle

   Dose: Cattle and Buffalo – 100 ml daily.

   Sheep and Goat – 50 ml daily.

4. *Uterolin* (Bioherbs Pharma) – 450 ml and 900 ml pack

   Dose: Cattle and Mare – 90-150 ml.

   Ewe and Doe – 30-50 ml.]

   Twice daily for a week.

   In retained placenta the dose should be repeated 3 hourly till the foetal membranes are expelled. Uterolin should be reached soon after parturition (calving).

5. *Replanta* (Indian Herbs) – 100 g cartoon, poly bag of 500g and 1 kg

   Dose: Cattle and Buffalo – 50-60 g.

   Mare – 30-40 g.

   Ewe and Doe – 8-12 g.

   Administer twice daily orally mixed with jaggery or feed for 3-6 days to ensure early involution of uterus. Administer one double dose orally soon after parturition and repeat single dose after every six hours till the placenta is shed completely within 24 hours.

6. *Uterocare* (*Excell*) – 500 g

   Dose: Large animal – 100 g twice daily for 2 days followed by 100 g once daily for 2 days.

7. *Uterotone Liquid* (Cattle Remedies) – 250 ml, 450 ml and 900 ml.

   Dose: 100-125 ml twice daily orally for 4 days.

8. *Utrift Liquid* (Indian Herbs)

   Dose: Cattle, Buffalo and Mare – 100 ml.

   Sheep and Goat – 50 ml.

   Administer twice on the first day soon after parturition and then repeat once daily for 3 days.

19.15 MASTITIS CARE : INTRA MAMMARY INFUSION TUBES

Indication

Acute and chronic mastitis in lactating and dry cows, buffaloes and milch goats.

Trade Names

1. *Pendistrin-SH* (Sarabhai Zydus) – 6 ml collapsible tube

   Composition: Procaine penicillin, streptomycin, sulphamerazine and hydrocortisone combine pack.

   Dose: Acute mastitis – 1 tube every 12 hours for 5-6 instillations.

   Chronic mastitis – 1 tube every 12 or 24 hourly for 2-3 days.

2. *Vetclox Plus Tube* (Sarabhai Zydus)

   Composition: Intrammary infusion tube contains Ampicillin + Cloxacillin for lactating cows and buffaloes.

Dose: Acute mastitis – 1 full tube (syringe) into each affected/suspected quarter after stripping off the milk at 12 and 48 hours interval.

Chronic mastitis – 1 tube every 12 to 24 hours interval.

3. *Floclox-L* (Vetnex)

   Composition: Intramammary infusion tube containing Cloxacillin sodium equivalent to 200 mg Cloxacillin.

   Dose: Infuse 1 syring per quarter. Repeat the treatment every 48 hours till complete cure.

4. *Cobactan-LC* (Intervet) – Packs cointain 3 intramammary syringes

   Composition: Broad spectrum anti-infective for the treatment of clinical mastitis in cattle and buffalo. It has outstanding activity against both Gram (+ ve) and Gram (-ve) organisms.

5. *Mammitel tube* (Intas) – 10 g syringe

   Each syringe contains Colistin sulphate 500,000 IU and Cloxacillin sodium 200 mg.

   Dose: 1 syringe per affected quarter at 12 hours interval, 3-4 times by intrammary route.

6. *Mastijet Fort* (Intervet) – 8 g injection (Box of 20 injections)

   Composition: For intramammary infusion for bovines during lactation.

   Each syringe contains Tetracycline HCl 200 mg, Neomycin base 250 mg, Bactracin 2000 IU and Prednisolone 10 mg.

   Dose: One injection per affected quarter every 12 hours. Total treatment is 4 administrations.

7. *Tilox Tube* (Wockhardt) – 5 g tubes

   Composition : Ampicillin + Cloxacillin.

   Dose: 1 tube per affected quarter at 12 hourly interval for 3-4 days.

8. *Mastrip* (Dabur Ayurvet)

   It is for milk examination to detect both clinical and subclinical mastitis.

9. *Mastilep Gel* (Dabur) – 50 g and 100g tubes

   Topical herbal gel for control of mastitis. Mastitis can be treated at subclinical stage using Mastilep.

   Dose: To use locally by liberal application on teats and under twice daily for 7 days.

10. *Dermanol Gel* (Indian Herbs) – 25 g tube

    A non greasy, non staining unique herbal cream for support to mastitis infusion therapy. Topically support for all control of microbes on teats and udder, strengthen the udder and teat canal barrier, actively promotes healing of mastitis affected lesions, effectively control inflammation and pain without any side effect.

11. *Wisprec* ™*Cream* (Natural Remedies) – 25 g tube

    Cream based, pleasant fragrance, non-staining, non-irritant, easily washable multispectrum, dermatological and anti-inflammatory cream.

    Use: In mastitis as a supportive topical anti-inflammatory to reduce pain and swelling.

19.16 HERBAL VETERINARY MEDICINE

19.16.1 Herbal Digestive and Stomachic

Indication

An appetite stimulant and digestive tonic.

Poor digestion, indigestion, hypophagia, primary and secondary anorexia, ruminal stasis, loss of appetite induced by digestive disturbances, dietetic errors, flatulence, chronic dyspepsia and in any gastro-intestinal disturbance.

Trade Names

Herbal Digestive and Stomachic Powders

1. *Herbogastrin* (Vetmed) – 100 g, 200 g and 1 kg poly packs

   Dose: Horse, Cattle and Buffalo – 40 g twice daily for 12 days.

   Sheep and Goat – 10-15 g.

   Calf, Colt, Heifer and Pig – 20-25 g.

2. *Rumibest* (TTK) – 200 g, 500g and 1 kg pack

   Dose: Cattle, Buffalo and Horse – 30-50 g BID, Sheep and Goat – 10-15 g BID Camel – 200 g twice daily.

3. *Himalayan Batisa* (Indian Herbs) – 100 g, 200 g, 400 g and 1 kg packs

   Dose: Horse, Buffalo and Cow – 40-60 g.

   Colt, Heifer, Pig and Calf – 20-30 g.

   Sheep and Goat – 10-15 g.

   Dog and Piglet – 3-5 g.

4. *Digestovet Powder* (Vets Farma) – 200 g, 500 g and 1 kg packs

   Dosage: Large animal – 50-100 g once daily for 2-3 days.

   Small animal – 15-25 g once daily for 2-3 days.

5. *Antiflat* (Charak Pharmaceutical) – 100 g pack

   Dose: Large animal – 15-25 g BID

   Small animal – 8-10 g BID.

6. *Digestone Powder* (Anuya) – 100 g pack

   Dose: Horse, Cow and Adult pig – 20-40 g.

   Sheep and Goat – 10-15 g.

   Dog – 3-4 g.

7. *Suruchi Powder* (KAP) – 50 g and 250 g packs
   Dose: Cow, Buffalo and Horse – 5-10 g BID.
   Calf, Colt, Pig, Sheep and Goat – 3 g BID for 5 days.
8. *Ruchamax* (Ayurvet) – 15 g, 60 g, 225 g and 1 kg packs
   Dose: 15 g orally twice daily for 3-5 days.
9. *Natural Batisa* (Natural Remedies) – 50 g single dose pouch.
   Dose: During disease conditions 50 g BID for 3 to 5 days with jaggery; as digestive tonic 50 g once every alternate day.
10. *H.B. Strong* (Indian Herbs) – 10 g sachet
    Dose: Cow and Buffalo – 10 g (1 sachet),
    Calf and Heifer – 5 g (½ sachet),
    Sheep and Goas – 2.5 g (1/4th sachet), once or twice daily with jaggery (as electuary).
11. *Appetonic* (Indian Hebs) – 100 g pack
    Dose: Cattle and Buffalo – 40 g BID; Sheep and Goat – 15-20 g BID.
12. *Catone Powder* (Cattle Remedies) – 100 g, 200 g, 400 g, 1 kg and 5 kg packs
    Dose: Cattle and Buffalo – 50 g BID.
    Horse and Mule – 30-40 g BID.
    Sheep and Goat – 10-15 g BID.
13. *Aryan Batisa* (Natural Herbs) – 100 g, 200 g, 400 g and 1 kg packs
    Dose: Cattle, Buffalo, Horse and Mule – 40-60 g
    Sheep and Goat – 10-15 g.
    Camel and large animals – 100 g, three times a week or on alternate day.
14. *Lomatich-DS* (Legend) – 100 g and 200 g.
    Dose: Small animal – 24 g BID.
15. *Maha Batisa Hajmi* (Pearl Chemical) – 200 g and 500 g
    Dose: Large animal – 40-60 g orally BID.
    Small animal – 15-30 g orally BID daily for 5-7 days orally as electuary.
16. *Ruchipro Powder* (Angels) – 100 g and 500 g packs
    Dose: Large animal – 50-100 g/day.
    Small animal – 25-30 g/day.
17. *Ruchi Chatni* (Kapila) – 100 g and 200 g packs
    Dose: Cattle – 50 g orally BID as electuary twice daily.
    Buffalo and Horse – 50-100 g.
    Small animal – 20-25 g orally BID.
18. *Aahar* (Kapila) – 100 g, 500 g and1 kg packs
    Dose: Large animal 25-50 g orally BID
    Small animal 15-25 g BID.

19. *Levucell-SC* (Venky's)

    Dose: Cow and Buffalo – 5-10 g daily.

    Calf, Goat and Sheep – 2.5-5 g daily.

20. *Enrumen* (Kapila) – 100 g pack

    Dose: Cow and Buffalo – 5-10 g daily

    Goat and Sheep – 2.5-5 g daily.

21. *Rumento Plus* (Crill) – 15 g sachet

    Dose: Large animal 1 sachet BID

    Small animal ½ sachet BID.

22. *Rumizyme Powder* (Arosol) – 25 g, 100 g, 250 g and 500g packets

    A unique herbal rumenatonic, appetizer and digestive as well as liver tonic. Stimulates appetite, boost digestive enzymes formation, corrects liver function, protects animal from anorexia, general debility and helps to prevent liver dysfunctions.

    Dose: Large animal – 20-25 g twice daily with feed.

    Small animal – 10 g twice daily with feed.

    Poultry/Swine – 1 kg/tone of feed.

23. *Rumicare* (Intervet) – 125 g sachet

    Composition: Calcium propionate – 60 g, Methionine – 5 g, Picrorhiza dry extract – 250 mg, Cobalt gluconate – 40 kg, Vitamin B_6 – 40 mg and Dextrose anhydrous – 535 g.

    Indication: Bloat, digestive disorders, hypoglycaemic condition in cattle, calves, sheep and goats.

    Dose: Adult cattle – 125 g sachet twice daily at 12 hours interval in ½ to 1 litre drinking water.

    Young cattle -½ sachet (62-63 g) twice daily, drench with ½ -1 litre water.

    Sheep and Goat – 1/4th sachet (31-32 g) once daily, drench with ½ to 1 litre drinking water.

Liquid Stomachic and Carminatives

24. *Herbogastrin Liquid* (Vet Med) – 200 ml bottle

    Dose: Large animal – 50 ml twice daily.

    Small animal – 25 ml twice daily.

    In severe and acute conditions the dose may be doubled.

25. *Anox Liquid* (Oxen Lab) – 100 ml, 200 ml, 500 ml and 5 litres packs

    Dose: Cattle and Buffalo – 50 ml daily for 7 days.

    Calf, Sheep and Goat – 20-30 ml daily for 7 days.

    Dog – 10 ml daily for 7 days.

26. *Carmigen* (Nugen) – 100 ml, 200 ml, 450 ml and 5 litres packs

    Having digestive and antibloat enzymes.

Dose: Buffalo – 50 ml twice daily.

Cattle – 40 ml orally twice daily.

Calf – 20 ml orally twice daily

Sheep and Goat – 10-15 ml orally BID.

27. *P-Zyme Vet* (Oxford Gems) – 100 ml, 200 ml and 450 ml packs

    Dose: Cattle and Buffalo – 40-50 ml orally BID.

    Calf, Sheep and Goat – 10-15 ml orally BID.

28. *RS-Zyme* (R.S. Pharmaceutical) – 100 ml, 200 ml and 450 ml packs

    Dose: Cattle – 20-25 ml/day.

    Sheep and Goat – 10-15 ml/day.

    Dog – 10 ml/day.

29. *Digecon* (Pharmacon) – 100 ml, 200 ml, 450 ml and 5 litres packs

    Dose: Cattle, Buffalo and Horse – 20-50 ml twice daily.

    Calf, Sheep and Goat – 10-15 ml orally BID.

    Dog – 10 ml twice daily.

Stomachic Bolus (Rumenotoric Bolus)

30. *Rumbion Bolus* (Indian Herbs) – 4 boli strip

    Dose: Cattle and Buffalo – 2 boli twice daily for 2-3 days.

    Sheep and Goat–1 bolus twice daily for 2-3 days.

31. *Surüchi Bolus Vet* (KAP) – 5 g bolus

    Dose: Cattle, Buffalo and Horse – 1 bolus twice daily for 5 days.

    Calf, Colt, Pig, Sheep and Goat – ½ bolus once daily for 5 days.

32. *Rumexon Forte Bolus* (Kumaon Herbs)

    Dose: Cattle and Buffalo 2-4 boli daily 2-3 days.

    Sheep and Goat – 1 bolus BID daily 2-3 days.

33. *Flora Boost Bolus* (Excell) – 4 boli strip

    Composition: Each bolous provides Live yeast culture 3 g, Amino acids 2 g and Liver extract 5 mg.

    Dose: Cattle, Buffalo and Camel – 1-2 boli daily for 5 days.

    Calf, Sheep and Goat – ½-1 bolus daily for 4-5 days.

34. *Go-Feed Bolus* (Legend) – Blister of 4 boli

    Composition: Contains live yeast culture, copper sulphate, dried ferrous sulphate, cobalt chloride, zinc sulphate, lactobacillus, mag. sulph, sodi bicarb and liver extract.

    Dose: Cattle and Buffalo -2 boli twice daily for 4 days.

    Calf, Sheep and Goat – 1 boli daily for 4 days.

35. *Floratone Bolus* (Concept) – Strips of 4 boli

    Dose: Cattle, Buffalo and Horse – 4 boli to be given at an interval of 12 hours (full course 12 boli).

Calf, Sheep, Goat, Dog – 1bolus to be given at an interval of 12 hours (full course of 3 boli).

36. *Bovirum Bolus* (Sarabhai Zydus) – 4 boli strip

    Dose: Cattle and Buffalo – 3-4 boli/day for 4 days.

    Caution: Use only for ruminants and provide plenty of drinking water to the treated animals.

37. *Rumentas* (Intas) – Strips of 4 boli

    Dose: Cattle and Buffalo – 2 boli twice daily for 2-3 days by oral route.

38. *Ecotas Bolus* (Intas)–Strip of 8 boli in a unit cartoon.

    Dose: Cattle and Buffalo – 2 boli daily orally for 4 days.

39. *Yeasacc Bolus* (Vetnex) – 4 boli strip

    Dose: Cattle and Buffalo – 2 boli daily orally for 4 days.

40. *Provisac Bolus* (Vetcare) – 4 boli strip

    Dose: Cattle and Buffalo – 1-2 boli BID orally for 3-4 days.

    Sheep and Goat – ½-1 bolus BID orally for 2-3 days.

41. *Instafeed-FS* (Bee Tee Pharma) – 4 boli in a strip

    A combination of yeast, Vitamin B-complex, Methionine, Copper and Cobalt.

    Dose: Cattle and Horse – Full course of 12 boli. Repeat 4 boli 3 times at 12 hours interval.

    Calf, Sheep and Goat – Full course of 3 boli. Repeat 1 bolus 3 times at 12 hours interval.

    Dose may be doubled in case of severe acidosis with flatulence.

42. *Pashubhog Boost Bolus* (Oxen Lab)–4 boli in a strip

    Composition: Bolus having live yeast culture with amino acids.

    Dose: Large animal – 2 boli orally BID for 2-3 days.

    Small animal – ½ to 1 bolus orally BID for 2-3 days.

43. *Biovest Bolus* (Vets Farma)–2 boli in blister pack

    Dose: 1-2 boli daily for large animal.

    ½–1 bolus daily for small animal.

44. *Biotone* (Bioherbs) – 100 g, 200 g, 400 g and 1 kg packs

    It is a true herbal probiotic and stomachic powder for all digestive disorders.

    Indication: Indigestion, flatulence, dyspepsia, anorexia, atony of stomach, faecal impaction, metabolic disorders and constipation.

    Dose: Sheep and Goat – 15-25 g.

    Horse and Cattle – 40-70 g.

    Orally twice daily in water, feed or gruels.

45. *Biotone Fs Bolus* (Karnataka Antibiotics) – 4 boli strip
    Dose: Large animal – 2 to 3 boli/day for 3-5 days.
    Small animal – ½ to 1 boli per day for 3-4 days.
46. *Feed-on-Bolus* (AFC) – Blister of 2 boli
    Dose: Large animal – 1-2 boli daily.
    Small animal – 1 bolus daily.

19.16.2 Antiflatulents (Antizymotics)

19.16.2.1 Anti Bloat Suspension (Oral Liquid) Medicines

Indication

The preparation contains simethicone which is indicated as a powerful antibloat suspension.

The medicines of this group are used for all types of tympany and frothy bloat.

Trade Names

1. *Brisil* (Brihans) – 115 ml bottle
   Composition: Simethicon – 1 per cent w/v.
   Dose: Large animal – 100-115 ml.
   Small animal – 15-25 ml.
2. *Tympex* (Vets Farma) – 100 ml bottle
   Composition: Simethicone – 1 per cent w/v.
   Dose: Cattle and Buffalo – 100 ml orally as drench.
   Sheep and Goat – 20 ml orally as drench.
3. *Blotonil* (Jeps) – 100 ml bottle
   Composition: Each 100 ml contains Silica in Dimethicone 1 per cent w/v and Arachis oil – 10 per cent w/v.
   Dose: Cattle and Buffalo – 100-200 ml at one time and can be repeated if necessary. Drench or through a stomach tube. Intra ruminal injection can also be given if necessary.
4. *Bloatcon* (Pharmacon) – 100 ml bottle
   Composition: Each 10 ml contains Simethicone – 400 mg, Aluminium hydroxide – 600 mg, Magnesium hydroxide – 300 mg and Sorbitol – 50 mg.
   Dose: Cattle and Buffalo – 100 ml twice daily.
   Sheep and Goat – 20 ml twice daily with a 6 hours gap.
5. *Bloatosil Suspension* (Wockhardt) – 100 ml bottle
   Composition: Each 100 ml contains Silica in Dimethicone – 1 per cent and Arachis oil 5 per cent.
   Dose: Cattle and Buffalo – 100 ml at a time by drenching.
   Sheep and Goat – 20 ml.
   By intra ruminal injection or by oral route.

6. *Gastina* (GSK) – 100 ml bottle

   A super quality anti-bloat liquid.

   Composition: Simithicon – 1 per cent, Dil oil – 0.5 per cent

   Dose: Cattle – 100 ml orally BID till symptoms disappear.

   Sheep and goat – 25 ml orally.

7. *Tynpex Liquid* (Prashanti Formulations) – 100 ml bottle

   Composition: Silica in Dimethicon (1 per cent w/v).

   Dose: Cattle – 50-100 ml orally BID.

   Sheep and Goat – 25 ml orally BID.

8. *Blotena* (Bioherbs) – 100 ml and 200 ml bottles

   Herbal formulation having Hing (*Ferula foetida*), Laser (*Allium sativum*), Kamila (*Mallotus philippinensis*) and Nosadar (Ammonium chloride).

   Dose: Sheep and Goat – 50 ml

   Horse and Cattle – 50-100 ml.

   In acute tympanitis smaller doses should be repeated at short intervals and 25 ml liquid may be injected intraruminally for quick relief.

9. *D-Bloat Liquid* (Indian Herbs) – 100 ml bottle

   Indicated for quick relief from bloat or tympany and for comprehensive management of frothy and for comprehensive management of frothy and gaseous bloat. It has got antifrothing, defrothing, antizymotic, carminative, antacid and digestive stimulant actions.

   Dose: Cattle – 50-100 ml orally BID.

   Sheep and Goat – 20-30 ml orally BID.

10. *Blotinox Liquid* (Cattle Remedies) – 100 ml and 450 ml bottles

    Dose: Cattle and Buffalo – 100 ml orally.

    Horse and Mule – 50-100 ml orally.

    Sheep and Goat – 50 ml orally.

    For quicker relief Blotinox liquid can be injected intraruminally.

19.16.2.2 Herbal-Anti Bloat/Anti Tympany Preparation (for prompt relief of Tympany or Bloat)

Trade Names

Herbal Liquid Anti-Flatulent/Anti-Bloat Preparations

1. *Afanil* (Ayurvet) – 100 ml bottle

   Dose: Large animal – 50 ml twice daily for 2 days

   Small animal – 25 ml twice daily for 2 days.

2. *Tyrel* (Natural Remedies) – 100 ml bottle

   Dose: Large animal – 100 ml

Small animal – 50 ml.

Administer one full dose orally or intraruminally and repeat if necessary.

Herbal Powder Anti-Flatulents/Antibloat Preparations

3. *Timpol Powder* (Indian Herbs) – 100 g, 400 g and 1 kg packs

   Dose: Horse, Cattle and Buffalo – 80 g.

   Colt, Heifer and Calf – 40 g.

   Sheep, Goat, Adult pig – 20-25 g.

   Timpol should be given alone or mixed with Magnesium sulphate – 150-400 g.

4. *Afron Powder* (Bootic Bhawan) – 100 g and 1 kg packs

   Dose: Cattle and Buffalo – 50 g to be mixed with ½-1 litre luke warm water and drenched.

5. *Gasnil Powder* (Vetmed) – 100 g pack

   Dose: Horse, Cattle and Buffalo – 50-100 g mixed in ½–1 litre luke warm water to be drenched carefully.

   Colt, Heifer and Calf – 40-50 g.

   Sheep and Goat – 20-25 g.

6. *Girtona Powder* (Anuya) – 100 g and 1 kg packs

   Dose: 50 g powder to be mixed with ½-1 litre of luke warm water and to be drenched carefully.

7. *N-Blot-06* (Natural Remedies) – 100 g and 1 kg packs

   An ideal antizymotic and antifrothing agent that checks excessive fermentation and gas formation.

   Dose: Horse, Cattle and Buffalo – 80 g.

   Calf, Colt and Heifer – 40 g.

   Sheep and Goat – 20-25 g.

   Dog and Piglet – 3-5 g.

8. *Timpanimal Powder* (Arosol) – 100 g and 200 g packs

   Dose: Cattle and Buffalo – 50 g orally BID.

   Calf, Sheep and Gota – 25 g orally BID.

9. *Papazyme Forte Vet Powder* (Angel's Group) – 100 g box

   Dose: Small animal – 15-20 g twice daily.

   Large animal – 25-50 g twice/thrice daily.

   In Tympany 100 g at a time and repeat after 12-24 hours.

   Anti Bloat Bolus

10. *Bloatinorm Bolus* (Excell)

    Composition: Each bolus contains Simethicone – 150 mg (treats frothy bloat), Dried Aluminium Hydroxide – 500mg (treat acidosis), Magnesium hydroxide – 1200 mg (acts as laxative) and Algeric acid – 300 mg (treats impaction).

Dose: Large animal – 2 boli twice daily. In acute conditions 4 boli at a time.

Small animal – 1 bolus twice daily. In acute condition 2-4 boli at a time.

11. *Acinil Bolus* (Excell)

    Dosage – Large animal – 2 boli twice daily.

    Small animal – 1 bolus twice daily.

19.16.3 Herbal Liver Tonic

Indication

For enhancing hepatic functions, effective management of liver disorder, hepatic dysfunctions, jaundice, hepatitis, adjunct therapy along with anthelmentics, flukicides and other chemical therapy, anorexia and off fed, general unthriftiness and debility, to strengthen stressed and sluggish liver during convalescence.

Trade Names

Herbal Liver Tonic (Liquid Preparation)

1. *Livsee* (Legend) – 100 ml, 200 ml, 500 ml, 1 litre and 5 litres

   Dose: Calf – 10 ml daily for 3-5 days.

   Large animal – 50 ml daily for 3-5 days.

2. *Vetliv Liquid* (Vetmed) – 200 ml in pet bottle

   Dose: Small animal – 20-30 ml twice daily with water.

   Large animal – 50 ml daily for 3-5 days.

3. *Zigbo Oral Liquid* (Natural Remedies) – 300 ml, 1 litre and 5 litres can/bottle

   Dose: Large animal – 30 ml once daily.

   Small animal – 10 ml once daily.

4. *Nuliv* (Nugen Pharma) – 200 ml, 450 ml and 1 litre bottle and 5 litres in jar

   Dose: Cattle and Buffalo – 10-20 ml twice daily for 8-10 days.

   Calf, Sheep and Goat – 5-10 ml twice daily for 8 to 10 days.

   Poultry (100 birds) – Broiler 5 to 10 ml from 2nd week to 6th week.

   Grower and Layer 15 ml for 10 days.

5. *Yakrifit Oral Liquid* (Ayurvet) – 250 ml bottle and 1 litre jar

   Dose: Large animal – 30-50 ml twice daily for 5-7 days.

   Small animal – 10-15 ml twice daily for 5-7 days.

   It treats liver dysfunction and improves productivity.

6. *Hepasol* (Enlag Labs) – 100 ml

   Dose: Cattle and Buffalo – 30-50 ml twice daily.

   Pig, Sheep and Goat – 15 ml twice daily.

Dog – 10 ml twice daily.

Poultry – 20 ml daily for 100 birds.

7. *Brotone Tonic* (Glaxo SmithKline) – 120 ml and 500 ml bottle

Tonic of liver extract and yeast extract.

Dose: Large animal – 40 ml for 3 days.

Small animal – 10 ml for 4 days.

Pig – 5-10 ml BID.

8. *Livosprin* (Sprindles Formulations) – 100 ml, 200 ml, 450 ml, 1 litre and 5 litres

An unique herbal liver protective for poultry and livestock.

Dose: Large animal – 30-50 ml BID.

Small animal – 10-15 ml BID

Poultry – 20 ml daily for 100 birds.

9. *Livovit* (Bery and Bery Vet) – 200 ml, 500 ml and 5 litres

Dose: Large animal – 30-50 ml daily.

Calf, Sheep, Goat and Dog – 5-10 ml daily.

Poultry – Chicks 5 ml daily/100 birds, Layers 20 ml daily/100 birds and Broiler 10 ml daily/100 birds.

10. *Tefroli Syrup* (TTK) – 120 ml, 500 ml and 4.5 litres

Dose: Cattle and Horse – 10-15 ml twice daily for 5-7 days.

Sheep, Goat and Pig – 5-10 ml twice daily for 5-7 days.

Cat and Dog – 5-10 ml twice daily for 5-7 days.

11. *Livluv Vet* (Marvet) – 100 ml, 200 ml, 500 ml, 1 litre and 5 litres

Dose: Large animal – 50 ml OD for 3-5 days.

Small animal – 10 ml OD for 3-5 days.

12. *Livcare Concentrate* (Kapila)–100 ml and 450 ml bottle

Dose: Cattle and Horse – 301-40 ml twice daily.

Calf, Sheep and Goat – 15-20 ml twice daily.

Dog – 5-10 ml twice daily.

Poultry – Broiler 1st to 2nd week – 3 ml/100 birds.

3rd to 4th week – 4 ml/100 birds.

5th week onwards – 6 ml/100 birds.

13. *Liv-100 Liquid* (Aerosol) – 500 ml, 1 litre and 5 litres

It acts as hepatoprotective and hepatogenerative medicine. It inhibits hepatic microsomal lipid peroxidation, supports reticuloendothelial systems, aids biotransformation of drugs and toxins and improves hepatocytes protein synthesis.

Dose: Cattle, Buffalo and Horse – 40 ml twice daily.

Sheep, Goat, Calf, Foal and Pig – 20-25 ml twice daily.

Poultry – Chicks (100 birds) 5 ml daily, Growers 10 ml daily, Layers and Breeders – 15 ml daily.

14. *Livodex Liquid* (Oxen Lab) – 250 ml, 500 ml, 1 litre and 5 litres

    A herbal liver tonic for animal and poultry.

    Dose: Cattle and Buffalo – 30-40 ml daily.

    Calf and Heifer – 30-40 ml daily.

15. *Livcon Syrup* (Pharmacon) – 500 ml and 5 litres

    Dose : Cattle and Buffalo – 30-40 ml daily.

    Calf, Sheep and Goat – 15-20 ml daily.

16. *Lifer Liquid* (Vets Farma) – 200 ml, 500 ml, 1 litre, 2 litres and 5 litres

    Composition: Iron, liver extract and vitamin B-complex.

    Dose: Cattle and Buffalo – 40 ml twice daily.

    Sheep, Goat, Pig and Calf – 15-20 ml twice daily.

17. *Livozyme-Fe Liquid* (Marion Pharma) – 200 ml, 500 ml, 1 litre and 5 litres

    Dose: Chicks – 10 ml/100 birds per day.

    Broilers and Layers – 25-50 ml/100 birds per day.

    Pig – 30-40 ml twice daily.

    Cattle and Horse – 30-40 ml twice daily.

    Dog – 5-10 ml twice daily.

Herbal Liver Tonic (Powder Preparation)

18. *Livgrow Powder* (Natural Herbs) : 100 g cartoon and 1 kg polybag.

    Dose: Cattle, Buffalo and Horse – 40-60 g.

    Calf, Colt and Pig – 15-20 g.

    Sheep and Goat – 8-12 g.

    Dog and Piglet – 3-5 g.

    Administer orally once or twice daily with feed for 10 days or more till complete recovery.

19. *Enliv* (Pfizer) – 100 g pack

    Dose: Cattle, Buffalo and Horse – 40-50 g.

    Calf, Foal and Pig – 20-25 g.

    Sheep and Goat – 10-15 g.

    Orally twice daily as electuary for 10 days or more till complete recovery.

20. *Vetliv* (Vetmed) – 100 g and 200 g

    Dose: Large animal 50 g twice daily.

    Small animal 25 g twice daily for 15 days as electuary.

21. *Liv-100 Powder* (Aerosol) – 1 kg, 5 kg and 25 kg bag
    Dose: Cattle, Buffalo and Horse – 25-30 g/day.
    Camel – 30-40 g/day.
    Calf, Colt and Pig – 10-15 g/day.
    Sheep and Goat – 5-10 g/day.
    Poultry – 250 g per tone of feed.
22. *Livol* (Indian Herbs) – 100 g cartoon, polybag of 1 kg and 5 kg
    Dose: Cattle, Buffaloe and Horse – 40-60 g
    Calf, Heifer, Colt and Pig – 15-20 g
    Sheep and Goat – 8-12 g
    Dog and Piglet – 3-5 g
    Orally once or twice daily with feed or as electuary for 10 days or more till recovery.
23. *Pashubhog Powder* (Oxen Lab) – 250 g and 500 g pack
    Dose: Large animal – 30-50 g daily BID.
    Small animal – 10-15 g orally BID.
24. *Livogel Powder* (Angel group) – 300 g
    Dose: Small animal – 10-15 g twice daily.
    Large animal – 20-30 g twice daily.
25. *Liv-100 Bolus* (Arosol)– 4 boli strip x 10 strip
    Dose: Cattle and Buffalo – 1-2 boli Orally BID for 5 days.
    Sheep and Goat – 1 bolus BID

19.16.4 Herbal Cough Mixture (Expectorant)

Indication

Cough and Cold, Laryngitis, Bronchitis, Pneumonia, Coryza and other non-specific respiratory affections.

Trade Names

1. *Caflon* (Indian Herbs) – 100 g and 1 kg packs
   Dose: Cattle, Horse and Buffalo – 30-40 g
   Colt, Calf, Sheep, Goat and Pig – 5-12 g
   Dog and Piglet (15-60 days) – 2-4 g orally in *gur*/treacle/warm water 2-3 times a day
   Poultry – 0-5-1 per cent in feed.
2. *Bronto* (Anja) – 100 g pack
   Dose: Cattle and Horse – 10-14 g
   Sheep and Goat – 2-3 g
   Pig and Dog – 3-4 g

3. *Coughdon Powder* (Vets Farma)
   Dose: Horse, Cow and Buffalo – 30-40 g
   Colt, Calf, Sheep, Goat and Pig – 5-10 g
   Dog and Piglet – 2-4 g twice daily.
4. *Cufgo* (Bhartiya Bootee Bhawan) – 100 g and 1 kg packs
   Dose: Horse and Cattle – 30-40 g
   Calf -10-15 g
   Sheep and Goat – 10 g
   Pig – 15-20 g
   Dog – 2-4 g.
5. *Biocuf* (Bioherbs Pharma) – 100 g pack
   Dose: Sheep and Goat – 10-15 g BID as electuary.
   Buffalo, Cattle and Horse – 20-30 g BID as electuary.

19.16.5 Galactogogue - for Better Milk Production

Indication

Improves milk yield, fat content and breeding efficiency, clinical and post parturient agalactia, lactation difficulties after diseases like FMD, Mastitis, Milk fever, retention of placenta *etc.*

Trade Names

Galactogogue Bolus

1. *Dugdhdan Bolus* (Cattle Remedies) – 8 x 6 boli box
   Dose: Cow and She buffalo – 4 boli twice daily.
   Doe and Ewes– 2 boli twice daily.
   Full dose to be given for 10 days.
2. *Payapro Bolus* (Ayurvet) – 4 boli in aluminium strip
   Herbal galactogogue bolus optimizes lactational yield, restores milk yield in lactational problems.
   Dose: 4 boli orally once daily for 10-15 days.
3. *Maxi Milk Bolus* (Sarabhai Zydus) – Strips of 4 boli
   Dose: Cattle and Buffalo–1-2 boli orally BID for 10-25 days.
4. *Milkoplex Bolus* (Rakesh Pharma)
   Dose: Cow and Buffalo – 1-2 boli twice a day.
5. *Utromilk* (Arosol) – 500 ml and 1 litre
   Herbal ecbolic uterine tonic with galactogogue action.
   Dose: Large animal – 50-60 ml orally twice on 1st day of parturition.
   Small animal – 10-20 ml BID on 1st day of kidding/lambing followed by OD for 3 to 5 days.

6. *Galog* (Indian Herbs) – 300 g cartoon

   Herbal galactogogue, restores, regulates and optimizes milk production.

   Dose: Cow and Buffalo – 50 g once daily for 17 days.

   Ewe and Doe – 10-15 g once daily mixed with *gur* or treacles.

7. *Boon-O-Milk* (Aries Agrovet) – 450 g and 1 kg jar

   Composition: It contains six non hormonal galactogus.

   Dose: Cattle and Buffalo – 15 g daily for 15 days.

8. *Milkotone* (Vetmed) – 500 g and 1 kg packets

   Ayurvedic/herbal galactogogue.

   Dose: Cattle and Buffalo – 25 g orally BID.

   Ewe, Doe and Sow – 10-15 g orally BID.

   It should be used consecutively for 10 days.

9. *Rasol* (BBB) – 100 g and 200 g

   Used as a galactogogue.

   Dose: Cow and She buffalo – 20-40 g orally BID for 10-30 days.

10. *Lactovet Powder* (Rakesh Pharmaceuticals) – 500 g packet

    Dose: Cow and Buffalo – 50 g daily.

11. *Milk Max* (Ethicare) – ½ kg and 1 kg pack

    Dose: Cattle and Buffalo – 50 g daily in feed.

12. *Milk Fit* (Natural Remedies) – 100 g pack

    Herbal milk booster and cattle feed supplement indicated for agalactia, hypogalactia and in lactation difficulties after FMD, metritis and mastitis.

Non-Herbal Milk Increaser

13. *Protivet Liquid* (Angels group) – 220 ml bottle and 5 litre jar

    Dose: For milch animal 40 ml twice daily for 12 days.

    For Ewe and Doe – 20 ml once daily for 15 days.

14. *Tonavit Liquid* (Angels group) – 450 ml, 170 ml and 5 litre jar

    It is a multi action liquid enzymes, vitamins and galactogogue.

    Dose: Small animal – 15-20 ml twice daily.

    Large animal – 30-40 ml twice daily for 10 days.

19.16.6 Herbal Antistress Medicine

Indication

The antistress, adaptogenic and immunomodulator herbal preparations. These are used to minimize the effect of disease stress, calving stress, extreme weather stress and all other stressful conditions.

Trade Names

1. *Stenot* (Natural Remedies) – 300 ml and 1 litre bottle
   Dose: Large animal – 30-50 ml/day depending upon severity of stress.
   Small animal – 15-20 ml/day depending upon severity of stress.
2. *Stenot Bolus* (Natural Remedies)–10 boli strip
   Dose: Large animal – 1-2 boli per day depending upon severity of stress.
   Small animal – ½ -1 bolus per day depending upon severity of stress.
3. *Hygest Bolus* (Natural Remedies) – 6 boli strip
   Dose: In Ketosis/Acidosis – 2 boli once daily a week before and 2 weeks after parturition.
4. *Groviplex Liquid* (Virbac AFC) – 500 ml and 5 litres jar
   Composition: B-complex, Lysine and Choline.
   Dose: Large animal – 100 ml daily; Calf – 20 ml daily.
5. *Kafcare* (Kapila) – 250 g poly pack.
   Composition: Vitamin $AD_3B_2B_{12}K$, calcium, phosphorus, iron, copper, cobalt, manganese, zinc, sulphur, iodine, lysine, methionine and choline chloride.
   Dose: Calf upto 4 months – 10 g daily.
   Calf above 4 months – 15 g daily.
6. *B-Com Forte* (Pearls chemicals)
   Dose: Cattle and Horse – 30-50 ml
   Calf, Sheep, Goat and Pig – 10-20 ml daily.
7. *Concitone* (Concept)–100 ml and 450 ml bottle
   Dose: Cattle and Buffalo – 20-25 ml once daily.
   Calf, Sheep and Goat – 10 ml once daily.
   Dog – 5 ml once daily.
8. *Dinosol* (Pharmacon) – 50 ml, 100 ml, 200 ml and 500 ml bottle
   Dose: Cattle – 10 ml twice daily.
   Calf – 5 ml twice daily.
   Dog – 5-10 ml BID.
9. *Vitadhan* (Ayurvet) – 60 ml and 300 ml bottle
   Composition: Herbal liquid vitamin supplement. It assures calcium and phosphorus absorption and utilization and ensures maximum production.
   Dose: Cattle and Buffalo – 10-20 ml daily.
   Calf – 10 ml daily.
10. *Vitamix Liquid* (Oxen Lab)–30 ml, 60 ml and 500 ml
    Composition : Liquid of Vitamins A, E, D_3 and B_{12}.
    Dose: Cattle and Buffalo – 10-15 ml daily.
    Calf – 5 ml daily.
    Sheep and Goat – 3-5 ml daily.

11. *Vimeral Liquid* (GSK) – 30 ml, 60 ml, 100 ml, 500 ml and 1 litre
    Dose: Large animal – 10 ml daily
    Small animal – 5 ml daily.
    Pig – 2-3 ml daily.
12. *Vetkal-B$_{12}$* (Sarabhai Zydus) – 100 ml, 500 ml, 1 litres, and 5 litres
    Dose: Cattle, Buffalo and Horse – 100 ml daily.
    Calf – 20 ml BID.
13. *Aminoplex* (Excell Aahar) – 20 ml, 500 ml and 100 ml
    Dose: Cattle and Horse – 30-50 ml
    Calf, Sheep, Goat and Pig – 10-20 ml.
    Dog – 5-10 ml.
14. *Magalvit Powder* (Care-O-Vet) – 100 g container
15. *Stressvit* (Excell) – 60 ml and 500 ml
    Dose: Cattle and Buffalo – 10 ml daily for 6 days.
    Calf, Sheep and Goat – 5 ml daily for 6 days.
16. *Vetral Liquid* (Vets Farma) – 30 ml, 60 ml, 100 ml, 500 ml and 1 litre
    Composition: Vitamin AD$_3$ E and B$_{12}$.
    Dose: Cattle and Buffalo – 20-25 ml
    Calf, Sheep and Goat – 5-10 ml
    Poultry – 20 ml/100 birds.
17. *Ambiplex Syrup* (Brihans) – 60 ml, 120 ml, 500 ml, 1 litre and 5 litres
    Vitamins with amino acids
    Dose: Cattle, Buffalo and Horse – 30-50 ml
    Calf, Sheep, Goat and Pig – 10-20 ml for 7-10 days.
    Dog – 5-10 ml 7-10 days in every month.
    Poultry for 100 birds – Chick 5-6 ml, Broiler 8-10 ml.
18. *Viselam* (Brihans) – 50 ml, 210 ml, 500 ml and 1 litre bottle
    A liquid feed supplement having vital vitamins AD$_3$EB$_{12}$ and folic acid, selenium and tryptophan along with essential amino acids for livestock and poultry.
    Dose: To be given as such or through drinking water.
    Cattle, Buffalo and Horse – 10-15 ml.
    Poultry for 100 birds – Chicks 5 ml, Grower/Broiler – 7.5 ml and Layer – 10 ml for 7-10 days.
19. *Plexiven* (Adven Pharma) – 100 ml, 500 ml and 5 litres
    Dose: Cattle and Buffalo – 15-25 ml BID.
    Calf, Sheep, Goat and Pig – 5-10 ml twice daily.

20. *Vitall* (Nugen) – 100 ml, 500 ml, 450 ml, 1 litre and 5 litres
    Dose: Calf – 10 ml, Cattle – 20 ml, Buffalo – 25 ml.
21. *Recovit* (Brihans)–30 ml, 120 ml, 500 ml and 1 litre
    Oral liquid Vitamins with optimum concentration of Vitamin AD_3B, C and B_{12}.
    Dose: Large animal 3-5 ml, Small animal – 1-2 ml.
    Poultry (for 100 birds) – Chicks 1-2 ml, Grower/Broiler 2-3 ml, Layer – 4-5 ml.
22. *Nubplex* (Nugen Pharma) – 100 ml, 200 ml, 450 ml and 5 litres
    Composition: Liquid Vitamin B-Complex with lysine, methionine and cobalt.
    Dose: Calf, Dog, Foal, Sheep and Goat – 5-10 ml.
    Cattle and Buffalo – 15-25 ml.
    Poultry (for 100 birds) – 15-20 ml.
23. *Livolysin* (Pharma Convet) – 100 ml, 200 ml, 450 ml, 1 litre and 5 litres
    Dose: Calf – 10 ml, Cattle – 20 ml, Buffalo – 25 ml, Poultry – 20 ml/100 birds.
24. *Enrovit* (Enlag Lab) – 30 ml, 60 ml, 100 ml and 500 ml
    Composition: Ideal feed supplement with Vitamin AD_3E and B_{12}.
    Dose: Cattle 5 ml daily for 7 days; Poultry – 5-10 ml/100 birds.
25. *Bery Plex* (Bery and Bery Vet) – 200 ml, 500 ml, 1 litre and 5 litres
    Dose: Horse, Cattle and Buffalo – 30-50 ml twice daily.
    Poultry – Chick 10 ml/100 birds, Broiler and Grower 15 ml/100 birds; Layer/Breeder – 20 ml/100 birds.
26. *Megaboost Liquid* (Vets Farma) – 500 ml, 1 litre and 5 litres pack
    Composition: A unique blend of Ca, P, Vitamin D_3 and B_{12}, stomachich extract and iron (Ferric ammonium citrate).
    Dose: Large animal 50 ml twice daily; Small animal 20 ml twice daily.
    Poultry – Chick 10 ml/100 birds, Broiler/Layer 20-50 ml/100 birds per day.
27. *Lysovit* (Oxford Gem) – 200 ml, 450 ml, 1 litre bottle
    Dose: Cattle and Buffalo – 30-50 ml BID; Small animal – 15-20 ml/BID.
28. *Bery Plex-PF* (Bery and Bery Vet) – 200 ml, 500 ml, 1 litre and 5 litres
    Dose: Cattle, Buffalo and Horse – 30-50 ml twice daily.
    Calf, Sheep and Goat – 20 ml twice daily.
    Poultry – Chicks 10 ml/100 birds, Broiler/Grower – 15 ml/100 birds.
29. *Plexcon* (Vetcon) – 200 ml, 450 ml and 1 litre
    Composition: An ideal tonic containing Vitamin B-complex with B_{12}.
    Dose: Large animal – 30-40 ml OD; Small animal – 15-20 ml OD.

30. *Retisol* (Vetcon) – 100 ml, 200 ml and 500 ml

    Composition: A multivitamin formulation or feed supplement with Vitamins A, D_3, E and B_{12}.

    Dose: Large animal – 15-20 ml BID; Small animal – 50-10 ml BID.

31. *Actoral-H* (Bery and Bery Vet) – 30 ml, 60 ml and 500 ml

    Composition: Vitamin AD_3E B_{12} and H – Essential vitamins liquid feed supplement with Biotin.

    Dose: Cattle, Buffalo and Horse – 10-15 ml/animal daily.

    Dog, Sheep and Goat – 5 ml per animal per day.

32. *Multisol Special* (Pearl Chemicals) – 30 ml, 60 ml and 120 ml bottle

    Composition: Vitamins A, D_3, E, B_{12} and K.

    Dose: Large animal – 10 ml twice daily.

    Small animal – 5 ml twice daily.

33. *Maplex Liquid* (Marion Pharma) – 10 ml, 200 ml, 500 ml and 1 litre

34. *Sharkoferol Vet* (Alembic)

    Composition: Iron oxide, Calcium gluconate, Vitamin A, D_3, B_1, B_2 and Niacinamide.

    Dose: Cattle and Calf – 10-15 ml, Dog and Cat – 5-10 ml OD.

19.16.7 Antiseptic Herbal Dressing Oil

Indication

For external use only in wounds (surgical wounds, traumatic wounds, lacerated wounds, broken horn, bite wounds, sores and fissures, yoke gall, gangrenous and ulcerated wounds, infected wounds, septic wounds, maggoted wounds), cuts, burns, scalds, foot lesions in FMD, ring worm, eczema, dermatomycosis and mange infestation. It provides antiparasitic, antibacterial, antifungal and antiseptic action, resolving swelling and pain.

Common Content

Neem oil, Eucalyptus oil, Turpentine oil, Chalmogra oil, Linseed oil, Karanja oil.

Use

Apply liberally twice or thrice daily in the affected areas after proper cleaning of the wound by cotton swab or spray.

Trade Names

1. *Dresol* (Kapila) – 50 ml, 100 ml, 1 litre and 5 litres
2. *Dressogen* (Nugen Pharma) – 50 ml and 100 ml in bottle
3. *Dressit* (Oxford Gems) – 50 ml and 100 ml bottle
4. *RS Oil* (RS Pharmaceuticals)- 50 ml and 100 ml bottle
5. *Cure Oil* (Bery and Bery Vet) – 50 ml and 100 ml bottle

Composition: Turpentine oil – 10 per cent, Eucalyptus oil – 3 per cent, Chalmogra oil – 2 per cent, Camphor – 5 per cent, Karanja oil – 6 per cent, Neem oil Q.S.

6. *Bactecon* (Pharmacon) – 50 ml, 100 ml and 1 litre bottle
7. *Saf Oil* (Legend) – 50 ml and 100 ml bottle.
8. *Himax Lotion* (Indian Herbs) – 100 ml bottle
9. *Dermanol* (Vetmed) – 30 ml and 50 ml
10. *Dressol* (Cattle Remedies) – 100 ml bottle
11. *Skinovet Skin Oil* (Angel's Group) – 100 ml and 450 ml

19.16.8 Herbal Ointments

Broad Spectrum Multipurpose Gels/Ointments for Wound Management

Indication

Wounds, burns, scalds, dermatological disorders, FMD foot lesions, foot rot, contagious ecthyma, eczema, infected wounds, maggoted wounds, ulcerated wounds, Dermatomycosis, herbal cream for support in mastitis infusion therapy.

Trade Names

1. *Sorin Ointment* (Vetmed)

   It is an anti bacterial, antifungal, antiseptic, anti-inflammatory, antiparasitic, demulcent and anodyne.
2. *Dressoment Ointment* (Nugen) – 25 g, 50 g tubes

   Herbal ointment for external use.
3. *Himax Ointment* (Indian Herbs) – 50 g tube and tin of 1 kg
4. *Himax-D Ointment* (Indian Herbs) – 25 g tube for dogs (pets)
5. *Charmil Ointment* (Dabur Ayurvet) – 25 g, 50 g squeeze tubes

   Apply once or twice daily after cleaning of the area till complete recovery.
6. *Inflagel Ointment* (Neospark drugs) – 25 g and 1 kg

   It contains multi action skin gel for external use only.
7. *Skinoment Gel* (Zeev Care Industries) – 50 g tube

   Multiaction skin gel for external use only.
8. *Topicure Gel* (Natural Remedies)

   Multipurpose herbal gel trusted for topical cure of all types of wounds including maggot wounds, FMD lesions, foot rot, Dermatomycosis, surgical wounds, deep penetrated and widespread wounds.
9. *Dermanol Cream* (Indian Herbs)

   Antimicrobical, miticidal, anti-inflammatory and vulnerary cream.
10. *Scavon Gel* (Himalayan Drugs)

    Antimicrobial, miticidal, anti-inflammatory and vulnerary exam.

11. *Dressona Ointment* (Bioherbs)

    Herbal ointment for wounds.

12. *Lorexane Ointment* (GSK) – 50 g and 100 g tube

    Composition: Gama Benzine Hexachloride.

    Acriflavin – 15 parts, Gammaxene – 15 parts, Vaseline 80 parts and Cetrimide 0.45 per cent w/w.

13. *Helax Ointment* (Boo teesa Pharma)

    Herbal fly repellent and wound healing ointment.

14. *Wisprec Cream* (Natural Remedies) – 25 g tube

    A multispectrum cream to treat skin disorders due to bacteria, fungi, mites *etc.*

    Use: To apply locally BID.

15. *Zinc Oxide Ointment*

    Composition: Zinc oxide – 15 parts + Vaseline – 85 parts.

16. *Dressol-FR Gel* (Cattle Remedies) – 50 g tube

    The broad spectrum antiseptic fly repellent gel.

17. *Skinoment Ointment* (Arosol) – 25 g tube

    Use: To apply eternally twice daily.

19.16.9 Non-Herbal and Herbal Aerosol Spray for Topical Wound Cure

Indication

Antibacteiral, antifungal and miticidal medicines. Recommended for surgical and FMD wounds, ring worm, dermatomycosis, myasis, traumitic wounds, mange infestation, maggoted wounds, flies and other infested wound *etc.*

Use

Spray liberally twice daily.

Trade Names

1. *Lorexane Spray* (GSK)
2. *Topicure Spray* (Natural Remedies) – 75 ml and 250 ml Spray Can
3. *Skin Heal Spray* (Nadian Herbs)
4. *D'mag Spray* (Intas) – 50 ml and 100 ml Spray Can (for canine)
5. *Scavon Spray* (Himalaya Drug) – 120 ml Can

19.16.10 Non-Hormonal Herbal Heat Inducer

High Power Herbal Heat Inducing Capsules

Indication

These medicines help to induce ovarian function, action similar to gonadotrophins, help to release hormones for inducing ovulatory oestrus, and ensure efficient breeding. May be used in anoestrus due to non-functional ovary and or non-specific reasons, delayed maturity due to non-specific reasons in heifers *etc.*

Dose

Cows, Buffalo, Mare and Heifer – 3 capsules daily x 2days.

Ewe, Doe and Dog – 2 capsules daily x 2 days.

Watch for estrous in next 10 days and repeat on 11th and 12th day, if required.

In case of repeat breeding condition repeat the dose on 6th and 7th day and if required repeat again on 17th and 18th day @ 3 capsules daily.

Trade Names

1. *Sajani* (Sarabhai Zydus) – 6 cap sachet
2. *Prajana* (Indian Herbs) – 6 cap pouch
3. *Janova* (Ayurvet) – 6 boli strip.
4. *Exapar* (Ayurvet)
5. *Gestaforte Bolus* (TTK) – Cartoon of 5 strips of 4 boli each
6. *Ovatone Capsule* (Legend) – 6 capsules in a strip
7. *Estrona Forte* Bolus (Rakesh Pharmaceuticals) – 10 boli pack

   It regulates estrus cycle, acts as uterine antiseptic and anti-inflammatory.

   Dose: Cow and Buffalo – 1 bolus daily for 10 days.
8. *Banjhna* (Bharatiya Bootee)

   Dose: For introduction of ovulatory heat in anoestrous cases,

   Small cow and buffalo – 3-4 caps orally.

   Large cow and buffalo – 4-6 caps orally.

   If the animal does not come in heat within 24 hours, repeat next dose.
9. *Heatasole Capsule* (Arosol Pharmaceuticals) – Blister pack of 6 caps strip

   A unique non-hormonal herbal heat inducer.

   Dose: 2 caps daily x 3 days.
10. *Bucofert Bolus* (Natural Remedies) – Pack of 6 boli

    It is an oestrus inducer bolus with power of phytoestrogen. It induces ovulatory oestrus in dairy animals for improving the overall breeding efficiency.

    Dose: 2 boli once daily orally for consecutive 3 days. If no or weak sign of heat occurs within 10 days, repeat the aforesaid dose.

19. 16.11 Herbal Immunomodulator

1. *Restoball* (Ayurvet) – 500 ml bottle and 1 litre jar

   It is an herbal immunomodulator, antistressor and rejuvenator.

   Dose: Cattle and Buffalo 50 ml twice daily for 5-10 days.

2. *Lackpro Syrup* (Angels Group) – 450 ml and 1 litre jar

   Dose: Small animal 15-20 ml twice daily for 10 days. Large animal 20-30 ml twice daily for 10 days.

19.17 MINERAL MIXTURES

19.17.1 Common Mineral Mixtures

Indication

Mineral deficiency, low milk production, poor and emaciated health, weak calf at birth. Improper digestion and assimilation, improved fertility, higher productivity, early maturity, healthy offsprings.

Trade Names

1. *Kcmin* (Kapila) – 1 kg poly pack and 50 kg bag

   Dose: Cattle and Buffalo – 25 g daily.

   Calf, Sheep and Goat – 5-15 g daily.
2. *Kalmin-L* (KAP)–1 kg poly pack

   Dose: Cattle and Buffalo – 28 g daily.

   Calf, Sheep and Goat – 5-15 g daily.
3. *Minerex-L Powder* (Excell) -1 kg pack

   Unique mineral mixture with lactobacillus, lysine and methionine.

   Dose: Cattle and Buffalo – 25-30 g daily.

   Small animals – 5-10 g daily.
4. *Grovimin Forte* (Pharmacon) – 500 g pack

   Mineral feed supplement for livestock and poultry, balanced with all essential minerals.

   Dose: Cattle, Buffalo and Horse – 20-30 g daily.

   Calf, Sheep, Goat and Pig – 10-15 g daily.
5. *Minfa* (Intas) – 1 kg and 10 kg poly bag

   Chromium enriched mineral mixture useful in improving milk production, overall growth, development and enhances reproductive performances.

   Dose: Cattle and Buffalo – 30-50 g daily; Calf 10 g daily.

   Mixing ratio for cattle feed: 1 kg to be mixed in 100 kg feed.
6. *Calmin Powder* (Cattle Remedies) – 1 kg poly bag

   Fights mineral deficiency with oral dosing 25 g twice daily for 20 days for cattle and buffalo and improves fertility.
7. *Magacal Powder* (Indian Herbs)–1 kg pack

   For optimum bone mineralization and to prevent calcium and phosphorus deficiency.
8. *Grogold Powder* (Vets Farma) – 400 g and 800 g

   Dose: Cattle and Buffalo – 20 g once daily.

9. *Ranmix* (Vetnex) – 1 kg packet
   Dose: Cattle and Buffalo – 25-30 g orally OD.
   Calf, Sheep and Goat – 5-10 g orally OD.
10. *Calmin* (Cattle Remedies) – 1 kg and 5 kg bag
    Dose: Large animal – 25-30 g daily; Small animal 6-10 g daily.
11. *Animin Powder* (Vets Farma) – 1 kg and 10 kg pack
    Dose: Large animal 30-60 g orally daily; Small animal 10-15 g orally daily.
12. *Profimin Powder* (Vets Farma) – 1 kg pack
    Composition: Minerals + amino acids.
    Dose: Large animal – 25 g once daily, Calf – 12 g daily.
13. *Minimix Powder* (Oxen Labs) – 1 kg and 5 kg pack
    Dose: Large animal 30-50 g orally per day per animal; Small animal 10-15 g orally per day per animal.
14. *Minerin Powder* (Vetmed)
    Dose: Large animal – 20 g twice daily with feed, atleast for 7-10 days.
    Small animal – 10 g twice daily with feed.
15. *Minerex Forte Powder* (Excell) – 250 g, 1 kg and 2.5 kg pack
    Composition: Mixture of vitamin AD_3K and B_{12} with minerals.
    Dose: Large animals 25 g daily; Small animal 10 g daily.
16. *Grovicon* (Pharmacon) – 1 kg pack
    Composition: Mineral feed supplement for livestock and poultry, provides all essential minerals.
    Dose: Cattle, Buffalo and Horse – 20-30 g daily.
    Calf, Sheep, Goat and Pig – 10-15 g daily.
17. *Encalmin Forte* (Enlag Labs) – 500 g, 1 kg and 2.5 kg
    Dose: Cattle, Buffalo and Horse – 25-30 g daily.
    Sheep, Goat and Pig – 10-20 g daily.
18. *Orcal-P Granules* (TTK) – 250 g, 500 g and 12.5 kg bag
    Composition: Calcium, Phosphorus and D_3 combination.
    Dose: Cattle and Horse – 30-50 g daily; Sheep, Goat and Pig – 10 g daily for 10 days.
19. *Agrimin Forte* (GlaxoSmithkline) – 500 g and 1 kg
    Dose: Cattle and Buffalo – 25 g orally OD 5 kg per day.
    Sheep and Goat – 5-10 g daily OD.
20. *Gynaecon* (Pharmacon) – 10 g
    Dose: Cattle, Buffalo, Heifer and Mare – 5-10 g twice daily.
    Sheep, Goat and Pig – ½ tsf twice daily.

21. *Lactivey* (Alved) – 500 g, 1 kg and 2.5 kg pack
    Unique mineral mixture with lactobacillus, lysine and methionine.
    Dose: Cattle and Buffalo – 25-30 g daily; Small animal – 5-10 g daily.
22. *Estromin* (Nugen)–500 g and 1 kg pack
    It contains essential minerals for anoestrus and silent heat.
    Dose: Heifer, Cow and Buffalo – 20-25 g once daily.
23. *Neocal-C* (Kapila) – 100 g poly pack and 400 g cartoon
    Dose: Cattle and Horse – 40-50 g BID.
    Calf, Sheep, Goat and Pig – 15-25 g BID.
24. *Totalmin* (Vetcon) – 500 g, and 1 kg
    Dose: Cattle and Buffalo – 25-30 g orally OD.
    Sheep and Goat – 10 g orally OD.
25. *Krishmin-Forte* (Pharmacon)–1 kg pack
    Mineral mixture with amino acid for livestock and poultry.
    Dose: Cattle, Buffalo and Horse – 20-30 g daily.
    Calf, Sheep and Goat – 10-15 g daily.
    Poultry – 5 g per kg feed.
26. *Ayumin-V* (Ayurvet) – 500 g and 1 kg pack
    Dose: Cattle and Buffalo – 30-35 g once daily for 15 days.
27. *Uniselit* (Ayurvet) – 10 g sachet
    It is an antioxidant trace mineral supplement.
    Dose: 10 g (1 sachet) daily for 15 days.
28. *Agrimin Powder* (GlaxoSmithkline) – 1 kg and 10 kg bag
    Dose: Large animal – 30-36 g daily; Small animal – 10-15 g daily.

19.17.2 Mineral Mixtures with Vitamins

Indication

Impaired nutrition, protein-vitamin imbalance, depressed production, retarded growth, nutritional disorders, improper assimilation, anoestrous, repeat breeding, and compromised immunity.

Trade Names

1. *Vitromin* (Kapila) – 500 g, 1 kg poly pack and 2.5 kg poly jar
   An ideal protein, vitamin, mineral readymix feed supplement for livestock.
   Dose: Cattle and Buffalo – 30-40 g daily.
   Sheep, Goat and Pig – 15-20 g daily.
   Duck and Poultry – 2.5-3 g/kg feed.
2. *Kem Trace Dry* (Kemin) – 500 g, 1 kg and 25 kg pack
   A blend of organic trace minerals with viable yeast and vitamins.

Dose: Cattle and Buffalo – 25 g daily (in severe deficiency condition 50 g/day).

3. *Nutrimin Forte* (Arosol)–1 kg, 6 kg and 25 kg poly bag.
   Unique, finely blended ideal vitamins and mineral mixtures.
   Dose: Small animal – 10-20 g daily.
   Large animal – 25-50 g daily
4. *Minovit Forte* (Pearls Chemicals) – 500 g and 25 kg pack
   Dose: Large animal – 25-30 g daily.
   Small animal – 5-10 g daily.
5. *C-Min Forte Plus* (C-care) – 500 g, 1 kg, 5 kg and 20 kg packs
   Special feed supplement for animals balanced with minerals, vitamins, amino acids and live yeast culture.
   Dose : Livestock – Mixing 1 kg/100 kg feed.
   Small animal – 15 g per day.
   Large animal – 25-30 g per day.
6. *Minerex Fort Powder* (Excell) – 250 g, 1 kg and 2.5 kg packs
   Dose: Large animal – 25 g daily.
   Small animal – 10 g daily.
7. *Vitaprotin DS* (Pharmacon) – 25 g, 500 g, 1 kg and 2.5 kg packs
   Dose: Cattle, Buffalo and Horse – 20-30 g OD.
   Calf, Sheep and Goat – 50-75 g daily.
8. *Concimin* (Concept) – 250 g, 1 kg and 2.5 kg packs
   Dose: Cattle, Buffalo and Horse – 15-20 g daily.
   Calf, Sheep and Goat – 5-10 g daily.
   Poultry – 2.5 kg/ton feed.
9. *Minadex-C Powder* (AFC) – 50 kg bag
   Dose: 2 kg in 100 kg cattle feed or 100 g daily for milch cattle, 25 g for small cow, 50 g for adult and dry cow.
10. *Ayumin-V* (Ayurvet) – 500 g, 1 kg and 5 kg bag
    Dose: Cattle and Buffalo – 30-50 g daily for 15 days.
11. *Alvite-M* (Alembic) – Poly bag of 1 kg and 2.5 kg
    Dose: Adult Cattle, Buffalo, Mare – 25 g/day.
    Calf and Heifer – 5-15 g/day.
    Sheep and Goat – 3-5 g/day.
12. *Lactivet Powder* (Alved) – 500 g, 1 kg and 5 kg packs
    Composition: Vitamins A, D_3, E, Mn, Zn, Co, P and Cu.
    Indication: Vitamins and mineral deficiencies.

Dose: Cow and Buffalo – 25 g daily, Heifer – 15 g daily, Breeding bull – 30 g daily.

13. *Biomin Powder* (Bioherbs) – 500 g and 1 kg packets
    Dose: Cattle and Buffalo – 3 g orally once daily.
    Calf, Sheep and Goat – 15-25 g orally once daily.
14. *Hylactin Powder* (Jeps) – 500 g and 1 kg packs
    Composition: Vitamins A, D_3, E, Cu, Co, Mn, Zn, Iodine.
    Dose: Large animal – 30-40 g, Young stock – 10-20 g.
15. *Minamil* (Brihans) – 500 g and 1kg
    It is a combipack of 10 vital vitamins and essential minerals for poultry and livestock.
    Dose: Cattle, Buffalo and Horse – 20-25 g.
    Calf, Sheep and Goat – 5-10 g.
    Pig and Foal – 5-10 g.
    Poultry – 20-30 g/100 birds.
16. *Complemin Fort* (Nugen) – 50 g, 1 kg and 5 kg poly bags
    A powder feed supplement of essential minerals and vitamins.
    Dose: Calf – 10 g, Cow – 25 g, Buffalo – 40 g, Foal – 20 g, Horse – 40 g, Pig – 5 g, Sheep and Goat – 10-15 g.
    Poultry mixing ratio – Broiler and Layer feed – 25 g/100 kg feed, Starter feed – 250 g/50 kg feed.
17. *Proteimin fort* (Oxford Gem)–500 g and1 kg packet
    Combipack of essential vitamins and minerals improves food digestibility, stimulates growth and production, corrects fertility problems, and maintains acid base balance.
    Dose: Cattle and Buffalo – 25-50 g, Calf, Sheep and Goat – 10-15 g.
18. *Encalmin forte* (Enlag lab) – 500 g, 1 kg and 2.5 kg
    Complete mineral mixture withproteins and vitamins.
    Dose: Cattle, Buffalo and Horse – 25-30 g daily.
    Sheep, Goat, Pig and Dog – 10-20 g daily.
19. *Nutrimin* (Arosol Pharmaceuticals) – 1 kg, 5 kg and 25 kg poly bags
    Dose: Cattle and Buffalo – 25-30 g OD.
    Sheep and Goat – 10 g OD.
20. *Bestamin Gold* (Vet Care) – 1 kg pack
    Composition: It contains metho chelated minerals, vitamins and methionine.
    Dose: Cattle and Buffalo – 50 g OD
    Sheep and Goat – 10 g OD.

19.17.3 Vitamins-Minerals Mixtures for Better Milk Production

Indication

For better quality and quantity milk, assisting in milk let down.

Trade Names

1. *Nutrisaac* (Vetcare) – 1 kg packet
   Dose: Lactating cow/buffalo 100 g/head/day orally.
2. *Lactin* (Kapila) – 500 g poly pack
   Composition: Ca, P, Vit. A, D_3, E, B_{12} and Herbs.
   Dosage: Cattle and Buffalo (Lactating) – 25-30 g daily.
   Small animal (Doe, Ewe and Sow)– 5-10 grams daily.
3. *Nutro Cal Dry* (Kemin) – 100 g, 1 kg, 5 kg and 25 kg
   Composition: Composed of propionates, organic form of Cu, Zn and Ca.

   Improves feed intake and blood glucose level, provides molecular energy, prevents ketosis, enhances milk production by improving the nutrient reserves.

   Dose: 50-100 g per animal per day for 3 days as supportive therpy during the treatment of off fed conditions and ketosis.
4. *Kem Trace Dry* (Kemin) – 500 g and 1 kg
   A blend of of organic trace minerals with viable yeast and vitamins. It increases milk yield and milk fat, supply high bioavailable trace minerals, replenishes deficiency of minerals.

   Dose: Large animal – 25 g/day.
5. *Lactomore* (Marion Pharma) – 500 g and 1 kg packs
   Dose: Cattle and Buffalo – 30-50 g OD, Doe and Ewe-15 g BID.
6. *Milchey* (Novartis)–100 tablets bottle
   A multiherbal preparation.
   Dose: 15 tabs twice a day on 1st day.
7. *R.S. Protein Forte* (R.S. Pharma)
   Dose: Cattle and Buffalo – 25-30 g; Sheep, Goat, Calf – 10-20 g.
8. *Care-Plus* (C-Care) – 1 litre, 5 litres and 20 litres jar
   A power for milk improving production, liquid animal feed supplement with calcium, phosphorus, Vit. A, D_3, B_{12}, minerals and essential botanicals.

   Dose: Cattle and Horse – 50 ml twice daily,

   Calf – 20 ml twice daily.

   Sheep, Goat, Dog and Sow – 10 ml twice daily.
9. *Milchend* (Legends) – 250 g pack
   It is a high milk yield formula balanced with vitamins, minerals and amino acids.

Dose : Large animal – 25 g per day.

Small animal – 5 g per day.

10. *Calcistrength* (Brihans) – 1 kg and 2.5 kg bags

    Composition: Calcium and phosphorous in 2 : 1 ratio with vitamin AD_3E and trace minerals and yeast powder.

    Dose: Cattle, Buffalo and Horse – 20-25 g daily with feed or with treacle.

11. *Biobloom* (Sarabhai Zydus) – 250 g and 1 kg

    Dose: Lactating animal – 15 g/day.

12. *Orcal-P Granules* (TTK) – 25 g, 500 g and 12.5 kg bags

    The bone calcium and productivity booster.

    It improves milk quality, milk fat per cent and augment milk yield, hastens fracture healing, reduces occurrence of milk fever, reduced uterine inertia, improves recovery from milk fever.

    Dose: Cattle and Horse – 30-50 g daily

    Sheep, Goat and Pig – 10 g daily

    Dog and Cat – 30-50 g daily

    For 10 days continuously in a month.

13. *Chelated Milmor Forte* (Novartis) – 1 kg packet

    It improves milk yield and increase fat percentage in milk, optimizes growth, improves fertility, ensures healthy calf, bring about better hard health.

    Dose: Cattle and Buffalo – 25-30 g daily.

    Calf, Sheep and Goat – 10-15 g daily.

14. *Leptaden Vet Tabs* (Alarsin) – 100 and 1000 tabs

    Ayurvedic medicine contains Kamboji and Jeevanti which initiates milk secretion, increase milk production and regulates milk discharge in small and large ruminants.

    Dose: Large animal – 10-15 tabs BID for 1-2 weeks then 10 tabs daily for 10 days.

15. *Milk Max* (Ethicare) – 1kg and 10 kg bags

    Dose: Adult Cattle and Buffalo – 25-30 g/daily orally or 1 kg/100 kg concentrate feed.

16. *Galog* (Indian Herbs) – 250 g and 1 kg pack

    Dose: Cow, Buffalo and Mare – 50 g daily for 15 days orally.

    Sheep and Goat – 10-15 g daily for 15 days.

17. *Berymin Forte* (Bery and Bery Vet) – 500 g, 1 kg, 3 kg and 5 kg bags

    It is a combipack of vitamins and minerals mixture (a balanced nutripack)

    Dose: Small animal – 10-15 g OD

    Large animal – 40-50 g OD.

18. *Cattle Mix* (Perals Chemicals) – 1 kg polybag
    Composition: It contains all types of essential minerals for cattle.
    Dose: 30-75 g for cattle.
19. *Ranmix Total* (Vetnex) – 1 kg pack
    Dose: Cattle and Buffalo – 30-40 g orally once daily.
20. *Super Care Liquid-365* (Excell)- 1 litre and 5 litre
    Dose: Large animal 100 ml daily for 10 days.
    Small animal 50 ml daily for 10 days.
21. *Hilak* (Ayurvet) -1 kg pack
    It increases milk production and fat per cent, and improves reproductive efficiency and health.
    Dose: 50-200 g per day or 50 g/5 litres milk production per day.
22. *Lactomax-AD$_3$* (Arosol Pharmaceuticals) – 250 ml, 500 ml and 1 litre bottle
    Dose: Cattle and Buffalo – 50 ml BID.
    Small animal – 15-20 ml BID.

19.17.4 Oral Calcium Syrup (Tonic)/Supplement

Indication

To replenish calcium drained through milk, to supplement the requirement of calcium and phosphorus for health and productivity, to meet the higher demand of calcium during gestation period and lactation, to minimize episodes of metabolic disorders, to improve foetus health, to prepare dam for better lactation, to tone up reproductive system and to optimize inter calving period.

19.16.4.1 Herbal Preparation

Indication

Enhance vital metabolic activities, act as immunomodulant, antistress, improve milk yield, mastitis, foetal growth, tone up reproductive system.

Trade Names

1. *Phytocal* (Natural Remedies) -1 lit. can and 5 litres Can
   Calcium supplement fortified with herbs for better milk production.
   Dose: Large animal – 100 ml, Small animal – 50 ml.
2. *Calshakti* (Intas) – 500 ml, 1 litre, 5 litres and 7.5 litres plastic jar
   Dose: Cattle and Buffalo – 100 ml OD
   Calf – 40 ml OD,
   Sheep and Goat- 10 ml OD.
3. *Calcimal Special Gel* (Oxen Labs) – 500 ml, 1 litre and 5 litres
   Composition: Not truly herbal, having calcium, phosphorus, Vitamin D$_3$ and B$_{12}$, Cobalt chloride, Jevanti, Satavari in gel form.
   Dose: Cattle and Buffalo – 100 ml orally daily.

Calf – 30 ml OD.

Sheep and Goat – 10-20 ml orally daily.

4. *Caldhan-V* (Ayurvet) – 1 litre and 5 litres jar

   Composition: Calcium and phosphorus supplement with Vitamin D_3 and B_{12} helps in improving milk yield in lactating animals and helps in better growth and production.

   Dose: Cattle and Buffalo – 50 ml twice daily.

5. *Cal More* (Indian Herbs) – 500 ml, 1 litre jerrycan and 5 litres jerrycan

   Composition: Formulation of calcium, phosphorous, Vitamin D_3 and Vitamin B_{12} for higher milk production and optimum body growth.

   Dose: Cattle and Buffalo – 50 ml orally BID.

   Small animal – 15-20 g BID.

6. *Capsola Gold* (Vetnex) – 1 litre, 2.5 litres and 5 litres

   Composition: Oral calcium rich in herbs for enhancement of milk production.

   Dose: Lactating cows and buffalo – 50 ml orally twice daily.

7. *Ossomin Vet* (TTK) – 200 ml, 450 ml bottle and 4.5 litres jerrycan

   Dose: Calf – 5 ml; Heifer – 10 ml; Adult Cow/Buffalo – 20 ml; Pregnant Cow and Buffalo – 30 ml orally daily.

19.17.4.2 Non-Herbal Calcium Oral Tonic

Indication

For production, reproduction, augmentation of lactational yield, ensures strong bones, teeth, cartilages, strong shelled egg production.

Trade Names

1. *Calphos D_3 liquid and bolus* (Excell) – 1 liter and 5 litres and 4 boli per strip

   Dose: Liquid

   Cattle and Horse – 100-120 ml daily for 8-10 days.

   Dog: 10-20 ml daily for 8 to 10 days.

   Bolus

   Large animal – 1-2 boli OD for 5 days.

   Small animal – ½- 1 bolus OD for 8-10 days.

2. *Calcimal suspension* (Oxen lab) – 500 ml, 1 litre and 5 litres

   Composition: Calcium with Vitamins D_3 and B_{12}.

   Dose: Cattle and Buffalo – 50-100 ml.

   Calf, Sheep, Goat and Pig – 20-30 ml daily.

   Dog – 5-10 ml daily.

   Poultry – 50-100 ml for 100 birds.

3. *Calciforte Syrup* (Nugen Pharma) – 200 ml, 500 ml, 1 litre and 5 litres

   A crystal clear calcium syrup enriched with iron and cobalt.

Dose: Livestock

Cattle – 50 ml, Buffalo – 70 ml, Calf – 5 ml, Pup – 10 ml, Adult dog and Cat – 20-25 ml.

Poultry

Chicken – 10 ml/100 chicks, Layer – 50 ml/100 birds, Broiler and Growers – 20 ml/100 birds.

4. *Calphos Plus* (Bery and Bery Vet) – 500 ml, 1 litre and 5 litres jar

   Composition: Calcium, Phosphorus, Vitamin A, D_3 and B_{12}.

   Dose: Cattle, Buffalo, Horse and Camel – 100 ml daily.

   Dog, Calf, Goat and Sheep – 20-50 ml daily.

   Layers birds – 100 ml/100 birds OD.

5. *Calphos-12* (Bery and Bery Vet) – 500 ml, 1 litre and 5 litres

   It is an ideal productive tonic, contains Ca, P with Vitamin D_3 and B_{12}.

   Dose: Cattle, Buffalo and Horse – 100 ml daily.

   Calf, Dog, Sheep and Goat – 10-20 ml daily.

   Grower and Broiler – 50 ml/100 birds, Layer – 100 ml/1000 birds.

6. *Calcimilk* (Pharmacon Vet) – 100 ml, 450 ml, 1 litre and 5 litres jar

   Dose: Small animal – 10-25 ml/animal BID for 10 days.

   Poultry – 50 ml/100 birds.

7. *Care Plus* (C-Care)

   It is a liquid animal feed supplement with Ca, P, Vitamins A, D_3 and B_{12}, minerals and essential botanicals.

   Dose: Dog, Calf, Sheep and Goat, Foal – 10 ml twice daily.

   Chick/Broiler – 10 ml daily (100 birds), Grower (100) – 25 ml daily, Layer (100) – 50 ml daily.

8. *Calcizin Syrup* (Nugen Pharma) – 200 ml, 500 ml, 1 litre and 5 litres

   Dose: Cattle – 50 ml, Buffalo – 70 ml, Calf – 25 ml, Sheep and Goat – 15 ml.

   Dog and Cat – 20 ml, Pup – 10 ml OD.

9. *Mifex Oral* (Novartis) – 1 litre and 5 litres jar

   Oral liquid medicine rich in calcium, magnesiuum, phosphorus, vitamins A, D_3 and B_{12}.

   Dose: Large animal 100 ml daily, small animal 25 ml per day.

10. *Encal-12* (Enlag Labs) – 50 ml, 1 litre and 5 litres

    Composition: Calcium, phosphorus with Vitamins D_3 and B_{12}.

    Dose: Cattle – 50-100 ml daily, small animal – 10-20 ml daily.

11. *Calcicon* (Vetcon) – 500 ml and 1 litre

    A non-sediment calcium oral tonic.

    Dose: Cattle and Buffalo – 50 ml orally BID, Calf, Sheep and Goat – 20-25 ml orally daily.

12. *Vita Calci Plus* (Oxford Gems) – 200 ml, 500 ml, 1 litre and 5 litres
    Dose: Cattle and Buffalo – 50 ml orally BID.
    Calf, Sheep and Goat – 15-20 ml orally BID.
13. *Calrin Plus* (Vetcon) – 500 ml and 1 litre
    Dose: Cattle and Buffalo – 40-45 ml orally BID.
    Calf, Sheep and Goat – 15-20 ml orally BID.
14. *Encal Plus* (Enlag Lab) – 100 ml, 500 ml and 1 litre
    Dose: Cattle and Buffalo – 40-50 ml BID
    Poultry – Chicks15 ml/100 birds; Grower and Broiler 20-30 ml/100 birds; Layer 30-40 ml/100 birds per day.
15. *Capsola* (Vetnex) – 500 ml, 1 litre, 2.5 litres and 5 litres
    Dose: Cattle and Buffalo – 50 ml orally BID
    Calf, Sheep and Goat – 20 ml orally BID.
16. *Megaboost* (Vets Farma) – 500 ml, 1 litre and 5 litres
    A unique blend of calcium, phosphorus, Vitamin D_3 B_{12} and stomach extract liquid feed supplement for livestock and poultry.
    Dose: Large animal – 50 ml twice a day.
    Dog – 10 ml twice a day.
    Broiler and Layer (100 birds) – 20-50 ml; Chicks (100 birds) 10 ml per day.
17. *Ostovet* (GSK) – 500 ml, 1 litre and 5 litres
    Dose: Cattle and Buffalo – 50 ml orally BID (100 ml OD)
    Calf, Sheep and Goat – 15-20 ml orally BID.
18. *Calvin-DS* (Pearl Chemicals) – 100 ml, 450 ml, 1 litre and 5 litres
    Dose: Cattle and Horse – 50 ml twice daily.
    Calf, Sheep and Goat – 15-20 ml twice daily.
    Poultry – Chicks 10 ml/100 birds, Growers – 25 ml/100 birds, Layers – 50 ml/birds.
19. *Ostovet Forte Liquid* (Virbac-APC)
    Dose: For high yielding cattle 100 ml mixture of Ostovet Forte + Vimeral 10 mg/day.
20. *Calsagar* (Indian Immunologicals) – 500 g pack
    Animal feed pellets containing calcium, phosphorus and Vit. D3.
    Dose: Lactating Cow and Buffalo – 50-80 g/day/animal.
    Dry adult and growing animal 25-30 g once daily.
21. *Cal-K* (Karnataka Antibiotic) – 100 ml, 200 ml, 500 ml and 5 litres
    Composition: Calcium, Phosphorus, Vitamins D_3, B_{12}, Vitamin-C and Manganese Dose: Small animal – 10 ml per animal daily for 7 days.
    Large animal – 50 ml/per animal daily for 5-7 days.

22. *Orical Oral* (IBC) – 1 litre and 5 litres
    Dose: Cattle and Buffalo – 40-50 ml daily per animal.
    Small animal – 15-20 ml daily per animal.
23. *Super Care Liquid* (Excell) – 1 litre and 5 litres
    Dose: Cattle and Buffalo – 100 ml daily for 10 days.
    Calf, Sheep and Goat – 50 ml daily for 10 days.
24. *Calcicare* (Brihans) – 100 ml, 500 ml, 1 litres and 5 litres
    Dose: Cattle and Buffalo and Horse – 40-50 ml daily.
    Calf, Sheep, Goat and Pig – 15-20 ml daily.
    Dog – 5-10 ml daily.
25. *Calfosvet Liquid* (Vets Farma) – 500 ml, 1 litre, 2 litres and 5 litres
    Composition: Ca, P, Vitamin D_3 and B_{12}.
    Dose: Cattle and Buffalo – 40-50 ml BID daily for 10-15 days.
    Calf, Sheep and Goat – 15-20 ml orally BID for 10-15 days.
26. *Ascal* (Alembic) – ½ litre, 1 litre and 5 litres
    Dose: Cattle and Buffalo – 100 ml daily for one week.
    Calf, Sheep and Goat – 25-30 ml daily for one week.
27. *Cal-Lactose* (Angel's Group) – 450 ml, 120 ml and 5 litres jar.
    Composition: Concentrate Calcium + Phosphorus + Vitamins D_3 and B_{12} + Protein + Sorbitol.
    Dose: Small animal -15-20 ml twice daily for 7 days.
    Large animal – 30-50 ml twice daily for 7 days.
28. *Cadisol-DC* (Sarabhai Zydus) – 100 ml, 500 ml, 1 litre and 5 litres jar
    Dose: Cattle, Buffalo and Horse – 50 ml orally twice daily for 10-15 days.
29. *Calcivet Liquid* (Marion Pharma) – 500 ml, 1 litre and 5 litres
    Composition : Oral calcium tonic.
    Dose: Cattle and Buffalo – 40-50 ml orally BID.
    Calf, Sheep and Goat – 15-20 ml orally BID.

19.18 REPRODUCTION FORMULA

19.18.1 Non-Hormonal Preparation

Indication

Treats anoestrus condition, corrects repeat breeding, corrects suppressed or delayed oestrus and conception, silent heat, early embryonic death due to mineral deficiency. Helps to maintain peak production.

Trade Names

1. *Repromin Dry* (Kemin) – 250 g and 500 g pack

Dose: Repeat breeders 25 g daily for 30 days (20 days for regular oestrus and 10 days after insemination)

Anoestrous animals – 25 g daily for 20 days.

2. *Gynaecon* (Pharmacon) – 100 g pack

   Dose: Cattle, Buffalo, Horse, Heifer (Max) – 5-10 g twice daily for 10-15 days.

   Sheep, Goat and Pig – ½ t.s.f. twice daily.

   Dog and Cat ½ t.s.f. twice daily.

3. *Estromin* (Nugen Pharma) – 500 g and 1 kg packet

   Dose: Cattle and Buffalo – 25 g once daily for 10-15 days.

   Heifer – 20 g OD

   Doe, Ewe and Sow – 10 g OD for 10-15 days.

4. *Gynotone Vet Powder* (Angels Group) – 30 g box

   Dose: Small animal 15-20 g twice daily.

   Large animal – 25-30 g twice daily.

5. *Heatasole Capsule* (Arosol Pharmaceuticals) – 6 cap strip

   Dose: Cattle, Buffalo – 2 cap BID x 3 days.

6. *Bestamin Gold* (Vetcare)–1 kg pack

   Composition: Methochelated minerals, stable vitamins fortified with bypass methionine complex. It improves fertility as well as productivity.

   Dose: Cattle and Buffalo – 30-40 g OD for 10-15 days.

   Small animal – 10-15 g OD for 10 days.

7. *Mintrus Caplets* (Ayurvet)

   Composition: Herbal trace minerals caplets enriched with selenium.

   Dose: 1 caplet daily from 1-20 days (for anoestrous and repeat breeding).

8. *Nutrisacc Bolus* (Vetcare) – 30 boli tin (Having bioactive chromium).

   Dose: Cattle and Buffalo

   Anoestrous – 2 boli BD for 15 days.

   For higher conception rate – 2 boli BD for 7-15 days after AI.

9. *Gesta Forte Bolus* (TTK) – 4 bolus strip.

   It is an ideal heat inducer and fertility promotes.

   Recommendation : Anoestrum – 4 boluses daily for 5 days.

   Repeat breeder – 4 boluses daily for 5 days from 17th day of previous oestrum.

   Delayed ovulation – 2 boluses daily for 10 days from 12th day of previous estrum.

   Underdeveloped genetilia and delayed puberty.

10. *Minotas Bolus* (Intas)–5 g bolus

    Composition: Trace mineral bolus with yeast.

    Dose: Cattle and Buffalo – 2 boluses daily for 2 weeks.

    Sheep and Goat – 1 bolus every alternate day for 2 weeks.

11. *Estromin Bolus* (Adven Pharma)

    Composition: Trace mineral bolus enriched with selenium and vitamin-E.

    Dose: Cattle and Buffalo – 2 boluses daily for 2 weeks.

    Sheep and Goat – ½ bol-daily for 2 weeks.

12. *Minerex Bolus* (Excell) – Strip of 4 boli.

    Composition: Each bolus provides 7 trace minerals and vitamins A, D_3 and E.

    Dose: 1 bolus daily for 7-10 days.

13. *Cyclomin-7 Bolus* (Concept)

    Composition: Each bolus is comprised of slow release preparation containing Co, Zn, Iodine, Mn, Cu, Fe and Se.

    Dose: Adult Cattle and Buffalo – 1 bolus per week.

    Calf and Heifer – ½ bolus once in a week.

14. *Flomin-C Bolus* (IBC)

    Dose: Cattle and Buffalo – 1-2 boli OD for 10 days.

    Heifer – 1 bolus Once daily orally for 10-12 days.

15. *Bioplex High Five* (Vetnex)

    Offers better fertility solutions.

    Dose: Cattle and Buffalo – 1-2 bolus once daily for 10-15 days.

16. *Bucomin-E* (Natural Remedies) – Pack of 10 capsules.

    Composition: Synergestic combination of 7 trace minerals enriched with Vitamin E.

    Dose: Cows and Buffalo – 1 caplet

    Sheep, Goats and Pig – ½ caplet

    Administer caplet orally with *gur* or flour for 10 consecutive days.

17. *Livozyme-Fe Bolus* (Marion Pharma) – Strip of 4 boli

    A unique and unparallel formula of Vitamins, minerals, probiotics, enzymes, calcium, protein, selenium and liver extract.

    Dose: Large animal – 1 to 2 bolus per day.

    Small animal – ½ to 1 bolus per day for 7 days or as advised by veterinarian.

18. *Arogen Bolus* (Arosol Pharmaceuticals) – 20 boli phoil

    Composition: Essential trace minerals with vitamin – E for fertility management.

    Dose: Large animal – 1-2 bolus BID.

    Small animal -1 bolus BID.

19.18.2 Vaginal Pessuries (for uterine treatment)

Indication

In endometritis, pyometra, metritis, chronic uterine infection, retention of placenta, after management of dystocia, repeat breeding cases as vaginal pessuries.

Trade Names

1. *Cotrimal Bolus* (Alembic) – 4 bolus strip

   Composition: Sulphamethoxazole – 1250 mg + Trimethoprim – 250 mg.

   Dose: 1) I/U irrigation with 2 boli dissolved in 1 litre water.

   Afer parturition 2 boli inserted deep I/U once.

   In any uterine infection 1-2 boli inserted deep into the uterus of the animal for 3-5 days.

2. *Furea Bolus* (Pfizer)

   Composition: Nitro Furazone 60 mg+ Urea 6 g

   Dose: Cow, Buffalo and Mare – 2 to 4 boli into the affected and normal uterine horns. Based on severity repeat treatment after 24 hours.

3. *U-Trox Bolus* (Vets Farma)

   Composition: Nitrofurazone – 60 mg + Urea – 6 g.

   Dose: 2-4 boli into each horn of the uterus, repeat after 24 hours.

4. *Uren Vet Bolus* (Dey's Vet) – (Bolus of Nitrofurazone and urea)

   Dose: 2-4 boli into the affected and normal uterine horn based on severity of infection.

5. *Furex Bolus* (Excell)

   Composition: Nitrofurazone and Urea bolus.

   Dose: 2-4 boli into each horn based on severity, can be repeated after 24 hours.

6. *Curacin-OZ Liquid* (Vets Farma) – 60 ml

   Composition: Ofloxacin + Tinidazole. It is used as potent antibacterial and antiprotozoal agent or substance. Used as a powerful I/U cleansing liquid.

7. *Lixen IU Bolus* (GSK) – (Agrivet Farm Care) – 2 boli strip

   Composition: Cephalexin – 750 mg + Urea – 2.5 g.

   Dose: 2 boli to be given for I/U indication.

8. *C-Floxfluterine Bolus* (Intas) – Strip of 2 boli

9. *C-Flox-TZ bolus*

   Composition : Each bolus contains Ciprofloxacin HCl – 1500 mg and Tinidazole – 1800 mg.

   Dose: Cattle and Buffalo – 1-2 bolus I/U daily for 2-3 days.

10. *Iodovet Bolus* (Excell) – strip of 6 boli.

    Composition : Povidone iodine – 600 mg.

    Dose: 1-2 boli I/U.

11. *Otrim Bolus* (Excell) – Strip of 4 boli.

    Dose: 2-4 boli I/U per day for 3 days.

12. *Duaprim* (Brihans)- Cotrimoxazole I/U bolus.

    Composition: Metronidazole – 1 g + Furazolidone – 200 mg.

    Dose: Large animal I/U administration – 1-2 boli daily 2 to 3 days.

    Small animal – I/U administration – ½ to 1 bolus daily for 2-3 days.

19.18.3 Intra Uterine Medicines – for Effective Uterine Wash Antibiotics/Antibacterials/Antiseptics

Indication

Uterine infections like Cervicitis, Endometritis and Pyometra.

Trade Names

1. *Ledexin Vet* (Legend) – 20 g sachet

   Composition: Cephalexin – 7.5 per cent w/w.

   Dose: One sachet to be dissolved in 50 ml and to be infused through I/U route.

2. *Lixen IU* (Glaxo) – 60 ml bottle

   Composition: Cephalexin Dry Suspension – 4.0 g/60 ml.

   Direction for use: Add water up to the mark on the bottle, and shake properly. This make 60 ml suspension for single use (through IU route).

3. *C-Flox Uterine* (Intas) – 50 ml vial

   Composition: Each ml contains Ciprofloxacin 40 mg.

4. *Curacin -OZ* (Vets Farma) – 50 ml pack

   A powerful intrauterine cleansing liquid with potent antibacterial – Ofloxacin and Antiprotozoal (Ornidazole).

5. *Enrocin – IU* (Vetnex) – 45 ml vial (5 per cent).

   Composition: Each ml contains Enrofloxacin 50 mg.

   Dose: 2.5-5 mg/kg body weight by I/U route.

6. *Iodomet Powder* (Excell) – 5 g powder

   It is one of the most effective uterine washes. After reconstitution each 30 ml contains Povidone Iodine – 10 per cent w/v and Metronidazole – 2 per cent w/v.

   Dose: 30 ml IV infusion, may be repeated after 24-48 hours.

   Administration: 5 g Iodomet to be dissolved in 30 ml water.

19.19 ECTOPARASITICIDES

The commonly used ectoparasiticides are Deltamethrin, Cypermethrin and Flumethrin *etc.*

These drugs exert potent knock down and killing effect on ectoparasites, reduce ectoparasitic stress that improve productivity, helps to maintain healthy skin, lustrous and glossy body coat and prevents transmission of vector borne diseases.

Indication

Ticks, Mites, Lice and Flies.

Trade Names

A) Deltamethrin

1) *Lysetik Liquid* (TTK) – 15 ml and 50 ml packs

Administration and Dosage: Either as spray or as dip.

Parasites	*Spray or Dip*	*Topping up*	*Application*
Ticks	2ml/lit. of water	3ml/lit. of water	Twice in 15 days
Lice/Keds	1ml/lit pf water	1.5ml/lit. of water	Single
Flies/Fleas	2ml/lit. of water	3ml/lit. of water	Single
Mites	4ml/lit. of water	6ml/lit. of water	Twice in 8 days

For farm house – 2 ml/litre of water for 20 sq m area.

2) *Megacide Vet* (Venky's Livestock) – 15 ml, 50 ml and 1 litre

Composition: Each ml contains Deltamethrin 17.5 mg (Deltamethrin – 1.75 per cent EC).

Directions for use

Parasites	*Spray or Dip*	*Topping up*	*Application*
Ticks	2 ml/1 litre water	3 ml/1 litre water	Twice in 15 days
Mites	4 ml/1 litre water	6 ml/1 litre water	Twice in 8 days
Lice/Keds	1 ml/1litre water	1.5 ml/1 litre water	Single
Fleas/Flies	2 ml/1 litre water	3 ml/1 litre water	single

3) *Butox* (Intervet) – 15 ml and 50 ml aluminum bottle

Each ml contains Deltamethrin BP – 12.5 mg.

Administration: To be used as spray, dip or dip charging/topping up.

Dose

Particulars	*Spray or Dip Charging*		*Topping up*	
Ticks	25.0 ppm	2 ml/litre of water	37-50 ppm	3.0 ml/litre of water
Lice	12.5 ppm	1 ml/litre of water	2.8-75 ppm	1.5 ml/litre of water
Mites	50.0 ppm	4 ml/litre of water	75 ppm	6.0 ml/litre of water
Flies	25.0 ppm	2 ml/litre of water	37-50 ppm	3.0 ml/litre of water

4) *Oral Ivermectin*

Vide section 19.5.7 of the Drug Index.

B) Cypermethrin

It is highly effective against ticks, fleas, mites, lice and flies.

5. *Ektomin* (Novartis) – 15 ml, 50 ml and 1 litre bottle

   Composition: Cypermethrin high Cis 10 per cent w/v.

   Dose: 1-2 ml per litre of water for application on body of the animal and repeat after 3-4 weeks.

6. *Cyprol* (Intas) – 15 ml and 50 ml bottle

   Composition: Each ml contains Cypermethrin high Cis – 100 mg.

   Dose: Livestocks 1 ml/litre of water.

   Animal Housing 20 ml/litre of water.

7. *Citox* (Oxen Lab) – 15 ml, 50 ml and 1 litre bottle

   Composition: Cypermethrin 10 per cent E.C.

   Dose: Livestocks 1 ml/litre of water.

   Animal housing 20 ml/litre of water (spray)

8. *Clinar* (GSK) – 5 ml, 15 ml and 50 ml bottle

   Composition: Cypermethrin Hi Cis – 10 per cent w/v ; each ml contains Cypermethrin 100 mg.

   Dose: Livestocks 1-2 ml/litre of water. In heavy infestation, it is desirable to repeat application after 1 hour.

   For effective control – add 20 ml clinar liquid in 5 litre of water. Animal housing 20 ml/litre water and spray in shed.

9. *Tikkil* (Indian Immunologicals) – 15 ml and 50 ml bottle

   Composition: Cypermethrin High Cis 10 per cent w/v.

   Cattle – 5 ml/litre water – Back line spray (or 5 litre/animal).

   Sheep and Goat – 1 ml/litre water, dip initial charge and replenishment.

   Camel – 1 ml/litre water – whole body spray and dip initial charge and replenishment.

   Poultry – 1 ml/60 litres water (spray mixtures for 1000 birds).

   Dog – 1 ml/litre water – whole body spray or wash.

C) Fenvalerate

It is also very good acaricidal agent.

10. *Tickomax* (Vetnex) – 15 ml and 50 ml

    Composition: Each ml contains Fenvalerate 20 per cent EC.

    Dose: Livestock – 5-6 ml/litre water for external use.

D) Flumethrin

It is used for control and management of all tick species, mites, flies and fleas.

11. *Flupor* (Vetnex) – 30 ml and 100 ml bottle

    Composition: Each ml contains 10 mg Flumethrin.

    Dosage and administration: Apply evenly along mid line of back from front of shoulder to tail head.

    Dose: 1 ml/10 kg body weight.

12. *Batycolpour on Drop* (Pfizer)

    Composition: Each ml contains Flumethrin 10mg.

    Apply along mid line of back from front of shoulder to tail head.

E) Other Ectoparasiticidals

13. *Neocidol* – 30 ml

    Composition: Diazinon

    Dose: 2-3 ml/litre of water by dip or bath.

14. *Taktic-5 per cent* (Intervet) – 25 ml

    Composition: Amitraz

    Dose: 6-10 ml/litre of water.

15. *Taktic-12.5 per cent* (Intervet) – 50 ml

    Composition: Each ml contains Amitraz – 125 mg.

    Dose: 2-3 ml/litre of water.

    For ticks Cattle and Buffalo – 2 ml/litre of water.

    Pig, Sheep and Goat – 4 ml/litre

16. *RIDD 12.5 per cent*–6 ml

    Composition: Amitraz

    Dose: 2-3 ml/litre of water.

17. *Cythion* – 60 ml

    Composition: Malathion

    Dose: 10 ml/litre of water.

18. *Sumicidon* – 100 ml bottle

    Composition: Fenvalerate

    Dose: 5 ml/litre of water.

19.20 VACCINES AND VACCINATION

Vaaccines are health products that trigger protective immune responses in animals so as to prepare them to fight future infections from disease causing agents. Some can lesson the severity of the diseases and other can prevent infection altogether. Animals should be vaccinated to protect them from many highly contagious and deadly diseases. Use of vaccines can prevent death and disease of animals. Traditionally vaccination is done annually. However, some vaccines induce immunity that lasts less than one year, whereas other may induce immunity that lasts well beyond one year.

Classification of Vaccines

Vaccines may be divided in to two groups, *viz.*, Core vaccines and Non-core vaccines.

Core vaccines: HS, BQ, Anthrax, FMD in cattle and some other herbivores. Rabies, Canine distemper, Canine parvovirus, Canine hepatitis in canines *etc.*

Non-core vaccines: Enterotoxanaemia, Canine kennel cough and other vaccines.

Vaccines are generally of two types, *viz.*,

1. Live vaccine
2. Killed/attenuated vaccine

Risk of Vaccination

Adverse responses are infrequent with annual vaccination. Risk factors can be minimized by carefully selecting vaccines on the basis of animals' need and choosing appropriate injection site and dose. In the face of contagious disease epidemic vaccination should be restricted *e.g.* FMD.

Commercial Vaccines Available in the Market

19.20.1 FMD Vaccine

1. *Bovilis FMDV Gel* (Intervet) – 10 ml and 30 ml vials

   It is an inactivated FMD vaccine with concentrated antigens adjuvanted with aluminium hydroxide gel and saponin. It contains a mixture of virus genotypes O, A and Asia-I.

   Dose: Cattle and Buffalo 2 ml SC

   Sheep and Goat – 1 ml SC

2. *Bovilis Clovax* (Intervet) – 10 ml (5 doses) and 30 ml (15 doses)

   Inactivated FMD vaccine with concentrated antigens adjuvanted with mineral oil. The vaccine contains a mixture of FMD virus serotypes O, A and Asia-1.

   Dose: Cattle and Buffalo – 2 ml by IM.

   Sheep and Goat through IM route.

3. *Foot and Mouth Disease vaccine* (Intervet) – 100 ml vial (50 doses)

   Inactivated Foot and Mouth Disease vaccine with concentrated antigens adjuvanted with mineral oil. The vaccine contains a mixtures of FMD virus serotypes O, A and Asia-1.

   Dose: Cattle and Buffalo – 2 ml

   Sheep and Goat – 1 ml

   Administration by IM injection.

4. *Raksha-Ovac* (Indian Immunologicals) – 30 ml and 100 ml vials

   Foot and Mouth Disease (oil adjuvanted vaccine) inactivated tissue culture with a mixture of FMD virus serotypes O, A and Asia-1.

Dose: Cattle, Buffalo and Calf – 2 ml SC.

Sheep and Goat – 1 ml SC.

Schedule of vaccination: Primary vaccination at 4 months of age.

First revamination – 9 months after primary vaccination.

Revaccination – Annual.

5. *Raksha FMD vaccine* (Indian Immunologicals) – 30 ml vial

   Raksha FMD vaccine contains tissue culture FMD vaccine with a mixture of FMD virus serotypes O, A and Asia-1.

   Dose: Cattle, Buffalo and Calf – 2 ml SC.

   Sheep and Goats – 1 ml SC.

   Schedule of vaccination: Primary vaccination at 4 months of age.

   First Revaccination – 9 months after primary vaccination.

   Revaccination – Annual.

19.20.2 Sheep Pox Vaccine

1. *Raksha-SP* (Indian Immunologicals) – 50 doses in glass vial + Diluent

   It is a living viral vaccine derived from cell cultures infected with an attenuates strain of sheep PVR virus. Romaninan sheep PVR virus. Romanian sheep for other strain is used.

   Dose: 1 ml of reconstituted vaccine.

   Schedule of vaccination: Age of vaccination – 3 months. Advisable to vaccinate after lambing season or during the onset of breeding season.

19.20.3 PPR (Peste Des Petits Ruminants) Vaccine for Sheep and Goat

1. *PPR vaccine* (IVRI/IAH/VB, Kolkata) – 100 doses (Freeze dried vaccine)

   A live attenuated homologous vaccine. It can be used after dissolving the vaccine in sterile diluent *e.g.* chilled NSS.

   Dose: 1 ml of reconstituted vaccine by SC route.

2. *Raksha-PPR* (Indian Immunologicals) – 25, 50 and 100 doses + sterile diluments.

   It is a freeze dried live attenuated homologous PPR vaccine. Surgri strain is used to prepare the vaccine having 10^3 TCID 50/dose.

   Dose: 1 ml of reconstituted vaccine by SC route at neck region.

19.20.4 HS Vaccine

1. *Raksha HS Vaccine* (Indian Immunologicals) – 100 ml (50 doses)

   Recommended for prophylactic vomination against cattle and buffaloes. It is a formaldehyde inactivated culture pasteurella multocida adsorbed on aluminum hydroxide gel.

   Dose: Cattle and Buffalo – 2 ml by SC injection.

Schedule of vaccination: Primary vaccination at six months of age.

Revamination – annually.

2. *Bovilis HS vaccine* (Intervet) – 50 ml vial (25 doses)

   H.S. vaccine containing inactivated *Pasteurella multocida* organisms adsorbed on aluminium hydroxide gel as an adjuvant used for prophylaxis against H.S.

   Dose: Cattle, Buffalo and calf – 2 ml by SC route.

   Schedule of vaccination: Age at primary vaccination 6 months and above.

   Revaccination – annually.

19.20.5 Combined HS and BQ Vaccine

1. *Raksha HS + BQ combined vaccine* (Indian immunologicals) – 90 ml (30 doses)

   Formaldehyde inactivated cultures of *Pasteurella multocida* and *Clostridium chauvoei* adsorbed on aluminum hydroxide gel. It is used for prophylactic vaccination against HS and BQ in cattle and buffaloes.

   Dose: Cattle, Buffalo and Calf – 3 ml SC.

2. *HS and BQ vaccine* (Biomed) – 100 ml (25 doses)

   Dose: Cattle, Buffalo and Calf – 4 ml SC.

3. *Bovilis HS BQ vaccine* (Intervet) – 50 ml vial (250 doses)

   Combined HS and BQ vaccine indicated for prophylaxis against HS and BQ of cattle and buffaloes.

   Dose: Cattle, Buffalo and Calf – 2 ml by S C route only.

   Schedule of vaccination: Primary vaccination – at the age of 6 months and above.

   Revaccination – annually.

19.20.6 Combined HS and FMD Vaccine

1. *Raksha Biovac* (Indian Immunologicals) – 30 ml vial

   FMD and HS oil adjuvant vaccine. The vaccine contains FMD inactivated antigens O, A and Asia-1 strains and formaldehyde inactivated *Pasteurella multocida* culture. It is homogenized to form a homogenase oil emulsion.

   Dose: Cattle and Buffalo – 3 ml IM.

   Schedule of vaccination: Primary vaccination at 4 months.

   Revaccination after 9 months of 1st vaccination.

2. *Raksha Triovac* (Indian Immunogiologicals) – 30 ml vial

   It is a combined vaccine contains FMD, HS and BQ oil adjuvant vaccine.

   Dose: Cattle and Buffalo – 3 ml.

   Schedule of vaccination: Primary vaccination at 4 months of age.

   Revaccination – First revaccination after 9 months. Subsequent revaccination – annually.

19.20.7 Enterotoxaemia Vaccine

1. *Raksha-ET* (Indian Immunologicals) – 100 ml vial

   It contains inactivated culture of an aerobically grown contains inactivated culture of an aerobically grown *Clostridium perfringens* type-D organism adjuvanted with aluminium hydroxide gel. It is recommended for enterotoxaemia in sheep and goats.

   Dose: Sheep and Goat – 2 ml SC

   Schedule of vaccination: Primary vaccination – 4 months age and above.

   Revaccination – annulally.

2. *Bovilis-ETV* (Intervet) – 10 ml (50 doses)

   It is an inactivated Enterotoxaemia vaccine containing toxoid of *Clostridium perfringerns* (Type-D). It is indicated for prophylaxis against pulpy kidney disease (Enterotoxaemia caused by *Cl. perfringens* type-D)

   Dose: Sheep and Goat – 2 ml SC.

   Schedule of vaccination: Primary vaccination 4-6 weeks age. Booster after 3-6 weeks of primary vaccination. Revaccination – 6 months interval.

19.20.8 Multicomponent Clostridial Vaccine

1. *Bovilis Mev* (Intervet) – 50 ml vial (25 doses)

   Composition

   Cl. perfringens type-B toxoid

   Cl. perfringens type-D toxoid

   Cl. perfringens type-C toxoid

   Cl. oedematiens type-B toxoid

   Cl. septicum toxoid, absorbed with aluminium hydroxide gel as at adjuvant.

Indication

For prophylaxis against enterotoxaemia (pulpy kidney disease), struck, lamb dysentery, black disease and braxy (malignant oedema).

Dose: Sheep and Goats – 2 ml SC orally.

Schedule of vaccination: Primary vaccination at the age of 4-6 weeks in lambs born to vaccinated ewes; and 1 week of age in lambs born to unvaccinated ewes.

Booster – After 3-6 weeks of primary vaccination. Revaccination – at 6 months interval.

19.20.9 *Brucella abortus* Vaccine

1. *Bmvax* (Indian Immunologicals) – 5 doses freeze dried vaccine + d iluent 10 ml.

   It is a live bacterial vaccine prepared with *Brucella abortus* (strain19). Keep the reconstituted vaccine on ice.

   Dose: Female calves of cattle and buffalo – 2 ml SC. Male calves should not be vaccinated. Do not vaccinate the pregnant animals.

19.20.10 Viral Vaccine–Canine Range

1. *Nobivac DHPPI* (Intervet) – 1 ml Single dose vial

   Combined vaccine against parvo, canine distemper, canine adeno virus and canine parainfluenza. The vaccine contained live attenuated strains of CPV, CD, canine adeno virus type-2 and canine para-influenza virus (Cornell strain).

   Dose: Reconstitute the freeze dried vaccine with Nobivac solvent and use by SC route.

2. *Nobivac Puppy DP* (Intervet) – Single dose vial

   Canine parvo and Canine distemper combined vaccine. It is a live attenuated virus vaccine contains canine parvo virus (CPV) and canine distemper virus (CDV).

   Dose: 1 ml by SC injection.

   Reconstitute one vial of Nobivac pupply DP in one vial of Nobivac solvent.

3. *Nobivac Corona* (Intervet)–Single dose vial + solvent

   Canine Corona virus vaccine. Each dose contains inactivated canine corona virus with a polymeric adjuvant.

   Dose: Inject 1ml of Nobivac Corona by SC route at the age of 4-6 weeks age followed by booster at 8 weeks of age and 12 weeks of age. Revaccination – annually.

4. *Vanguard CV* (Pfizer) – 1 ml dose vial

   Canine Corna virus vaccine.

   Schedule of vaccination: Primary vaccination at 6 weeks of age. Annual revaccination is recommended dose IM or SC. Don't vaccinate unhealthy and pregnant bitches.

5. *Duramune CVK* (Fort-Dodge) – 1 ml vial (Single dose pack)

   Killed canine corona virus vaccine for immunization of dogs against canine corona virus.

   Dose: 1 ml SC or IM.

   Schedule of vaccination: Primary vaccination at 17 weeks or above. Booster at 2-3 weeks after primary vaccination. Repeat annually.

6. *Megavac CC vaccine* (Indian Immunologicals) – Single dose pack

   Inactivated tissue culture vaccine.

   Dose: 1 ml SC or IM.

   Schedule of vaccination: Primary vaccination at 8-9 weeks age. Booster at 12 weeks. Repeat annually.

7. *Nobivac-C* (Intervet)

   Killed or inactivated canine corona virus vaccine.

   Dose: 1 ml SC or IM.

   Schedule of vaccination: Primary vaccination at 8-9 weeks age. Booster at 12 weeks. Repeat annually.

8. *Nobivac Rabies* (Intervet) – 1 ml and 10ml vials

   It is used for active immunization of healthy dogs, cats, sheep, goats, horses and in principle all the healthy mammals against rabies.

   Dose: 1 ml / animal by SC or IM.

   Schedule of vaccination: Primary vaccination Dog, Cat and Ferrets at 3 months of age.

   Revaccination at 3 years interval. Annual revaccination at endemic areas.

9. *Raksha Rab* (Indian Immunologicals) – 1 ml, 5 ml and 10 ml vials

   Rabies veterinary vaccine, inactivated (Cell culture). It contains tissue culture rabies compound.

   Dose: Dog, Cattle, Sheep, Camel and all other species – 1 ml by SC or IM route.

   Schedule of vaccination: Prophylaxis – at 3 months of age and above.

   Post exposure regimen – 1st dose on '0' day, 2nd dose on 3rd day, 3rd dose on 7th day, 4th dose on 14th day, 5th dose on 28th day, 6th dose on 90th day.

10. *Vanguard – 5L* (Pfizer) – Single dose (Vanguard-5 + Leptoferm-C-1 ml)

    It is used for the protection against Canine distemper, Infectious canine hepatitis (ICH) caused by CAV-1, canine parainfluenza, *L. canicola, L. icterohaemorrhagica*.

11. *Vanguard Plus 5CVL* (Pfizer)

    This is combined vaccine prepared on canine cell line gives protection against CD, ICH, CAV-2, Canine Parvo, Canine Parainfluenza, Leptrospira and canine corona.

    Dose: Freeze dried portion (*i.e.* Vanguard plus 5/L) can be reconstituted with 1 ml of sterile cold distilled water if desired or can be reconstituted with IM canine corona virus vaccine and injection through SC route.

12. *Megavac-6* (Indian Immunologicals)– 1 ml vial (Single dose pack)

    Tissue culture vaccine against CD, ICH, Canine Parvo virus and Leptospirosis.

    Dose: 1 ml SC.

    Schedule of vaccination: Primary vaccination at 8-9 weeks. Second (Booster) - 12 weeks.

    Revaccination annually.

13. *Candur DHL + P* (Intervet) – Single dose pack

    Against distemper, hepatitis, Leptospirosis, and Parvovirus infection.

    Administration by IM or SC.

    Primary vaccination: 7-9 weeks; Booster 12-14 weeks, Repeat – annually.

14. *Megavac DHRL* (Indian Immunologicals) – Single dose pack

    Aquous vaccine against CD, ICH (Type – II ICH), rabies, *L. canicola* and *L. icterohaemorrhagica.*

    Primary vaccination – 8-9 weeks; Second at 12 weeks.

19.20.11 Viral Vaccine – Feline Range

1. *Nobivac Tricat* (Intervet) – Single dose vial

   Indicated vaccine against FHV (Feline Herpes virus), FCV (Feline Calci virus) and Feline pan leucopaenia virus.

   Dose: Reconstitute one vial Nobivae Tricat in one vial of Nobivac solvent and inject by SC route.

   Schedule of vaccination: Basic vaccination either at 9 or 12 weeks of age or 12 and 15 weeks of age, then annual or by bi-annual vaccination.

Part – VI

Miscellaneous Information Pertaining to Veterinary Practice

Chapter 20

Common Instruments/Equipment Used in Veterinary Practice

The most common instruments/equipment used in veterinary practice are enlisted below. The instruments are arbitrarily grouped for ease of presentation. The specification and approximate price of each of the instruments/equipment are given in this chapter. The price might vary due to several factors. However, one may get an idea about the price of various items from the given information. This list of instruments/equipment especially helps in establishing/running a Veterinary Dispensary/Clinic.

Sl.No.	*Name*	*Specification*	*Unit/Pack*	*Price (Rs.)*
	Common items required for veterinary practice			
1.	Nylon syringe, sterilizeable	2 ml	1	4.00
		5 ml	1	5.00
		10 ml	1	7.00
		20 ml	1	8.00
		30 ml	1	9.00
		50 ml	1	10.00
2.	All Glass syringe, ISI marked	2 ml	1	35.00
		5 ml	1	45.00
		10 ml	1	50.00
		20 ml	1	75.00

Contd...

Sl.No.	Name	Specification	Unit/Pack	Price (Rs.)
3.	Veterinary metal syringe, Roux type	2 ml	1	55.00
		5 ml	1	85.00
		10 ml	1	95.00
		20 ml	1	130.00
4	Veterinary metal syringe, Artho type	2 ml	1	85.00
		5 ml	1	115.00
		10 ml	1	135.00
		20 ml	1	155.00
5	Automatic syringe	30 ml with adjustable dose of 1-5 ml	1	550.00
6	All Glass syringe, Tuberculosis		1	90.00
7	Luer Lock syringe with metal tip	2 ml	1	50.00
		5 ml	1	60.00
		10 ml	1	75.00
		20 ml	1	95.00
8	Hypodermic Needle Luer Mount	No. 18x1" or 1½" for large animal	10/packet	15.00
		No. 15, 16, 17 x 1½" for large animal	10/packet	20.00
		For small animal	10/packet	12.00
		For Tuberculosis or Insulin	10/packet	12.00
		No. 15, 16 x 3"	10/packet	160.00
		No. 15, 16 x 4"	10/packet	200.00
		No. 15, 16 x 6"	10/packet	400.00
9	Hypodermic Needle Record Mount	No. 18 x 1½"	10/packet	20.00
		No. 15, 16 x 1½"	10/packet	25.00
10	Hypodermic Needle	For small animal	10/packet	20.00
11	Surgical gloves	No. 6½, 7, 8 (unsterilized, superior quality)	Box of 25 pairs	275.00
		No. 6½, 7, 8 (sterilized, superior quality)	Box of 25 pairs	300.00
12	Blood taking needle	For blood specimen	1	110.00
13	Biopsy needle	Superior quality	1	350.00
14	Veterinary clinical thermometer		Box of 10	175.00
15	Digital clinical thermometer		1	110.00
16	Veterinary stethoscope, Litman type	Super deluxe quality	1	450.00

Contd...

Sl.No.	Name	Specification	Unit/Pack	Price (Rs.)
17	Veterinary diagnostic kit	Complete in a carrying bag for field work	1 set	2500.00
18	Dispensing Scale with weight		1	275.00
19	Medicine spatula	Stainless steel	1	50.00
20	Pestle and Mortar, metallic	Small	1	200.00
		Medium	1	300.00
		Large	1	400.00
21	Pestle and Mortar, glass	2 oz	1	70.00
		4 oz	1	90.00
		8 oz	1	120.00
		16 oz	1	150.00
	General Surgical Instruments/Items required for Veterinary Dispensary/Clinic			
22	Artery Forceps, Straight/Curved	12.5 cm	1	60.00
		15 cm	1	70.00
		20 cm	1	90.00
		25 cm	1	120.00
		30 cm	1	140.00
23	Dressing Scissors, Straight/Curved	12.5 cm	1	55.00
		15 cm	1	65.00
		20 cm	1	85.00
24	Mayo's Scissors, Straight/Curved	6½"	1	80.00
		7½"	1	90.00
		8½"	1	110.00
		10"	1	160.00
25	Halstead Mosquito Artery Forceps, Straight/Curved	5"	1	65.00
		6"	1	80.00
26	Dissecting Forceps, Plain (non-toothed)	12.5 cm	1	20.00
		15 cm	1	25.00
		20 cm	1	35.00
		25 cm	1	50.00
27	Dissecting Forceps, Rat toothed	12.5 cm	1	20.00
		15 cm	1	25.00
		20 cm	1	40.00
		25 cm	1	65.00
28	Allies Tissue Forceps	15 cm	1	85.00
		20 cm	1	100.00

Contd...

Sl.No.	Name	Specification	Unit/Pack	Price (Rs.)
29	Micro fine Forceps		1	75.00
30	Needle Holder	15 cm	1	70.00
		20 cm	1	85.00
		Mathew's Universal Standard size	1	150.00
31	B P Handle	No. 3 or 4	1	20.00
		No. 7	1	30.00
32	B P Blade	No. 10, 11, 12, 15, 20, 21, 22, 23, 24	Box of 100	200.00
33	Towel clip	Cross action	1	25.00
34	Towel clamp	Backhau's	1	65.00
35	Veterinary Scalpel	Standard size	1	20.00
36	Veterinary Syme's Abscess knife	Standard size	1	20.00
37	Suture Removing Scissors		1	100.00
38	Bandage/Gauge Cutting Scissors		1	150.00
39	Suture Needle, Cutting/Non-cutting	For large animal	Packet of 6	20.00
	and Straight/Curved/Half circle	For small animal	Packet of 6	20.00
40	Suture Needle for stitching small organs		Packet of 6	25.00
41	Suture Needle for internal tissue		Packet of 6	30.00
42	Nylon suture	Gut reel	1	25.00
		Hank	1	5.00
43	Silk reel, 22 m	No. 1/0, 2/0, 3/0. 1, 2	1	70.00
44	Razor for animal		1	60.00
45	Dressing probe with eye	15 cm	1	10.00
		20 cm	1	15.00
		25 cm	1	20.00
		30 cm	1	25.00
46	Amputation knife	15 cm	1	75.00
		20 cm	1	100.00
		25 cm	1	135.00
47	Amputation saw		1	125.00
48	Surgeon gown	Made of green cloth	1	250.00
49	Surgeon cap	Made of white or green cloth	1	20.00
50	Surgeon mask	Made of white or green cloth	1	15.00
51	Surgeon face mask	Disposable	100 pieces	200.00
52	Surgeon cap	Disposable	100 pieces	300.00
53	Duster Cotton	Medium size	1	15.00
		Large size	1	25.00

Contd...

Sl.No.	Name	Specification	Unit/Pack	Price (Rs.)
	Livestock Farm Equipment			
	Items for Cattle/Buffalo			
54	Ear tag, brass button type with number	22 mm	1	12.00
	or code engraved for cattle/buffalo	16 mm	1	10.00
55	Ear tag applicator for cattle/buffalo	For 22 mm or 16 mm ear tag	1	200.00
56	Ear tag with number or code printed for cattle/buffalo	Polyplast with brass pin point easy to insert	1	20.00
57	Ear tag applicator for above ear tags for cattle/buffalo		1	600.00
58	Ear tag, strip type, engraved with Serial No. for cattle/buffalo	Aluminium made	100 pieces	400.00
59	Ear tag applicator for above ear tags for cattle/buffalo		1	150.00
60	Tattooing set, four spaced, with one set of numbers 0 to 9 and letter A to Z	Aluminium made	1	1500.00
61	Spare Number set 0 to 9, for tattooing		1 set	200.00
62	Spare Letter set A to Z, for tattooing		1 set	400.00
63	Tattooing ink		50 ml	15.00
	Tattooing ink		500 ml	150.00
64	Cold Branding Iron 0 to 9		1 set	1000.00
65	Cold Branding Iron A to Z		1 set	2500.00
66	Hot Branding Iron 0 to 9		1 set	800.00
67	Hot Branding Iron A to Z		1 set	2000.00
68	Branding ink		500 ml	150.00
69	Ear Notching Pliers		1	250.00
70	Dehorner	Electric with wire and plug	1	160.00
		Non-electric	1	100.00
71	Drenching bottle, aluminium		1	75.00
72	Catheter	Single channel	1	40.00
		Double channel	1	60.00
73	Intrauterine catheter	Disposable	1	7.00
		Metallic	1	80.00
74	Trocar and Canula	Wooden handle	1	50.00
		Metal handle	1	100.00
75	Cattle probang		1	190.00
76	Mouth gag	Wooden	1	70.00
		Metal	1	230.00
		Brass	1	1100.00

Contd...

Sl.No.	Name	Specification	Unit/Pack	Price (Rs.)
77	Stomach tube, rubber	For cattle	1	125.00
		For calf	1	50.00
78	Tooth rasp for cattle		1 set	160.00
79	Tooth chisel with guard		1	230.00
80	Rumenotomy set		1	2100.00
81	Rumen fluid extraction pump		1	1700.00
82	Hoof trimmer		1	90.00
83	Hoof cutter		1	200.00
84	Hoof testing forceps		1	400.00
85	Castrator	19" for large animal	1	2500.00
86	Hair clipper for large animals		1	575.00
87	Razor for animals		1	50.00
88	Scrubbing body brush		1	50.00
89	Animal catcher for holding violent animals		1	500.00
90	Metal detector, hand hold with rechargeable batteries		1	5700.00
91	Metallic chain for cow/bull/buffalo		1	240.00
92	Cotton rope	½" diameter x 10 meter length with both ends bounded	1	150.00
		1" diameter x 10 meter length with both ends bounded	1	225.00
93	Manila rope	½" diameter x 10 meter length with both ends bounded	1	150.00
		1" diameter x 10 meter length with both ends bounded	1	300.00
94	Jute rope	½" diameter x 10 meter length with both ends bounded	1	95.00
		1" diameter x 10 meter length with both ends bounded	1	190.00
95	Bull leader with long stick		1	350.00
96	Bull nose punch		1	450.00
97	Bull nose ring	Copper	1	85.00
		Aluminium	1	40.00
		Brass	1	85.00
98	Bull holder with thumb		1	60.00

Contd...

Sl.No.	*Name*	*Specification*	*Unit/Pack*	*Price (Rs.)*
		Items for Teat Care		
99	Milk siphon with rounded tip	Self retaining and adjustable	1	20.00
100	Teat slitter with concealed blade		1	85.00
101	Teat tumor extractor with three rings		1	75.00
102	Teat dilator with screw		1	60.00
103	Teat dilator, HUB type, for use in toughness of milking	Thin HUB, specially designed to insert in the teat easily	1	20.00
104	Teat knife Maclean's		1	40.00
105	Teat scissors		1	90.00
106	Micro fine teat forceps		1	50.00
107	Teat holding forceps		1	70.00
108	Teat plug	Simple, plastic	100 pieces	100.00
		Bulbous, plastic	1	3.00
		Bulbous, metallic	1	20.00
		Self retaining type, metallic	1	20.00
109	Teat injection tube for medicine		1	20.00
110	Milk sucking preventor to prevent calf for sucking milk		1	180.00
111	Mouth shutter for calf to prevent calf for sucking milk and to protect teat sore		1	30.00
112	Teat instrument set	Complete with 9 items in a zip type pouch	1 set	300.00
		Complete with 18 items in a zip type pouch	1 set	550.00
		Items for Milk Testing		
113	Milk butyrometer	Corning glass, 0-10%, ISI marked	1	25.00
114	Lock stopper for milk butyrometer	Gerber type, ISI marked	1 dozen	42.00
115	Regulating pin for Lock stopper	Aluminium made	1	7.00
116	Milk pipette 10.75 ml		1	12.00
117	Tilt measure 10 ml for acid, with rubber cork, without bottle	Glass	1	12.00
		Plastic	1	10.00
118	Tilt measure 1 ml for alcohol,	Glass	1	12.00
	with rubber cork, without bottle	Plastic	1	10.00
119	Lactometer	ISI marked	1	120.00

Contd...

Sl.No.	Name	Specification	Unit/Pack	Price (Rs.)
120	Dairy thermometer, stem type, mercury/alcohol filled		1	12.00
121	Richmond scale for SNF calculation		1	300.00
122	Gerber centrifuge machine for milk fat testing, hand driven, solid construction, perfect alignment with ball bearing	12 tests capacity	1	1400.00
		24 tests capacity	1	1500.00
123	Gerber centrifuge machine for milk fat testing, electrically operated, AC 50 cycles, ¼ HP motor, single phase 220/230 volts with switch, indicator lamp, cord plug pin, fitted in heavy iron base pan	12 tests capacity	1	4500.00
		24 tests capacity	1	5000.00
124	Gerber centrifuge machine for milk fat testing, electrically operated, AC 50 cycles, ¼ HP motor, single phase 220/230 volts with switch, indicator lamp, cord plug pin, fitted in heavy iron base pan, with timer and brake	12 tests capacity	1	6300.00
		24 tests capacity	1	6500.00
125	Butyrometer stand cum shaker	Plastic made, capacity 12	1	80.00
		Plastic made, capacity 24	1	120.00
		Aluminium made, capacity 12	1	125.00
		Aluminium made, capacity 24	1	135.00
126	Pipette stand	Round shape, aluminium made, capacity 12	1	90.00
		Horizontal shape, wooden, capacity 12	1	175.00
		Polyplast, capacity 12	1	180.00
127	Milk sample bottle with cap, plastic	50 ml	1	3.00
		75 ml	1	4.00
		100 ml	1	5.00
128	Milk collection tray	Stainless steel	1	1500.00
129	Brush for cleaning milk sample bottle, nylon bristles		1 dozen	24.00
130	Brush for cleaning milk pipette, nylon bristles		1 dozen	18.00
131	Brush for cleaning butyrometer, nylon bristles		1 dozen	18.00
132	Milking pail	Stainless steel	1	3500.00
	Milk can	Stainless steel, 20 litres capacity	1	3700.00
		Stainless steel, 40 litres capacity	1	4000.00
		Aluminium, 40 litres capacity	1	3500.00

Contd...

Sl.No.	Name	Specification	Unit/Pack	Price (Rs.)
133	Milk testing kit for adulteration check		1	3300.00
134	Amyl alcohol, milk testing quality	400 ml	1	75.00
	Items for Poultry Section			
135	Leg bands, Serial Number engraved		100 pieces	200.00
136	Wing bands, Serial Number engraved		100 pieces	200.00
137	Automatic vaccinator for RD		1	350.00
138	Automatic vaccinator for Fowl pox		1	350.00
139	Electric debeaker	Complete with stand	1	4000.00
140	Spare blade for debeaker		1	500.00
141	Egg candler/tester, electrically operated		1	750.00
142	Egg weighing balance	1 to 100 g	1	800.00
143	Bird weighing balance		1	1000.00
144	Chick feeding tray		1	120.00
145	Egg tray, plastic	30 eggs capacity	1	35.00
146	Clipping scissors for clipping wings of birds		1	100.00
147	Infra red lamp with stand for brooding		1	600.00
148	Sprayer for pest control,	3½ litres	1	1300.00
	manually operated	6 litres	1	1500.00
		9 litres	1	1800.00
		12 litres	1	2000.00
149	Hygrometer to check humidity		1	600.00
150	Poultry sexing light		1	800.00
151	Chick feeder, plastic	2 kg capacity	1	100.00
152	Grower feeder, plastic	8 kg capacity	1	300.00
153	Poultry feeder, round, plastic	10 kg capacity	1	350.00
154	Poultry feeder, large size, plastic	14 kg capacity	1	450.00
155	Chick drinker, plastic		1	100.00
156	Grower drinker, plastic		1	200.00
157	Cage chick drinker, plastic		1	50.00
158	Automatic poultry drinker, plastic		1	400.00
159	Chick drinker stand		1	40.00
160	Grower drinker stand		1	50.00
161	Nipple drinking system for cages		1	35.00
162	Cage mat	13x13"	1	40.00
		23x14.5"	1	60.00
163	Gas brooder without thermostatic control		1	7500.00

Contd...

Sl.No.	Name	Specification	Unit/Pack	Price (Rs.)
164	Gas brooder with thermostatic control to be attached with LPM cylinder		1	10500.00
165	Hot air blower, electrically operated to control winter temperature		1	1000.00
166	Poultry vaccine carrier, polyplast, unbreakable, with hanging straps with ice cubes to maintain required temperature		1	1000.00
167	Disposable gloves, polythene, up to wrist length to handle dead birds and to mix feed		100 pieces	100.00
168	Pollution Face mask		1	75.00
169	Poultry Post Mortem set	Complete with instruments in a zip pouch	1	500.00
170	Poultry diagnostic kit	Complete in a bag suitable for poultry farm	1	2000.00
171	Poultry Post Mortem tray		1	900.00
172	Poultry Post Mortem table, top covered with stainless steel sheet		1	8000.00
	Items for Sheep and Goat Section			
173	Castrator for goat/sheep	9"	1	2000.00
174	Trocar and Canula for goat/sheep		1	50.00
175	Hair clipper, manual		1	750.00
176	Hair clipper, electrically operated		1	10000.00
177	Clipping scissors		1	100.00
178	Dosing syringe for goat/sheep		1	500.00
179	Drenching pipe for goat/sheep, plastic		1	35.00
180	Mouth gag for goat/sheep		1	50.00
181	Ear tag strip type with serial number engraved, aluminium made, for goat/sheep		100 pieces	350.00
182	Ear tag applicator for strip type ear tags for goat/sheep		1	150.00
183	Ear tag button type with number code engraved, brass made, for goat/sheep		1	9.00
184	Ear tag applicator for button type ear tags for goat/sheep		1	180.00
185	Delivery hook for goat/sheep		1	175.00
186	Intra uterine catheter for goat/sheep		1	50.00
187	Delivery forceps for goat/sheep		1	1000.00
188	Vaginal speculum, metallic, for goat/sheep		1	300.00
189	Artificial vagina with metal valve for semen collection for goat/sheep		1	275.00
190	AI catheter metallic for goat/sheep for insemination liquid semen		1	80.00

Contd...

Sl.No.	Name	Specification	Unit/Pack	Price (Rs.)
	Items for Pig Section			
191	Pig holder for catching pigs		1	475.00
192	Mouth gag for pig		1	250.00
193	Delivery hook for pig		1	200.00
194	Intra uterine catheter for pig		1	90.00
195	Delivery forceps for pig		1	1000.00
196	Tooth cutting forceps for pig		1	200.00
197	Vaginal speculum for pig		1	400.00
198	Vaginoscope with light arrangement for pig		1	800.00
199	Ear tag strip type with serial number engraved, aluminium made, for pig		100 pieces	350.00
200	Ear tag applicator for strip type ear tags for pig		1	150.00
201	Ear tag button type with number code engraved, brass made, for pig		1	9.00
202	Ear tag applicator for button type ear tags for pig		1	180.00
	Items for Equine Section			
203	Mouth gag for horse		1	1000.00
204	Mouth gag right or left jaw for horse		1	450.00
205	Stomach tube for horse		1	140.00
206	Catheter for horse	Metallic	1	100.00
		Polythene	1	40.00
207	Balling gun with spring for horse		1	350.00
208	Hoof cutter set for horse		1	1800.00
209	Tooth rasp set for horse		1	175.00
210	Dandy brush for horse		1	80.00
211	Muzzle for horse		1	900.00
212	Anti-kicking device for horse		1	280.00
213	Hobbles casting hitching/master		1	600.00
214	Hair clipper for horse	Manual	1	700.00
		Electrically operated	1	10000.00
216	Horse shoe		1	90.00
217	Halter for horse		1	750.00
218	Riding saddle for horse, complete with blanket and peddle		1	7000.00
219	Pole saddle for horse, complete with blanket		1	7000.00

Contd...

Sl.No.	Name	Specification	Unit/Pack	Price (Rs.)
220	Riding bridles single/double for horse		1	1000.00
221	Driving bridles for horse		1	900.00
222	Harness saddle for horse		1	6000.00
223	Harness collar for horse		1	650.00
224	Harness crupper for horse		1	200.00
225	Head rope for horse		1	150.00
226	Hoof chisel for horse		1	350.00
227	Hoof gauge for horse		1	350.00
228	Trachea tube for horse		1	500.00
229	Vaginal speculum for horse		1	800.00
230	Vaginoscope with light arrangement for horse		1	1300.00
231	Autopsy set for horse		1	5000.00
	Items for Dogs			
232	Mouth gag Gray's		1	350.00
233	Mouth gag for pups		1	450.00
234	Mouth gag for dog with adjustable blade		1	900.00
235	Stomach tube for dog		1	55.00
236	Enema syringe, rubber		1	60.00
237	Delivery hook for dog		1	175.00
238	Whelping forceps	9"	1	150.00
239	Whelping forceps	12"	1	200.00
240	Vaginal speculum for dog		1	300.00
241	Vaginoscope with light arrangement for dog		1	800.00
242	Rectal speculum for dog	Without light arrangement	1	180.00
		With light arrangement	1	800.00
243	Grooming brush for dog		1	125.00
244	Claw nipper for dog		1	150.00
245	Mouth shutter for dog		1	150.00
246	Dog chain, choak neck		1	175.00
247	Dog collar		1	150.00
248	Tracking harness for dog		1	115.00
249	Tracking lease for dog		1	115.00
250	Cross body belt, leather made, for dog		1	400.00
251	Rubber ball for dog		1	40.00
252	Artificial bone for dog		1	35.00
253	Metallic comb		1	120.00

Contd...

Sl.No.	Name	Specification	Unit/Pack	Price (Rs.)
254	Dog coat	Small size	1	250.00
		Medium size	1	350.00
		Large size	1	400.00
255	Uterine dressing forceps		1	130.00
256	Uterine sponge forceps		1	135.00
257	Intrauterine catheter for bitch		1	40.00
258	Ear forceps for dog		1	50.00
259	Eye speculum for dog		1	230.00
260	Throat forceps for dog		1	225.00
261	Dog catcher		1	530.00
262	Tail docking scissors for pups		1	120.00
263	Canine tooth extraction forceps		1	175.00
264	Canine dental scaler		1	60.00
265	Canine dental probe		1	45.00
266	Canine dental chisel	Straight/Angular	1	170.00
267	Canine autopsy set		1 set	2000.00
268	Weighing scale for pups		1	900.00
	Gynaecological/Obstetrical items			
269	Obstetrical set for large animals		1	600.00
270	Dystocia set for large animals		1	1800.00
271	Foetotomy set in a sterilizable box		1	2500.00
272	Hook set with calving rope for extracting dead/live foetus		1	60.00
273	Delivery hook for large animals		1	150.00
274	Delivery hook for small animals		1	150.00
275	Uterine dilator for large animals		1	500.00
276	Obstetric chain	30"	1	100.00
		60"	1	125.00
277	Prolaps clamp	3"	1	60.00
		4"	1	70.00
		7"	1	140.00
278	Uterine sponge forceps	16"	1	225.00
		20"	1	300.00
279	Uterine flushing curette		1	115.00
280	Cervix dilator for large animals		1	600.00
281	Cannula for puncturing ovarian cyst		1	160.00
282	Uterine biopsy needle		1	280.00
283	Intraterine catheter, metal for large animal		1	80.00
284	Intrauterine catheter, disposable for large animal		1	7.00

Contd...

Sl.No.	Name	Specification	Unit/Pack	Price (Rs.)
	Items for Artificial Insemination			
285	AI gun French medium design to be used with 0.5 ml straw		1	90.00
286	AI gun French mini design to be used with 0.25 ml straw		1	135.00
287	Universal AI gun French method to be used with 0.5 ml or 0.25 ml straw		1	160.00
288	Universal AI gun French method to be used with 0.5 ml or 0.25 ml straw, with locking system		1	260.00
289	Spare Sealing ring for above guns	Plastic made	100 pieces	100
290	AI gun German design to be used with 0.3 ml straw		1	50.00
291	Spare Sealing ring for above guns		1	3.00
292	Gun container for French design gun, plastic		1	100.00
293	Gun container for French design gun, metallic		1	300.00
294	Gun container for German design gun, plastic		1	15.00
295	AI sheath French medium design to be used with 0.5 ml straw		Pkt of 50	50.00
296	AI sheath French mini design to be used with 0.5 ml straw		Pkt of 50	60.00
297	AI sheath for universal gun		Pkt of 50	60.00
298	AI sheath German design gun		Pkt of 50	70.00
299	Sheath container, PVC to hold 50 nos.		1	35.00
300	Spare stopper for above container		1	5.00
301	Sheath container, metallic to hold 50 nos.		1	530.00
302	French medium design AI straw 0.5 ml		100 pieces	100.00
303	French mini design AI straw 0.25 ml		100 pieces	150.00
304	German design AI straw 0.3 ml, both side open without sealing balls		100 pieces	30.00
305	Sealing balls for German design AI straw 0.3 ml		100 pieces	17.00
306	AI gloves up to shoulder length	Disposable	100 pieces	200.00
307	AI gloves latex rubber up to arm length		1 pair	65.00
308	Straw cutting scissors		1	60.00
309	Straw holding twizer	12"	1	50.00
310	Straw holding forceps with serrated jaw	10"	1	130.00
311	Thawing flask		1	50.00

Contd...

Sl.No.	Name	Specification	Unit/Pack	Price (Rs.)
312	Stainless steel tray for keeping sterilized AI items		1	550.00
313	Thawing box rectangular, rexin covered, fitted with zip		1	100.00
314	Goblet for French medium straws	Plastic, 35x118 mm	1	5.00
		Plastic, 65x118 mm	1	7.00
		Aluminium, 35x118 mm	1	16.00
		Aluminium, 65x118 mm	1	25.00
315	Goblet for French mini straws	Plastic, 12x118 mm	1	3.00
		Aluminium, 12x118 mm	1	15.00
316	Goblet for German straw	Plastic, 35x60 mm	1	4.00
		Plastic, 65x60 mm	1	6.00
		Aluminium, 35x60 mm	1	16.00
		Aluminium, 65x60 mm	1	25.00
317	Goblet holding forceps	10"	1	290.00
		12"	1	350.00
		14"	1	400.00
318	Goblet stand for French design	35x118 mm	1	50.00
		65x118 mm	1	60.00
319	Goblet stand for German design		1	65.00
320	Identification tag with flap for goblet		1	10.00
321	Lifter for Jumboo LN_2 specially designed		1	350.00
322	Dip stick for LN_2	Graduated, polyplast 75 cm	1	30.00
		Graduated, polyplast, 100 cm	1	40.00
		Stainless steel, 100 cm	1	260.00
		Aluminium, 100 cm	1	200.00
323	LN_2 pouring spout fitted with jet		1	500.00
224	Protective gloves to handle LN_2	12"	1	85.00
		14"	1	100.00
		16"	1	150.00
325	Protective goggles while working with LN_2		1	650.00
326	Rubber ring for LN_2 cylinder	300 mm	1	375.00
		380 mm	1	475.00
		440 mm	1	550.00
		470 mm	1	575.00
		490 mm	1	650.00

Contd...

Sl.No.	Name	Specification	Unit/Pack	Price (Rs.)
327	Trolley for LN_2 cylinder		1	850.00
328	Disposable mask while working with LN_2		1	140.00
329	Disposable cap while working with LN_2		1	260.00
330	Artificial vagina Danish model with metal valve with raised rim at both ends	12"	1	500.00
	for bull, made of synthetic rubber	14"	1	550.00
331	Semen collection tube, amber colour, graduated	10 ml or 15 ml	1	18.00
332	Air blower for AV for giving air pressure		1	40.00
333	Insulating bag for carrying semen vial, collection tube, rubber linners and cones, made of foam leather		1	60.00
334	Semen storage vial, polyplast,	2 ml	1	3.00
	autoclavable	5 ml	1	4.00
		10 ml	1	5.00
335	AV brush for cleaning AV		1	18.00
336	Gum boot assorted size		1	650.00
337	Thermos flask, stainless steel	500 ml capacity	1	700.00
		1000 ml capacity	1	800.00
338	Ice box insulated, polyplast	16.5 litres capacity	1	1200.00
	Laboratory Equipment/Glass wares/Polyplast wares			
339	Laboratory compound microscope with Eye piece 5x, 10x, 15x (any two), objective 10x, 45x and 100x Oil immersion, complete in a carrying box		1	5000.00
340	Laboratory compound microscope with light arrangement		1	7000.00
341	Binocular Research Microscope with binocular head and light arrangement		1	11000.00
342	Water bath with stirrer, electrically operated fitted with thermostatic control	Size 22x15x10 cm	1	12000.00
343	Hot air oven, electrically operated, thermostatically controlled, Elements are placed at bottom, out body of mild steel with duce painted	45x45x45 cm (with inner chamber aluminium made)	1	10000.00
		35x35x35 cm (with inner chamber aluminium made)	1	8000.00
		45x45x45 cm (with inner chamber stainless steel made)	1	15000.00
		35x35x35 cm (with inner chamber stainless steel made)		12000.00

Contd...

Sl.No.	Name	Specification	Unit/Pack	Price (Rs.)
344	Bacteriological incubator, electrically operated, thermostatically controlled, heating elements are placed at bottom, double walled with inside chamber made of aluminium or stainless steel sheet and out body of mild steel with duce painted, the door has glass viewing window	45x45x45 cm (with inner chamber aluminium made)	1	11000.00
		35x35x35 cm (with inner chamber aluminium made)	1	9000.00
		45x45x45 cm (with inner chamber stainless steel made)	1	15000.00
		35x35x35 cm (with inner chamber stainless steel made)	1	11000.00
345	Glass ware drier, electrically operated for drying the laboratory glass ware by blower force air through 12 pipes fitted with heating element, with powerful motor, ON/OFF switch		1	6000.00
346	Digital pH meter		1	8000.00
347	Pipette drier, electrically operated		1	7000.00
348	Slide carrying table for 20 slides		1	130.00
349	Slide cabinet, made of wooden with	For 500 slides	1	3700.00
	aluminium fitting for 3x1" slides	For 1000 slides	1	4500.00
		For 2000 slides	1	8500.00
350	Analytical balance, sensitivity 0.1 mg, capacity 200 g		1	3750.00
351	Test tube, made of heat	10x75 mm	1	3.00
	resistance glass	12x100 mm	1	4.00
		15x125 mm	1	5.00
		25x100 mm	1	9.00
		25x150 mm	1	10.00
352	Test tube holder		1	7.00
353	Spirit lamp, brass		1	100.00
354	Test tube stand, aluminium for 24 test tubes		1	100.00
355	Conical flask, made of heat	100 ml	1	90.00
	resistance glass	250 ml	1	150.00
		500 ml	1	175.00
		1000 ml	1	300.00
356	Conical flask with screw cap,	100 ml	1	40.00
	made of polyplast	250 ml	1	60.00
		500 ml	1	100.00

Contd...

Sl.No.	Name	Specification	Unit/Pack	Price (Rs.)
357	Volumetric flask, flat bottom, wide mouth, made of heat resistance glass	100 ml	1	150.00
		250 ml	1	175.00
		500 ml	1	225.00
		1000 ml	1	400.00
358	Volumetric flask, polyplast	100 ml	1	125.00
		250 ml	1	160.00
		500 ml	1	250.00
359	Measuring cylinder, graduated, made of heat resistance glass	50 ml	1	285.00
		100 ml	1	335.00
		250 ml	1	555.00
		500 ml	1	670.00
360	Measuring cylinder, polyplast	25 ml	1	50.00
		50 ml	1	65.00
		100 ml	1	95.00
		250 ml	1	125.00
		500 ml	1	185.00
		1000 ml	1	500.00
361	Laboratory spatula	6"	1	18.00
		8"	1	25.00
362	Petri dish		Box of 12	550.00
363	Beaker, polyplast	50 ml	1	18.00
		100 ml	1	20.00
		250 ml	1	35.00
		500 ml	1	60.00
		1000 ml	1	130.00
364	Reagent bottle, polyplast, wide mouth	60 ml	1	35.00
		125 ml	1	40.00
		250 ml	1	75.00
365	Measuring jug, polyplast	250 ml	1	40.00
		500 ml	1	45.00
		1000 ml	1	80.00
		2000 ml	1	125.00
366	Petri dish 90 mm disposable		1	12.00
367	Funnel with long stem, polyplast	50 mm	1	7.00
		75 mm	1	10.00
		100 mm	1	18.00
368	Dessicator vacuum	150 mm	1	1800.00
		200 mm	1	2575.00

Contd...

Sl.No.	Name	Specification	Unit/Pack	Price (Rs.)
369	Cetrifuge tube, conical or round bottom with screw cap, polyplast	10 ml	1	17.00
		15 ml	1	21.00
		50 ml	1	36.00
370	Test tube stand, polyplast	For 96 test tubes	1	550.00
	Miscellaneous Items			
371	Dust bin, plastic with pedal		1	200.00
372	Dispensing scale with weight	Large size	1	600.00
373	Spring balance, dial type	100 kg capacity	1	900.00
		50 kg capacity	1	750.00
		10 kg capacity	1	250.00
374	Counter Scale Balance	Weight range 10 g to 5 kg	1	1500.00
375	Tray with cover, enameled	8x6"	1	250.00
		8x10"	1	350.00
		12x10"	1	400.00
376	Dissecting tray	12x10"	1	400.00
377	Jug, graduated and enameled	500 ml	1	300.00
		1000 ml	1	350.00
		2000 ml	1	700.00
378	Mug, enameled	12 cm (1 litre capacity)	1	100.00
379	Kidney tray, enameled	8"	1	100.00
		10"	1	125.00
		12"	1	150.00
380	Funnel, enameled	3"	1	140.00
		4"	1	220.00
		6"	1	275.00
		8"	1	415.00
381	Bucket with cover, enameled	10"	1	350.00
		11"	1	450.00
		12"	1	500.00
382	Surgical tray, stainless steel	8x6"	1	275.00
		10x8"	1	400.00
		12x10"	1	600.00
383	Kidney tray, stainless steel	10"	1	115.00
		12"	1	160.00
384	Autoclave, vertical with stainless steel inner and outer body, fitted with pressure gauze, heavy lid and double safety valve	20x12"	1	12000.00

Contd...

Sl.No.	Name	Specification	Unit/Pack	Price (Rs.)
385	Dressing drum, stainless steel, seamless		1	700.00
386	Oxygen cylinder, complete with flow meter, tubing, key trolley *etc.*	40 cft capacity	1	7000.00
387	Saline stand with heavy base		1	750.00
388	Instrument and Dressing Trolley with stainless steel shelves		1	7000.00
389	Stool with three legs, revolving, stainless steel top		1	750.00
390	Stool with four legs, revolving, stainless steel top		1	950.00
391	Operation Table for small animals and dogs with upper top covered with stainless steel and remaining body spray painted	Size: 4 ft x 2 ft x 32"	1	8000.00
392	Operation Table for large animals and dogs with upper top covered with stainless steel and lower top metal	Size: 5 ft x 2½ ft x 32"	1	13000.00

Items for Establishment of a Training Centre

Sl.No.	Name	Specification	Unit/Pack	Price (Rs.)
393	Xerox Machine		1	70000.00
394	LCD Projector and Polythene Screen		1	72000.00
395	Laptop		1	72000.00
396	Desktop Computer with Table and Chair		1	35000.00
397	Laser-jet Printer (B and W)		1	7000.00
398	UPS 3 KV		1	30000.00
399	Digital camera		1	23000.00
400	Audio System with microphone, speaker		1 set	30000.00
401	White Board, Marker and Eraser		1 set	2500.00
402	Generator set and its accessories		1	65000.00
403	A.C. Machine and accessories		1	70000.00
404	Display Notice Board		1	5000.00
405	Furnished Lecture Room with 40 armed writing chairs		1	100000.00
406	Wooden platform, 1 ft height		1	20000.00
407	Podium (for delivering speech on dias)		1	20000.00
408	Steel Almirah		4 nos.	50000.00
409	Steel rack		2 nos.	10000.00
410	Steel Wall Photoframe and photograph		20 pieces	50000.00
411	Table on dais for 5 members		1 set	25000.00
412	Aqua Guard (water purifier)		1 set	10000.00

Photographs Pertaining to Diagnosis of Diseases

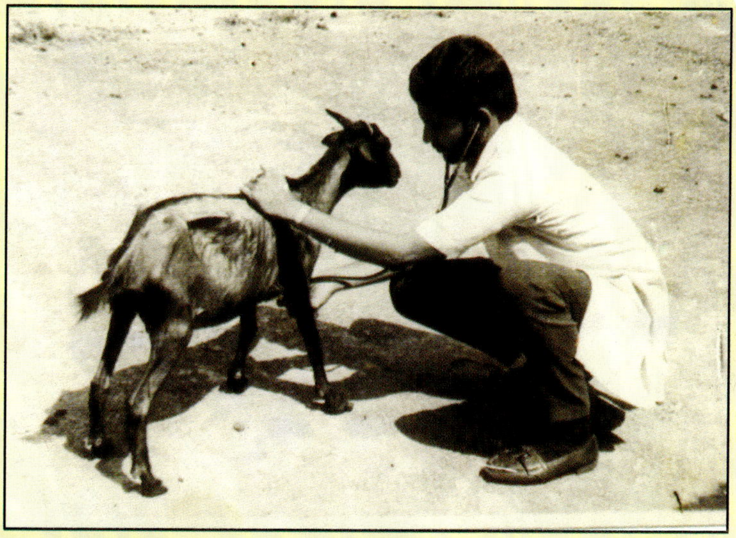

Figure 1: Auscultation by use of stethoscope

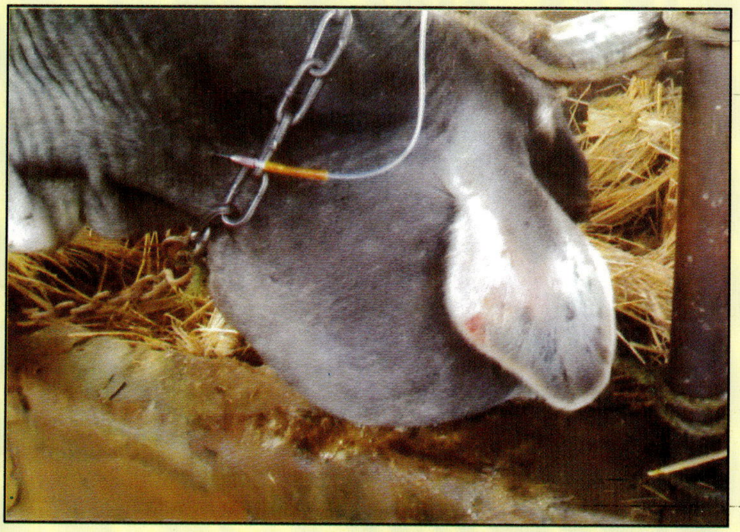

Figure 2: Acute Haemorrhagic Septicaemia showing severe throat and sub mandibular oedema in a cow

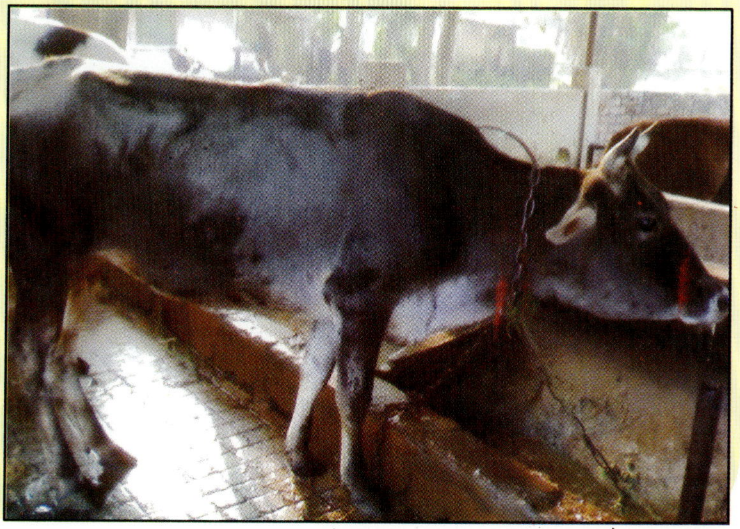

Figure 3: Clinical case of Haemorrhagic Septicaemia in a crossbred cow showing salivation and submandibular oedema (Early stage of H S)

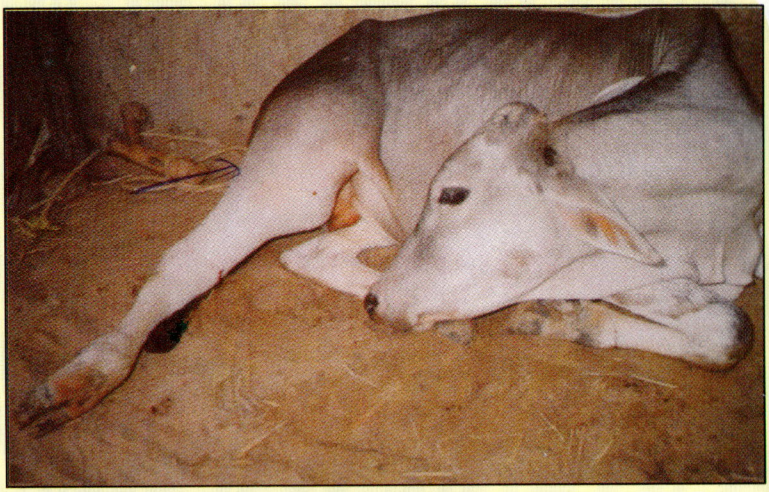

Figure 4: Black Quarter in a male calf affecting left hind limb

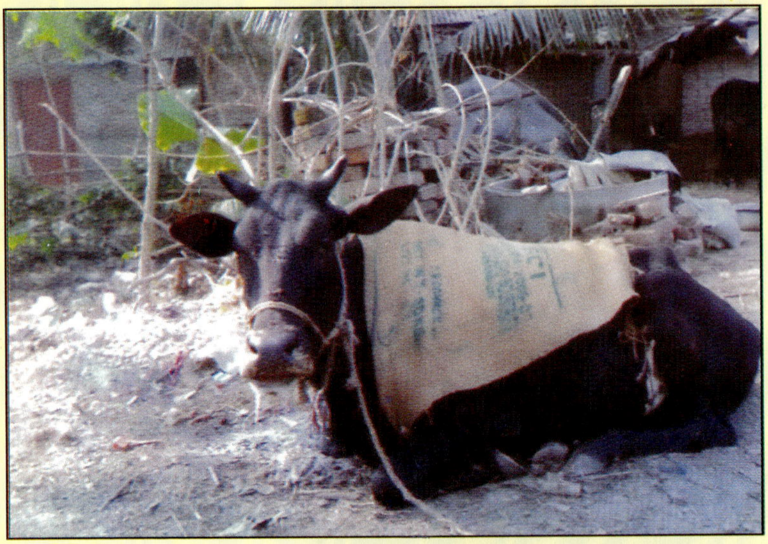

Figure 5: Sever FMD in a crossbred cow showing salivation

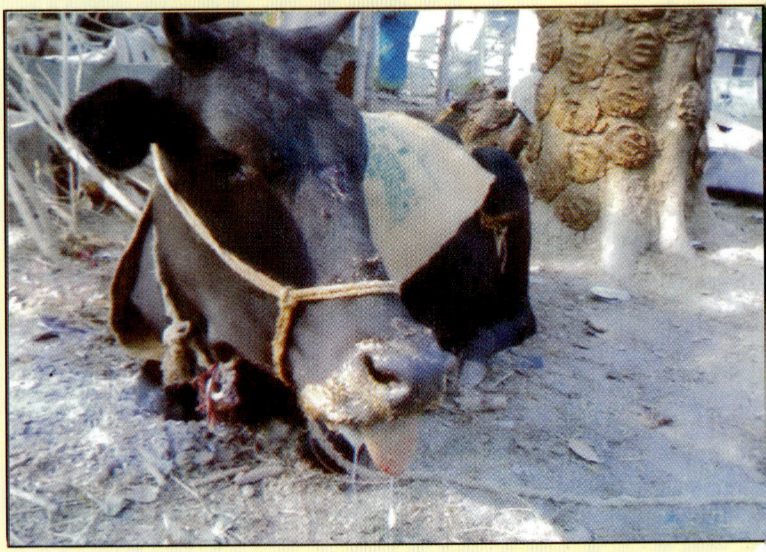

Figure 6: Glossal paresis owing to severe FMD infection and ulceration on tongue with tongue protrusion

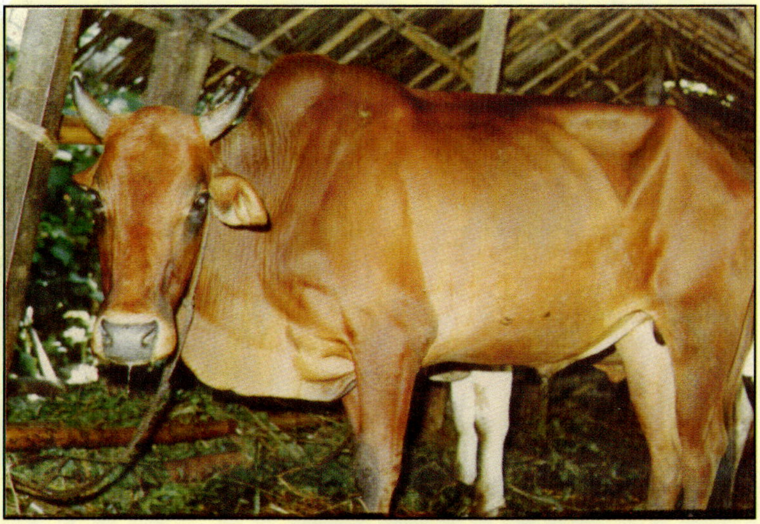

Figure 7: Hilly bullock suffering from FMD showing salivation

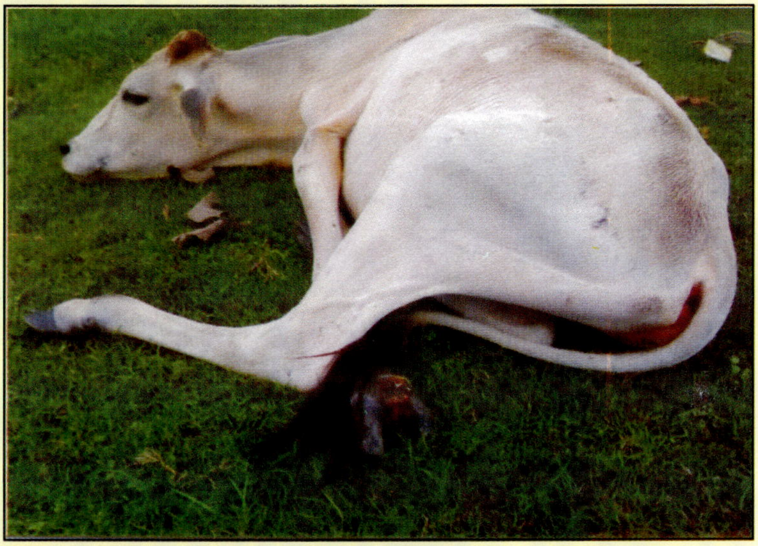

Figure 8: Post FMD complication in a calf showing interdigital ulceration and magotization

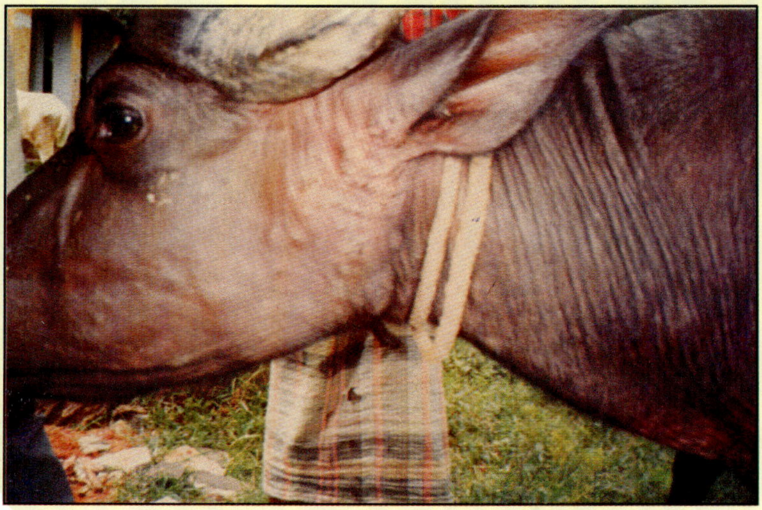

Figure 9: Buffalo pox with pock lesions on the base of the ear and face

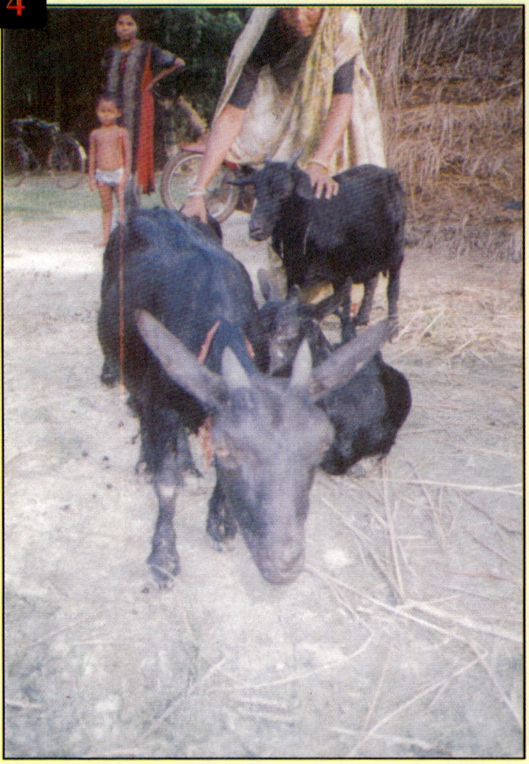

Figure 10: Bengal goats suffering from Goat Pox

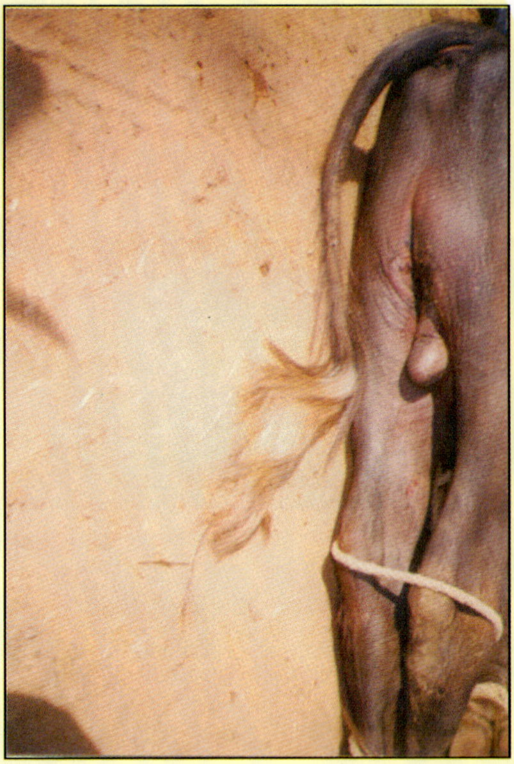

Figure 11: Buffalo pox infection showing pox lesion at inguinal and perigenital area

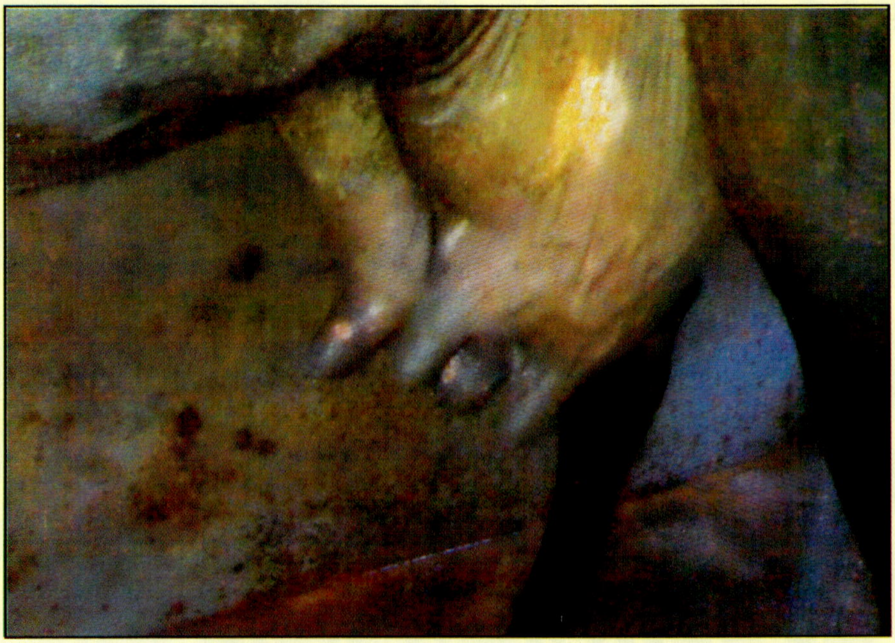

Figure 12: Cowpox with udder and teat lesions (vesicles and ulcers)

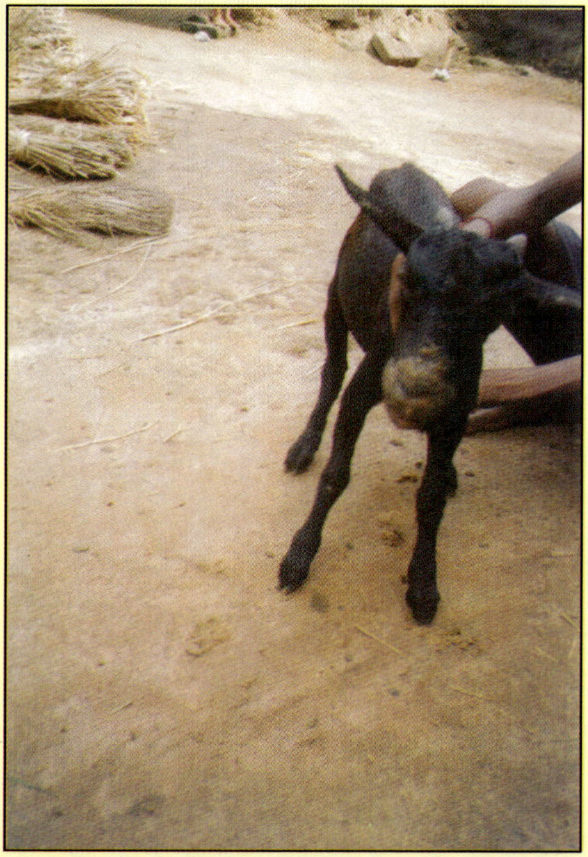

Figure 13: Contagious Ecthyma (Scabby mouth/Sore lip) in a goat

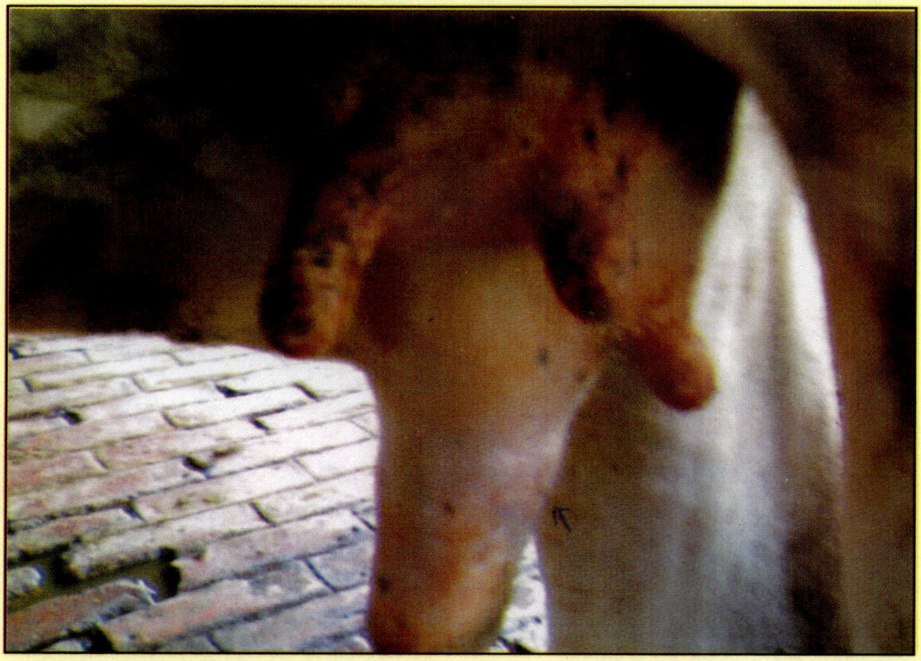

Figure 14: Chronic Mastitis in a dry cow affecting single teat leading to gangrene

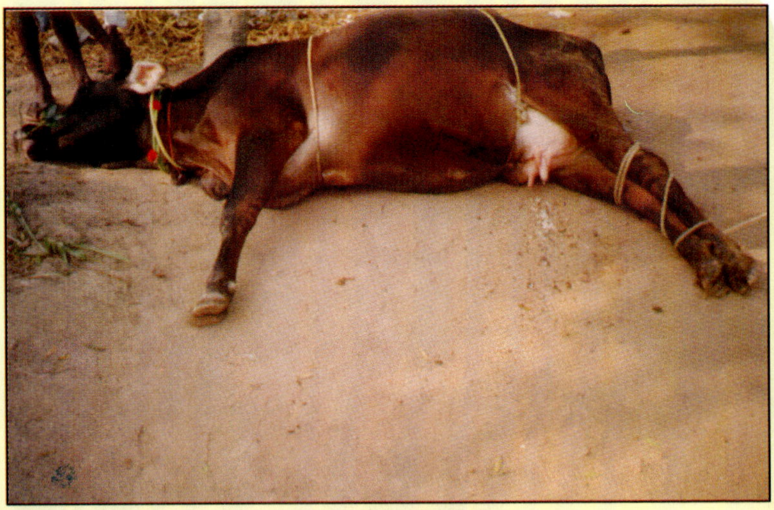

Figure 15: Mastitis showing release of coagulated milk in the form of paste

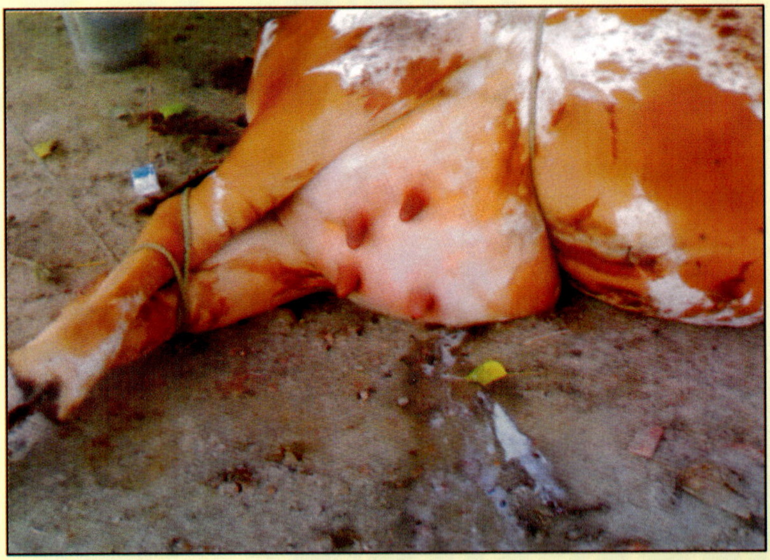

Figure 16: Mastalgia and Mastitis in a lactating cow

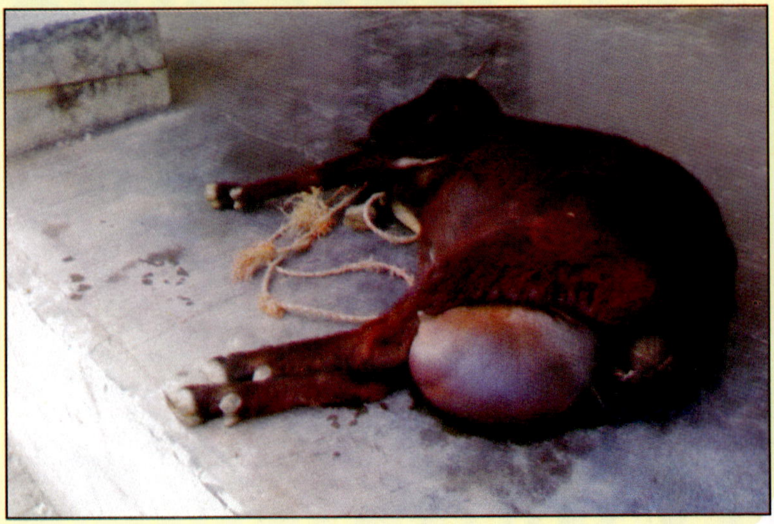

Figure 17: Acute Mastitis in a Bengal Goat with cyanotic changes in affected quarter leading to gangrene

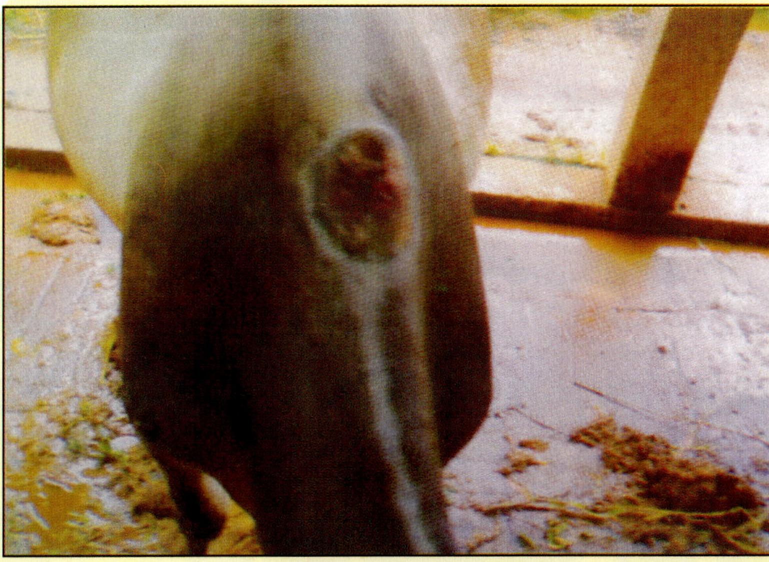

Figure 18: Humpsore in a bullock

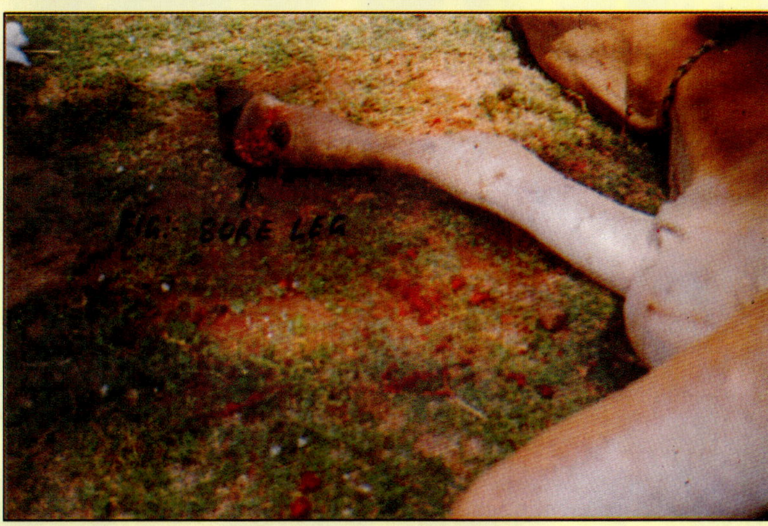

Figure 19: Foot sore due to Stephano-filariasis

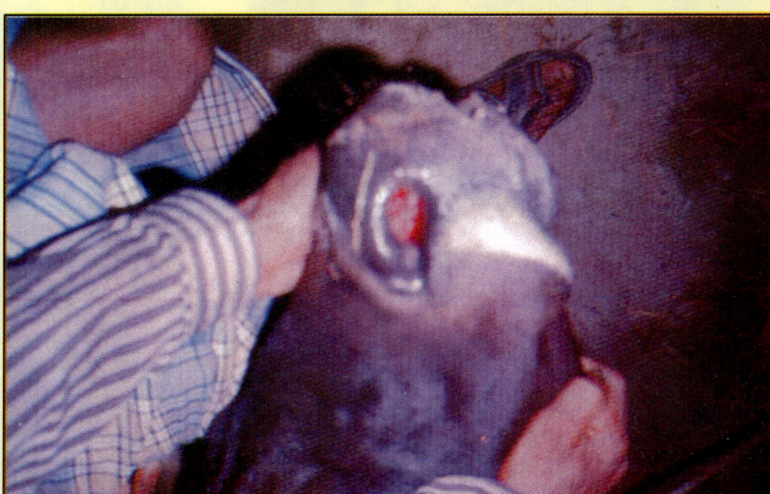

Figure 20: Nasal Granuloma in a cow

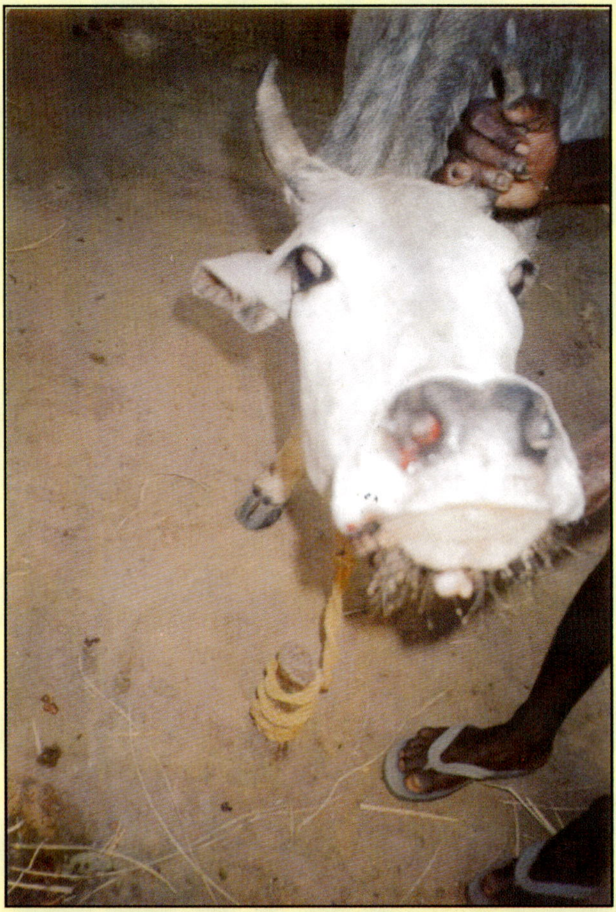

Figure 21: Nasal granuloma with oozing of blood from nostril of a bullock

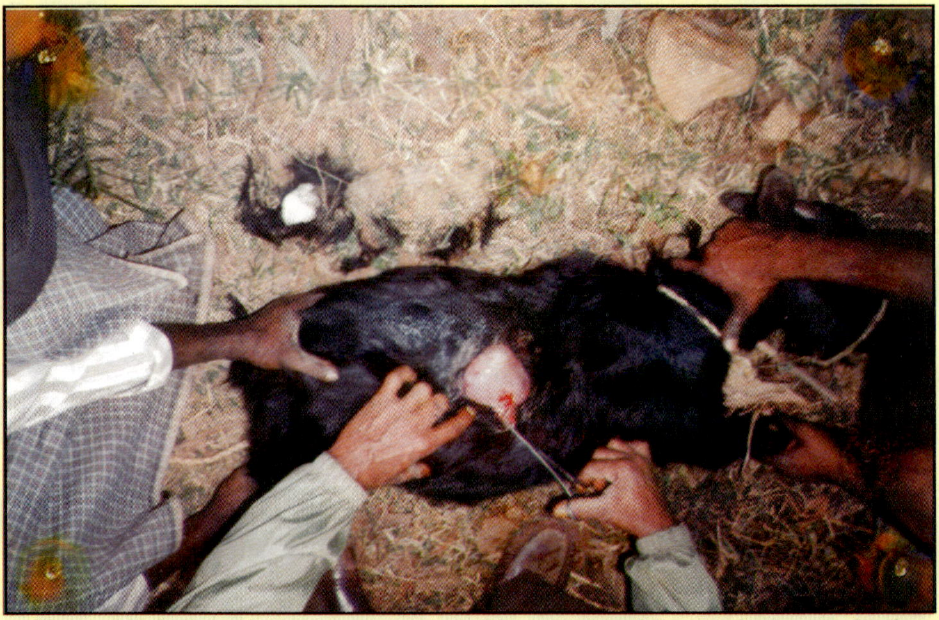

Figure 22: Solitary Coenurus gaigeri cyst in a goat and its surgical ennucleation

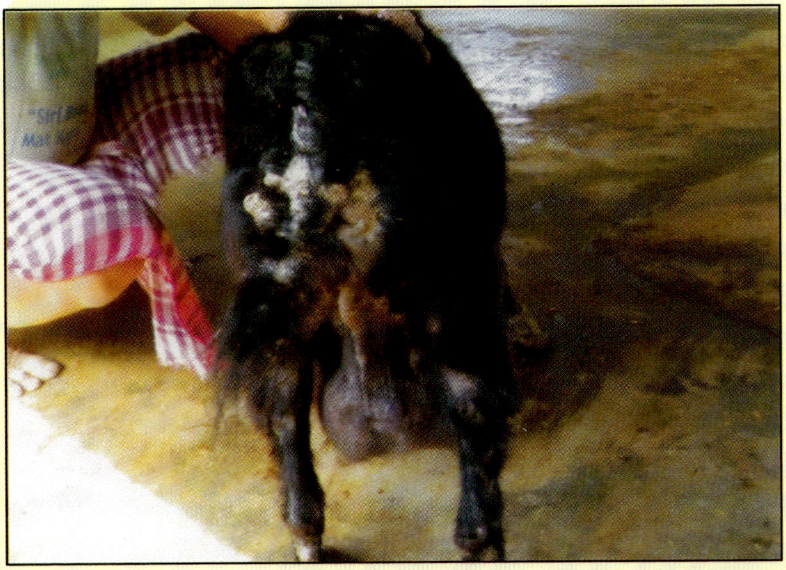

Figure 23: Generalised Scabies in Black Bengal doe

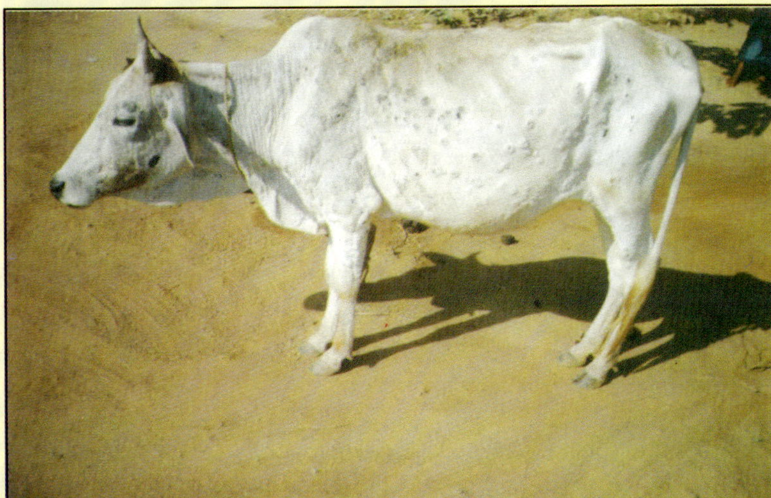

Figure 24: Generalized Mange infestation in a heifer

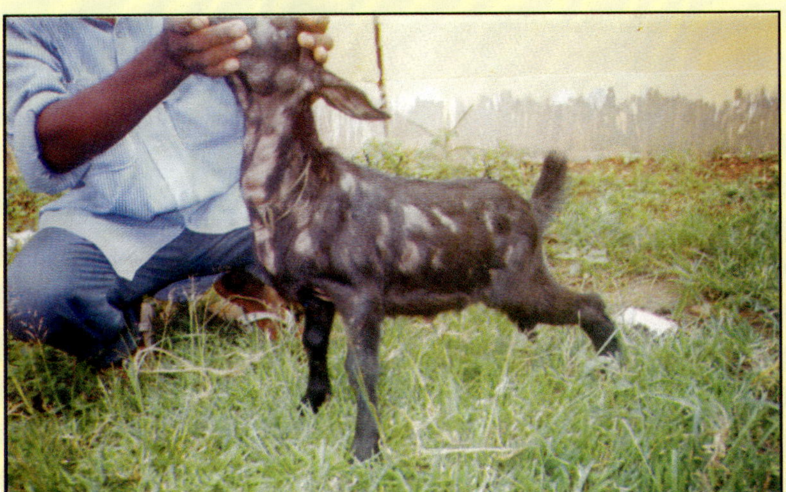

Figure 25: Mange infestation in a goat

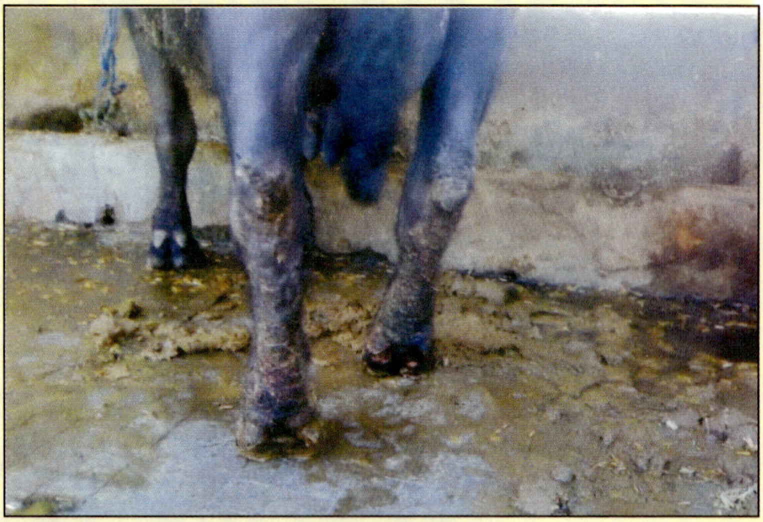

Figure 26: Mycotic dermatitis affecting hind limbs of a buffalo

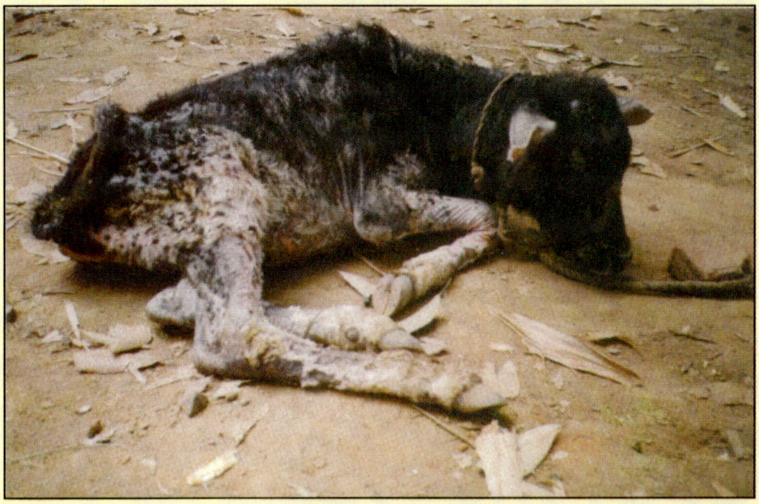

Figure 27: Chronic extensive dermatitis in a calf showing alopecia, wrinkling, thickening and scale formation

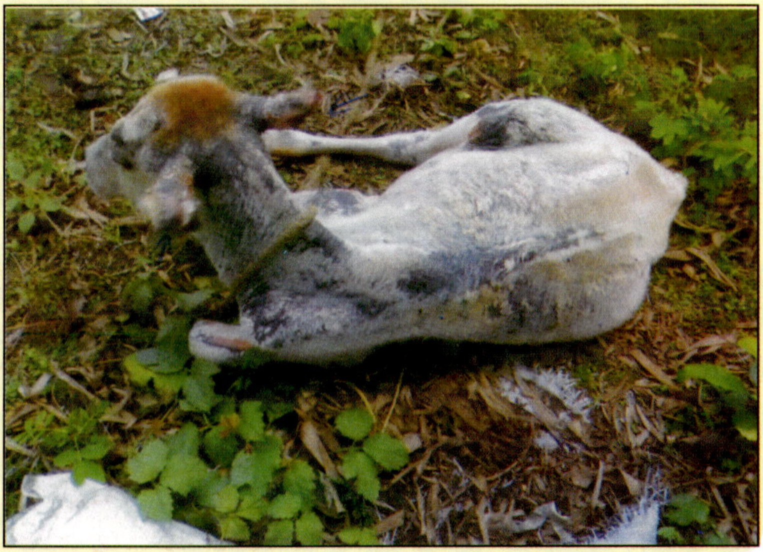

Figure 28: Photosensitization with extensive skin lesions and ear gangrene

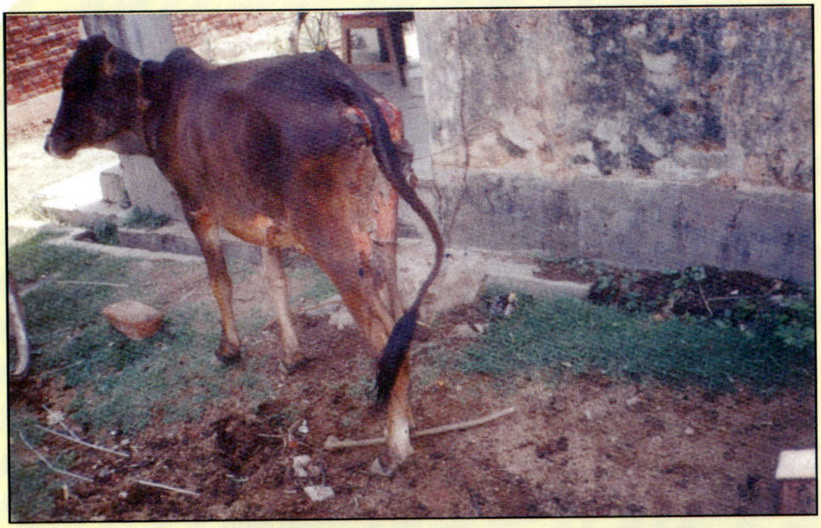

Figure 29: *Lantana camera* poisoning with skin sloughing in a cow

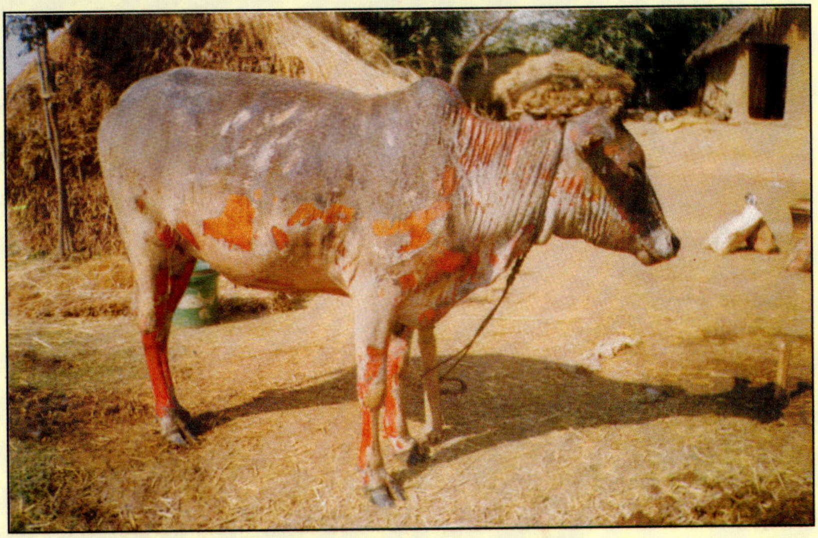

Figure 30: Extensive thermal burn in a bullock

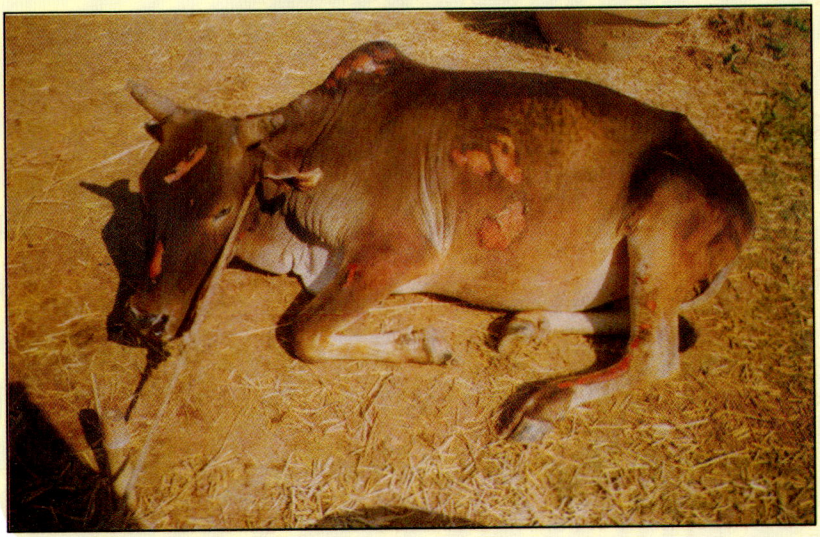

Figure 31: Thermal burn in a bullock

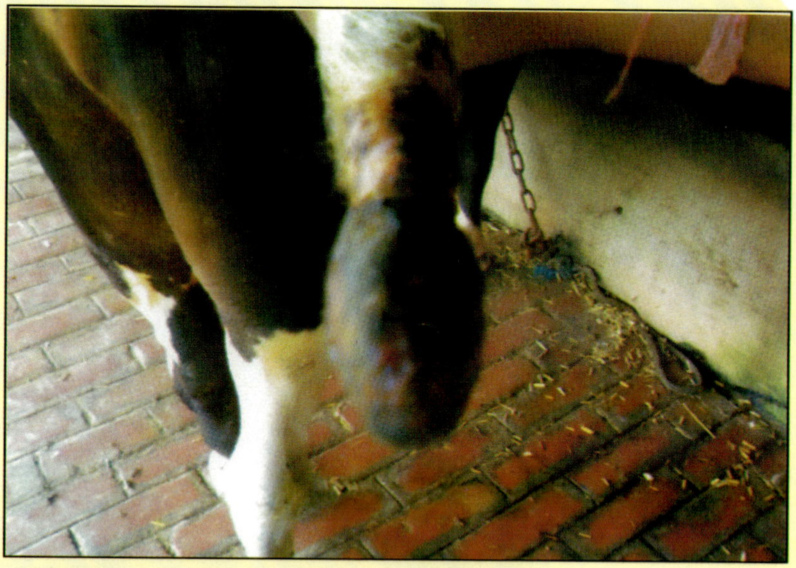

Figure 32: Tail gangrene in a cow

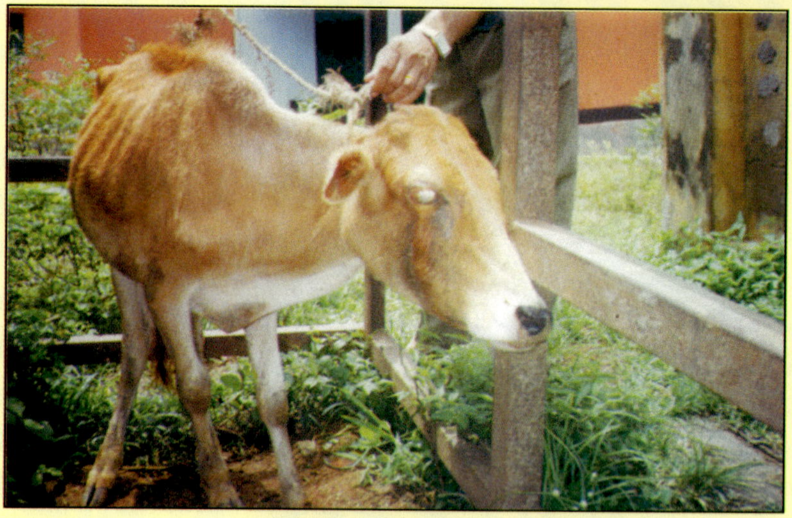

Figure 33: Corneal ulceration and damaged eyeball in a calf

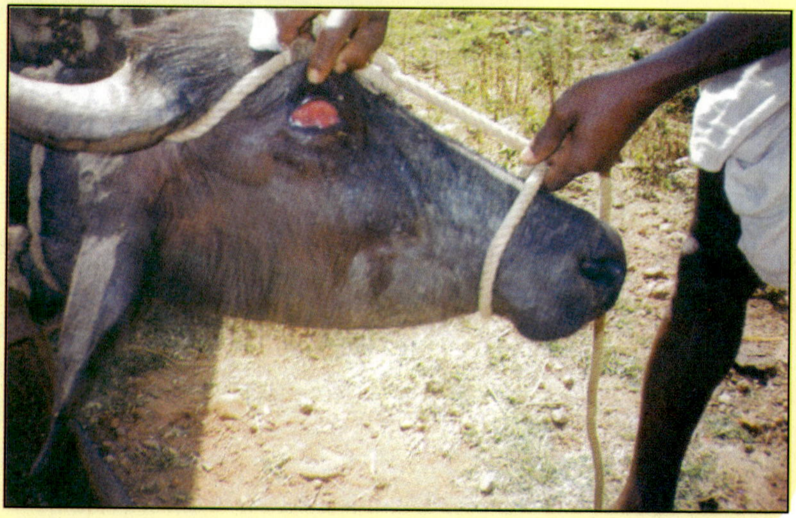

Figure 34: Conjunctivitis with profuse lachrymation in a buffalo

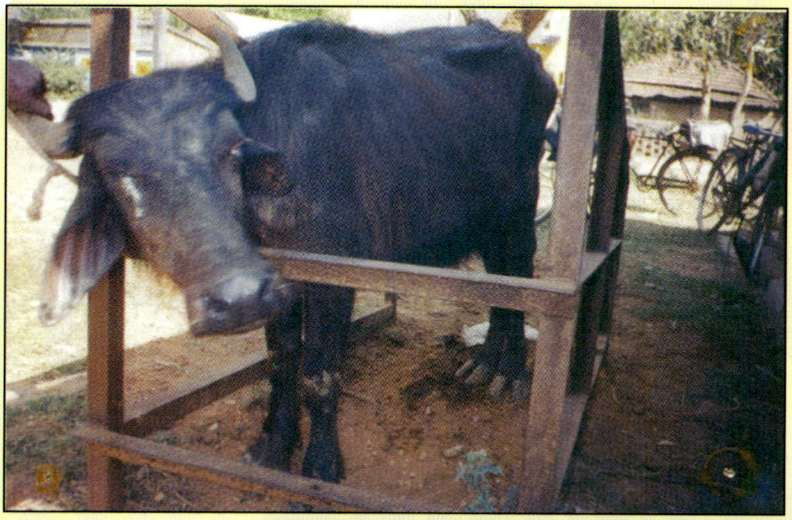

Figure 35: Mucopurulent ocular discharge with conjunctivitis in a buffalo bullock (Ophthalmic infection)

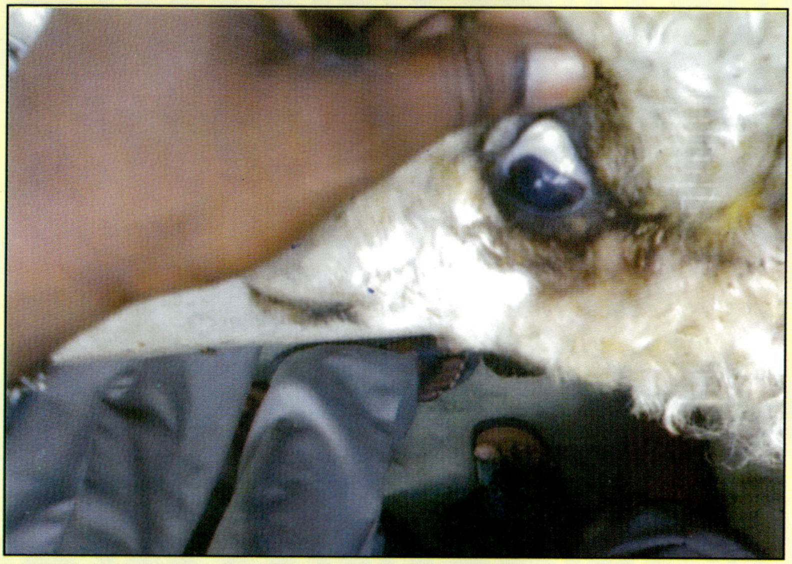

Figure 36: Severe anaemia in a lamb

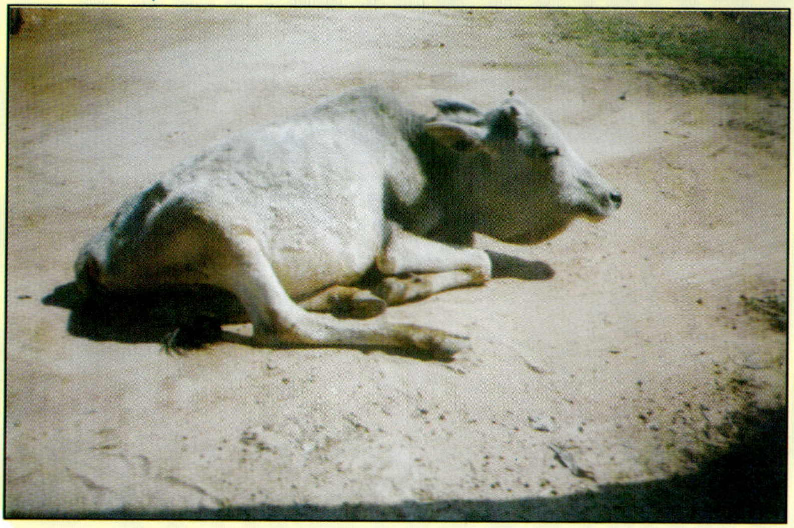

Figure 37: Calf showing facial oedema, sub mandibular oedema (Bottle jaw) and anaemia

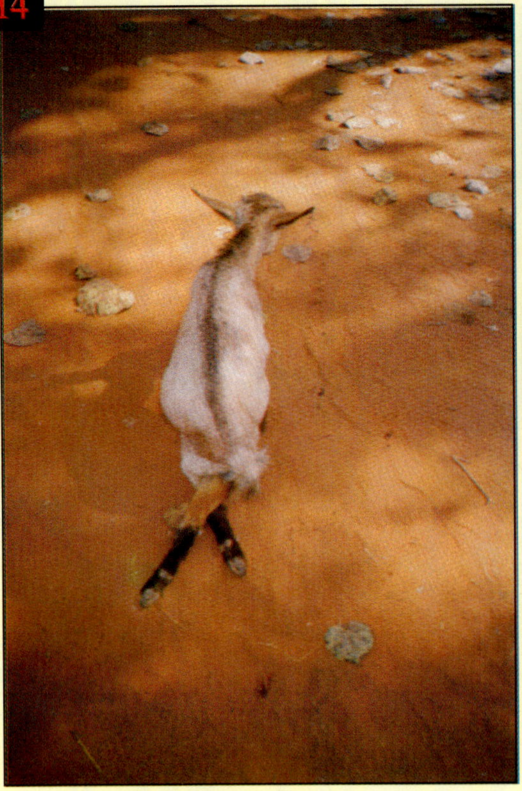

Figure 38: Posterior paralysis in a goat

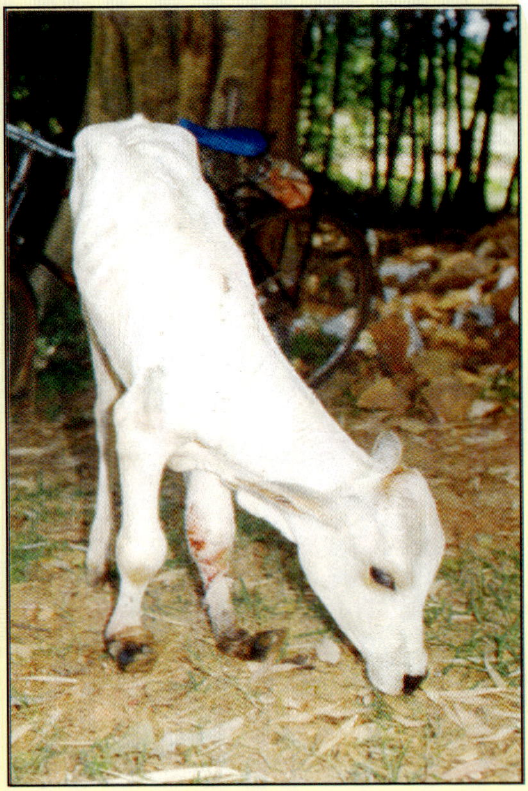

Figure 39: Arthritis with gangrenous foot in a calf

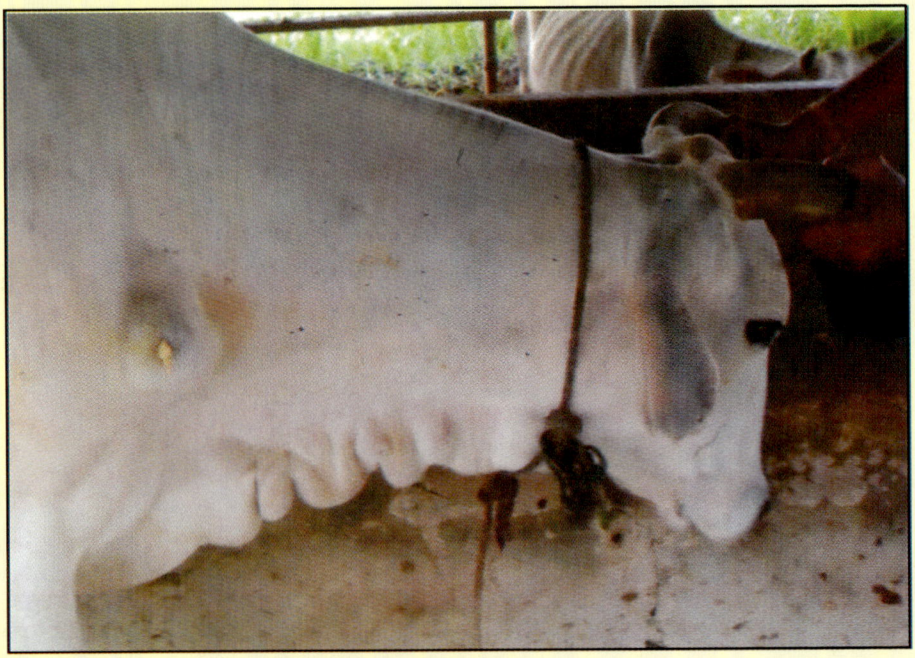

Figure 40: Multiple abscess in a cow

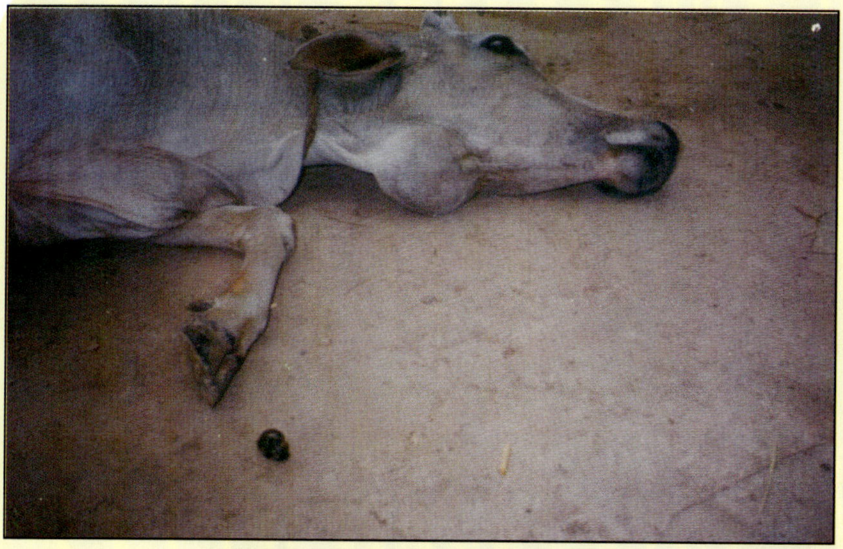

Figure 41: A big sized ripened abscess on the throat of a cow

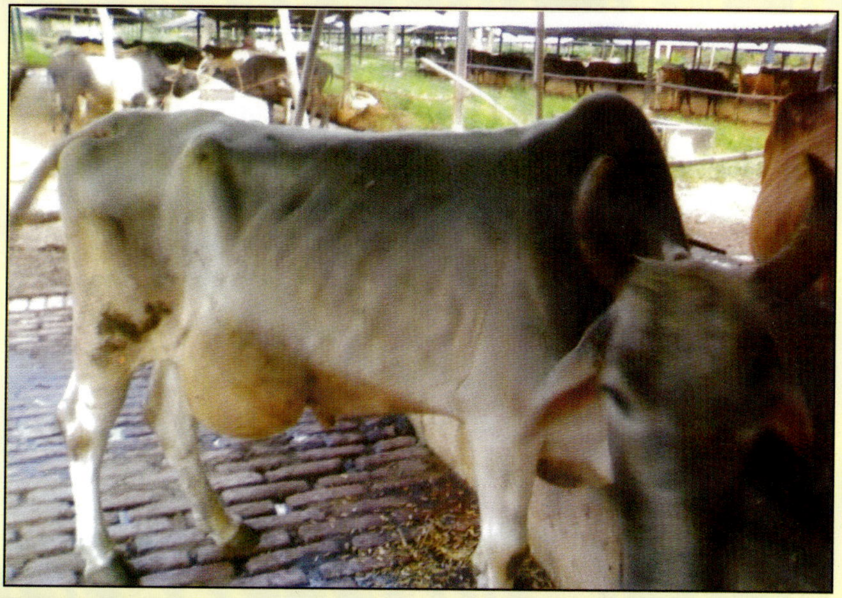

Figure 42: A very big size abdominal hernia in a cow

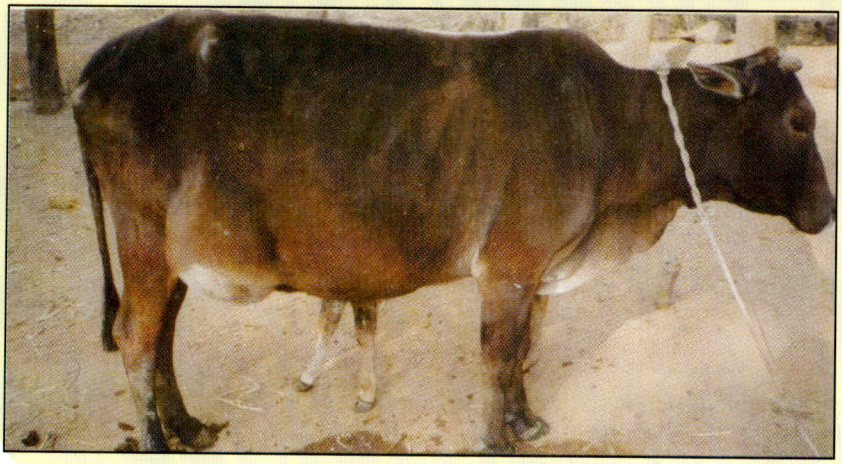

Figure 43: Abdominal hernia in a cow

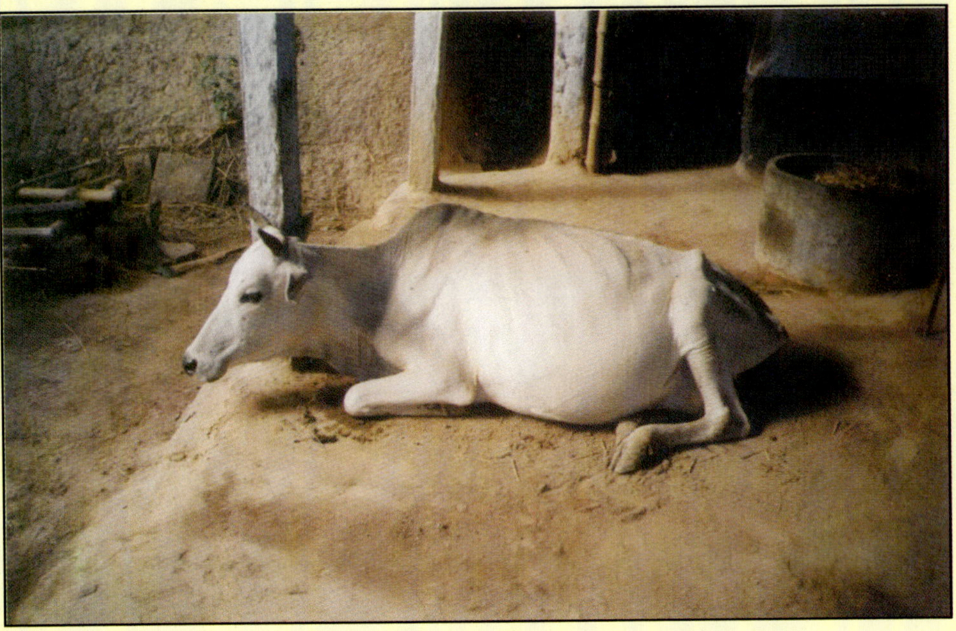

Figure 44: Recurrent Bloat (Impaction) in an indigenous cow with grave prognosis

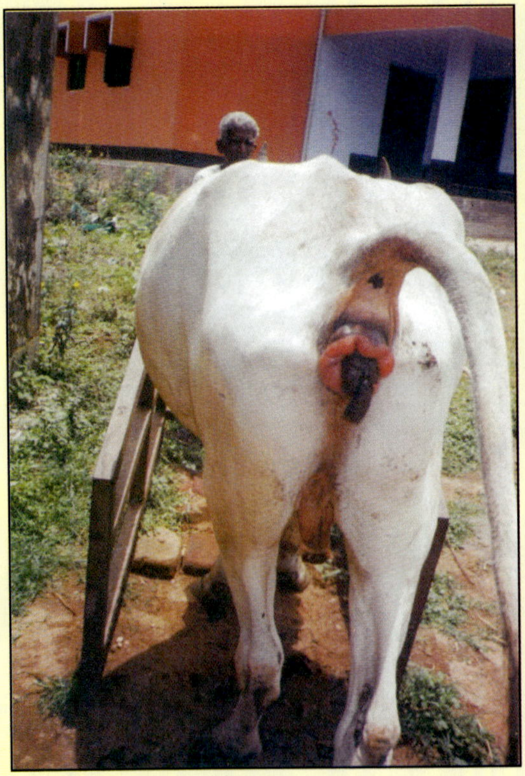

Figure 45: Constipation with anorectal oedema in a bullock

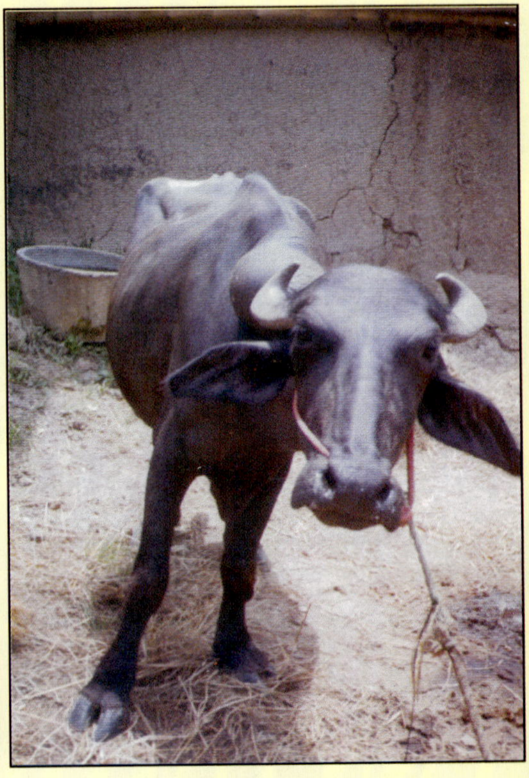

Figure 46: Chronic yoke gall in a buffalo bullock

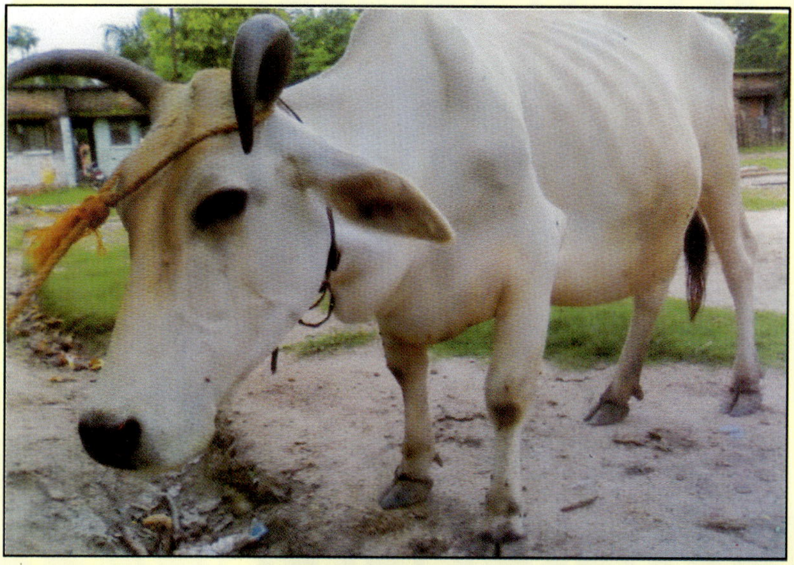

Figure 47: Traumatic reticulo pericarditis (TRP) showing brisket and ventral oedema in a cow

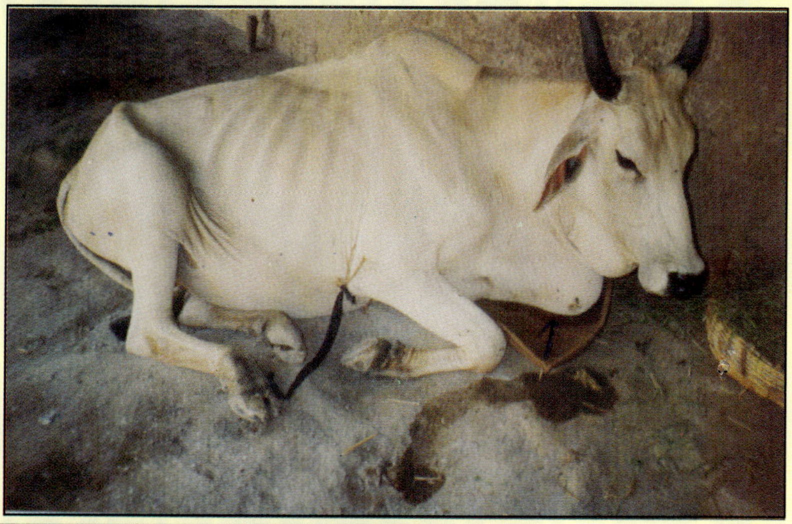

Figure 48: Traumatic reticulo pericarditis showing sternal and brisket oedema in a bullock

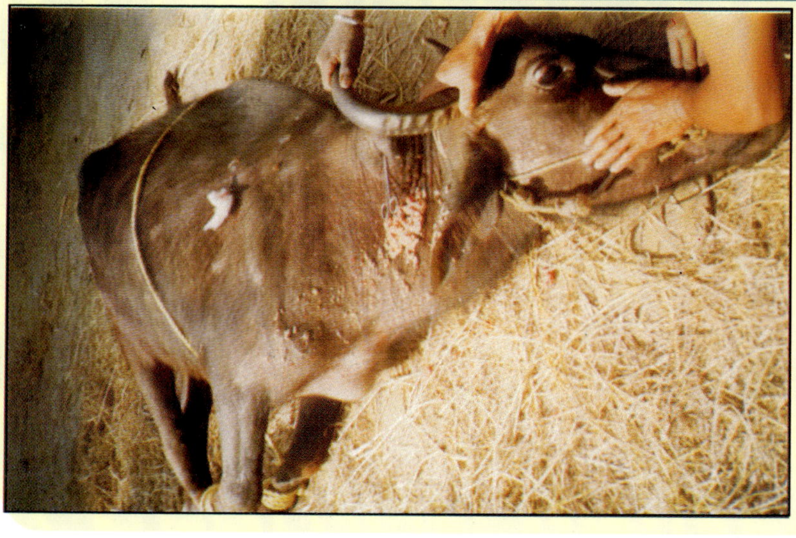

Figure 49: Yoke gall in a buffalo terminating in matured abscess and its operation

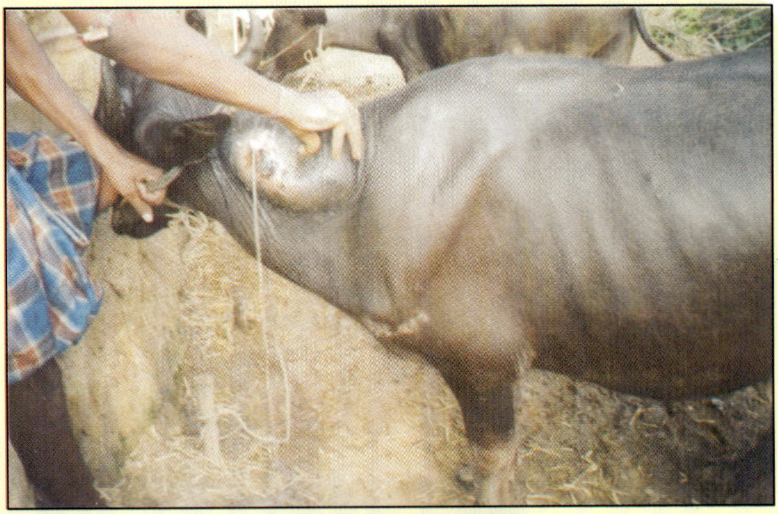

Figure 50: Yoke gall terminated into abscess in a buffalo

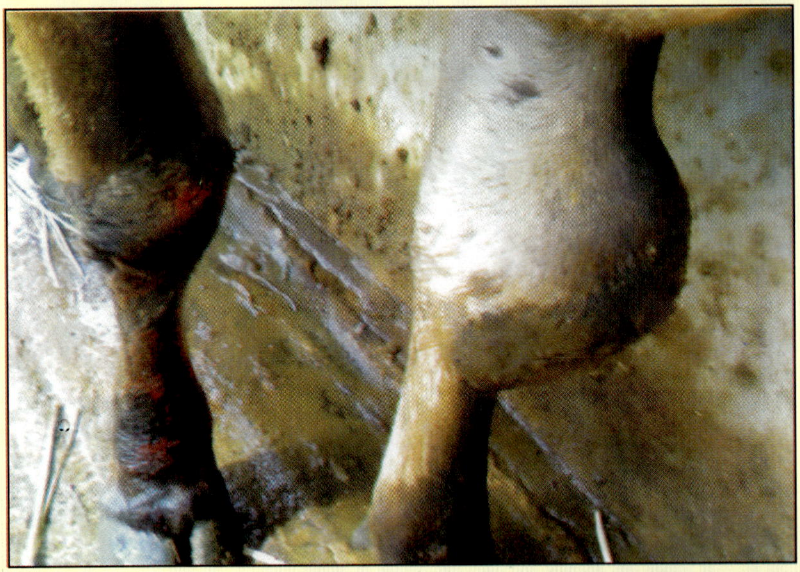

Figure 51: Knee hygroma and bursitis in a cow

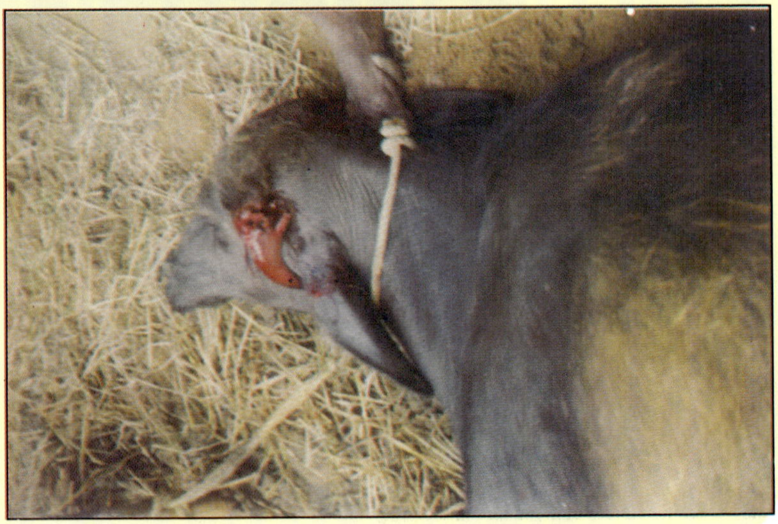

Figure 52: Broken horn in a young buffalo (Avulsion of Horn and complete fracture)

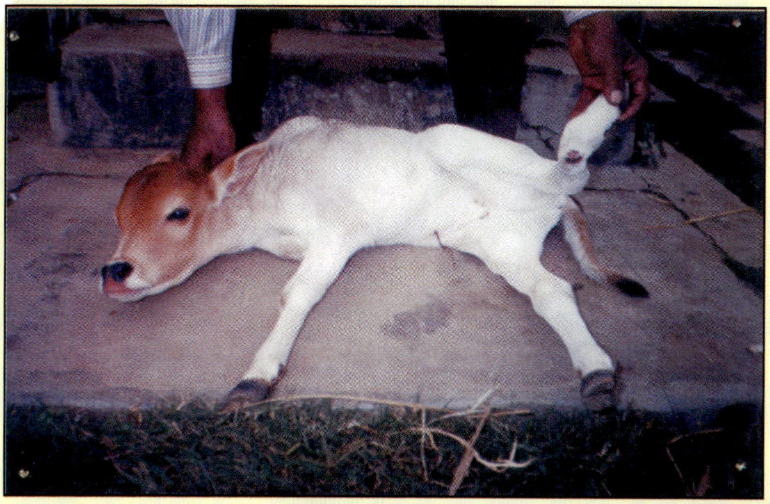

Figure 53: Fractured limb with open wound in a calf

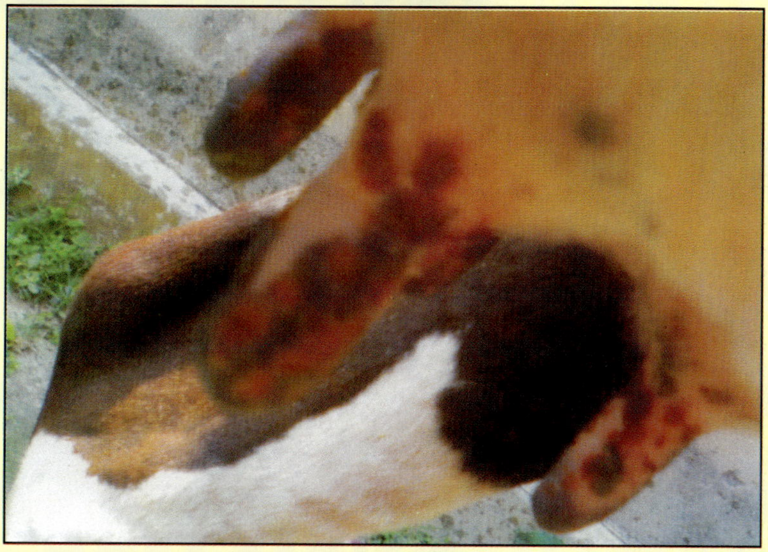

Figure 54: Bovine ulcerative mammilitis (affected teats showing ulceration)

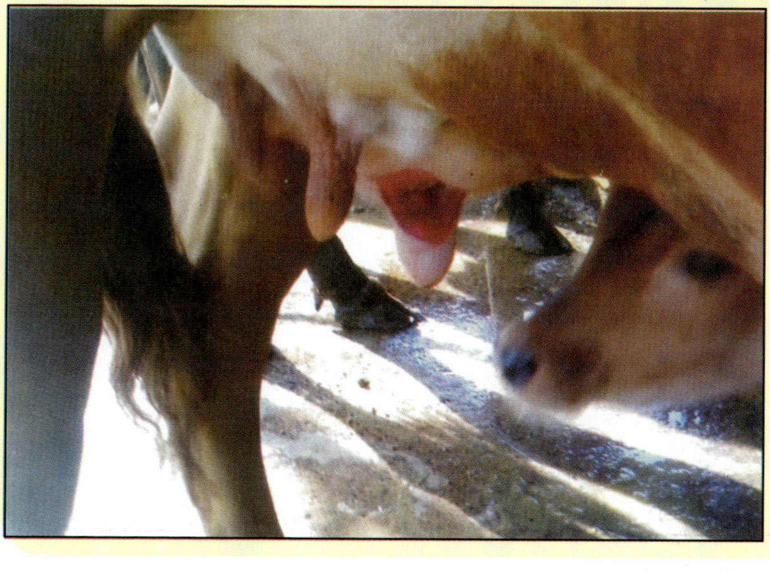

Figure 55: Ulcerative Thelitis in a cow (Raw ulcerative mammilitis in a cow)

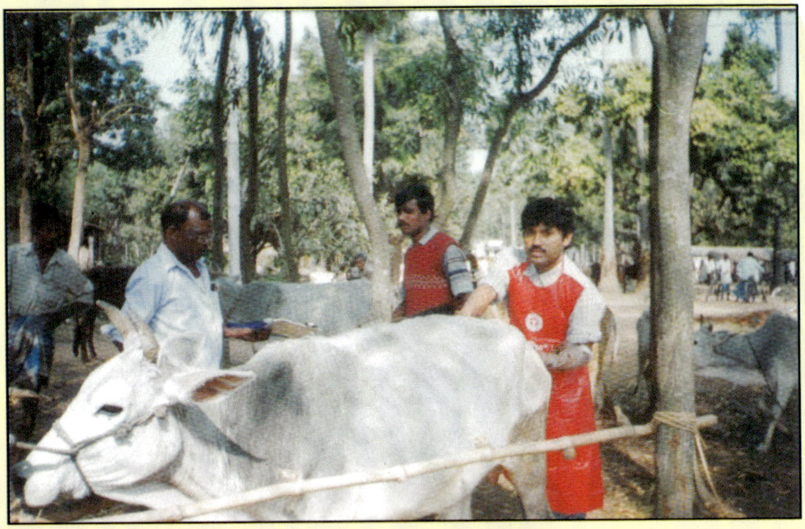

Figure 56: Per rectal Gynaecological examination in progress

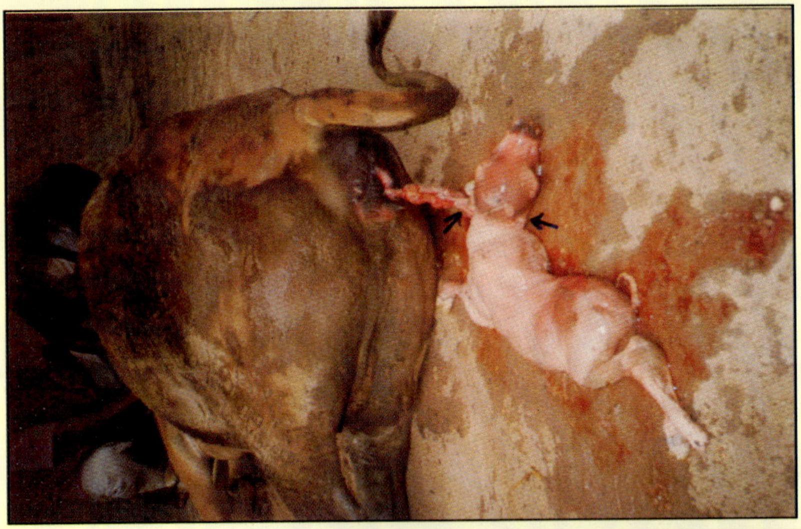

Figure 57: Abortion in a cow due to cord strangulation on foetal neck

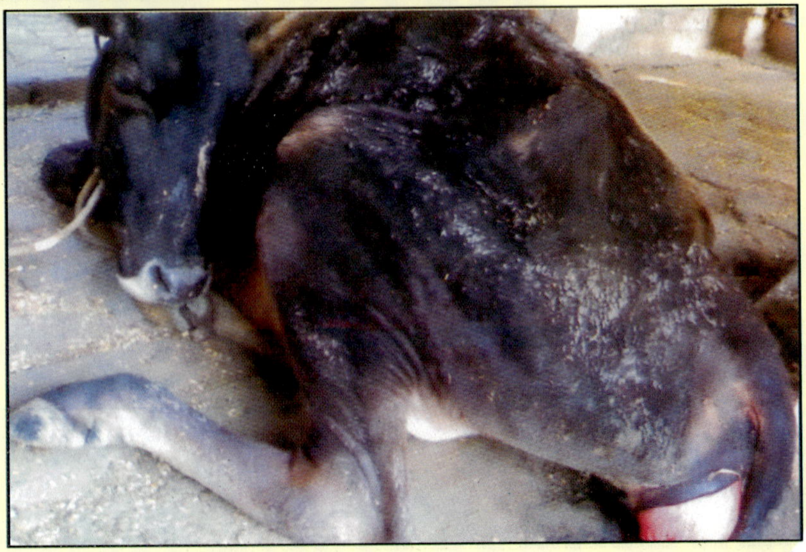

Figure 58: Post parturient hypocalcaemia with genital prolapse

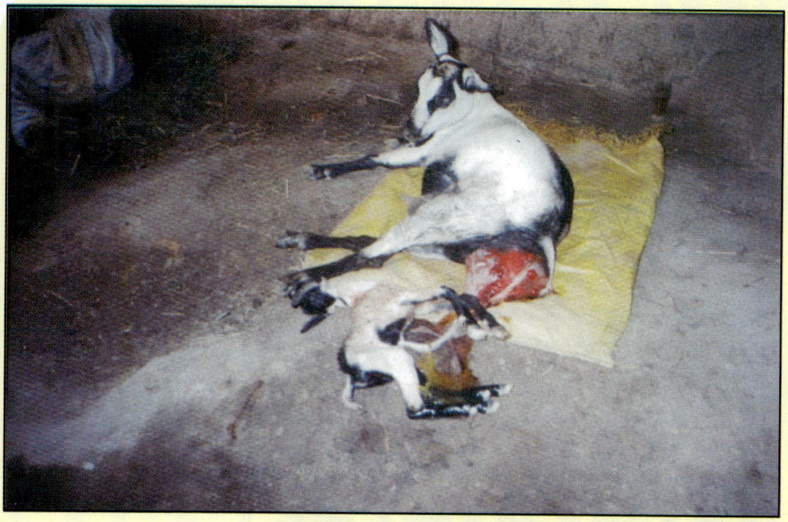

Figure 59: Kidding with prolapsed uterus

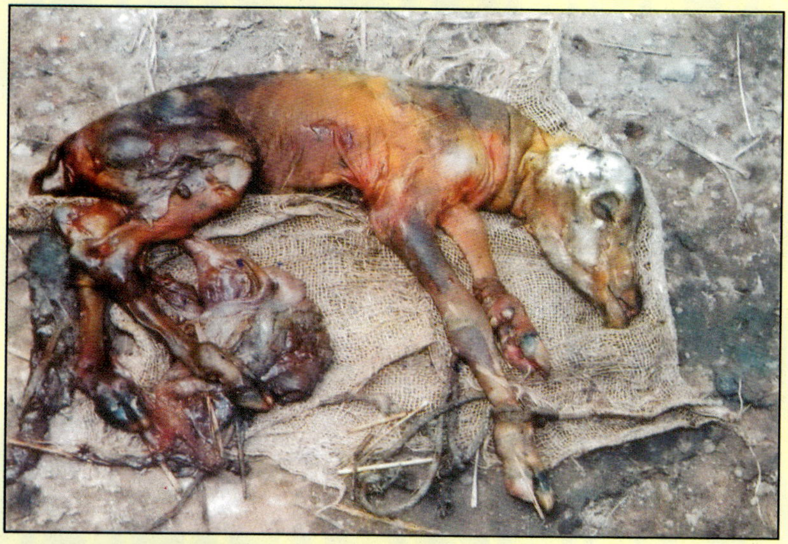

Figure 60: Mummified bovine foetus removed per vaginum from a crossbred cow (Haematic foetal mummification)

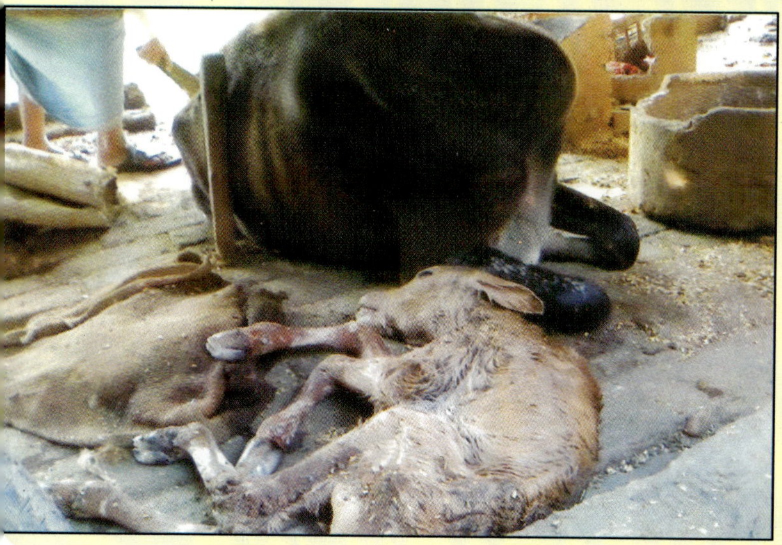

Figure 61: Per vaginal delivery of a dead calf from a crossbred peri-parturient

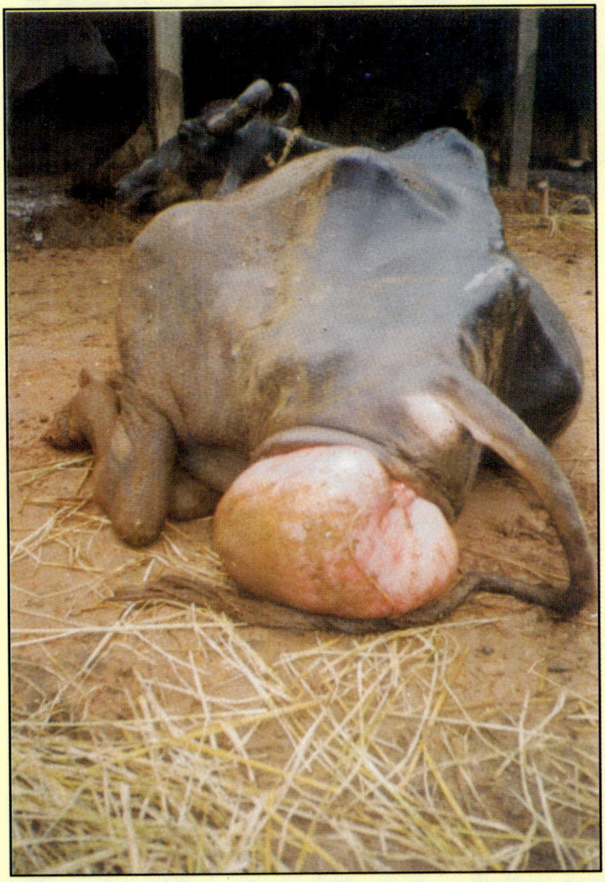

Figure 62: Prepartum cervicovaginal prolapse (Gravid uterus) in a she buffalo

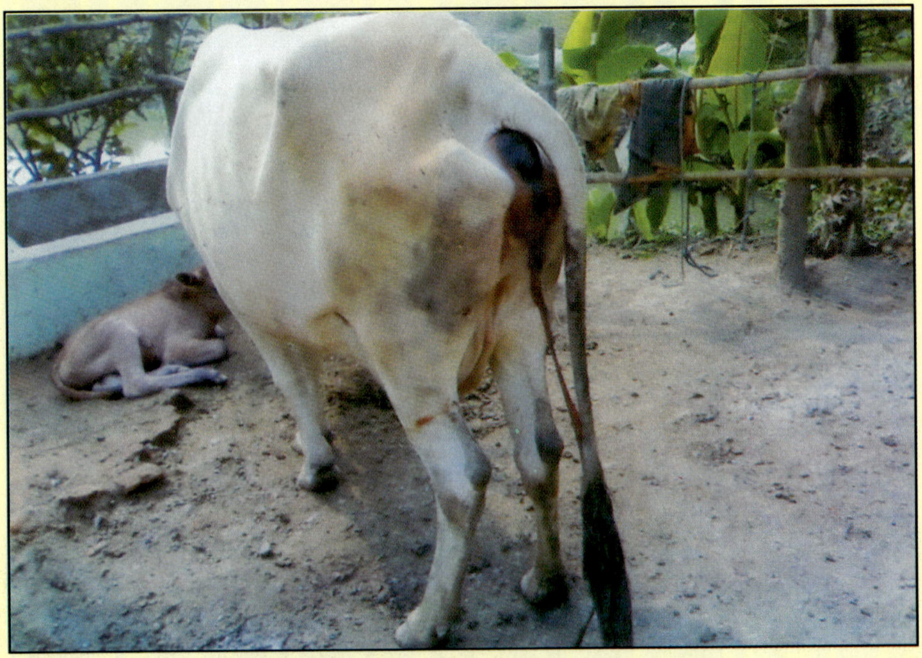

Figure 63: Retention of placenta in a cow

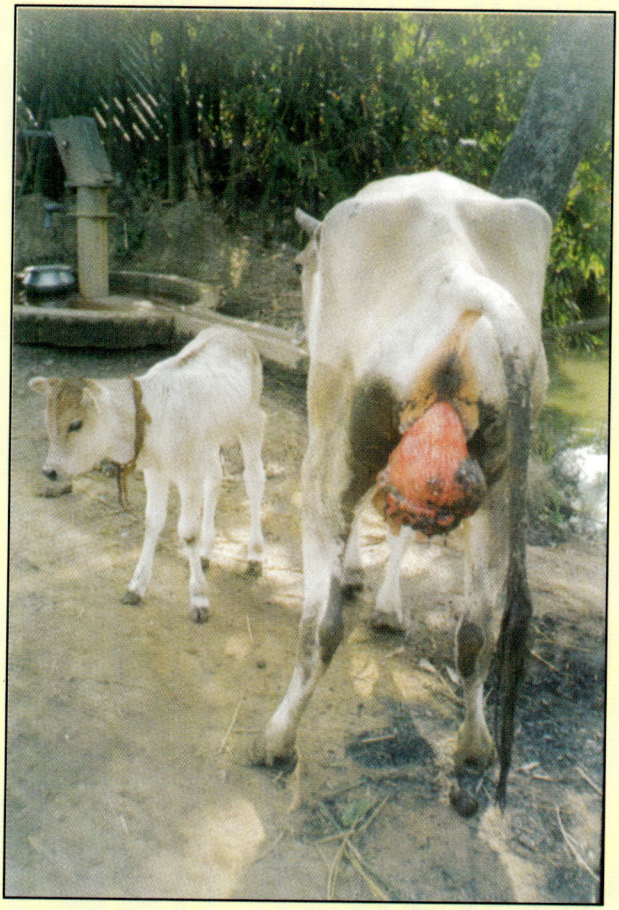

Figure 64: Recurrent post partum cervico vaginal prolapse in a crossbred cow

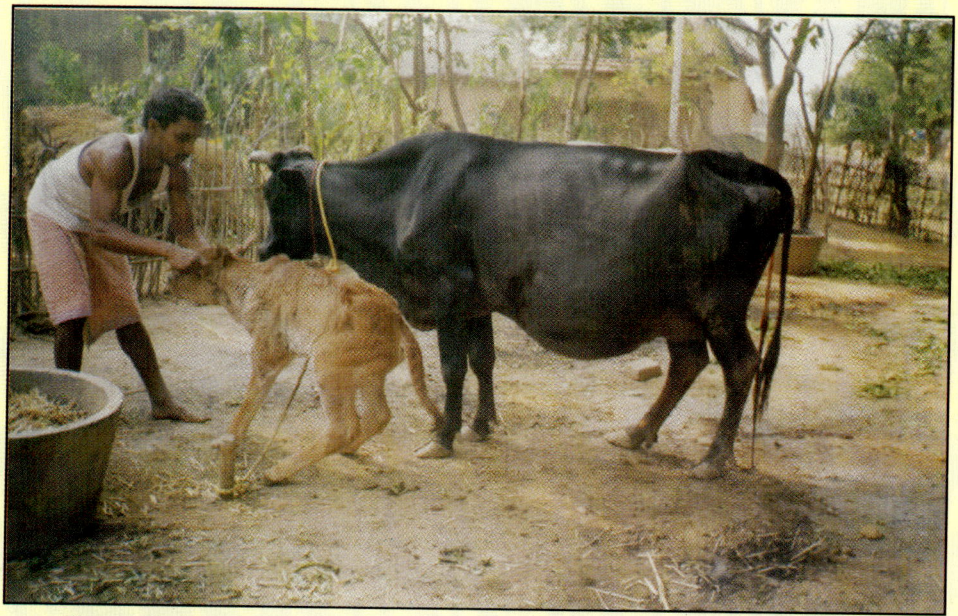

Figure 65: Retention of placenta in a crossbred cow (48 hrs after calving)

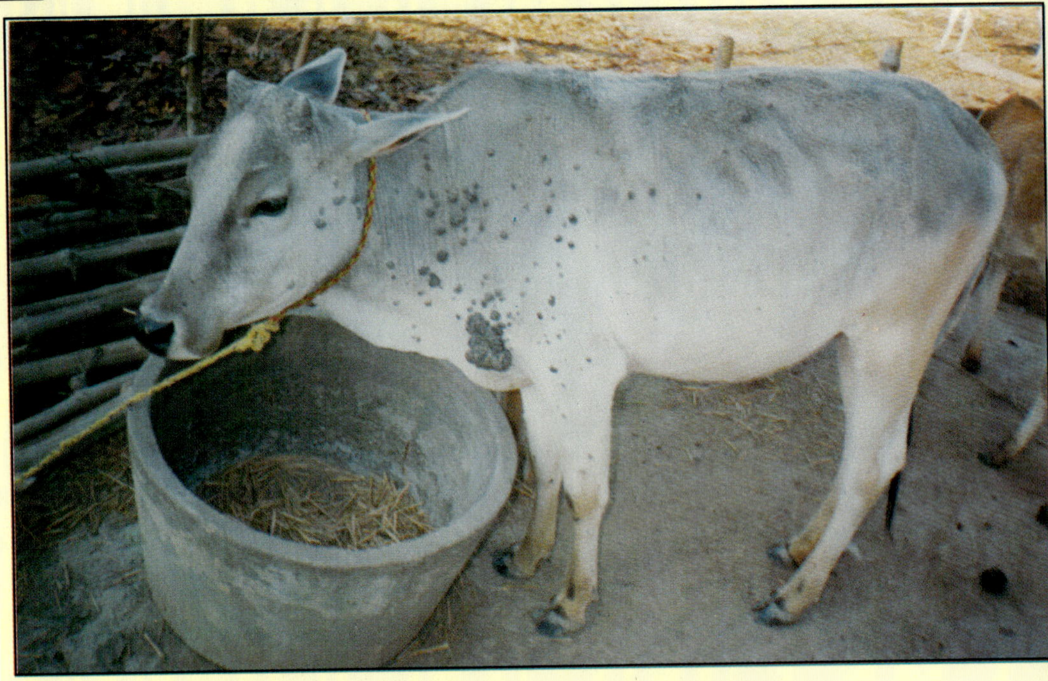

Figure 66: Warts (Bovine cutaneous papilomatosis)

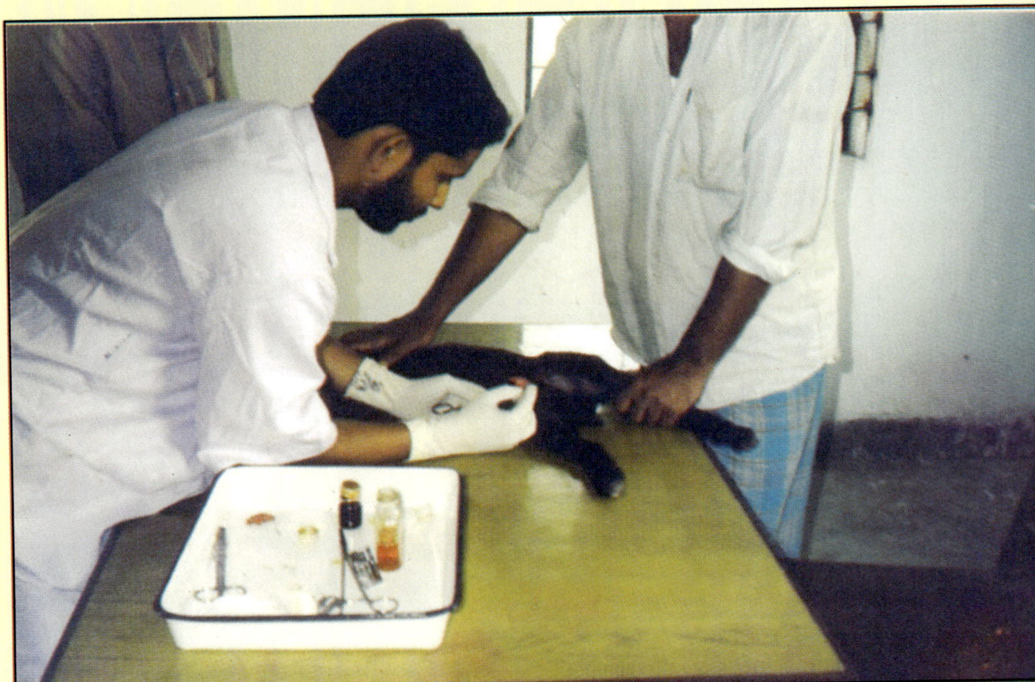

Figure 67: Castration of kid by open method

Chapter 21
Proforma of Various Certificates

21.1 CERTIFICATE OF SOUNDNESS OF ANIMAL

This is to certify that I have this day.. examined the animal described below at the request of Sri...
....

Description of the animal:

Species..............................Breed..Pedigree...

Sire........................ Dam....................................Age/Date of birth............................ Sex................

Weight.................... Colour.................. Height................... (in cm/hands)

Identification marks/No., if any.............................

In my opinion, the above described animal is sound/unsound (if unsound, form of unsoundness is to be mentioned) at this moment.

....

Place: *Signature of the Veterinary Officer*

Date: *(Stamp of designation and address)*

Registration No.

NB: The fitness certificate and soundness certificate are synonymous.

21.2 CONSENT FORM FOR SURGERY

Description of the animal:

Species............................. Breed.................................... Age............................ Sex....................

Weight................... Colour..................Identification marks/No., if any................................

I, the undersigned, do hereby declare that I am the owner/duly authorized agent for the owner of the above described animal, and that all the complications and risk involved in anaesthesia and/or surgery have been explained to me. I, therefore, willingly give my consent for the operation to be performed and will not hold the veterinary doctor (name and address)

....

....

and his/her assistant(s) responsible for any mishap.

Place: *Signature of the owner/*

Date: *duly authorized agent for the owner*

Name:

Address:

NB: For doing any kind of surgery, the risk for the same should be intimated clearly to the owner/duly authorized agent, and the above note should get signed by the owner/duly authorized agent before doing any operation.

21.3 CONSENT FORM FOR EUTHANASIA

Description of the animal:

Species............................. Breed.................................... Age............................ Sex....................

Colour.................................Identification marks, if any..

I, the undersigned, do hereby certify that I am the owner/duly authorized agent of the owner of the above described animal, that I do hereby give the veterinary doctor (name and address)...

....

and his/her assistant(s) full and complete authority to destroy and dispose of the said animal in whatever manner the veterinary doctor or his/her assistant(s) shall deem fit, and I do hereby forever release the said veterinary doctor or his/her assistant(s) from any and all liability for so destroying the animal. I do also certify that to the best of my knowledge the said animal has not bitten any person or animal during the last 15 days, and has not been exposed to rabies.

Place: *Signature of the owner/*

Date: *duly authorized agent for the owner*

Name:

Address:

....

(To be filled by the Veterinary Doctor)

Type and method of euthanasia:..

Method of disposal of carcass:...

....

Place: *Signature of the Veterinary Officer*

Date: *(Stamp of designation and address)*

Registration No.

[NB: Euthanasia means painless death. It is described in detail in chapter 17, section 17.8.11.]

21.4 PROFORMA FOR POST MORTEM REPORT

Description of the animal:

Species.............................. Breed.................................... Age............................ Sex.....................

Weight.................... Colour..................Identification marks/No., if any.................................

Necropsy Findings:

The animal died on (date):................................ Necropsy done on (date):...........................

Time of necropsy done:..................... Place (where necropsy conducted):...........................

Sufferings before death: Ailed from (date) ....to ....

Clinical Diagnosis, if any:...

Tentative diagnosis:..

External Examination of the Carcass:

Appearance –

Visible mucosae –

Secretions -

Excretions –

Internal Examination of the Carcass:

1. *Alimentary System:*

Mouth –	Oral/buccal cavity –	Pharynx –
Stomach –	Rumen –	Reticulum –
Omasum –	Abomasum –	
Small intestine –	Liver –	Gallbladder –
Pancreas –	Spleen –	Large intestine –
Peritoneum –		

2. *Respiratory System:*

Nasal cavity –	Nostrils –	Larynx –
Trachea –	Thyroid –	Lungs –
Pleura –	Pleural sac –	

3. *Urogenital System:*

Kidney –	Urinary Bladder –	Ureter –

In case of Male:

Scrotum –	Testicle –	Penis –
Penile Urethra –		

In case of Female:

Vulva –	Vagina –	Cervix –
Uterus –	Ovary –	Pelvic Organs –

4. *Cardio Vascular System:*

Thoracic cavity –	Diaphragm –	
Pericardium –	Heart –	Auricles (L/R) –
Ventricles (L/R) –		
Aorta –	Arteries –	Veins –
Lymph Nodes –		

5. *Musculo skeletal system:*

Fracture –	Trauma –	Laceration –
Myopathy –	Dislocation –	Luxation –
Osteopathy –		

6. *Brain/Central Nervous System:*

Skull –	Cerebrum –	Cerebellum –
Meninges –	Cranium –	CSF –

Collection of materials for:

(a) Laboratory investigation –

(b) Histopathological examination –

(c) Forensic examination –

Diagnosis (as per necropsy):..

....

Signature of the Autopsy Surgeon

Registration No. and Office Seal/Address

21.5 PROFORMA FOR SENDING SAMPLES TO LABORATORY

Description of the animal:

Species............................ Breed.................................. Age........................... Sex....................

Weight................... Colour.................Identification marks/No., if any...............................

Disease suspected..

Name and Address of the Owner:...

....

Material to be examined in respect of...

Sent to laboratory (name and address)...

....

on (date)...................................... by................................ (mode – special messenger/post).

Date of P M Examination done.. No. ....

Hours post death...................................... preservatives used...

....

Place: *Signature of the Veterinary Officer*

Date: *Name:*

Address:

NB: The specimen (organ) should represent the active lesion along with some healthy portion for histopathological examination. The organ should be cut in to 0.5 cm thick pieces and preserved in 10 per cent formalin solution approximately 10 times the volume of the specimen.

21.6 PROFORMA OF FIT CERTIFICATE FOR SLAUGHTER

This is to certify that I have this day... examined the animal described below and that I consider the animal to be fit/unfit for slaughter.

(1) Name and address of the owner:

(2) Description of the animal:

Species............................Breed.................................Pedigree...

Sire...................... Dam..................................Age/Date of birth...................... Sex............

Weight.................. Colour................ Height.................. (in cm/hands)

Identification marks/No., if any...........................

If unfit for slaughter, reasons should be given...

....

....

Place: *Signature of the Veterinary Officer*

Date: *(Stamp of designation and address)*

21.7 PROFORMA OF CERTIFICATE FOR TRANSPORT OF DOG

This is to certify that I have personally examined the animal, described below, of Sri/ Smt..., S/O, D/O Sri... resident of.. to the best of my ability and satisfaction, and that the animal shows/does not show evidence of any infectious and/or contagious disease at this moment.

Description of the animal:

Breed.................................Pedigree.. Sire.......................

Dam...................................Age/Date of birth....................................... Sex................

Weight................... Colour................. Height.................. (in cm)

Identification marks/No (if any)...

Registration No. (if any)...

Language used with the animal:...

Feeding system followed:..

The animal is pregnant/not pregnant (if pregnant, stage of pregnancy is to be mentioned)...

The animal is vaccinated against the following diseases:

(*i*) Rabies on (date)...

(ii) Canine Distemper on (date)..

(*iii*) Infectious Canine Hepatitis on (date)...................................

(*iv*) Parvo Virus Infection on (date)..

(*v*) Leptospirosis on (date)..

(*vi*) Others...

Test conducted:

(i) Clinical examination...

....

(*ii*) Laboratory examination (Haematological/Biochemical/Faecal/Urine analysis/X-ray/ECG *etc.*)..

....

In my opinion, the animal is found/not found positive for disease..................................

....

I,.., sign this certificate this day...

of................................ month.................................. year.................................. (in words).

....

Place: *Signature of the Veterinary Officer*

Date: *(Stamp of designation and address)*

21.8 RECORD CARD FOR VACCINATION

Name and Address of the Owner:..

....

Description of the animal:

Breed.................................Pedigree..Sire.................................

Dam.................................Age/Date of birth...............................Sex.................................

Weight...............................Colour...........................Height....................................(in cm)

Identification marks/No (if any)..

Date	*Name of Vaccine (and Manufacturer)*	*Batch No. and Expiry Date*	*Route of Administration*	*Next Due Date*	*Signature of Veterinarian*

21.9 RECORDING OF A CASE HISTORY

1. **OPD No./Animal No.** .... **Date**...
2. Name and Address of Owner..

   ....
3. Brief History...
4. General condition of the animal..
5. Clinical Examination...

   ....
6. Sample Collected..
7. Laboratory findings...

8. Diagnosis..

9. Treatment suggested..

....

10. Follow up report (if any)..

....

Attended by..

....

....

Chapter 22
Miscellaneous Information

22.1 IMPORTANT PHYSIOLOGICAL NORMS AND LONGEVITY OF VARIOUS ANIMALS

Species	*Body Temperature*		*Respiration Rate (Nos./min)*	*Pulse rate (Beats/min)*	*Average Longevity (Years)*
	°C	*°F*			
Cattle	38.6	101.5	20–25	50–60	20
Buffalo	36.8 (winter)– 39.4 (summer)	98.2 (winter)– 103 (summer)	15–20	40–50	15
Sheep	38.9	102	20–30	70–80	12
Goat	39.1	102.5	20–30	70–80	15
Pig	39.2	102.6	10–20	70–90	18–20
Rabbit	39.6	102.7	158	180	12
Fowl	41.1	106	15–30	300	
Horse	37.8–38.5	100–101.3	8–12	38–42	20–30
Camel	35.0–38.6	95–101.5	5–12	30–50	45
Dog	37.5–39.0	99.5–102.2	14–24	80–90	10–15
Cat	38.0–39.5	100.4–103.1	20–30	110–130	12
Elephant	35.0–36.4	95.0–97.5	6–9	28–40	60
Monkey	38.3	101.0	20	100	

NB: *Conversion of Celsius (°C) to Fahrenheit (°F) and vice versa:*

35°C is equal to 95°F. For each 1°C increase or decrease, 1.8 is to be added or subtracted respectively, to express the temperature in Fahrenheit.

Celsius (C) to Fahrenheit (F): °C x 9/5 + 32 = °F

Fahrenheit (F) to Celsius (C): °F – 32 x 5/9 = °C

2.2 IMPORTANT PHYSIOLOGICAL DATA OF COMMON LABORATORY ANIMALS

Parameters	*Mice*	*Rat*	*Guinea Pigs*	*Hamster*		*Rabbit*
				Syrian	*Chinese*	
Birth weight (g)	1–1.5	6.5	70–100	20	–	50–70
Adult body weight (g)	30–40	250	800	80–90	35–40	1500–5,500
Daily feed consumption (g)	5–6	15–20	45–50	10–15	10	200–250
Age at first matting (months)	1.5–2.0	2.5–3.0	3.0	2–3	2–3	6–7
Age suitable for experimentation (months)	1.5	1.5	3	1	1	6
Heart rate/minute	350–750	310–500	250–400	315–410	310–420	150–300
Respiratory rate/minute	85–230	70–180	70–110	35–130	30–125	40–60
Blood volume (per cent of body weight)	7–10	5–7	6–12	6–9	6–10	5–8
Sex ratio (Male : Female)	1 :3	1 : 5	1 : 6	1 : 1	1 : 1	1 : 6
Life span (years)	1.5–2.54	2–3	3–5	2–3	2–3	5–6
Gestation period (days)	20–21	21–27	65–67	16	21	31–32
Litter size	7–12	8–10	3–4	5–7	4–5	6–8
Age at weaning (weeks)	3 wks	3 wks	2–3 wks	3–5 wks	3	7
Weaning weight (g)	10–15g	40–50	150–240	35–45	8–10	800–1500
Reproductive life (years) after 1st mating	1	1	2	1.5	1	3
Litters/year	8–10	7	4–5	10	7	4–5
No. of pairs of mammary glands	5	5	1	6–7	4	3–4
Total RBC x 10^{12}/L	7–11	7–10	5–7	6–7	–	5–7
Total WBC x 10^{9}/L	4–12	5–15	7–14	7–10	–	6–12
Average body temperature (°C)	37	38	39	39	–	40

22.3 NORMAL HAEMATOLOGY OF ANIMALS

Species	*RBC (million/ cu. mm.)*	*WBC (thousand/ cu. mm.)*	*Platelets (thousand/ cu. mm.)*	*Haemo-globin (g%)*	*Haematocrit/ PCV (%)*	*ESR (mm/hr)*	*Clotting time (min)*
Cattle	5–10 (7.5)	4–12 (7.9)	350	8.5–13.5 (11)	28–42 (35)	0–3	5
Buffalo	5.0–7.3 (6.65)	5–10	–	9.0–12.9 (10.8)	30–36 (33)		–
Sheep	8.5–13.5 (10.8)	4–12 (7.4)		9.3–14.8 (11.5)	27–43 (35)	0–3	–

Contd...

Species	*RBC (million/ cu. mm.)*	*WBC (thousand/ cu. mm.)*	*Platelets (thousand/ cu. mm.)*	*Haemo–globin (g%)*	*Haematocrit/ PCV (%)*	*ESR (mm/hr)*	*Clotting time (min)*
Goat	8–18 (15)	4.5–13.0 (8.9)	2500	8.8–13.8 (11.3)	25–40 (34)	2–2.5	–
Pig	5.0–8.5 (6.8)	11–22 (17.1)	403	8.3–12.7 (10.4)	32–46 (40)	1–1.4	–
Fowl	3.24	9.8	254	13.5	40	1.4	–
Horse	6.9	5.1	176	12–14	33.4	6	6.75
Dog	5.5–9.5 (6.2)	8–14 (9.5)	155	10–16 (13)	37–55 (45)	5–20 (10)	8.6
Cat	5–10 (7.5)	5.5–19.5 (12.5)		8–15 (12)	25–45 (33)	–	–
Man	5.4	5.1	214–360	15–16	44	8.3	6.17

* Blood constituents are liable to show markedly different values depending upon methodology employed.

Source: Various published literatures.

Figures within brackets are average data.

22.4 NORMAL SERUM BIOCHEMISTRY OF ANIMALS

Species	*Protein (g %)*	Glucose *(mg/ 100 ml)*	Total Cholesterol *(mg/100 ml)*	Bilirubin *(mg/ 100 ml)*	Calcium *(mg/ 100 ml)*	Phosphorus *(mg/ 100 ml)*	Iron *(mg/ 100 ml)*
Cattle	7.6	40–70	50–230	0.2–0.5	10.5–12.25	3.2–8.4	57–162
Buffalo	6.8	50–70	–	0.3–0.4	10.8	6.0	300
Sheep	5.2	40–60	100–150	0–0.4	9.0–12.25	2.9–7.4	166–222
Goat	6.2	45–50	55–200	0–0.1	9.25–11.5	4.0–9.7	150
Pig	7.4	65–95	100–250	0–0.4	9.0–13.25	4.6–10.2	91–199
Fowl	–	5.9	58–94	–	9–12	–	–
Horse	6.72	2.5	96.8	–	12–13.4	–	–
Dog	6.1–7.8	2.1	100–250	0.1–0.6	9.8–11.6	2.8–5.1	–
Cat	5.4–7.0	2.3	95–135	–	8.22	–	–
Man	7.5	2.4	150–250	–	9–11	–	–

* Blood constituents are liable to show markedly different values depending upon methodology employed.

Source: B. Prasad (1992) and various published literatures.

22.5 PHYSIOLOGICAL NORMS OF SOME ZOO ANIMALS IN CAPTIVITY

Species	*Gestation Period (days)*	*Body Temperature*		*Average Longevity (Years)*
		(°C)	*(°F)*	
Tiger	103–112	38–39	100.4–102.2	20–25
Lion	110–112	38–39	100.4–102.2	25–30
Leopard	93–105	38–39	100.4–102.2	21
Cheetah	91–95	38–39	100.4–102.2	15
Chimpanzee	216–261	37.2	99	50 or more
Orangutan	275	37	98.6	35 or more
Gorilla	251–289	37.2	99	40
Bear	155–245*	37.5–38	99.5–100.4	20–30
Deer	200**	38	100.4	15–18
Zebra	330–365	37–38	98.6–100.4	25–28
Elephant	630–660	36.4	97.5	40–50

*Variable depending upon time of implantation.

** Variable with species.

Source: L M Acharjyo (1983), Heinz-George Klos and E M Lang (1983) and other literatures.

22.6 LIST OF TERATOGENIC DRUGS

Drug/Chemical	*Organ/System Affected*
Tetracycline	Teeth, skeleton
Corticosteroid	Palate, limb, oedema
Griseofulvin	Brain, palate, skeleton
Androgen	Masculinization
Folic acid antagonist (aminopterin, pyrimethamine)	Embryo toxic
Perbendazole	Brain, kidney, skeleton, limbs

22.7 LIST OF DRUGS CONTRA-INDICATED IN LACTATION

Drug/Chemical	
Androgen	Oestrogen (high dose)
Atropine	Phenylbutazone
Antithyroid drugs	Reserpine
Chloramphenicol	Sulphonamides
Ergotamine	Tetracycline
Lithium	Vitamin A, D (high dose)

22.8 LIST OF DRUGS SAFE IN LACTATION

Drug/Chemical	
Ampicillin	Insulin
Antacids	Iron
Antihistamines	Kanamycin
Chlorpromazine	Lincomycin
Codeine	Morphine
Digoxin	Nitrofurantoin
Erythromycin	Paracetamol
Folic acid	Penicillin
Frusemide	Phenothiazine
Gentamycin	Salicylates
Ibuprofen	Streptomycin

22.9 LIST OF POTENTIALLY HAZARDOUS DRUGS IN PREGNANCY

Drug/Chemical	
Aminoglycosides	Metronidazole
Amphotericin B	Nitrofurantoin
Chloramphenicol	Polymyxins
Fluoroquinolones	Sulphonamides (long acting)
Griseofulvin	Tetracyclines
Ketokonazole	Trimethoprim

22.10 LIST OF POTENTIALLY HAZARDOUS DRUGS IN NEONATES

Drug/Chemical	
Aminoglycosides	Polymyxins
Chloramphenicol	Sulphonamides
Fluoroquinolones	Tetracyclines
Nalidixic acid	Trimethoprim
Nitrofurantoin	

22.11 LIST OF DRUGS NOT RECOMMENDED IN PARTICULAR SPECIES OF ANIMALS

Species of Animal	*Drugs Not Recommended*
Cat	Paracetamol (Acetaminophen), Levamisole, Ascabiol lotion ®
Rabbit	Lincomycin, Clindamycin, Penicillin group (especially Ampicillin), Spiramycin, Tylosin, Erythromycin and Oleandomycin.
Epileptic patient	Phenothiazine transquilizers

22.12 RELATIVE PRODUCTION EFFICIENCIES AND ECONOMY OF DIFFERENT MEAT PRODUCING ANIMALS

Animals	*Gestation Interval (Months)*	*No. of Offspring per Dam per Year*	*Marketing Age (Weeks)*	*No. of Crops per Year*	*Feed Conversion Efficiency (FCR)*	*Per cent of Protein Conversion Efficiency*
Beef cattle	36	1	52	1	5	6.0
Sheep	18	1	52	1	5.4	3.0
Swine	15	25	26	2	2.5	12.0
Broiler	6.5	140	6	7.5	1.9	21.0
Rabbit	6.5	36	10	5	2.5	5.0
Fish	12	10,000*	52	1	2.5	4.0

*: Less 1 per cent is viable at market age.

22.13 CONTENTS OF A VETERINARY EMERGENCY KIT

Medicines

Injections: Coramine, Adrenaline, Atropine sulphate, Largactil, Siquil, Prednisolone acetate, Dexona, Paracetamol, MP3 (Meloxicam-Paracetamol), Nimovet (Nimesulide), Pethidine, Penicillin, Tetracycline.

Intravenous fluids: Normal saline, Dextrose 5 per cent, Destrose 10 per cent, Ringer's lactate, Calcium borogluconate.

Others: Tr. Iodine, Povidone iodine, Potassium permanganate, Dettol, Savlon, Liquid paraffin, Sodibicarb, *etc.*

Other Requisites

Syringe with needle of assorted size (2 ml, 5 ml, 10 ml, 20 ml, 50 ml), Suturing needle (assorted size), Nylon thread, Catgut (assorted size), Cotton, Gauge, Bandage, Scissors, Scalpel, Forceps, Artery forceps, Stomach tube, Catheter, Intravenous set, Trocar and Canula, Gloves, Torch *etc.*

References

Acharjyo, L M (1983) General Principles of Health Care and Disease Management of Wild Animals and Birds in Captivity. Silver Jubilee Souvenir, Assam State Zoo and Botanical Garden, Assam.

Bandyopadhyay, S K, Bhattachartta, B, Roy Choudhury, R and Basu, S (2007) Text Book of Veterinary Gynaecology, Artificial Insemination, Obstetrics and Assisted Reproduction, Kalyani Publishers, New Delhi.

Chakrabarty, A, Ray, S K and Sahoo, N (2004) Text Book of Veterinary Ethics and Jurisprudence, Kalyani Publishers, New Delhi.

Das, S K (2005) Hand Book of Veterinary Practitioners, Kalyani Publishers, New Delhi.

Ganti, G A (1983) Veterinary Clinical Pathology, CBS Publishers and Distributors, Delhi.

Garg, R and Nagori, M K (2004) VETNDEX, NBS Publishers and Distributors, Bikaner, Rajasthan.

Ghosh, N. (2006) Rabbit Production, Diseases and Treatment, 1st Bengali edition, Kalyani Publishers, New Delhi.

Ghosh, N. (2008) Animal Production, Diseases and Treatment, 2nd Bengali edition, Kalyani Publishers, New Delhi.

Ghosh, N. (2008) Goat Production, Diseases and Treatment, 2nd Bengali edition, Kalyani Publishers, New Delhi.

Ghosh, N. (2009) Poultry Farming, 1st Bengali edition, Kalyani Publishers, New Delhi.

Ghosh, N. (2011) Poultry Science and Practice – A Text Book, 1st edition, International Book Distributing Co. (Publishing Division), Lucknow.

Heinz-George, K and Lang E M (1983) Hand Book of Zoo Medicines, Van Nostrand Reinhoid Co., New York.

Kumar, A (2002) Veterinary Surgical Techniques, Vikas Publishing House Pvt Ltd, New Delhi.

Pandey, D N (1996) Veterinary Practitioner's and Pet Lover's Handbook for Dogs and Cats, 1st edition, International Book Distributing Co. (Publishing Division), Lucknow.

Patri, S and Matham, V K (2009) Vet's Ready Reckoner, New India Publishing Agency, New Delhi.

Prasad, B (1992) Veterinary Clinical Diagnostic Technology, CBS Publishers and Distributors, Delhi.

Prasad, B (1997) Veterinary Pharmaceuticals, 4th edition, CBS Publishers and Distributors, Delhi.

Sapre, V A (2003) A Handbook for Veterinary Physician, 15th edition, International Book Distributing Co. (Publishing Division), Lucknow.

Index of Animal Diseases

Abscess *228*
Actinobacillosis *152*
Actinomycosis *152*
Acute bloat *65*
Acute Pulmonary Emphysema *219*
Agalactia *215, 272*
Amphistomes *186*
Amputation of horn *294*
Amputation of tail *288*
Anaemia *207*
Anaplasmosis *173, 190*
Anoestrus *264*
Anorexia *209*
Anthrax *38, 148, 235*
Anuria *86*
Arsenic poisoning *144*
Arthritis *108, 111*
Ascarids *180*
Atresia ani 52, 287
Avulsion of Horn *230, 294*

Babesiosis *174, 190*
Bacterial diseases *147*
Balanoposthitis *92*
Black Quarter *148, 235*
Bloat *64*
Blood in Milk *216*
Blue Tongue *40, 161, 191*
Botulism *153*
Bovine ketosis *130*
Broken horn *229*
Bronchitis *76*
Brucellosis *38, 150, 190, 235, 435*
Burn *314*
Burns and Scalds *225*

Caesarean operation *290*
Calcium deficiency *197*
Calf scours *97*
Cardiac arrest *94*
Castration *286*

CBPP (Contagious Bovine Pleuro Pneumonia) *39, 154*

CCPP (Contagious Caprine Pleuro Pneumonia) *39, 155*

Cestodes *186*

Chlorinated hydrocarbon poisoning *141*

Choke *58*

Chronic bloat *66*

Cobalt deficiency *202*

Coccidiosis *176*

Colibacillosis *153*

Colic *59*

Congestive cardiac failure *95*

Conjunctivitis *115*

Constipation *207*

Contagious Ecthyma *166*

Copper deficiency *200*

Corneal opacity *117*

Cutaneous Papillomatosis *167*

Cuts and Wounds *222*

Cyanide poisoning *145*

Cystitis *90*

Diarrhoea *205*

Diseases caused by ectoparasites *190*

Diseases of blood *96*

Diseases of cardiovascular system *93*

Diseases of eye *115*

Diseases of liver *73*

Diseases of locomotor system *107*

Diseases of nervous system *100*

Diseases of reproductive system *81*

Diseases of skin *118*

Diseases of urinary system *86*

Distomiasis *104*

Downers syndrome *132*

Ectoparasitism *190*

Eczematous dermatoses *120*

Enteritis in Sheep and Goat *212*

Enterotoxaemia *155, 435*

Ephemeral Fever *160, 191*

Epilepsy *105*

Epileptic seizure *105*

Epistaxix *79*

Euthanasia *295, 462*

Fascioliasis *184*

Fatty cow syndrome *137*

Fever *204*

First Aid in Bleeding *222*

Foetal maceration *85*

Foot and Mouth Disease / FMD *40, 158, 234, 235, 432*

Foreign body syndrome *94*

Fracture *226*

Gastro-intestinal worms *181*

Grain poisoning *62*

Haematuria *88*

Haemoglobinuria *87*

Haemorrhage *97*

Haemorrhagic Septicaemia / HS *149, 235, 433*

Heart worm *183*

Heat stroke *97*

Hepatitis *74*

Hernia *291*

Hog Cholera *171*

Hook worm *183*

Horn Fracture *229*

Horn Injuries *224*

Hydrophobia *169*
Hypodermatosis *123*
Hypogalactia *272*
Hypomagnesaemia *135*
Hypovitaminosis-A *194*

Icterus *73*
Incordination of gait *101*
Infantile tetany *112*
Infectious diseases *232*
Iodine deficiency *201*
Iron deficiency *201*
Jaundice *73*

Keratitis *116*
Kerato conjunctivitis *116*

Lact acidosis *62*
Lantana camera poisoning *145*
Laryngitis *76*
Lead poisoning *142*
Leptospirosis *38, 156*
Listeriosis *39, 155*
Lumpy Jaw *152*
Lung worm *182*

Macro mineral deficiency *197*
Manganese deficiency *202*
Mange *123, 310, 312*
Mastitis *39, 270*
Medial pattelar dysmotomy *287*
Mercury poisoning *143*
Metabolic diseases *126*
Metritis-Pyometra *202*
Micro / trace mineral deficiency *198*
Milk fever *127, 129*
Mineral deficiency diseases *197*
Mites *124*
Motor disturbances *102*
Mycoplasma in Calves *215*
Myopathy *110*
Myositis *110*

Nasal Schistosomiasis *186*
Neonatal Calf Diarrhoea *213*
Neonatal Calf Pneumonia *214*
Nephritis *89*
Nitrates and Nitrites poisoning *143*
Nodular worm *183*

Oedema *99*
Oliguria *86*
Organophosporus poisoning *141*
Osteomalacia *113*
Osteoporosis *114*
Otitis *117*

Parakeratosis *123*
Paralysis *102, 104*
Paralysis, radial nerve *112*
Paramphistomiasis *185*
Parasitic diseases *179*
Paratuberculosis *39, 156*
Parotitis *57, 221*
Parturient Paresis *127, 217*
Penile retraction *293*
Pericarditis *93*
Peripheral circulatory failure *95*
Pest Des Petits Ruminants 165, 236
Pharyngitis *53*

Phosphorus deficiency *136, 197*
Photosensitization *121*
Pica *210*
Piroplasmosis *174*
Plant toxicity *145*
Pneumonia *78, 203*
Poisoning *139*
Polyencephalomalacia *196*
Polyneuritis *101, 195*
Polyuria *86*
Post parturient diseases *266*
Post-parturient haemoglobinuria *136*
Pox *163, 433*
PPR *165, 236*
Pre-parturient hypocalcaemia *130*
Prolapse of genetalia *269*
Protozoan diseases *173*
Pulmonary emphysema *77*
Pulmonary oedama *77*
Pyelonephritis *90*
Pyoderma *120*

Rabies *169*
Ranula *289*
Red urine *88*
Reproductive disorders *264*
Retention of placenta *266*
Retention of Urine *220*
Rhinitis *76*
Ricket *112, 113*
Rinderpest *160*
Ringworm *122, 310*
Rumen dysfunction *60*
Ruminal acidosis *62, 70, 71*
Ruminal Fermentative Disorders *68*

Salmonellosis in Calves *215*
Selenium deficiency *201*
Shock *97*
Simple indigestion *63, 211*
Snake Bite *230*
Snoring disease *80*
Sprain *109*
Sprain *313, 314*
Stomatitis *55*
String halt *287*
Surra *175*
Swine Fever *171*

Tail Gangrene *225*
Tapeworm
TB *151*
Tetanus 151
Thelitis *209*
Three days sickness *160*
Torticolis *220*
Tracheitis *76*
Trauma, brain *106*
Trypanosomiasis *175*
Tuberculosis *39, 151*
Tuleraemia *190*

Udder Oedema *?16*
Urea poisoning *144*
Urethral rupture *92*
Urinary calculi *292*
Urinary incontinence *91*

Urolithiasis 92, *292*
Urticaria *119*

Vagus indigestion *67*
Veneral diseases *81*
Viral diseases *158*

Whole milk tetany *136*
Wooden tongue *152*
Wound *223*

Yokegall *227*

Zinc deficiency *199*

Index of Generic and Trade Names of Medicines/Drugs Used in Veterinary Practice

The generic and brand names of the drugs/medicines described in the text of this book are alphabetically arranged in this section. The generic names and group names are inscribed in block capital letters. The trade names are provided with manufacturer/company name within bracket and inscribed in italic letters.

A3 Vet Bolus/Injection (*Brihans*) *362, 366*

A3 Vet Plus Injection (*Brihans*) *363*

Aahar (*Kapila*) *393*

Acinil Bolus (*Excell*) *399*

Aciphos Injection (*Excell*) *382*

Acriflavin *309, 313*

Actoral-H (*Bery & Bery Vet*) *409*

Adcelin Injection (*Virbac*) *374*

ADENOCHROME *372*

Afanil (*Ayurvet*) *398*

Afron Powder (*Bootic Bhawan*) *399*

Agrimin Forte (*GlaxoSmithkline*) *414*

Agrimin Powder (*GlaxoSmithkline*) *415*

Akayci Injection (*Brihans*) *337*

Alben Suspension (*Jeps*) *346*

ALBENDAZOLE *346*

ALBENDAZOLE AND IVERMECTIN COMBINED *348*

Albicon Bolus/Tab (*Pharmacon*) *347, 348*

Albogen Bolus/Tablet (*Nugen*) *347, 348*

Albomar Bolus/Suspension (*GSK*) *346, 347*

Albomr Micronised Tablet (*GSK*) *348*

Albonil tablet (*ACW*) *348*

Albopa Tab (*Pearl Chemicals*) *346, 347, 348*

Albovet Liquid (*Marion Pharma*) *341*

Alergo Injection (*Jeps*) *371*

Alincomycin Vet (*Alved*) 338
All Clear Bolus (*Vetcare*) 349
Alphos-40 Injection (*Alved*) 383
Alverin Injection (*Alved*) 353
Alverin Plus Injection (*Alved*) 353
Alvite-M (*Alembic*) 426
Alzonex Tablet/Bolus (*Neospark*) 348
Ambiplex Syrup (*Brihans*) 407
AMIKACIN *337*
Amikox Injection (*Oxen Labs*) 337
Aminocin Injection (*Neospark*) 337
Aminoglycosides *82*
Aminoplex (*Excell Aahar*) 407
Amix-250 Injection (*Daffodils*) 337
Ammonium carbonate *309*
Amoxirum Forte injection (*Agrivet Farm Care*) 322
AMOXYCILLIN + CLOXACILLIN *335*
AMOXYCILLIN *319, 322*
AMPICILLIN + CLOXACILLIN *324*
AMPICILLIN *319, 321*
Ampicillin injection (*Modern Lab*) 321
Ampixel Injection (*Excell*) 321
ANALGIN *365, 367*
Analgin Injection (*Oxen Labs*) 366
Analgon Suspension (*Wockhardt*) 347
Anicort Injection (*IBC*) 370
Animin Powder (*Vets Farma*) 414
Anistamin injection (*Intas*) 371
Anox Liquid (*Oxen Labs*) 394
ANTHELMINTICS *320, 346, 360*
ANTI BLOAT *398*
ANTI BLOAT SUSPENSION *397*
ANTI TYMPANY PREPARATION *398*
Antibac-C (*Oxford Gem*) 343
ANTIBIOTICS *321, 428*
ANTIDIARRHOEALS *344*
ANTIFLATULENTS *397*
ANTIFUNGAL *319*
Antihaemoprotozoans *319*
ANTIHISTAMINIC *370*
Antilar injection (*Reedson*) 371
ANTIMICROBIAL *82, 319, 428*
Antiprotozoal *319*
ANTISPASMODIC DRUG *367*
ANTISTRESS *405*
ANTIZYMOTICS *397*
Appetonic (*Indian Hebs*) 393
Arimox Injection (*Daffodils*) 325
Arogen Bolus (*Arosol*) 426
Arogesic-P Bolus (*Anol*) 367
Aryan Batisa (*Natural Herbs*) 393
Ascal (*Alembic*) 424
Ascaper (*Angels Group*) 361
Astrinex (*Vetmed*) 344
Atrima Bolus (*Prima Vet Care*) 341
Avermac Injection (*Oxen Labs*) 353
Avil Injection (*Intervet*) 372
Axefendol Suspension (*Alved*) 350
Ayumin-V (*Ayurvet*) 415

Bactecon (*Pharmacon*) 410
Bacteridox Injection (*Alved*) 341
Bacterisol Injection/Bolus (*Alved*) 340, 341
Baifidine (*BAIF*) 338
Bandykind plus (*Vetkind*) 348
Banif Bolus (*Brihans*) 349
Banjhna (*Bharatiya Bootee*) 412
Batycolpour on Drop (*Pfizer*) 431
B-Com Forte (*Pearls chemicals*) 406
B-Com-L Injection (*Wockhardt*) 379

Becknor Bolus (*Natural Remedies*) 344
Beejet Injection (*Vets Farma*) 376
Belamyl Injection (*Sarabhai Zydus*) 378
Benvet Bolus (*Cipla*) 347
Bery Plex (*Bery & Bery Vet*) 408
Berymin Forte (*Bery & Bery Vet*) 419
Bestamin Gold (*Vetcare*) 417, 425
Betade Injection (*Bee Tee Pharma*) 374
Betphos Injection (*Bee Tee Pharma*) 383
Biobloom (*Sarabhai Zydus*) 419
Biocuf (*Bioherbs Pharma*) 404
Biomex Forte Injection (*IBC*) 378
Biomin Powder (*Bioherbs*) 417
Bion-12 Vet Injection (*Morvel*) 377
Bioplex High Five (*Vetnex*) 426
Biostamin Inj. (*IBC*) 371
Biostrep Injection (*Vetnex*) 333
Biotone (*Bioherbs*) 396
Biotone Fs Bolus (*Karnataka Antibiotics*) 396
Biotrim DS (*Vetnex*) 342
Biotrim Injection (*Vetnex*) 340
Biovest Bolus (*Vets Farma*) 396
Bistrepen Injection (*Alembic*) 332
Bleed Check Injection (*Bee Tee Pharmaceuticals*) 372
Bloatcon (*Pharmacon*) 397
Bloatinorm Bolus (*Excell*) 399
Bloatosil Suspension (*Wockhardt*) 397
Blotena (*Bioherbs*) 398
Blotinox Liquid (*Cattle Remedies*) 398
Blotonil (*Jeps*) 397
Bmvax (*Indian Immunologicals*) 435
Bolin Injection (*Merind*) 366
Boon-O-Milk (*Aries Agrovet*) 405
BORIC ACID 313
Bothcillin injection (*Oxen Labs*) 325
Botropase injection (*Juggat*) 372
Bovilis Clovax (*Intervet*) 432
Bovilis FMDV Gel (*Intervet*) 432
Bovilis HS BQ vaccine (*Intervet*) 434
Bovilis HS vaccine (*Intervet*) 434
Bovilis Mev (*Intervet*) 435
Bovilis-ETV (*Intervet*) 435
Bovirum Bolus (*Sarabhai Zydus*) 396
Bovoplex-C Injection (*Indian Immunologicals*) 379
Brandocillin Injection (*Intas*) 321
Briben Suspension/Bolus (*Brihans*) 346, 347
Brical Injection (*Brihans*) 379
Brimdin Injection (*Brihans*) 338
Brisil (*Brihans*) 397
Brisone Injection (*Brihans*) 369
Britax Injection (*Brihans*) 333
Brivit Injection (*Brihans*) 374
Bronto (*Anja*) 403
Brotone Tonic (*Glaxo SmithKline*) 401
BRUCELLA ABERTUS VACCINE 435
BT Flox-TZ Tablet (*Bee Tee Pharma*) 343
Btoxfen Bolus (*Bee Tee Pharma*) 350
Btplex-C Injection (*Bee Tee Pharma*) 376
Bucofert Bolus (*Natural Remedies*) 412
Bucomin-E (*Natural Remedies*) 426
Butagesic-K (*Concept*) 364
Butox (*Intervet*) 429

Cadex Injection (*CRIL*) 369
Cadisol-DC (*Sarabhai Zydus*) 424
Caflon (*Indian Herbs*) 403
Cal More (*Indian Herbs*) 421
Calbim Injection (*GSK*) 382

Calborol Injection (*Novartis*) *381*

Calcicare (*Brihans*) *424*

Calcicat Injection (*Cattle Remedies*) *381*

Calcicon (*Vetcon*) *422*

Calciforte Syrup (*Nugen Pharma*) *421*

Calcimag Injection (*Cattle Remedies*) *382*

Calcimal Special Gel/Injection/Suspension (*Oxen Labs*) *380, 420, 421*

Calcimal-CBG (*Oxen Labs*) *381*

Calcimilk (*Pharmacon Vet*) *422*

Calcinet Injection (*Excell*) *380*

Calcistrength (*Brihans*) *419*

CALCIUM BORO-GLUCONATE *381*

CALCIUM GLUCONOLACTOBIONATE WITH VITAMIN D_3 E B_{12} *380*

CALCIUM LEVULINATE *379*

CALCIUM SYRUP/SUPPLEMENT *420, 421*

CALCIUM, MAGNESSIUM AND DEXTROSE INJECTION *381*

Calcivet Liquid (*Marion Pharma*) *424*

Calcizin Syrup (*Nugen Pharma*) *422*

Caldhan-V (*Ayurvet*) *421*

Calfosvet Liquid (*Vets Farma*) *424*

Calgonate Injection (*Indian Immunologicals*) *381*

Cal-K (*Karnataka Antibiotic*) *423*

Cal-Lactose (*Angel's Group*) *423*

Calmax Injection (*Vetnex*) *381*

Calmax-M (*Vetnex*) *382*

Calmin (*Cattle Remedies*) *414*

Calmin Powder (*Cattle Remedies*) *413*

Calphos D_3 liquid/bolus (*Excell*) *421*

Calphos-12/Plus (*Bery & Bery Vet*) *422*

Calrin Plus (*Vetcon*) *423*

Calsagar (*Indian Immunologicals*) *423*

Calshakti (*Intas*) *420*

Calvib Injection (*GSK*) *381*

Calvin-DS (*Pearl Chemicals*) *423*

Camphor *309, 313*

Candur DHL + P (*Intervet*) *437*

CANINE VACCINE *436*

Capsola/Gold/Injection (*Vetnex*) *380, 421, 422*

Care Plus (*C-Care*) *418, 422*

Carmigen (*Nugen*) *394*

Carron oil *309, 314*

Castor oil *309*

Catcillin Injection (*CRIL*) *321*

Catechu *309*

Catlo Genta (*CRIL*) *336*

Catlox Injection Vet (*Cattle Remedies*) *325*

Catone Powder (*Cattle Remedies*) *393*

Cattle Mix (*Perals Chemicals*) *420*

Cavit Injection (*Brihans*) *375*

Cefavet Injection (*Excell*) *333*

Ceflax powder (*Neospark*) *329*

Cefloxen-Vet Injection (*Tarun*) *328*

CEFOTAXIME *333*

CEFTIOFUR 331

Ceftivet Injection (*Vetnex*) *331*

CEFTRIAXONE *330*

CEPHALEXIN *328*

Cestophen Tablet/Suspension (*Pearls Chemical*) *356, 357*

Cflox Injection/Power Injection (*Intas*) *328*

C-Flox Uterine (*Intas*) *428*

C-Floxfluterine Bolus (*Intas*) *427*

C-Flox-TZ bolus (*Intas*) *427*

Charmil Ointment (*Dabur Ayurvet*) *410*

Chelated Milmor Forte (*Novartis*) *419*

Chirata *310*
CHLORAMPHENICOL *83, 333*
Chloramphenicol Injection (*Modern Labs*) *334*
Chloramphenicol Injection (*Nandini Med. Lab*) *334*
Chloramphenicol Sod. Succinate Inj (*KAP*) *334*
Chloraxin Injection (*Cipla*) *334*
Chlorazin Injection (*CRIL*) *371*
Chloril Vet Injection (*TTK*) 371
CHORIONIC GONADOTROPHIN *385*
Chorulon Injection (*Intervet*) *385*
Chromostat injection *372*
Cillox Injection (*Excell*) *325*
Cipla Ceft Vet Injection (*Cipla*) 330
Cipoxin Injection (*Oxen Labs*) *328*
CIPROFLOXACIN *319, 327*
Ciptas-TZ Suspension (*Intas*) *342*
Ciptec-Vet Injection (*Cipla*) *328*
Citarin-L (*Bayer*) *358*
Citox (*Oxen Lab*) *430*
Clinar (*GSK*) *430*
CLOMIFENE CITRATE *388*
Clomoxy Injection (*Brihans*) *335*
CLOPROSTENOL *387*
CLOSANTEL *351*
Clostenol Injection (*Sarabhai Zydus*) *387*
CLOSTRIDIAL VACCINE *435*
Clox Mox Injection (*Daffodils*) *335*
Cloxillin Injection (*Reedson*) *325*
Clozan Bolus/Tablet/Suspension (*Jeps Pharma*) *356*
C-Min Forte Plus (*C-care*) *416*
CNS depressants *104*
CNS Stimulants *103*
Cobactan-LC (*Intervet*) *391*
Complemin Fort (*Nugen*) *417*
Conampi Injection (*Concept*) *321*
Concimin (*Concept*) *416*
Conciplex Injection (*Concept*) *375*
Concitone (*Concept*) *406*
Conmectin Injection (*Concept*) *353*
Conmox Injection (*Concept*) *336*
CORTICOSTEROIDS *368*
Cotrimal Bolus (*Alembic*) *339, 427*
CO-TRIMOXAZOLE *340*
COUGH MIXTURE *403*
Coughdon Powder (*Vets Farma*) *404*
Cpm Vet injection (*Cipla*) *371*
Cufgo (*Bhartiya Bootee Bhawan*) *404*
Curacin -OZ/liquid (*Vets Farma*) *427, 428*
Curacin-O Bolus (*Vets Farma*) *343*
Curadex Vet Injection (*Concept*) *369*
Cure Oil (*Bery & Bery Vet*) *409*
Cyclin DT Bolus (*Excell*) *343*
Cyclix (*Intervet*) *387*
Cyclomin-7 Bolus (*Concept*) *426*
CYPERMETHRIN *430*
Cyprol (*Intas*) *430*
Cystorolin (*B & AHP*) *388*
Cythion (AHP) *431*

D'mag Spray (*Intas*) *411*
Dafochrome Vet injection (*Daffodills*) 372
Dafomol Injection (*Daffodills*) *362*
Damox Injection (*Daffodils*) *335*
D-Bloat Liquid (*Indian Herbs*) *398*
DELTAMETHRIN *429*
Dermanol (*Indian Herbs*) *391, 410*
Dermanol (*Vetmed*) *410*
DEWORMERS *346*

DEXAMETHASONE *369*
Dexo Injection (*Daffodil*) *370*
Dexona Injection (*Sarabhai Zydus*) *369*
Dexonil Injection (*Reedson*) *370*
Dextrolyte (*Enlag Lab*) *345*
Diadisco (*Bhartiya Bootee Bhawan*) *344*
Diagen (*Nugen*) *342*
Diardon Powder (*Vets Farma*) *344*
Diarex Tablet (*Himalaya*) *344*
Diarok (*Ayurvet*) *344*
DICHLOROPHEN *356*
Dicrysticin-S Large dose Injection (*Sarabhai Zydus*) *333*
DICYCLOMINE *367*
Digecon (*Pharmacon*) *395*
DIGESTIVE AND STOMACHIC *392*
Digestone Powder (*Anuya*) *392*
Digestovet Powder (*Vets Farma*) *392*
Diminazine diaceturate *177*
DINOPROST TROMETHIAMINE *388*
Dinosol (*Pharmacon*) *406*
Disovet-M Injection (*IBC*) *363*
Distonex Bolus/Tab/Suspension (*Neosprak*) *354, 355, 356*
Distrol Injection (*Oxen Lab*) *384*
DP-Loton Injection (*Vest Farma*) *385*
Dresol (*Kapila*) *409*
DRESSING OIL *314, 409*
Dressit (*Oxford Gems*) *409*
Dressogen (*Nugen*) *409*
Dressol (*Cattle Remedies*) *410*
Dressol-FR Gel (*Cattle Remedies*) *411*
Dressoment Ointment (*Nugen*) *410*
Dressona Ointment (*Bioherbs*) *411*
Duaprim Bolus/Injection (*Brihans*) *340, 342, 428*
Dugdhdan Bolus (*Cattle Remedies*) *404*
Duramune CVK (*Fort-Dodge*) *436*
Duraprogen (*Vet Care*) *385*
Dydistop Forte (*Oxen Labs*) *343*

E.R.S. Liquid (*Excell*) *345*
E-Care-Se Injection (*Vetcare*) *377*
ECBOLIC *389*
Ecotas Bolus (*Intas*) *396*
ECTOPARASITICIDES *428*
Ektomin (*Novartis*) *430*
Electra (*Sprindles Formulations*) *345*
Electra-C (*Jeps*) *345*
Electro Gen (*Nugen*) *345*
Electrocon (*Pharmacon*) *345*
ELECTROLYTES *345*
Electrovet (*Marion Pharma*) *345*
Emoxel Injection (*Excell-R*) *336*
Encal-12/Plus (*Enlag Labs*) *422, 423*
Encalmin Forte (*Enlag Labs*) *414, 417*
Endectin Bolus/Tab (*Excell*) *352*
Endex Bolus/Suspension (*Novartis*) *359, 360*
Endoban Suspension (*TTK*) *346*
Endoben Bolus (*TTK*) *347*
Enidex Injection (*Excel*) *369*
Enliv (*Pfizer*) *402*
Enrobact Injection (*Martin & Brown*) *327*
Enrobest Injection (*TTK*) *327*
Enrocin – IU (*Vetnex*) *327, 428*
Enrocin (*Vetnex*) *327*
Enrocip Injection (*Cipla*) *327*
Enrodac-10 Injection (*Sarabhai Zydus*) *327*
ENROFLOXACIN *319, 326*
Enrored Injection (*Reedson*) *327*
Enrovet Injection (*Vets Farma*) *327*

Enrovit (*Enlag Lab*) *408*
Enrox Injection (*Alembic*) *327*
Enrumen (Kapila) *393*
Enteromycetin Injection (*Deys Vet*) *334*
ENTEROTOXAEMIA VACCINE *435*
Epidosin Injection (*TTK*) *368*
Epidosin Vet Injection (*TTK*) *385, 389*
Esgipyrin-N Injection (*Sarabhai Zydus*) *367*
Estromin (*Nugen*) *415, 425, 426*
Estrona Forte Bolus (*Rakesh Pharmaceuticals*) *412*
ETHAMSYLATE *372*
Exact Injection (*Excell*) *330*
Exapar Liquid (*Ayurvet*) *389, 412*
EXPECTORANT *403*
Expell Suspension (*Excell*) *346*

Fascon Bolus (*Pharmacon*) *359*
Fasimec Suspension (*Novartis*) *352, 360*
Fasinex Bolus/Suspension (*Novartis*) *354*
Fazole Bolus (*Unichem*) *343*
Feed-on-Bolus (*AFC*) *397*
FELINE VACCINE *438*
FENBENDAZOLE *348*
Fentas Bolus (*Intas*) *348*
Fentas Plus Suspension (*Intas*) *359*
FENVALERATE *430*
Fenzole Bolus/Tablet (*Jeps*) *349*
Feroliv Injection (*Excell*) *375*
Fertitone Injection (*Bee Tee Pharma*) *384*
Fertizyl (*Intervet*) *388*
Fertophos (*Glaxo SmithKline*) *383*
Floclox-L (*Vetnex*) *391*
Flomin-C Bolus (*IBC*) *426*
Flora Boost Bolus (*Excell*) *395*
Floratone Bolus (*Concept*) *395*
Floxidin Injection (*Intervet*) *327*
FLUKICIDE *354*
Fluknide Suspension/Bolus (*Excell*) *356*
Flukodin –DS (*Arosol*) *359*
Flupor (*Vetnex*) *431*
Fluzic Bolus/Suspension (*Vetnex*) *354*
FMD VACCINE *432*
Folligon (*Intervet*) *386*
Foot and Mouth Disease vaccine (*Intervet*) *432*
Fortius injection (*Virbac*) *327*
Fumar Bolus (*Legend*) *343*
Furea Bolus (*Pfizer*) *427*
Furex Bolus (*Excell*) *427*

GALACTOGOGUE *404*
Galog (*Indian Herbs*) *405, 419*
Garlic *309*
Gasnil Powder (*Vetmed*) *399*
Gastina (*GSK*) *398*
Genprim Bolus (*Legend*) *342*
Genta Biotic Injection (*KAP*) *336*
GENTAMICIN *336*
Gentamicin Injection (*TTK*) *337*
Gentamycin Injection (*Vetcare*) *336*
Gentavet Injection (*Oxen Labs*) *336*
Gentax Injection (*DPL, Daffodills*) *336*
Gestaforte Bolus (*TTK*) *414, 425*
Ginger *310*
Girtona Powder (*Anuya*) *399*
GNRH *386*
Grogold Powder (*Vets Farma*) *413*
Grovicon (*Pharmacon*) *414*
Grovimin Forte (*Pharmacon*) *413*
Groviplex Liquid (*Virbac AFC*) *406*

Grow-UP (*Vetcon*) 345
Gynaecon (*Pharmacon*) 414, 425
Gynotone Vet Powder (*Angels Group*) 425

H.B. Strong (*Indian Herbs*) 393
HAEMOSTAT 372
HEAT INDUCER 411
Heatasole Capsule (*Arosol*) 412, 425
Helax Ointment (*Boo teesa Pharma*) 411
Helind Suspension (*Intas*) 359
Helmax (*Vetmed*) 361
Helmonil Powder/Tablet/Injection (*Alved*) 350, 351
Helmonil-C Injection (*Alved*) 358
Hepasol (*Enlag Labs*) 400
Hepatogen Injection (*Jeps*) 378
HERBAL VETERINARY MEDICINE 392
Herbogastrin (*Vetmed*) 392, 394
Hexanide Bolus (Zydus AHL) 355
Hilak (*Ayurvet*) 420
Himalayan Batisa (*Indian Herbs*) 392
Himax (*Indian Herbs*) 410
Hitek Oral Solution/Injection (*GSK*) 352, 353
Hivit Injection (*Vetnex*) 375
Hormo P_2 alpha (BCAHP) 388
HORMONES FOR FERTILITY 384
HS and BQ vaccine (*Biomed*) 434
HS VACCINE 434
Hygest Bolus (*Natural Remedies*) 406
Hylactin Injection/Powder (*Jeps*) 380, 417
Hyprogen Injection (*Reedson*) 385

Iliren Injection (*Intervet*) 387
IMMUNOMODULATOR 412
Inclox Injection (*Brihans*) 325
Inflagel Ointment (*Neospark*) 410
Inimox Injection (*Indian Immunologicals*) 335
Inj. F.P.P. (*Alembic*) 332
Inj. F.P.P. (*Sarabhai Zydus*) 332
Injection AC-Vet (*Intas*) 325
Injection AC-Vet Forte (*Intas*) 325
Injection AC-VET Max (*Intas*) 325
Injection Oxiprim (Oxen Lab) 340
Injection Vet Clox (*Sarabhai Zydus*) 325
Instafeed-FS (*Bee Tee Pharma*) 396
Intacal Injection (*Intas*) 381
Intacef Injection (*Intas*) 330
Intamox (*Intas*) 335
Intamycin (*Intas*) 323
Intamycin-LA (*Intas*) 323
Intavita Injection (*Intas*) 374
Intrim Bolus (*Intas*) 342
Intrim Forte Bolus (*Intas*) 342
Iodine ointment 309
Iodomet Powder (*Excell*) 428
Iodovet Bolus (*Excell*) 427
Isapgol 310
Ivectin Tablet/Injection (*Indian Immunologicals*) 352, 353
IVERMECTIN 351, 352
IVERMECTIN ORAL 351
Ivmasol-75 Injection (*Vetnex*) 351

Janova (*Ayurvet*) 412
Juramate Injection (*Vetcare*) 387

Kafcare (*Kapila*) 406
Kalbend Bolus (*KAP*) 347
Kalbend Tab (*Karnataka Antibiotics*) 348

Kalmin-L (*KAP*) 413
Kalmisol Injection (*Karnataka Antibiotic*) *351, 358*
Kampibiotic Injection (*Karnataka antibiotic*) 321
Kcmin (*Kapila*) 413
Kem Trace Dry (*Kemin*) 415, 418
Ketop Injection (*Alembic*) 364
KETOPROFEN 364
K-Flox Injection,Vet (*KAP*) 326
Kira Kill (*Oxen Labs*) 349
Kira Kill-DS (*Oxen Lab*) 349
Klox amp Injection (*KAP*) 325
Klozanide-L Bolus/Suspension (*KAP*) 360
Kriminth (*Bootees*) 361
Krishmin-Forte (*Pharmacon*) 415

Lactivet (*Alved*) 415
Lactivet Powder (*Alved*) 416
Lactomag injection (*Intas*) 381
Lactomax-AD_3 (*Arosol*) 420
Lactomore (*Marion Pharma*) 418
Lactovet Powder (*Rakesh Pharmaceuticals*) 405
Lavitone-H Injection (*TTK*) 375
Ledexin Vet (*Legend*) 428
Legenta Injection (*Legend*) 337
Lemasol-75 Injection (*Vetnex*) 358
Lemidine Bolus (*Legend*) 339
Lemilyte (*Legend*) 345
L-En-RO Injection (*Legend*) 327
Leptaden Vet Tabs (*Alarsin*) 419
Levadex Injection (*GSK*) 378
LEVAMISOLE 350, 357
Levoxy Bolus/Suspension (*Cattle Remedies*) 360
Levucell-SC (*Venky's*) 394
LH PREPARATION 385
Lifer Liquid (*Vets Farma*) 402
LINCOMYCIN 83, 337
Liv-100 Bolus/Liquid/Powder (*Arosol*) 401, 403
Livcare Concentrate (*Kapila*) 401
Livcon Syrup (*Pharmacon*) 402
LIVER EXTRACT WITH VITAMIN B-COMPLEX 377
LIVER TONIC 400
Livgrow Powder (*Natural Herbs*) 402
Livluv Vet (*Marvet*) 401
Livo-Bee Injection (*Marion Pharma*) 379
Livobex Injection (*TTK*) 378
Livodex Injection (*Oxen Lab*) 378, 402
Livogel Powder (*Angel group*) 403
Livol (*Indian Herbs*) 403

Livolysin (*Pharma Convet*) 408
Livosprin (*Sprindles Formulations*) 401
Livovit (*Bery & Bery Vet*) 401
Livozyme-Fe Bolus/Liquid (*Marion Pharma*) 402, 426
Livron Injection (*Vets Farma*) 378
Livsee (*Legend*) 400
Lixen Bolus/Powder (*GSK*) 329
Lixen IU (*Glaxo*) 427, 428
Lofac-M Bolus (*Legend*) 366
Lomatich-DS (*Legend*) 393
Lorexene Ointment/Spray (*GSK*) 411
Loxy bolus/injection (*Legend*) 323, 324
LUMETHRIN 430
Lutalyse Injection (*Novartis*) 388
Lutropin-V (*Vets Farma*) 385
Lysetic liquid (*TTK*) 429
Lysovit (*Oxford Gem*) 408

M.P.Con Bolus (*Pharmacon*) 366
Macef Injection (*Marion Pharma*) *331*
Maclox Injection (*Marion Pharma*) *326*
MACROLIDES *83*
Magacal Powder (*Indian Herbs*) *413*
Magnesium sulphate *309*
Maha Batisa Hajmi (*Pearl Chemical*) *393*
Malexin Powder (*Marion Pharma*) *329*
Mammitel tube (*Intas*) *391*
Maplex Liquid (*Marion Pharma*) *409*
Mastijet Fort (*Intervet*) *391*
Mastilep Gel (*Dabur*) *391*
MASTITIS CARE *390*
Mastox Injection (*Jeps*) *336*
Mastrip (*Dabur Ayurvet*) *391*
Maxi Milk Bolus (*Sarabhai Zydus*) *404*
M-Ceft Injection (*Alembic*) *331*
MEBENDAZOLE *349*
Mectin Injection (*Alembic*) *353*
Megaboost (*Vets Farma*) *408, 423*
Megacide Vet (*Venky's Livestock*) *429*
Megaclox Vet Injection (*Cipla*) *335*
Megalvit powder (*Care-O-Vet*) *407*
Megavac CC vaccine (*Indian Immunologicals*) *436*
Megavac DHRL (*Indian Immunologicals*) *438*
Megavac-6 (*Indian Immunologicals*) *437*
Melflam Vet Injection (*Cipla*) *362*
Melobest-P Injection (*TTK*) *364*
Melonex Bolus/Injection (*Intas*) *362, 366*
Melonex Plus Injection (*Intas*) *364*
Melonex Power Injection (*Intas*) *363*
Meloxi Injection (*Vets Farma*) *362*
MELOXICAM *362, 363, 366*
MELOXICAM WITH PARACETAMOL *363*
Menroflox -100 Injection (*Modern Lab*) *326*
Mercurocrome *309*
Meriquin Injection (*Merind*) *327*
METRONIDAZOLE *83*
Mifex Injection (*Novartis*) *382*
Mifex Oral (*Novartis*) *422*
Milchend (*Legends*) *418*
Milchey (*Novartis*) *418*
Milk Fit (*Natural Remedies*) *405*
Milk Max (*Ethicare*) *405, 419*
Milkoplex Bolus (*Rakesh Pharma*) *404*
Milkotone (*Vetmed*) *405*
Minadex-C Powder (AFC) *416*
Minamil (*Brihans*) *416*
MINERAL MIXTURES *413*
MINERAL MIXTURES WITH VITAMINS *415, 418*
Minerex (*Excell*) *413, 414, 416, 426*
Minerin Powder (*Vetmed*) *414*
Minfa (*Intas*) *413*
Minimix Powder (*Oxen Labs*) *414*
Minotas Bolus (*Intas*) *426*
Minovit Forte (*Pearls Chemicals*) *416*
Minthal Bolus (*Alembic*) *347*
Mintrus Caplets (*Ayurvet*) *425*
Miphocal Injection (*Indian Immunologicals*) *382*
Moxcell Injection (*Alembic*) *336*
MP3 Injection (*Vetnex*) *363*
Multisol Special (*Pearl Chemicals*) *409*
Munomycin forte injection (*Glaxo SmithKline*) *332*

Natural Batisa (*Natural Remedies*) *393*
N-Blot-06 (*Natural Remedies*) *399*
N-D Plex Forte-L Injection (*Nandini Lab*) *379*

Neblon Powder (*Indian Herbs*) *344*
Neem *310*
Nemasol Injection (*Jeps Pharma*) *351, 358*
Neocal-C (*Kapila*) *415*
Neocare Forte Powder (*Vetcare*) *335*
Neochlor Injection (*Vetcare*) *334*
Neocidol (*Novartis*) *431*
Neocyclin bolus (*Intas*) *324*
Neodox Bolus (*Vetcare*) *343*
Neomec Injection (*Intas*) *352*
NEOMYCIN *334*
Neoprofen Injection (*Vetnex*) *364*
Neozide Bolus/Suspension (*Intas*) *354, 356*
Neozide Plus Suspension (*Intas*) *359*
Nepoclox Vet (*TTK*) *326*
Nervine tonics *103*
Neurovet Injection (*Alved*) *376*
Neuroxin-12 Injection (*Sarabhai Zydus*) *377*
Nilzan Suspension/Bolus (*GSK*) *358*
NIMESULIDE + PARACETAMOL *367*
NIMESULIDE *364*
Nimodex (*Oxen Labs*) *365*
Nimovet Injection (*Indian Immunologicals*) *365*
Nimulite Plus (*Vets Farma*) *367*
Nimusulide Injection (*Daffodills*) *365*
Nobivac Corona (*Intervet*) *436*
Nobivac DHPPI (*Intervet*) *436*
Nobivac Puppy DP (*Intervet*) *436*
Nobivac Rabies (*Intervet*) *437*
Nobivac Tricat (*Intervet*) *438*
Nobivac-C (*Intervet*) *436*
Noworm Bolus (*Vets Farma*) *350*
NSAID *320, 361, 364, 366*
Nubplex (*Nugen Pharma*) *408*
Nuliv (*Nugen Pharma*) *400*
Nulox Vet Injection (*KAP*) *363*
Nutriliv Injection (*Vetcare*) *378*
Nutrimin (*Arosol*) *416, 417*
Nutrisaac (*Vetcare*) *418, 425*
Nutro Cal Dry (*Kemin*) *418*

Oestrovet (*Excell*) *388*
Okazan (*WPL*) *355*
Olgard Suspension (*Intas*) *359*
Omitax Injection (*Daffodils*) *333*
Omoxin Injection (*Oxen Labs*) *335*
Orcal-P Granules (*TTK*) *414, 419*
Orical Injection/Oral (*IBC*) *379, 424*
Oriprim Bolus (*Sarabhai Zydus*) *339, 341*
Oriprim Injection (*Sarabhai Zydus*) *340*
Orlox Injection (*Medivet*) *325*
Ossomin Vet (*TTK*) *421*
Ostovet (*GSK*) *423*
Otrim Bolus (*Excell*) *343, 428*
Ovatone Capsule (*Legend*) *412*
Oxaclin-LA (*Intervet*) *324*
Oxaclon-200 (*Arlgo Pharma*) *354*
Oxalgin-NP Injection/Bolus (*Zydus AHL*) *365, 367*
Oxcef Injection (*Oxen Labs*) *330*
OXFENDAZOL *350*
Oxillin Injection (*Oxen Labs*) *321*
Oxiprim Forte Bolus (*Oxen Lab*) *341*
OXYCLOZANIDE *354*
Oxyfen Suspension (*Arigo Pharma*) *350*
OXYTETRACYCLINE *82*
Oxytetracycline injection-LA (*Pfizer*) *323*
Oxyvet bolus (*Oxen Lab*) *324*

Oxyvet injection (*Oxen Lab*) 324
Oxyvet-LA injection (*Sarabhai Zydus*) 323

Pabadene Bolus (*Intas*) 340
Panacur Tablet/Bolus (*Intervet*) 349
Papazyme Forte Vet Powder (*Angel's group*) 399
PARACETAMOL 361, 363
Paracetol Injection (*Sarabhai Zydus*) 362
Paramol Injection (*Modern Lab*) 362
Parid Injection (*Vets Farma*) 353
Pashubhog Boost Bolus/Powder (*Oxen Lab*) 396, 403
Payapro Bolus (*Ayurvet*) 404
P-Depot Injection (*Sarabhai Zydus*) 385
Peflacin bolus (*Neospark*) 329
Peflacin powder (*Neospark*) 329
PEFLOXACIN 329
Pelox tablet (*Wockhardt*) 330
Pelwin tablet (*Wockhardt*) 330
Pendistrin-SH (*Sarabhai Zydus*) 390
PENICILLIN 82, 332
Pepper 310
Pepsid-C (*Concept*) 376
PGF_2 alpha 387
Phenimal Injection (*Oxen Lab*) 371
Phenimal-DS Injection (*Oxen Lab*) 371
Pheniramine Maleate Injection (*Intervet*) 371
PHENYL BUTAZONE 367
PHOSPHOROUS 382
Phytocal (*Natural Remedies*) 420
Pinkojet Injection (*Brihans*) 375
Pinkojet-L (*Brihans*) 378
Piperazin Hydrate Liquid (*Karnataka Antibiotics*) 357
Piperazine Adepate Powder (*KAP*) 357
Piperazine Hexahydrate (*TTK*) 357
PIPERAZINE HEXAHYDRATE 357
Piperazine Liquid (*GlaxoSmithKline*) 357
Plexcon (*Vetcon*) 408
Plexiven (*Adven Pharma*) 407
PMSG 386
Polyvet-B Injection (*Excell*) 377
Potassium permanganate 309, 313
PPR vaccine (*IVRI/IAH/VB, Kolkata*) 433
Prajana (*Indian Herbs*) 412
PREDNISOLONE 368
Prednisolone Acetate Injection (*Intervet*) 369
Predox Injection (*Oxen Lab*) 369
Profimin Powder (*Vets Farma*) 414
PROGESTERONE 384
Proteimin fort (*Oxford Gem*) 417
Protivet Liquid (*Angels group*) 405
Provisac Bolus (*Vetcare*) 396
Proxivet Injection (*Wockhardt*) 364
Pyramectin (*Bee Tee Pharma*) 360
P-Zyme Vet (*Oxford Gems*) 395

Quin Intas (Intas) 326
Quinapyramine 78
QUINOLONES 82
Quinrocin injection (*Neospark*) 327

R.C. Forte Injection (*Vetnex*) 325
R.S. Protein Forte (*RS Pharma*) 418
Rafox Plus (*Alved*) 358
RAFOXANIDE 358
Raksha Biovac (*Indian Immunologicals*) 434

Raksha FMD vaccine (*Indian Immunologicals*) *433*

Raksha HS + BQ combined vaccine (*Indian Immunologicals*) *434*

Raksha HS Vaccine (*Indian Immunologicals*) *433*

Raksha Rab (*Indian Immunologicals*) *437*

Raksha Triovac (*Indian Immunogiologicals*) *434*

Raksha-ET (*Indian Immunologicals*) *435*

Raksha-Ovac (*Indian Immunologicals*) *432*

Raksha-PPR (*Indian Immunologicals*) *433*

Raksha-SP (*Indian Immunologicals*) *433*

Ranbamicin Injection (*Vetnex*) *336*

Ranmix (*Vetnex*) *414*

Ranmix Total (*Vetnex*) *420*

Rasol (*BBB*) *405*

Receptal Injection (*Intervet*) *386*

Recovit (*Brihans*) *408*

Regain Bolus (*Excell*) *350*

Replanta (*Indian Herbs*) *390*

Repromin Dry (*Kemin*) *424*

Restoball (*Ayurvet*) *412*

Retisol (*Vetcon*) *409*

RIDD 12.5% *431*

Robatran Vet Bolus (*TTK*) *341*

ROS (*RS Pharmaceuticals*) *345*

RS Oil (*RS Pharmaceuticals*) *409*

RS-Zyme (*RS Pharmaceutical*) *395*

Ruchamax (*Ayurvet*) *393*

Ruchi Chatni (*Kapila*) *393*

Ruchipro Powder (*Angels*) *393*

Rumbion Bolus (*Indian Herbs*) *395*

Rumentas (*Intas*) *396*

Rumento Plus (*Crill*) *394*

Rumexon Forte Bolus (*Kumaon Herbs*) *395*

Rumibest (*TTK*) *392*

Rumicare (*Intervet*) *394*

Rumizyme Powder (*Arosol*) *394*

Saf Oil (*Legend*) *410*

Sajani (*Sarabhai Zydus*) *412*

Sancal Vet injection (*Novartis*) *380*

Scavon Gel/Spray (*Himalayan Drugs*) *410, 411*

Sharkoferol Vet (*Alembic*) *409*

SHEEP POX VACCINE *433*

Sirochrome Injection (*Albert David*) *372*

Skin Heal Spray (*Nadian Herbs*) *411*

Skinoment Gel (*Zeev Care Industries*) *410*

Skinoment Ointment (*Arosol*) *411*

Skinovet Skin Oil (*Angel's group*) *410*

Soda Phos Injection (*Vetnex*) *384*

Solampi injection (*Brihans*) *321*

Sorin Ointment (*Vetmed*) *410*

Spasgan Injection (*Oxen Labs*) *368*

Spasmonim Bolus (*Excell*) *368*

Spasmovet Injection (*Wockhardt*) *368*

Steclin bolus (*Sarabhai Zydus*) *324*

Stenot (*Natural Remedies*) *406*

STEROIDS *320*

STILBOSTEROL *384*

STREPTOPENICILLIN *332*

Stressvit (*Excell*) *407*

Stronic Injection (*Vetnex*) *378*

Styptocid Injection (*Stadmid*) *372*

SULBACTAM *330*

Sulcoprim Bolus/Powder (*Concept*) *341*

Sulfamin Injection (*Indian Immunologicals*) *338*

SULPHADIMIDIN *338, 339*

Sulphadimidine powder *309*

Sulphadimidine Sodium Injection (*Novartis*) *338*

Sulphaguanidine Guanidin Bolus (*Oxen Lab*) *339*

Sulphatrim Injection (*Vets Farma*) *340*

SULPHONAMIDES *82, 338*

Sulphur *309*

Sumicidon *431*

Super Care Liquid (*Excell*) *420, 424*

Suprazole Bolus/Suspension (*Vetnex*) *346, 347*

Suruchi Bolus/Powder (*KAP*) *393, 395*

Synchromate Injection (*Primavet*) *387*

Taenil (*Indian Herbs*) *361*

Taktic-5%/12.5% (*Intervet*) *431*

Tefroli Syrup (*TTK*) *401*

Terramycine injection (*Pfizer*) *323*

Tetracycline WSP Vet (*Intervet*) *324*

Tetravet bolus (*Marion VCL*) *324*

Tetzan Suspension/Bolus (*Jeps Pharma*) *359*

Thiacal Injection (*Wockhardt*) *381*

Tickomax (*Vetnex*) *430*

Tikkil (*Indian Immunologicals*) *430*

Tilox Tube (*Wockhardt*) *391*

Timpanimal Powder (*Arosol*) *399*

Timpol Powder (*Indian Herbs*) *399*

TINCTURE BENZOIN *309*

TINCTURE IODINE *309*

Tolzan F (*HPL*) *355*

Tolzan Plus (*Intervet*) *359*

Tolzan-F Suspension (*Intervet*) *355*

Tonavit Liquid (*Angels group*) *405*

Tonophosphan Injection (*Intervet*) *383*

Topical preparations *310*

Topicure Gel/Spray (*Natural Remedies*) *410, 411*

Totalmin (*Vetcon*) *415*

Toxen Injection (*Oxen Labs*) *333*

Toxol Injection (*Vesper*) *376*

T-Phos Injection (*Intervet*) *383*

Tranquilisers *104*

TRIAMCENOLONE *370*

Tribivet Injection (*Intas*) *376*

TRICLABENDAZOLE *354*

Trimafen Suspension/Bolus/Tab (*Pearls Chemical*) *356*

Trisa-VL (*Pearl Chemicals*) *342*

Trizol Bolus (*Jeps*) *341*

T-T-Cef Vet Injection (TTK) 331

Turmeric *309*

Turpentine oil *309, 313*

Tympex (*Vets Farma*) 397

Tynpex Liquid (*Prashanti Formulations*) *398*

Tyrel (*Natural Remedies*) *398*

Unimycin bolus (*Unichem*) 335

Unimycin Injection (*Unichem*) 334

Uniselit (*Ayurvet*) 415

Uren Vet Bolus (*Dey's Vet*) 427

Urimin Injection (*GSK*) 383

UTERINE TONIC 389

Uterocare (*Excell*) 390

Uterolin (*Bioherbs Pharma*) 390

Uterotone Liquid (*Cattle Remedies*) 390

Utrift Liquid (*Indian Herbs*) 390

Utrina Liquid (*Kumaon Herbs*) 389

Utrodex Injection (*Oxen Lab*) *3054*
Utromilk (*Arosol*) *404*
Utro-On (*Natural Herbs*) *389*
U-Trox Bolus (*Vets Farma*) *427*
Utrox DS Injection (*Neospark*) *323*
Utrox-LA injection (*Neospark*) *323*

VACCINES *431*
VAGINAL PESSURIES *427*
VALETHAMATE BROMIDE *368, 389*
Valvagen Bolus (*Pfizer*) *347*
Vanguard – 5L (*Pfizer*) *437*
Vanguard CV (Pfizer) *436*
Vanguard Plus 5CVL (*Pfizer*) *437*
Vectin Injection (*IBC*) *353*
Velminth Bolus/Suspension (*IBC*) *346, 347*
Ves Phos Injection (*Vesper*) *383*
Vesplex Forte (*Vesper Pharmaceuticals*) *376*
Vet Fen-B (*Indian Immunologicals*) *349*
Vet Fen-T (*Indian Immunologicals*) *349*
Veta-A Injection (*TTK*) *373*
Vetaceph Injection (*Vetcare*) *330*
Vetaceph Plus Injection (*Vetcare*) *331*
Vetaceph-TAZO Injection (*Vetcare*) *331*
Vetalgin Vet Injection (*Intervet*) *365*
Vetalog Injection (*Sarabhai Zydus*) *370*
Vetampin Injection (*Wockhardt*) *321*
Vetaxim Injection (*Cattle Remedies*) *333*
Vetclox Plus Tube (*Sarabhai Zydus*) *390*
Vetliv (*Vetmed*) *400, 402*
Vetmate Injection (*Vetcare*) *387*
Vetocort Injection (*Alembic*) *370*
Vetral Liquid (*Vets Farma*) *407*
Vimeral Liquid (*GSK*) *407*
Viselam (*Brihans*) *407*
Vita Calci Plus (*Oxford Gems*) *423*
Vitacept Injection (*Concept*) *374*
Vitade Injection (*Sarabhai Zydus*) *374*
Vitadhan (*Ayurvet*) *406*
Vitall (*Nugen*) *408*
Vitamin A Injection (*GSK/Legend*) *373*
VITAMIN B_1, B_6, B_{12} 376
VITAMIN-A *373*
VITAMIN-AD_3 *374*
VITAMIN-E *377*
VITAMINS B-COMPLEX *375, 411*
Vitamix Liquid (*Oxen Lab*) *406*
Vitamyl Injection (*Cipla*) *377*
Vitaprotin DS (*Pharmacon*) *416*
Vitromin (*Kapila*) *415*

Wisprec Cream (*Natural Remedies*) *392, 411*
Woktrin tablet (*Wockhardt*) *341*
Wolicyclin injection (*Wockhardt*) *323*
Wopell (*Indian Herbs*) *361*
Worm Herb (*Kapila*) *361*
Wormer Bolus (*IBC*) *347*
Wormer Tab (*Legend*) *348*
Wormin Tab/Powder (*Cadila*) *349*
Wormner Vet Suspension (*Legand*) *346*
Wormpar (*Oxen Lab*) *347*
Wormpar DS (*Oxen Lab*) *347*

X-Ceft Injection (*Alembic*) *332*
X-L Pex Injection (*Alved*) *376*
Xlplex Forte Injection (*Alved*) *376*
Xnel injection (*Pfizer*) *331*
Xyclofen Injection (*Excell*) *363*

Yakrifit Oral Liquid (*Ayurvet*) 400
Yeasacc Bolus (*Vetnex*) 396

Zanide Bolus/Tablet/Suspension (*Legend*) 354, 356
Zeet Injection (*Alembic*) 372
Zenliv-Fort Injection (*Tanen Pharmaceuticals*) 379
Zenvet (*Intas*) 351
Zigbo Oral Liquid (*Natural Remedies*) 400
Zinc oxide 309
Zinc Oxide Ointment 411
Zobid-M Injection (*Sarabhati Zydus*) 363
Zodex Bolus (*Concept*) 349
Zoonic (*Oxen Labs*) 355
Zycloz Bolus/Oral solution (*Sarabhai Zydus*) 351